CONCEPTS IN IMMUNOLOGY AND IMMUNOTHERAPEUTICS

2nd Edition

Editors
Jim Koeller, M.S.
Joseph A. Tami, Pharm.D.

Authors
Jeffrey C. Delafuente, M.S.
Suzanne M. Fields, Pharm.D.
Jeanne T. Flynn, Pharm.D.
Jim Koeller, M.S.
Karl K. Kwok, Pharm.D.
Kathleen D. Lake, Pharm.D.
Timothy R. McGuire, Pharm.D.
Karen I. Plaisance, Pharm.D.
Bonnie D. Purdy, Pharm.D.
Kelly A. Scott, Pharm.D.

American Society of Hospital Pharmacists
4630 Montgomery Avenue
Bethesda, MD 20814
301-657-3000

Made possible through a grant from Sandoz Pharmaceuticals Corporation

The information presented herein reflects the opinions of the author(s) and reviewer(s). It should not be interpreted as official policy of ASHP or as an endorsement of any product(s).

Produced by the American Society of Hospital Pharmacists' Educational Services Division and Special Projects Division.

ISBN: 1-879907-06-2

Contents

List of Tables

List of Figures

Preface

The biotechnology product explosion continues. There are 17 new products or indications currently approved for use in the United States by the Food and Drug Administration (FDA). There are also 14 products or new indications awaiting FDA approval. In addition, there are well over 100 other products in clinical trials throughout this country.

With this explosion of new technology, a single source of information to enhance the pharmacist's data base would be useful. Many pharmacy practitioners have never had a formal course in basic or applied immunology. However, in everyday practice they are finding it necessary to understand the functions of the immune system, its response to disease processes, and the mechanism by which it may be modulated to treat disease.

The rapid advances in immunology and recombinant DNA technology have obviously had an impact on the nature of medical publishing. This has become apparent in how quickly medical information becomes outdated. Although the first edition of *Concepts in Immunology and Immunotherapeutics* was just published in 1990, it has already become outdated because of the explosion in the advancement of science and clinical therapeutics. In this second edition of a self-study text that was written by pharmacists for pharmacists, all the chapters have been updated to reflect current knowledge. New information covering such topics as recently identified interleukins, clinical studies with colony-stimulating factors, solid-organ transplantation, monoclonal antibodies, molecular techniques for identifying HLA types, and agents for use in HIV-infected patients has been included.

The text is in two parts. Part 1 reviews the basics of immunology and its process, and Part 2 concentrates on the clinical application of these concepts for preventing and treating specific disease states. This self-study text is designed for practicing pharmacists, postgraduate trainees (e.g., residents, fellows) and for pharmacy students to be used as a primer or supplement to other texts.

Jim Koeller, M.S.
Joseph A. Tami, Pharm.D.
May 1992

Contributors

ASHP acknowledges the following people who contributed their time and expertise to the development of this text:

Daniel M. Canafax
University of Minnesota College of Pharmacy

Mary Ellen Carasiti
Rush-Presbyterian-Saint Luke's Medical Center

Daniel T. Casto
University of Texas Health Science Center, San Antonio

Maryann E. Davio
Rush-Presbyterian-Saint Luke's Medical Center

Andrew J. Donnelly
Rush-Presbyterian-Saint Luke's Medical Center

James W. Driver
Rush-Presbyterian-Saint Luke's Medical Center

Nora B. Flint
Rush-Presbyterian-Saint Luke's Medical Center

Deborah D. Fortado
Rush-Presbyterian-Saint Luke's Medical Center

Rodney J. Franey
University of Kentucky

John V. Gladish
Sandoz Pharmaceuticals Corporation

Susan Goodin
University of Kentucky

Mark D. Grebenau
Sandoz Pharmaceuticals Corporation

Rawley M. Guerrero
University of Utah Hospital

Anthony J. Infante
University of Texas Health Science Center, San Antonio

David S. Johnson
University of Maryland Cancer Center

Keith A. Krolick
University of Texas Health Science Center, San Antonio

John G. Kuhn
University of Texas Health Science Center, San Antonio

John T. Kung
University of Texas Health Science Center, San Antonio

Robert E. Lamb
Rush-Presbyterian-Saint Luke's Medical Center

Stan F. Lowe
American Society of Hospital Pharmacists

Wayne R. Melchior
Harper Hospital

Mary Beth Micallef
Harper Hospital

James R. Minor
National Institutes of Health

Marion T. Morton
Sandoz Pharmaceuticals Corporation

Christine M. Nimmo
American Society of Hospital Pharmacists

Pauravi B. Patel
Harper Hospital

Vana R. Prewitt
American Society of Hospital Pharmacists

Laura L. Schreiber
Rush-Presbyterian-Saint Luke's Medical Center

William Sgriccia
C.S. Mott Children's Hospital

Elizabeth M. Simonetti
American Society of Hospital Pharmacists

Marie A. Smith
American Society of Hospital Pharmacists

Peter V. Tortorici
Rush-Presbyterian-Saint Luke's Medical Center

Sharon L. Young
Rush-Presbyterian-Saint Luke's Medical Center

About This Pharmacy Continuing Education Program

For purposes of obtaining continuing education credit, this self-instructional text, *Concepts in Immunology and Immunotherapeutics, 2nd Edition,* has been divided into Part 1 and Part 2. Part 1 covers Chapters 1 through 5. You may earn .8 CEUs by successfully completing the CE test for *Concepts in Immunology and Immunotherapeutics, 2nd Edition,* Part 1. The ACPE number for Part 1 of the course in immunology is 680-204-9258. Part 2 of the course covers Chapters 6 through 11. The test for this segment is *Concepts in Immunology and Immunotherapeutics, 2nd Edition,* Part 2. You may earn 1.6 CEUs for Part 2. The ACPE number for Part 2 is 680-204-9259. Both tests and answer sheets are bound separately from this book.

The American Society of Hospital Pharmacists is approved by the American Council on Pharmaceutical Education as a provider of continuing pharmaceutical education.

How to Study *Concepts in Immunology and Immunotherapeutics*

Although this text is primarily designed as a self-study text for practicing pharmacists, it may also be used in pharmacy school curriculums as a primer or a supplemental text for self-study.

As you proceed through this text, you will find many of the basic concepts are illustrated with tables, charts, or figures for clarification. Terminology associated with immunology and immunotherapeutics is likewise essential to attaining the learning objectives, and you will find key words highlighted in the margins of the chapters. For easy reference, a list of abbreviations, a glossary, and an index are included in the back of the book.

You can make this text an effective self-study tool if you follow these suggestions:

1. Set a goal for completing the book and establish a schedule for studying without interruption or distractions. A library can be an ideal place to study.
2. Read the introduction and learning objectives in each chapter. These sections tell you why the chapter is important, what specific information you will be expected to know for answering the end-of-course questions, and how the chapter is organized.
3. Scan the chapter, noting the subject headings and key words.
4. Read the chapter, keeping the learning objectives in mind. Underline or highlight important passages and make notes in the wide margins.
5. Read the summary to review the main points of the chapter. Review anything that still seems unclear.
6. Answer the self-study questions to evaluate your understanding of the information and preparedness for the end-of-course questions.
7. Review information pertaining to any questions you answer incorrectly.
8. Expand your knowledge through readings suggested at the end of some of the chapters. Although you will not be tested on this information, such independent learning will add depth and detail to your understanding of immunology and immunotherapeutics.
9. Study with other pharmacists. Discuss and share perceptions.
10. Observe pharmacists working on issues related to immunology and discuss immunotherapeutics with them.

CHAPTER 1

Overview of the Immune System

Jeanne T. Flynn, Pharm.D.
Manager, Professional Services
AMGEN
Thousand Oaks, CA

Introduction

Immunology represents one of the fastest-growing areas in medicine today. Along with the rapid increase in knowledge of this area has come the development of unique and exciting immunomodulating drugs. Before clinicians can fully understand the activity of these new agents, they must develop a clear understanding of the basic functions of the immune system.

This chapter will provide a brief overview of the development and functions of the immune system and will introduce many topics that will be covered in greater detail in the following chapters. Emphasis will be placed on how the different components of the immune system interact in order to maintain the delicate balance required for a properly functioning immune system.

Learning objectives

This chapter should give the pharmacist a better understanding of the basics of the immune system and its various components, including monocytes, neutrophils, B- and T-lymphocytes, and the complement system. With this background, the pharmacist can then go on to master the specific aspects of the immune system covered in subsequent chapters. After reading this chapter, the learner will be able to—

- Describe the mechanisms of action of the nonspecific immune response.
- Describe the mechanisms of action of the specific immune response.
- Discuss the influence of antigen properties and structures on the relative immunogenicity of an antigen.
- Discuss the mechanisms of action of the complement system.
- Describe how pre- and post-natal development of the immune system influences immunogenic responses in infancy.

Chapter organization

This chapter presents introductory information about the innate and specific immune system responses with definitions and discussion of the components of each. The characteristics of specificity, memory, and tolerance of these components are described, followed by a discussion of factors that affect the immune mechanism. A full description and discussion is given to antigens and complement. Some undesirable effects of immunity are covered; the chapter closes with an overview of the development of the human immune system.

Suggested Preparation

No specific review is needed to understand this chapter. The following references may be helpful: References 1 (pages 30–43), 3, 6, and 10.

Immunity and Defense Mechanisms

The overall function of the immune system is to protect the host from any foreign material (antigen) both by recognizing the material as nonself and by eliminating or neutralizing this material. This overall function is accomplished through two separate yet interactive responses of the immune system, namely, the nonspecific (innate) and the specific (acquired) responses. This section outlines and compares the major functional activities of the nonspecific and specific immune responses.

Nonspecific (Innate) Immune Response

The nonspecific immune response consists of naturally occurring (innate) defense mechanisms. These responses are not directed toward a specific antigen (e.g., foreign material) and are therefore termed nonspecific. Consequently, these responses do not change or adapt upon reexposure to a foreign substance. Therefore, immunity is not conferred. In general, this functional division of the immune system is responsible for resisting penetration of microorganisms and other foreign agents, destroying foreign substances invading tissues, and eliminating toxic wastes.[1] These immune responses are the first line of defense against intrusive organisms or substances.[1,2]

First-line Defense. The first line of defense against invading organisms includes physical defenses and barriers, such as the skin, mucus, and respiratory cilia, and also biochemical defenses, such as lysozyme, gastric acid, and lactic acid.

The simplest defense against invading pathogens is the mechanical barrier provided by the skin, which is impenetrable by most organisms (Figure 1-1). The skin also undergoes epithelial cell turnover, which, along with substances present on skin (salt, lactic acid, and unsaturated fatty acids), aids in removing microbes.[3,4] Another defense against foreign invasion is the harshly acidic environment of the stomach followed by the

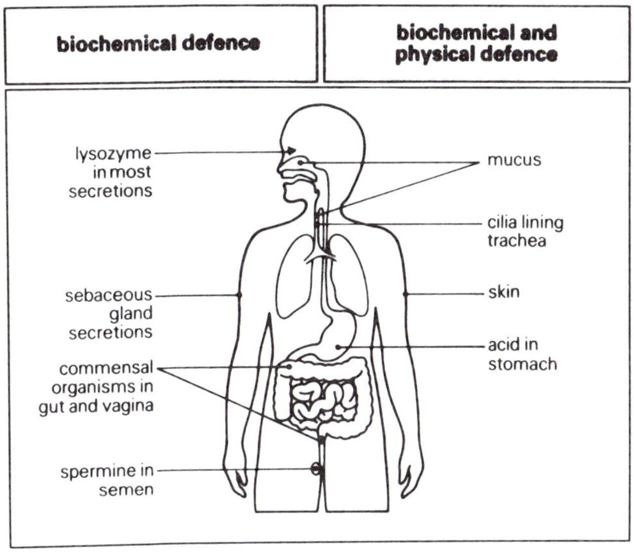

Figure 1-1. Protection against access by microorganisms

SOURCE: Reprinted with permission from Roitt IM, Brostoff J, Male DK, eds. Immunology. 2nd ed. London: Gower Medical Publications; 1989:1.4.

very alkaline environment of the small intestine. These environments together eliminate almost all pathogens from orally ingested substances. Yet another is the respiratory cilia, which sweep away inhaled substances.

Physical defenses

If a microorganism is able to gain access to the host, many additional first-line defense mechanisms work to aid in eliminating it. Mucus secreted by membranes lining inner surfaces of the body can trap foreign substances, inhibiting them from penetrating cells. Bile acids deconjugated by intestinal anaerobes inhibit many microorganisms. The small and large intestines are colonized with noninvasive bacteria, which compete with pathogens for nutrients. In addition, factors such as nonspecific inhibitors are released by various tissues.[4]

Biochemical defenses

Lysozyme is the most abundant and widespread of the various soluble bactericidal substances in the body.[3] It is present in high concentrations in urine, nasal mucus, tears, and saliva. Lysozyme, a muramidase, functions by cleaving a B-1,4-glycosidic bond in the cell wall of Gram-positive bacteria. (Although this same bond is present in Gram-negative bacteria, it is protected by the presence of lipid.[3])

Second-line Defense. Organisms that are able to survive the body's first lines of defense come up against the second lines of defense: inflammation, phagocytosis, and complement.

Inflammation. Inflammation is one of the most important components of the nonspecific immune response and is responsible for producing some of the classic signs and symptoms of infection. It is a complex series of events that occur in response to tissue injury as the host attempts to maintain homeostasis.[1] Upon injury, large quantities of vasoactive substances such as histamine (from mast cells in the skin that have been punctured) are released.[1] These substances induce vasodilation, increase local blood flow, and (by increasing vascular permeability) allow the release of fluid and protein, including fibrinogen, into the tissues. These effects may be prolonged by the release of additional substances 6 to 12 hours after injury. These additional substances include complement products as well as bradykinins and prostaglandins.[5] Fibrinogen aids the defense process by clotting extracellular and lymphatic fluid to delay spread of bacterial or toxic products.[1] The classic symptoms produced by these events include erythema (redness) from blood-vessel dilation, edema from the excess fluids in the soft tissues, and induration (swelling) from accumulation of fluid and cells.

Neutrophils

Within an hour of the start of inflammation, the endothelial cells become sticky because of the expression of adhesion molecules, and neutrophils, which are the major cell type present at the site of acute inflammation, begin to marginate and adhere to the endothelium (pavementing). Neutrophils comprise the largest percentage (60% to 70%) of white blood cells in the peripheral blood. The neutrophil is a phagocytic cell with granules that contain bactericidal substances, which are released upon phagocytosis.

Monocytes/ macrophages

Within 4 hours of the start of inflammation, mononuclear cells (monocytes) also migrate to the area of injury. Mononuclear phagocytes are composed of monocytes and macrophages. Monocytes are mobile leukocytes capable of phagocytosis. Once in the tissues, monocytes grow much larger and become tissue macrophages, which are distributed throughout the body and can survive for months or even years. This system of monocytes and macrophages has traditionally been called the reticuloendothelial system (RES). It was once thought that a major portion of the blood vessel endothelial cells could perform phagocytic functions. It is now known that they do not, and the RES has been renamed the mononuclear phagocyte system.[1,6]

Tissue macrophages are generally present in areas of the body that are easily exposed to infectious agents. They include the Kupffer cells in the liver sinuses, which protect against invasion by bacteria through the gastrointestinal tract; macrophages in the lymph nodes, which aid in destroying foreign particles not destroyed in local tissues; and the alveolar macrophages in the respiratory system.[7]

Phagocytes

Phagocytic cells are stimulated to mobilize to the site of injury by chemotactic factors such as some members of the complement system, damaged tissue, products of bacteria, and other inflammatory cells. After adhering to the endothelium, phagocytic cells, neutrophils, and, to a lesser extent, macrophages exhibit amoeboid movement and actively migrate through the endothelial wall by a process called diapedesis[1,2,5] (Figure 1-2). Once at the area of tissue damage or invasion, phagocytic cells adhere to the offending particle and ingest it.

Degranulation

Phagocytosis. Phagocytosis involves invagination of the plasma membrane of the phagocyte, uptake of the particle into the cytoplasm, and enclosure within a vacuole (phagosome). Opsonins such as complement and immunoglobulins increase the rate and quantity of particle uptake by making the particle more visible and susceptible to phagocytosis. Phagocytic cells have receptors that specifically recognize the exposed portion of these opsonins when they coat bacteria. Once the foreign particle is fully inside the cell, these phagosomes fuse with lysosome granules, causing the lysosomes to burst (degranulation) and release their hydrolytic enzymes, as well as other bactericidal substances. Associated with degranulation is an increase in the production of hydrogen peroxide and superoxide radicals, which kill the bacteria, allowing the lytic enzymes to digest them[1,3] (Figure 1-3). Much of the tissue damage associated with injury can be attributed to degranulation.

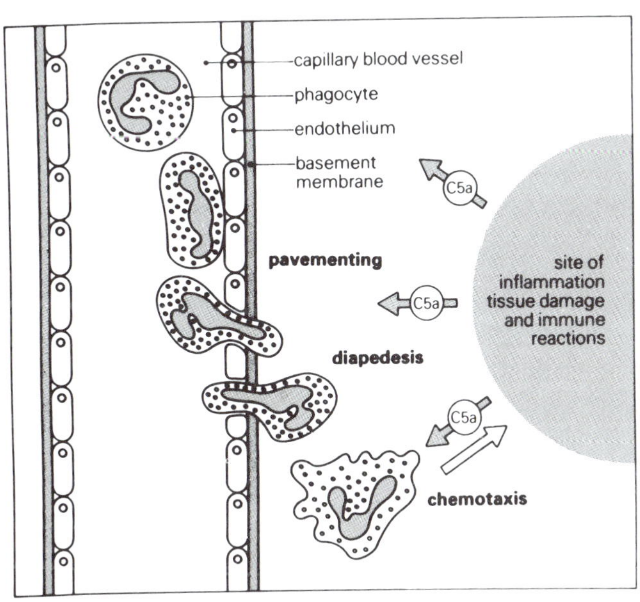

Figure 1-2. Steps in inflammation

SOURCE: Reprinted with permission from Roitt IM, Brostoff J, Male DK, eds. Immunology. 2nd ed. London: Gower Medical Publications; 1989:1.4.

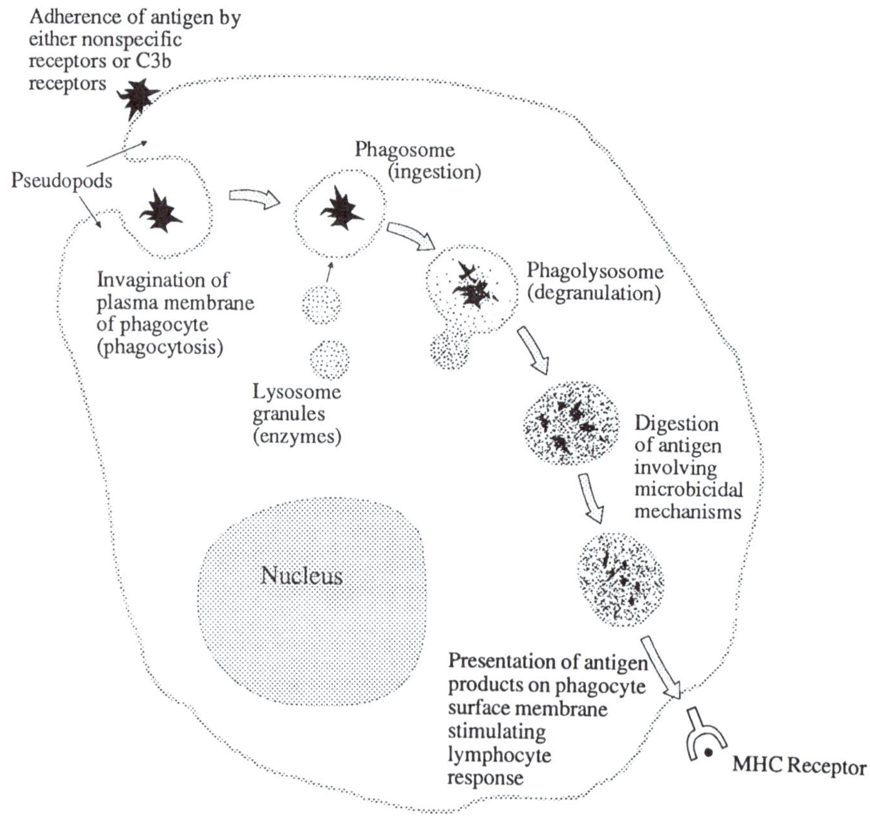

Figure 1-3. Phagocytosis

Complement. Complement (proteins that circulate in an inactive form) can be activated through either the classical or alternative pathway. Either pathway results in the production of many peptides, which are also involved in inflammation. The active forms of complement components C3 and C5 are known to stimulate histamine release, which increases vascular permeability, causing a pooling of cells necessary for immune activity. In addition, the active form of C5 results in a chemotactic response to neutrophils, monocytes, and macrophages, attracting them to the area of inflammation.[8]

Specific (Adaptive) Immune Response

When a host is invaded by a foreign substance, all components of the immune system participate to varying degrees. If the innate immune response fails to completely protect the individual from an antigenic challenge, the adaptive (or specific) immune components are called into play. In contrast to the nonspecific immune response, the specific immune response confers immunity (resistance to repeated exposures of the same antigen), primarily through the mechanisms of specificity and memory. In addition, the specific immune response is responsible for the development of tolerance.[3]

Memory and tolerance

Macrophages play a pivotal role in linking the two lines of defense of the immune system. B and T lymphocytes, the major mediators of the specific immune response, are rendered almost ineffective unless told what to do by macrophage or other antigen-presenting cells.[1,3,5] Macrophages are now known to function by processing the antigen into a form recognized by the components of the specific immune response and presenting the antigen to these components. In addition, macrophages produce and secrete a variety of biologically active factors that influence lymphocyte activity.

T Lymphocytes. T lymphocytes are the lymphocytes that are primarily responsible for cell-mediated immunity. This term was developed when it was realized that T lymphocytes themselves must be transferred from donor to recipient to confer this type of immunity. The cell-mediated arm of the immune system is primarily responsible for developing immunity to infections caused by microorganisms that live and multiply within the cells of the host, such as tuberculosis, smallpox, and toxoplasmosis. In addition, this system is responsible for delayed hypersensitivity reactions (see Chapter 4), most transplant rejection (see Chapter 9), tumor surveillance (see Chapter 10), and graft-versus-host disease (see Chapter 9).

Cell-mediated immunity

T lymphocytes develop from the pluripotent stem cells in the bone marrow as do the B lymphocytes, but, unlike B lymphocytes, they differentiate further in the thymus. Early in development, T cells develop surface markers and further differentiate to form distinct functional subpopulations. These subpopulations include suppressor T, helper T, and cytotoxic T cells, which are pivotal to the regulation of the immune response[9,10] (Figure 1-4). Once released from the thymus, T lymphocytes can be found in the bloodstream, lymph nodes, bone marrow, and spleen; they can live longer than 20 years.[9]

Differentiation

Besides performing those functions mentioned under cell-mediated immunity, T lymphocytes help regulate the effects of B cells, produce lymphokines and other mediators of the immune response, and link the nonspecific with the specific immune responses through their interaction with macrophage.[10] (For further discussion of T lymphocytes, see Chapter 2.)

B Lymphocytes. B lymphocytes are responsible for the function of the humoral arm of the immune system. *Humoral* means *of the fluids* and applies to this form of immunity because antibodies in the cell-free plasma

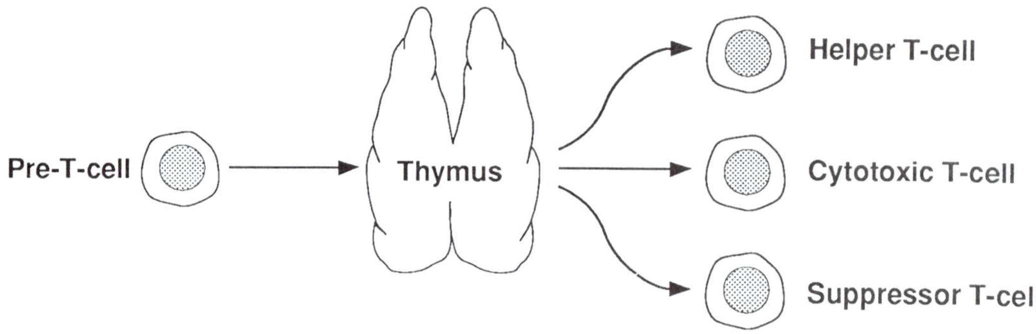

Figure 1-4. T-cell differentiation

SOURCE: Reprinted with permission from Paul WE. The immune system: an introduction. In: Paul WE, ed. Fundamental immunology. New York: Raven Press; 1984:11.

Humoral immunity

of one individual can transfer immunity to another. Humoral immunity provides a major defense against bacterial infections through the production of antibodies.

Differentiation

In birds, differentiation of B lymphocytes from the pluripotent stem cells occurs in the bursa of Fabricius. Mammals do not have a discrete organ for B-cell differentiation. Rather, these cells develop from lymphoid stem cells in the fetal liver from early in gestation. Further B-cell production is transferred to the bone marrow, where it continues during adulthood.[3] Upon leaving the bone marrow, B lymphocytes enter various lymphoid tissues throughout the body. Each B lymphocyte has on its surface membrane antibodies of the same single specificity it will produce when stimulated by the corresponding antigen. Once stimulated, B lymphocytes further differentiate into plasma cells that are dedicated to the mass production of antibody. Once antibody is secreted, plasma cells have a life span of 2 to 3 days.[9,10] (For further discussion of B lymphocytes, see Chapter 2.)

Antigenic determinants/ epitopes

Specificity. This term refers to the ability of a T or B lymphocyte to react exclusively to the presence of a particular molecular configuration (called antigenic determinant or epitope) of a substance, and not to react to other substances. Both T lymphocytes and antibodies have specificity; that is, they both can recognize only one antigen. Some antigens are shared by groups of unrelated species. For example, patients who develop antibodies against B-hemolytic streptococcal antigens run the risk of having these antibodies cross-react with antigens in their own cardiac tissue.

A single pathogen may have several different epitopes, each of which may evoke its own specific immune response. Since there are many thousand antigens that can be recognized by the immune system, each unique lymphocyte represents a minor part of the total. However, once a lymphocyte recognizes and reacts to an antigen, clonal expansion of those specific lymphocytes occurs. All the T lymphocytes or B lymphocytes produced with the same specificity against an antigen are collectively referred to as a clone[3,5,9] (Figure 1-5).

Clone

Memory. Memory is the property of evoking a more vigorous specific immune response upon reexposure to a particular antigen. This response is attributable to two processes. The first process is the proliferation (or clonal expansion) of both B and T lymphocytes specific to the antigen on first exposure. Some of these lymphocytes go on to form either antibodies or sensitized lymphocytes, which decrease with time. The second process occurs when other lymphocytes form a more persistent population of memory cells, which, upon later reexposure to the same antigen, greatly augment the specific immune response. Antibody development can be used as an example: In the primary immune response a lag time follows initial exposure to antigen before antibody is developed. Upon reexposure, the development of antibodies is much quicker and more intense[3,5] (Figure 1-6).

Clonal expansion

Tolerance. Immunologic tolerance develops when exposure of a host to an antigen, which normally results in an immune response, does not result in an immune reaction.[11,12] There is evidence for both T- and B-cell tolerance. Several mechanisms are involved in immunologic tolerance.

Clonal Abortion. In neonatal animals, tolerance can be easily induced. Some have suggested, therefore, that exposure of a developing lymphocyte to an antigen at some critical point may lead to deletion of that lymphocyte

Mechanisms of tolerance

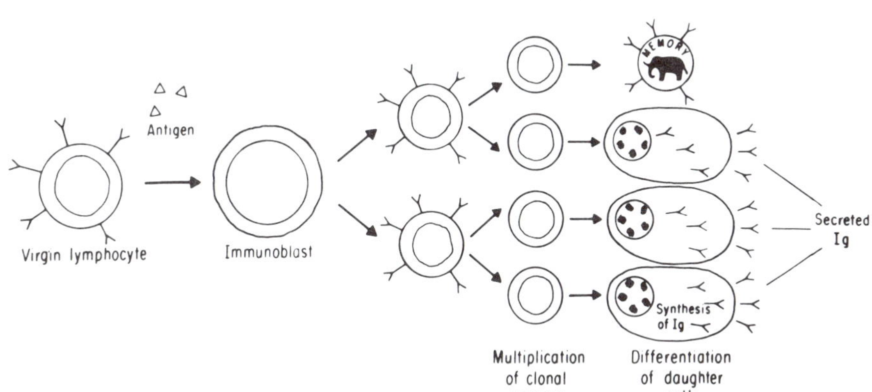

Figure 1-5. Clonal expansion of lymphocytes

SOURCE: Reprinted with permission from Widmann FK, ed. An introduction to clinical immunology. Philadelphia: F. A. Davis Company; 1989:19.

clone. This may be the mechanism used to destroy those lymphocyte clones specific for the body's own tissues. For example, when B and T cells are exposed to low concentrations of antigen while immature, cell maturity can be arrested. The result can be that the B or T lymphocyte is unable to respond to that antigen on subsequent exposure.[11,12]

Clonal Exhaustion. This effect occurs when B lymphocytes are repeatedly exposed to T-independent antigen. All the mature B lymphocytes capable of responding to this antigen are stimulated to differentiate so that no cells are left capable of responding when subsequently reexposed to the antigen.

Functional Deletion. B lymphocytes require T lymphocytes (helper T cells) to respond to T-dependent antigens. If the T lymphocytes are not available, then the B cells can be functionally deleted. In addition, if a very high dose of a T-independent antigen is presented to a B cell, too few B cells may be present to respond. T cells can be functionally deleted if one of the subsets of mature T cells is deleted, leading to loss of function.

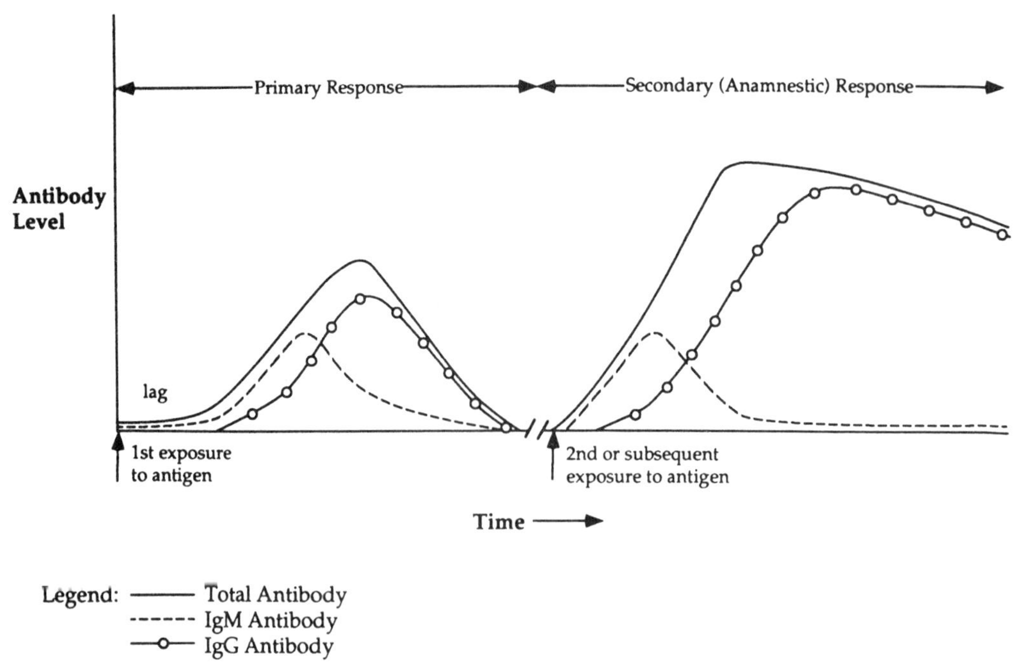

Figure 1-6. Graph of differences between primary and secondary antibody responses

SOURCE: Reprinted with permission from Miller LE, Ludke HR, Peacock JE, Tomar RH, eds. Manual of laboratory immunology. 2nd ed. Philadelphia: Lea and Febiger; 1991:1–25.

Antibody-forming Cell Blockade. This occurs when an excess of T-independent antigens bind and thereby block B-cell surface receptors. This binding of antigen subsequently interferes with antibody secretion.

T-cell Suppression. T-cell suppression occurs when suppressor T cells actively suppress other T-cell subsets or B cells.[11,12]

In addition to factors already mentioned, the genetic makeup of the individual, as well as the structure and route of administration of an antigen, has an effect on tolerance development.

Factors that Affect Immune Mechanisms

Genetic Factors. The entire immune system, including its proper development and the rate at which immune responsiveness matures, is an expression of genetic traits. Genes encode for immunoglobulins, major histocompatibility antigens, blood group antigens, T-cell receptors, and soluble mediators involved in the immune response. Alterations in this coding process can lead to immunodeficiency disorders, autoimmune disorders, and malignancy. Genetic variation among individuals helps to explain the variability in responsiveness to infections and vaccines. In addition, a thorough understanding of the genetic expression of histocompatibility antigens is required for successful transplantation.[13]

Age. Deficiencies of the immune system have been documented in the very young.[14,15] Immune deficiencies have also been found in the very old. The elderly are at increased risk of infection. Some of this decrease in immunity is secondary to other diseases, such as diabetes. More important, there is growing evidence that deficiencies in the immune system develop as the individual ages. This process is called immunosenescence. Specifically, the number and function of T cells have been found to decrease. In addition, abnormal antibody production and function have been documented. In contrast, phagocytosis does not appear to change with aging.[2,16]

Immunosenescence

Metabolic Factors. Three metabolic factors are known to affect the immune system: glucose, adrenal corticosteroids, and thyroid hormones. Patients with diabetes mellitus are at increased risk of infection, as are those with decreased function of the thyroid or adrenal glands. It is well known that patients treated with steroids are at increased risk for viral or bacterial infection.[17]

Environmental Factors. Individuals exposed to very crowded living conditions are more susceptible to infection. Increased exposure, as well as increased transmission of microorganisms, at least partially explains this susceptibility. In addition, malnutrition is often present in populations living in such conditions. The development of cell-mediated immunity can be impaired in malnourished infants.[17] In animals, malnutrition has resulted in defects in all immune components, including the nonspecific immune response. Anergy often accompanies malnutrition, as is shown by a lack of response to skin tests measuring responsiveness to common antigens to which patients have previously been exposed.[18]

Physiologic Factors. Many physiologic factors benefit the immune system: gastric juices, which, on account of their acidic pH, destroy many pathogenic bacteria after ingestion; normal urinary flow, which clears bacteria from the urinary tract; cilia, which help move bacteria and other substances out of the respiratory system; skin secretions, which contain lactic acid (known to be bactericidal) and saturated fatty acids (which may render the skin more resistant to fungi); and the bactericidal enzyme lysozyme, which is found in many cells and body fluids.[1,3]

Antigens and Antigenicity

This section describes the basics of the structure and properties of antigens. Emphasis is on those properties that increase the immunogenicity of an antigen.

Immunogens and antigens

An immunogen is defined as a substance that causes a detectable immune response (humoral, cellular, or both). Molecules to which antibodies bind are called antigens (antibody-generating).[3] The specific portion of the antigen molecule that combines with antibody is called the antigenic determinant, or epitope (Figure 1-7). All immunogens are antigenic, but the reverse is not always true—all antigens are not always immunogenic.[19] For example, penicillin, because of its low molecular weight, does not elicit an immune response (and therefore is not an immunogen) unless it is coupled with a carrier molecule. These low-molecular-weight compounds, referred to as haptens, are antigenic but not immunogenic.

Haptens

Classification of Antigens

Autoantigens

Immune reactions can occur against antigens that arise from within the host or from outside the host. Antigens that arise from within the host are termed autoantigens. Autologous antigens are self antigens that normally do not elicit an immune response. If a response is elicited, autoimmune diseases may result.[6] (See Chapter 6.)

Alloantigens

Immune responses against antigens from members of the same species as the host are considered alloimmune or homologous responses, and these antigens are termed alloantigens. Allogeneic antigens are genetically

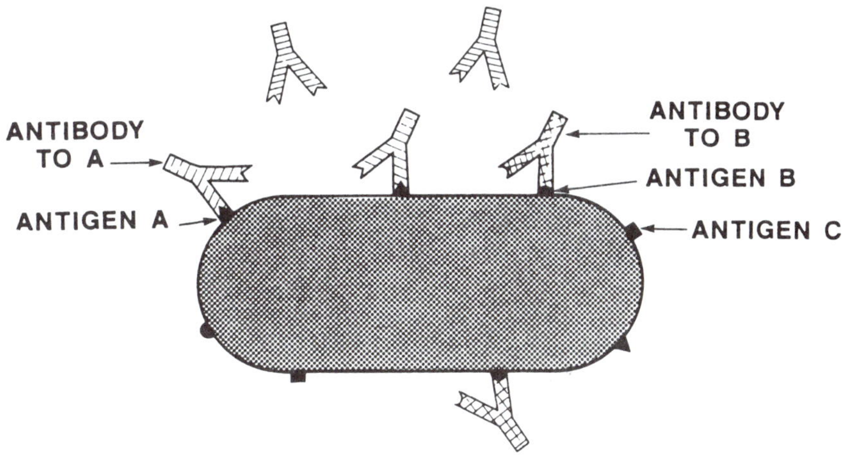

Figure 1-7. Antigens on the surface of a microbial cell

SOURCE: From Vickerstaff Joneja JM, Bielory L. Understanding allergy, sensitivity, and immunity. Copyright © 1990 by Rutgers, The State University.

determined and help distinguish individuals from one another. Examples of these antigens include the histocompatibility antigens and those found on blood cells and platelets. Immunization with these antigens can result in blood transfusion reactions or organ transplant rejections.[6] (See Chapters 3 and 9.)

Heteroantigens

Antigens from different host species are completely foreign. These antigens are heteroantigens, and responses directed against them are termed heterologous or xenogeneic (Table 1-1).

Structure of Antigens

Many antigens or immunogens have one or more antigenic determinants, or epitopes, which enable the body to distinguish them as being foreign. In fact, the more diverse structural characteristics are on a molecule, the more likely the molecule is to be antigenic. In addition to these sites, other structural features affect the immunogenicity of a particular antigen. The size of the antigen is one of the most important determinants. A molecule with a molecular weight of less than 10,000 rarely causes a clinically significant immune response unless it is attached to a hapten. Although the humoral immune system reacts to the hapten, cell-mediated responses generally occur against both the hapten and the carrier protein. In general, the more complex the antigenic structure, the more immunogenic it is. For example, proteins that are present in a polymeric or aggregated state are much more likely to induce an immune response than those in a monomeric form.[6,12] Furthermore, the accessibility of the antigen determinants may also

Table 1-1 Classification of Antigens

Source	Descriptive Term for Antigen	Descriptive Terms for Immune Response	Examples
Material from host	Autoantigen	Autoimmune Autologous	Antibodies to hormones Cellular attack on liver cells
Material from some other human	Alloantigen	Alloimmune Homologous Allogeneic	Antibodies to transfused blood cells Cellular attack on trans-planted organ
Material from plants, micro-organisms, chemicals, other animals	Heteroantigen	Heterologous Xenogeneic	Antibodies to bovine or porcine insulin Cellular response to poison ivy

SOURCE: Adapted with permission from Widmann FK, ed. An introduction to clinical immunology. Philadelphia: F. A. Davis Company, 1989:48.

affect their ability to elicit a response.[20] No one molecular configuration is immunogenic, but it is known that if the configuration of a particular antigen changes, the antibody may no longer be able to recognize it.[6,12,19]

Properties of Antigens

Several of the important physical properties of antigens have been discussed in terms of their structure. In addition, other physical and chemical properties, such as the sequence of amino acids present in a molecule or the mobility of the antigenic determinant of a molecule, can help establish the immunogenicity of a particular compound.[19] Proteins and carbohydrates elicit a greater antigenic response than lipids or nucleic acids. Hydrophilic molecules are more immunogenic than hydrophobic molecules.

Dose and Route of Administration of Antigens

Finally, the route and timing of administration and dose of the antigen have an impact on the antigenicity. In general, soluble antigens are more likely to result in an immune response when injected parenterally than when administered orally. Higher doses of antigen are also much more likely to result in an immune response than lower doses.[12]

Complement

In this section the interactions of complement with the other components of the immune system are emphasized. In addition, the harmful effects resulting from complement deficiencies are discussed.

The term *complement* describes a group or system of approximately 25 proteins that function to produce inflammation, opsonize foreign material for phagocytosis, and help mediate direct cytotoxicity.[21-23] The discovery of the complement system began in the late 1800s, when it was realized that the addition of fresh serum to a mixture containing specific antibody and a cellular antigen often resulted in cell death. The investigation to identify the biochemical basis of this cell death eventually led to the discovery of the complement system.[24]

Enzyme Cascade

The proteins that make up the complement system circulate in inactive forms until stimulated. These proteins consist of both functional and regulatory proteins. They are synthesized mainly in the liver and also, to some extent, by lymphocytes and monocytes.[21,22] Activation of the first of the proteins sets off a series of reactions known as the complement cascade. The three major steps in this cascade are the initiation of the cascade, amplification of the reactions, and membrane attack leading to cell death.[21] This cascade leads to the development of important biologic products that help the process of inflammation, opsonization, and cytotoxicity (see Table 1-2).

Three major steps

Classical Pathway

The complement cascade can be initiated or activated by either the classical or the alternative pathway (Figure 1-8). The classical pathway begins when complement is exposed to an antigen-antibody complex. This complex allows the C1q protein of the C1 complement unit to bind to two or more Fc regions of certain immunoglobulins, which sets off the cascade.[21,22]

Alternative Pathway

The alternative pathway was discovered when it was realized that a complement reaction could occur that does not depend on antigen-antibody complexation. This pathway is stimulated by sugar moieties in some yeast

Table 1-2 Biologic Effects of Complement Activation Products

Products	Biologic Activity
C3a	Contraction of smooth muscle Increase of vascular permeability Degranulation of mast cells and basophils with release of histamine Degranulation of eosinophils Aggregation of platelets
C3b	Opsonization of particles and solubilization of immune complexes with subsequent facilitation of phagocytosis
C3e	Release of neutrophils from bone marrow resulting in leukocytosis
C4a	Contraction of smooth muscle Increase of vascular permeability
C5a	Contraction of smooth muscle Increase of vascular permeability Degranulation of mast cells and basophils with release of histamine Degranulation of eosinophils Aggregation of platelets Chemotaxis of basophils, eosinophils, neutrophils, and monocytes Release of hydrolytic enzymes from neutrophils
C5a-des-arg	Chemotaxis of neutrophils Release of hydrolytic enzymes from neutrophils
Bb	Inhibition of migration and induction of spreading of monocytes and macrophages

SOURCE: Reprinted with permission from Kunkel SL, Ward PA, Caporale LH et al. The complement system. In: Bellanti JA, ed. Immunology III. 3rd ed. Philadelphia: W. B. Saunders Company; 1985:110.

and bacterial cell walls.[23] The alternative pathway initially bypasses the C1, C4, and C2 factors of the classical pathway but eventually converges with it, forming the membrane attack unit that leads to cell lysis.[23]

Regulatory Mechanisms of the Complement Cascade

Since the biologic products produced by the complement system are numerous and quite potent, the system is tightly regulated. Short half-lives and instability of key bonds represent one mechanism of regulation. In

Inhibitors

addition, some of the complement components are inactivated by proteolytic enzymes. Certain binding proteins bind to complement

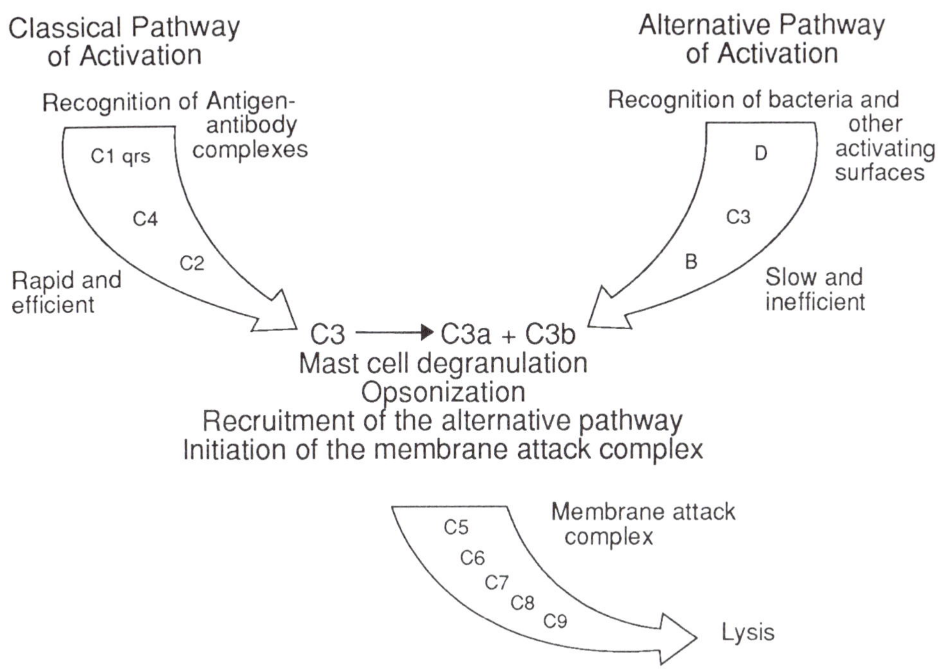

Figure 1-8. The complement system

SOURCE: Reprinted with permission from Paul WE. The immune system: an introduction. In: Paul WE, ed. Fundamental immunology. 2nd ed. New York: Raven Press; 1989:19.

components, thus making them more susceptible to still other proteins. C1 esterase inhibitor forms irreversible complexes with components of the classical pathway, thereby regulating activation of the pathway.[1]

Complement in Infections

Activators

Once microorganisms stimulate the production of specific antibodies, antigen-antibody complexes are formed. These complexes can activate complement, resulting in bacterial death. In addition, a variety of substances can activate the complement system without the assistance of antibody: yeast cell wall, lipopolysaccharide in bacterial cell walls, viruses, and fungi.

Complement Deficiencies

Complement deficiencies can be either congenital or acquired.[21] Acquired deficiencies are most often associated with immune complexes. As the disease progresses the deficiency gets worse, and vice versa. Insight into the role of complement has been gained from studying individuals with genetic deficiencies of complement. Inherited deficiencies of almost all complement components have been described, the most common being a deficiency in C2. Connective tissue disease has been strongly associated with deficiencies in the early complement proteins of the classical pathway; individuals with deficiencies in later components have increased susceptibility to neisserial infections. Finally, genetic deficiency of the C1 esterase inhibitor manifests itself as hereditary angioedema.[21] For a more complete list of complement deficiencies and their consequences, see Table 1-3.

Undesirable Consequences of Immunity

Alterations in the activity of the immune system can lead to harmful consequences for the host. Hyperresponses can lead to allergic reactions or autoimmune disease, and hyporesponses may lead to immunodeficiency disorders and malignancies.

Allergy and Hypersensitivity

Hyperresponses

If the immune system is in a state of overactivity, allergy or hypersensitivity may ensue. When a host is reexposed to an antigen, a boosting of the immune response occurs. When the antigen responsible is present in large amounts, or if specific immune responses are in a heightened state, then this secondary response can be excessive and may lead to host damage.[3] It is important to realize that the immune responses that lead to these excessive reactions are those normally used by the host to fight infection. (For further discussion of allergy and hypersensitivity, see Chapter 4.)

Autoimmunity

Most individuals recognize and tolerate self (autologous) antigens in contrast to nonself antigens. In autoimmunity, inappropriate processing of an antigen by the host's immune system may lead to an immune response against self antigens.[6] (See Chapter 6 for further discussion.)

Malignancy

Hyporesponses

It is known that organ tranplant recipients who require extensive use of immunosuppressive agents are at increased risk for certain neoplasms. In addition, patients with acquired immune deficiency syndrome have a high incidence of Kaposi's sarcoma and non-Hodgkin's lymphoma (see Chapter 8). Further, children born with immunologic deficiencies are at greater risk for developing malignancy than those with normal immune function.[24] (See

Table 1-3 Inherited Deficiencies in Complement and Complement-related Disorders

Deficient Protein	Observed Pattern of Inheritance at Clinical Level	Reported Major Clinical Correlates
C1q	Autosomal recessive	Glomerulonephritis, systemic lupus erythematosus
C1r	Probably autosomal recessive	Syndrome resembling systemic lupus erythematosus
C1s	Found in combination with C1r deficiency	Systemic lupus erythematosus
C4	Probably autosomal recessive (two separate loci, C4A and C4B)	Syndrome resembling systemic lupus erythematosus
C2	Autosomal recessive, HLA-linked	Systemic lupus erythematosus, discoid lupus erythematosus, juvenile rheumatoid arthritis, glomerulonephritis
C3	Autosomal recessive	Recurrent pyogenic infections, glomerulonephritis
C5	Autosomal recessive	Recurrent disseminated Neisseria infections, systemic lupus erythematosus
C6	Autosomal recessive	Recurrent disseminated Neisseria infections
C7	Autosomal recessive	Recurrent disseminated Neisseria infections, Raynaud's phenomenon
C8 β chain or C8 α-γ chains	Autosomal recessive	Recurrent disseminated Neisseria infections
C9	Autosomal recessive	None identified
Properdin	X-linked recessive	Recurrent pyogenic infections, fulminant meningococcemia

Table 1-3 (continued)

Deficient Protein	Observed Pattern of Inheritance at Clinical Level	Reported Major Clinical Correlates
Factor $\overline{D}$	?	Recurrent pyogenic infections
C1 inhibitor	Autosomal dominant	Hereditary angioedema, increased incidence of several autoimmune diseases
Factor H	Autosomal recessive	Glomerulonephritis
Factor 1	Autosomal recessive	Recurrent pyogenic infections
CR1	Autosomal recessive	Association between low numbers of erythrocyte CRI and systemic lupus erythematosus
CR3	Autosomal recessive	Leukocytosis, recurrent pyogenic infections, delayed umbilical-cord separation

SOURCE: Reprinted with permission from Frank MM. Complement in the pathophysiology of human disease. *N Engl J Med.* 1987;316:1528.

Chapter 10 for further discussion of the role of the immune system in tumor development.)

Complement-dependent Reactions Resulting in Injury

Autoantibodies

Complement-dependent reactions resulting in injury are known to be caused by at least two mechanisms: activation of complement by autoantibodies and activation by immune complexes. Autoantibodies are antibodies directed against host tissue, and complement activated by them will eventually result in destruction of host tissue. This phenomenon occurs in several diseases, including Goodpasture's syndrome, in which the antibodies are directed against glomerular basement membrane; myasthenia gravis, which results from the action of autoantibodies against acetylcholine receptors; and rheumatic heart disease, which involves cross-reactive antibodies attacking host cardiac tissue.[20]

Immune complexes

Immune complexes that are deposited or locally formed in the walls of small vessels and subsequently activate complement also result in host tissue injury. Examples of diseases in which this mechanism is involved in causing injury include rheumatoid arthritis, systemic lupus erythematosus, and myocarditis.[20]

Development of the Immune System

This section discusses the in utero and postnatal development of the immune system.

In Utero Maturation

Hematopoiesis

Both the nonspecific and the specific immune responses begin to mature in utero sometime during the second to third month of gestation.[14] Cells responsible for the proper function of the immune system descend from the hematopoietic pluripotent stem cell (HPSC), located in the yolk sac of the developing embryo. After migrating via the blood circulation to the fetal liver and spleen, these cells reside in the bone marrow, where hematopoiesis continues throughout life.[25]

Cell differentiation

Depending on the microenvironment present, development of the HPSC can lead to the production of either lymphoid stem cell or myeloid stem cell precursors. Differentiation of lymphoid stem cells evenutally leads to the production of the T and B lymphocytes, cells involved in the specific immune response. Myeloid stem cell precursors differentiate further into erythrocytes and platelets, as well as the cells responsible for the nonspecific immmune responses—the granulocytes (neutrophils, eosinophils, and basophils) and the monocytes and macrophages (Figure 1-9).

Phagocytic cell functions

The two major functions of the nonspecific immune response are inflammation and phagocytosis.[26] The cells primarily responsible for these functions are the granulocytes and the monocytes and macrophages, which develop early during gestation. Although adult numbers of neutrophils are found in peripheral blood long before birth, these cells do not function as phagocytes in early infancy to the extent that they do in adulthood.[14,15] The phagocytic function of neonatal monocytes appears to be equal to that seen in adults, but their function in processing and presenting exogenous antigens to cells of the specific immune response is clearly less.[14,15,27]

As can be seen from Figure 1-9, development of the lymphoid cell lineage proceeds down two different paths to produce either T cells or B cells. At approximately the seventh week of gestation in humans, some of the lymphoid stem cells from the circulation enter the thymus, where they are induced to differentiate into T (thymus-derived) lymphocytes.[14]

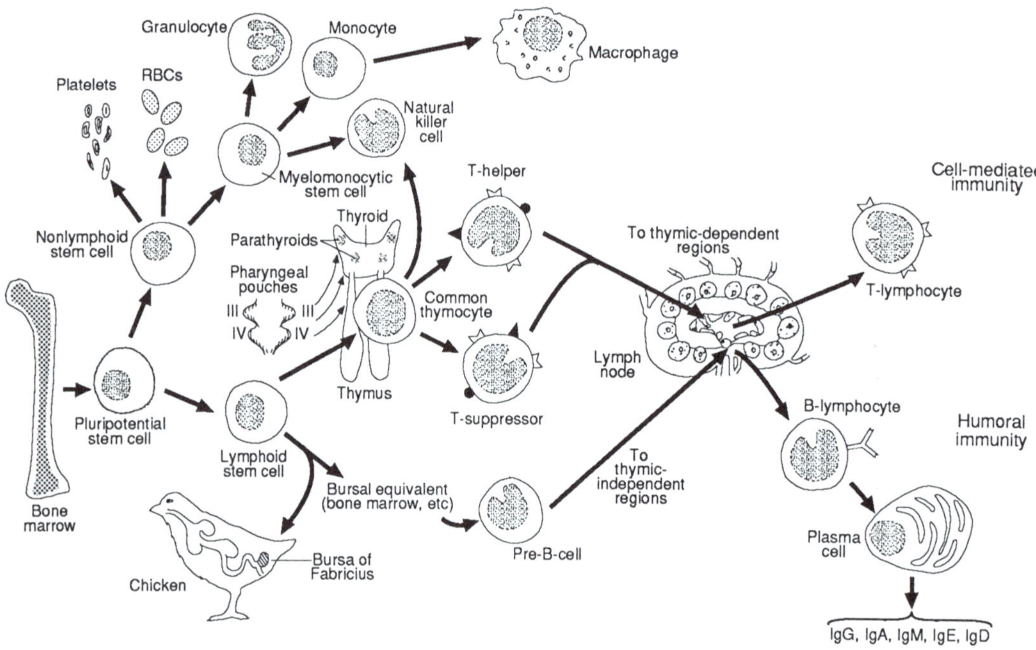

Figure 1-9. Schematic representation of ontogeny of immune response, showing differentiation of progenitor cells into hematopoietic and immunocompetent cells

SOURCE: Adapted with permission from Bellanti JA, Kadlec JV. General immunobiology. In: Bellanti JA, ed. Immunology III. 3rd ed. Philadelphia: W. B. Saunders Company; 1985:48.

T cells

The number of mature T cells in the fetus continues to rise during development and, by the time of birth, reaches a level that is near that of a normal adult or slightly higher. This increase is primarily due to a rise in the number of suppressor T cells.[15]

The function of T cells in utero and at birth has been found to be less than during adulthood. Some T-cell responses are difficult to determine because the most common methods used depend on previous sensitization. Approximately 2 weeks after thymic lymphopoiesis begins, fetal thymocytes become responsive to the T-cell mitogen phytohemagglutinin. In addition, there is evidence that cord blood T lymphocytes can respond to antigens to which the mother has been sensitized.[14] Whether maternal transfer of cell-mediated immunity provides protection to the fetus is unclear.[28]

B cells

B cells are primarily responsible for humoral immunity.[25] Humoral immunity is provided by circulating antibodies and serves as a major defense against bacterial infections. B cells are the precursors of antibody-producing cells.

Pre-B cells, the earliest form of these cells, are first found in the fetal liver by the eighth week of gestation. As soon as the bone marrow becomes functional it contains many pre-B cells, and it is the primary site of these cells in adults. These cells are rarely seen in the spleen, lymph nodes, or blood. Pre-B cells contain mu polypeptide chains in their cytoplasm but contain no antigen receptors (mu chain is the heavy chain of IgM). The next stage of B-cell differentiation is represented by a cell (the immature B lymphocyte) that expresses surface IgM receptors only. This cell is very susceptible to inactivation by antigen, a mechanism thought to be important to the development of tolerance. Between the 10th and 12th weeks of gestation, cells expressing immunoglobulins other than IgM on their surface appear; IgG-positive cells appear before IgD and IgA cells. By the 15th week of gestation, the distribution of different immunoglobulins on the B lymphocytes is similar to that of adults (Figure 1-10).[14] The steps in development shown in Figure 1-10 depend on antigen stimulation and result in plasma cells that manufacture antibodies of one particular immunoglobulin class directed against one specific antigen.

Plasma cells

Few plasma cells develop during gestation, both because of a delay in B-cell maturation in the fetus and because of the protection from antigens provided the fetus by the placenta. Adult levels of IgG are found at birth because of maternal transfer of this immunoglobulin across the placenta, beginning at approximately 32 weeks' gestation. In contrast, the levels of IgA, IgM, IgD, and IgE in the blood are low at birth; IgM is the highest, at 10% of normal adult levels.[14] Lower levels of immunoglobulins at birth (with the exception of IgG) partially explain the increased susceptibility of newborns to Gram-negative infections.[15]

Complement system

The complement system is a group of proteins that circulate in an inactive form until activated by either an antigen-antibody complex (classical pathway) or by bacterial and fungal polysaccharides (alternative pathway). During the first 5 to 6 weeks of gestation, proteins of the complement system start to be produced by the fetal liver. Levels of both classical and alternative pathway components are low in newborns, particularly in low-birthweight infants.[15] This low level of complement may contribute to the increased susceptibility of newborns to infections.

The development of the various components of the immune system has been discussed here as if each component developed separately. This view, however, is too simplistic. Just as the immune system is a complex system of checks and balances, so is its development. The full expression of an

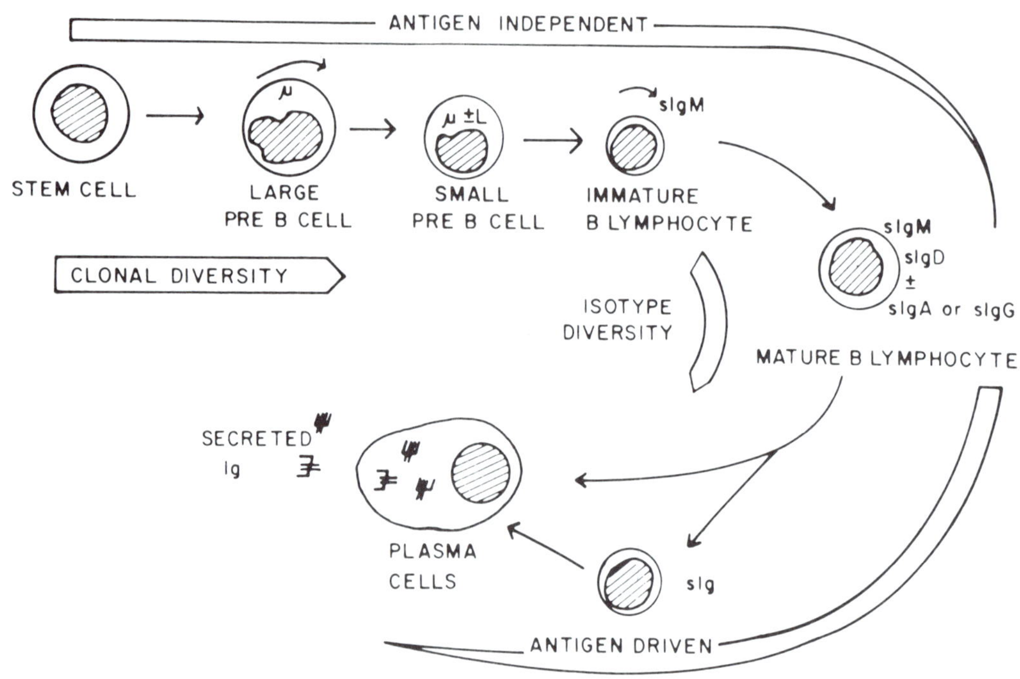

Figure 1-10. Developmental stages of B cells

SOURCE: Reprinted with permission from Lawton AR. Developmental stages of B cells. In: Twomey JJ, ed. The pathophysiology of human immunologic disorders. Baltimore: Williams and Wilkins; 1982:11-28.

immune response depends on the maturation of all the various components. In addition, the functional immaturity of the neonatal immune system may be related to immature cellular interactions rather than immature components. Deficiencies in cell-mediated or humorally mediated immunity in the neonate may be due to incompetent, immature, or absent T or B cells or macrophages, or to alterations in the balance of helper T and suppressor T cells.[14]

Postnatal Development

There is little information on the postnatal development of cell-mediated immunity. It is known that normal delayed hypersensitivity is present before the age of 1 year, but whether older infants' immunity to live microorganisms is equivalent to that of adults is still unclear.[29]

More is known about postnatal development of the humoral immune system. Levels of the various immunoglobulins generally increase after birth as a result of exposure to various antigens. One exception to this increase is IgG. The IgG present in the neonate at birth is primarily maternal and has a half-life of 20 to 30 days. Serum levels of IgG fall rapidly, the lowest levels occurring between the second and fourth months of life. Thereafter they increase, reaching adult levels by 4 to 6 years of age. Adult levels of IgM are usually reached by approximately 1 year of age, and adult levels of IgA by puberty[29] (Figure 1-11).

By the first 3 to 6 months of life, serum complement components of both the alternative and classical pathways reach adult levels.[29]

Summary

The function of the immune system is to protect the host from foreign substances by innate and specific immune defenses. The immune defense system includes physical and biochemical barriers, inflammation, and phagocytosis. If the foreign substance penetrates further and persists, specific immune responses are brought into action.

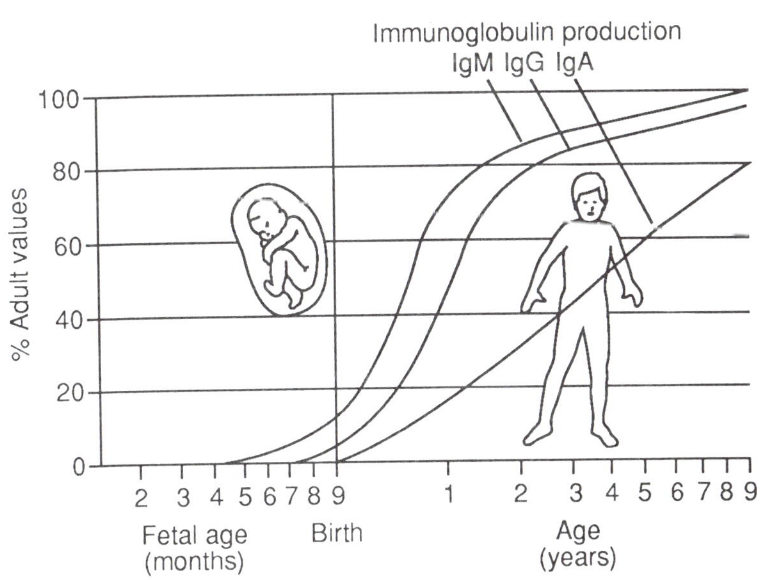

Figure 1-11. The development of serum immunoglobulins in the pre- and postgestational periods

SOURCE: Reprinted with permission from Goldman AS, Han Pong AJ, Goldblum RM. Host defenses: developmental and maternal contributions. *Advances in Pediatrics.* 1985;32:74.

Immunity is conferred by specific immune responses, including the development of antibodies, specialized lymphocytes, and lymphokines. These defenses are composed of two parts. The humoral arm of the immune system mainly fights infection by producing antibodies. The cell-mediated arm of the immune system attacks microorganisms that live intracellularly.

The complement system is a complex series of proteins that augments both the nonspecific and specific immune responses. Since uncontrolled complement reactions can be quite deleterious to the host, complement is a tightly regulated system. The important role that complement plays in the immune system is dramatized by the consequences of various acquired and congenital complement deficiencies.

The normally functioning immune system is a complex balance of many interacting components. Abnormal or deficient development of any one of the components can lead to deficiencies in all phases of the immune response.

References

1. James K. Mechanisms of the nonspecific immune response. In: Sheehan C, ed. Clinical immunology principles and laboratory diagnosis. Philadelphia: J. B. Lippincott Company; 1990:44–50.
2. Saltzman RL, Peterson PK. Immunodeficiency of the elderly. *Review of Infectious Diseases.* 1987;9:1127–35.
3. Male D, Roitt I. Adaptive and innate immunity. In: Roitt I, Brostoff J, Male D, eds. Immunology. 2nd ed. London: Gower Medical Publishing; 1989:1.1–1.10.
4. Vickerstaff Joneja JM, Bielory L, eds. Understanding allergy, sensitivity, and immunity. New Brunswick, NJ: Rutgers University Press; 1990:41–51.
5. Miller LE, Ludke HR, Peacock JE et al, eds. Manual of laboratory immunology. 2nd ed. Philadelphia: Lea and Febiger; 1991:1–25.
6. Widmann FK, ed. An introduction to clinical immunology. Philadelphia: F. A. Davis Company; 1989:44–61.
7. Paul WE. The immune system: an introduction. In: Paul WE, ed. Fundamental immunology. 2nd ed. New York: Raven Press; 1989:3–21.
8. Haynes BF, Fauci AS. The immune system. In: Wilson JD, Braunwald E, Isselbacher KJ, et al, eds. Harrison's principles of internal medicine. 12th ed. New York: McGraw Hill; 1991:76–86.
9. Scott DW, Barth RK. Lymphocyte development, differentiation, and function. In: Hoffman R, Benz EJ, Shattil SJ, et al, eds. Hematology basic principles and practice. New York: Churchill Livingstone; 1991:543–51.

10. Chen S-L. Mechanisms of the specific immune response. In: Sheehan C, ed. Clinical immunology principles and laboratory diagnosis. Philadelphia: J. B. Lippincott Company; 1990:30–43.
11. Howard J, Male D. Immunological tolerance. In: Roitt I, Brostoff J, Male D, eds. Immunology. 2nd ed. London: Gower Medical Publishing; 1989:12.2–12.11.
12. Fike DJ. Nature of antigens. In: Sheehan C, ed. Clinical immunology principles and laboratory diagnosis. Philadelphia: J. B. Lippincott Company; 1990:105–112.
13. Cook A. Genetic control of immunity. In: Roitt I, Brostoff J, Male D, eds. Immunology. 2nd ed. London: Gower Medical Publishing; 1989:11.1–11.9.
14. Lawton AR, Cooper MD. Development and function of the immune system. In: Stiehm ER, ed. Immunologic disorders in infants and children. 3rd ed. Philadelphia: W. B. Saunders Company; 1989:1–15.
15. Burgio GR, Ugazio AG, Notarangelo LD. Immunology of the neonate. *Current Opinion in Immunology.* 1990;2:770–7.
16. Ershler WB. Immune senescence. In: Graziano FM, Lemanske RF, eds. Clinical immunology. Baltimore: Williams and Wilkins; 1989:106–12.
17. Bellanti JA, Kadlec JV. Introduction to immunology. In: Bellanti JA, ed. Immunology III. 3rd ed. Philadelphia: W. B. Saunders Company; 1985:1–15.
18. Chandra RK. The relation between immunology, nutrition and disease in elderly people. *Age Ageing.* 1990;4(suppl):25–31.
19. Golub ES, ed. Immunology: a synthesis. Sunderland, MA: Sinauer Associates; 1987:17–35.
20. Kunkel SL, Ward PA, Caporale LH et al. The complement system. In: Bellanti JA, ed. Immunology III. 3rd ed. Philadelphia: W. B. Saunders Company; 1985:106–16.
21. Frank MM. Complement in the pathophysiology of human disease. *N Engl J Med.* 1987;316:1525–9.
22. Reid KBM. The complement system. In: Hames BD, Glover DM, eds. Molecular immunology. Eynsham, Oxford, England: IRL Press; 1988:189–236.
23. Frank MM, Fries LF. Complement. In: Paul WE, ed. Fundamental immunology. 2nd ed. New York: Raven Press; 1989:679–701.
24. Dawson M, Moore M. Tumour immunology. In: Roitt I, Brostoff J, Male D, eds. Immunology. 2nd ed. London: Gower Medical Publishing; 1989:18.1–18.17.
25. Sharp JG, Crouse DA, Purtilo DT. Ontogeny and regulation of the immune system. *Archives of Pathology and Laboratory Medicine.* 1987;11:1106–12.
26. Tami JA. Immunology for the clinical pharmacist. *Pharmacotherapy.* 1987;7(suppl 2):3s–6s.

27. Lydyard P, Grossi C: Development of the immune system. In: Roitt I, Brostoff J, Male D, eds. Immunology. 2nd ed. London: Gower Medical Publishing; 1989:14.2–14.9.
28. Pabst JF, Godel JC, Spady W et al. Transfer of maternal specific cell-mediated immunity to the fetus. *Clinical and Experimental Immunology*. 1987;68:209–14.
29. Goldman AS, Ham Pong AJ, Goldblum RM. Host defenses: development and maternal contributions. *Advances in Pediatrics.* 1985;32:71–100.

Self-Study Questions

1. What innate defense mechanisms work together to destroy almost all orally ingested pathogens?

   1. Acidic stomach and alkaline small intestine.

2. In what way do intestinal bacteria function as a first line of defense in protecting the host from pathogens?

   2. The noninvasive intestinal bacteria compete for the same nutrients needed by the pathogens.

3. Which of the following is principally responsible for cell-mediated immunity?

   A. Phagocytes.
   B. Macrophages.
   C. B lymphocytes.
   D. T lymphocytes.

   3. D

4. What is the term associated with the immune system's ability to mount an accelerated response upon reexposure to antigen?

   A. Memory.
   B. Phagocytosis.
   C. Specificity.
   D. Tolerance.

   4. A

5. Autologous antigens that elicit an immune response may cause autoimmune diseases.

   A. True.
   B. False.

   5. A

6. Which of the following elicits the greatest immunogenic response?

   A. Lipids.
   B. Nucleic acids.
   C. Carbohydrates.
   D. Hydrophobic molecules.

   6. C

7. B

7. How is the alternative pathway of the complement system usually activated?

   A. Antigen-antibody complexes.
   B. Polysaccharides in bacterial cell walls.
   C. Other proteins.
   D. Lymphokines.

8. Initiation of the cascade, amplification of the reactions, and membrane attack leading to cell death.

8. List the three major steps in the complement cascade.

9. 3 to 6 months.

9. How many months usually pass before a newborn's serum complement components of alternative and classical pathways reach adult levels?

10. 2nd, 4th; 4 to 6 years.

10. Serum levels of IgG in newborns reach their lowest between the _____and _____ months of life, reaching adult levels by ______________________.

CHAPTER 2

Cellular and Tissue Components of the Immune System

*Jim Koeller, M.S.**
Clinical Associate Professor, University of Texas
Oncology Clinical Specialist, Audie Murphy Hospital
San Antonio, TX

Introduction

Immunotherapy encompasses a range of therapies designed to manipulate the human immune system. These therapies include active and passive immunization, treatment with immunopotentiators and immunosuppressants, hyposensitization for allergic disorders, and bone marrow transplantation. In each of these immunotherapy processes, the cells and tissues of the immune system are called into action to achieve the desired immune response.

It has only been recently, however, that immunologic research has been able to provide advanced knowledge about the mechanism of action of the immune system's cells and tissues. This knowledge has led to the development of new drugs and therapies used for treating such illnesses as cancer, arthritis, and diabetes.

Understanding how the cells and tissue of the immune system function will help the pharmacist in establishing immune therapy goals and regimens and monitoring patient response. In later chapters, the knowledge gained from this chapter will assist the learner in understanding the effects of specific immunotherapy on the complex interactions of the immune system and its components. Appropriate cellular and tissue response to therapy is crucial to preventing disease, treating disease, and avoiding graft rejection.

Learning objectives

After reading this chapter, the learner will be able to—

- Describe the immunologic function of the mononuclear phagocytes.
- Describe the immunologic function of polymorphonuclear granulocytes.
- Discuss the mechanism of action of phagocytosis.
- Describe the immunologic function of T lymphocytes.

*The author wishes to acknowledge the contributions of Tracey A. Waddelow, Pharm. D., and Michael C. Sneller, M.D., to the development of this chapter.

- Describe the mechanism of action of B lymphocytes.
- Describe the functions of the lymphatic tissues of the immune system.

Chapter organization

This chapter first discusses myeloid and lymphoid cells and their roles in the innate and acquired immune responses. Phagocytosis is explained with descriptions of monocytes, macrophages, antigen-presenting cells, granulocytes, and platelets. A discussion of the T lymphocytes and their subpopulation markers follows. The characteristics and function of antibodies are discussed next. The chapter concludes with a description of the tissues of the immune system.

Suggested Preparation

Chapter 1 of this text should be read before reading this chapter. In addition, the reader may find the following references helpful.

- Bellanti JA, ed. Immunology III. Philadelphia: W. B. Saunders Company; 1985.
- Roitt IM, Brostoff J, Male DK. Immunology. 2nd ed. London: Gower Medical Publishing; 1989.
- Stites DP, Terr AI. Basic and clinical immunology. 7th ed. East Norwalk, CT: Appleton and Lange; 1991.

Nonspecific Cellular Components

Myeloid and lymphoid cells

Most of the immune system cells are white blood cells (WBCs) that originate in the bone marrow. WBCs are broadly categorized as myeloid or lymphoid cells. The myeloid cells are the major components of the nonspecific (or innate) immune response, and the lymphoid cells make up the specific (or acquired) immune response. When a foreign substance (antigen) is first introduced into the body, the nonspecific immune response, including phagocytosis and inflammation, is initiated. Subsequent exposure to the same antigen involves primarily the specific immune response, including memory B and T cells.

Myeloid cells grow to maturity in the bone marrow compartment. Lymphoid cells differentiate and mature in lymphatic tissues, including bone marrow and the thymus, the primary lymphatic tissues. Some of the lymphoid cells then circulate through the secondary lymphatic tissues such as the spleen and lymph nodes.

The maturation process of each of the different functional blood cells is depicted in Figure 2-1. Myeloid and lymphoid cell lines can develop from either the pluripotent or totipotent stem cell of the bone marrow. The entire

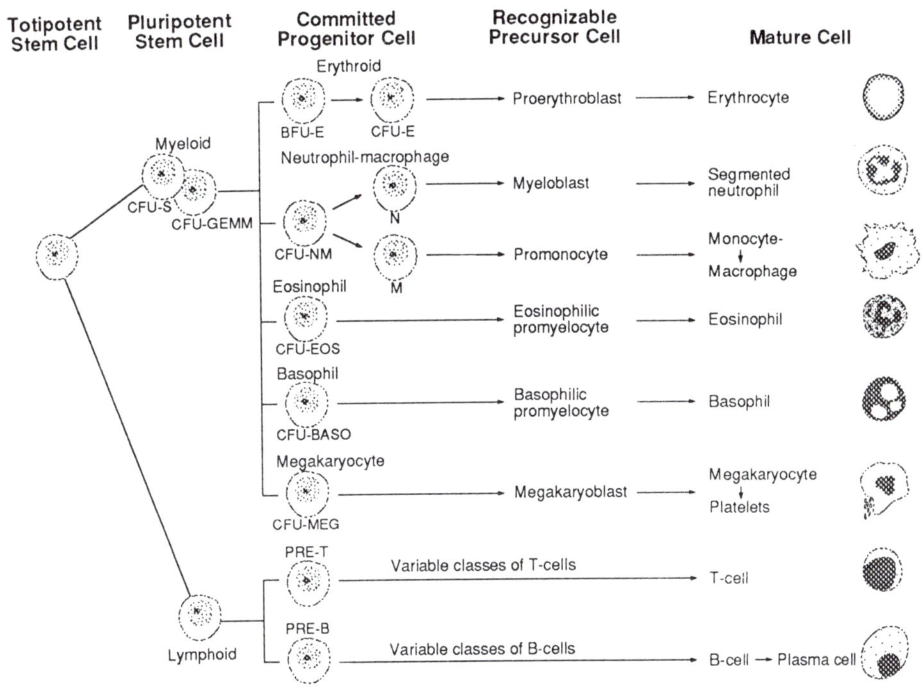

baso = basophil; BFU = burst-forming unit; CFU = colony-forming unit; E = erythrocyte; EOS = eosinophil; GEMM = granulocyte, erythrocyte, macrophage, monocyte; meg = megakaryocyte; NM = neutrophil/ monocyte; S = stem cell

Figure 2-1. Hematopoiesis—the process of blood cell maturation from the stem cells to the active, functional blood cell

SOURCE: Reprinted with permission from Chervenick PA. Hematopoiesis. In: Stein JH, ed. Internal medicine. 2nd ed. Boston: Little, Brown;1987:912.

hematopoietic cascade relies on the self-renewing capacity of the pluripotent stem cell. Stem cells, by definition, are all capable of self-renewal or differentiation. The process of hematopoiesis is influenced by growth factors such as the colony-stimulating factors (CSFs) as well as the marrow microenvironment.[1]

Six cell types are involved in the nonspecific immune response or myeloid family: mononuclear phagocytes (monocytes and macrophages), polymorphonuclear granulocytes (neutrophils), eosinophils, basophils, mast cells, and platelets.[2]

Phagocytosis

One hundred years ago the Russian zoologist Metchnikoff microscopically observed the result of introducing a rose thorn into starfish larvae (the larvae have no circulatory system and are almost transparent). The area became swollen from the visible movement of many cells to the puncture site. He theorized that the function of these mobile cells was to defend the organism by attacking the intruder.[3]

It is now known that even upon the first entry of a foreign substance, phagocytic cells take up and remove the antigen. All that is required during this first exposure of the antigen is recognition of the substance as nonself. Simple recognition, coupled with the fact that phagocytic cells do not bear antigen-specific receptors, explains the term "nonspecific immune response."

In the nonspecific immune response, the most active cells are the phagocytes, which are committed to destroying foreign particles (antigens). The activity of these cells is unchanged by their interaction with the antigen. Both mononuclear cells (macrophages) and polynuclear cells (neutrophils and eosinophils) are capable of phagocytosis.[4]

Process

The process of phagocytosis begins with stimulation of the phagocytic cell, which initiates the following series of cellular events. The phagocyte moves toward the foreign substance in a process called chemotaxis. The complement system, bacteria, lymphocytes, neutrophils, and cancer cells all produce chemotactic substances that attract the phagocytic cell to the foreign invader (see Figure 1-3, Chapter 1).[2-5]

Products of the complement system and of lymphocytes (immunoglobulin G) coat (opsonize) the antigen, facilitating chemotaxis (see Chapter 1) and phagocytosis. Specific complement receptors (CR1 and CR3) found on neutrophils and macrophages function to opsonize particles. These receptors multiply greatly as lymphokines and other chemotactic substances are released (see Chapter 1). The phagocyte then attaches to and engulfs the antigen with cellular projections (pseudopods), resulting in an intracellular vesicle containing the antigen. Enzymes are secreted into the vesicle to break down and inactivate the antigen. Finally, parts of this processed antigen may be deposited on the surface membrane of the phagocyte to enable lymphocytes to recognize and react to the antigen.[2-7] (See the discussion of major histocompatibility complex in Chapter 3.)

Mononuclear Phagocytes

Development

The function of monocytes and macrophages is based on size, cellular morphology, and location of each cell. Monocytes develop from the myeloid stem cell in the bone marrow and circulate through the bloodstream. Once the monocyte leaves the circulation and enters tissue it is called a macrophage. This transformation produces a cell 10 times the size of a monocyte. The macrophage has increased phagocytic capacity resulting from an increased supply of enzymes, lysosomes, and energy-producing mitochondria.

Macrophage types

There are two types of macrophage, fixed and wandering. The fixed macrophages are described according to their location in tissue: alveolar macrophages line the alveoli of the lung, histiocytes are in the connective tissues, littoral cells are in the spleen, microglial cells are in the brain, peritoneal macrophages patrol the abdominal cavity, mesangial cells are in the kidney, and Kupffer cells reside in the liver.[2,3,8] Wandering macrophages respond to infectious pathogens or invaders throughout the body.

The maturation process from pluripotent stem cell in the bone marrow to monocyte takes 7 days (Figure 2-2). Monocytes live in the circulation 2 to 3 days before they leave the bloodstream and enter tissue to become macrophages. Monocytes leave the blood vessel by a process known as diapedesis after they become adherent to the blood vessel wall. The migration of the monocyte into the tissues without the stimulation of inflammation is apparently a random event. The average turnover rate for the macrophages is 7 million cells per hour per kilogram of body weight. The life span of a macrophage is thought to be measured in months. Although macrophages are mature cells, they remain capable of cell division, a capacity neutrophils do not possess. Factors contributing to the death of these cells are yet unknown. One hypothesis is that an intense phagocytosis may lead to their demise through the uncontrolled release of enzymes and other chemicals directly into the cell's cytoplasm.[3,5,8,9]

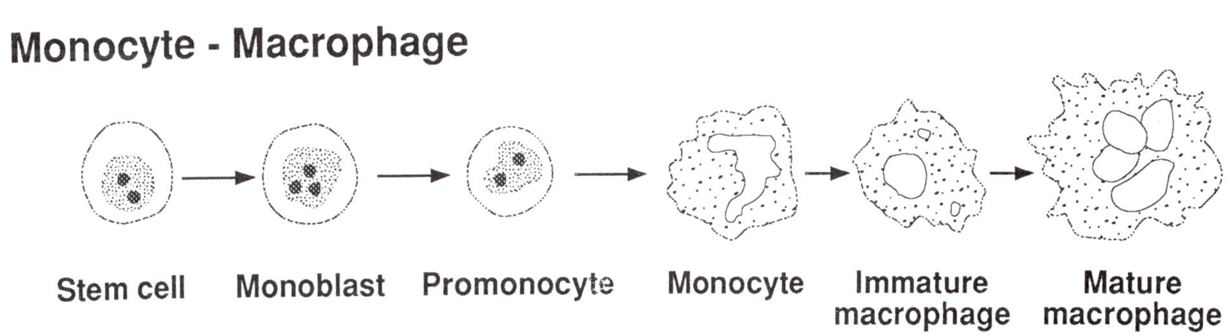

Figure 2-2. Mononuclear development

SOURCE: Reprinted with permission from Hutton JJ, Cline MJ. Hematopoiesis and the red cell. In: Stein JH, ed. Internal medicine. Boston: Little, Brown;1983:1470.)

The outer membrane of a macrophage moves constantly. It is studded with microvilli, which help attach the macrophage to antigen. The cell's interior has many small lysosomes containing digestive enzymes such as acid hydrolases and peroxidase. When released into the phagocytic vesicle, these enzymes kill the invading organism. Two receptors on the cell's outer membrane promote binding of the macrophage to the invader. Fc (crystallizable fragment) is the immunoglobulin receptor, and C3b the receptor for complement. There are other receptors on the macrophage membrane for lymphokines to facilitate communication among cells.[3,5,6]

Macrophage activation

A normal resting macrophage is activated by lymphokines such as interferon (IFN) gamma and granulocyte-macrophage colony-stimulating factor (GM-CSF), which are both released from T lymphocytes (see Chapter 10). Once activated, macrophages release tumor necrosis factor (TNF) and interleukin-1 (IL-1), resulting in a more efficient killing cell. The activated macrophage increases in size, develops more pseudopods, and is better able to adhere to the antigen surface.[5-8]

APCs

Macrophages also function as antigen-presenting cells (APCs) that process the antigen biochemically to a more immunogenic form and present it on the cell surface to be recognized by specific, sensitized T lymphocytes. This APC activity is expressed by macrophages bearing surface class II major histocompatibility complex (MHC) molecules (see Chapter 3). APCs initially activate helper T cells (discussed later in this chapter). The term APC is often used to designate a specific form of macrophage.

Other cell types that function as APCs are dendritic cells, B lymphocytes, and microglial cells. APCs are primarily located in the skin (Langerhans' cell), lymph nodes and spleen (follicular dendritic cell), central nervous system tissue (microglial cells), and thymus. Inside the lymph node, the APC is uniquely able to interdigitate with more than one T cell, resulting in a very efficient means of presenting antigen to many cells at once.[2,5,8]

Granulocytes

Granulocytes contain cytoplasmic granules that can be stained. The color, type, and number of the granules vary depending on the stage of cell growth and development. Generally, the granules contain enzymes used in cellular function. The granulocyte family comprises neutrophils, eosinophils, basophils, and mast cells.

Function and characteristics

Neutrophils. The primary function of neutrophils is to phagocytize foreign particles. These specialized WBCs make up 60% to 70% of the total WBC count. Mature polymorphonuclear granulocytes are released into the bloodstream after a 14-day process of developing from pluripotent stem cells in the bone marrow. Granulocytes reside in the bloodstream for approximately 7 hours before they enter the tissues, where they survive for an additional 1 to 3 days (Figure 2-3).[5,9,10] More than 100 billion neutrophils are produced each day.

Eosinophils. Eosinophils make up 1% to 3% of the total WBCs. Their granules are large and stain intensely red. They mature in the bone marrow for 3 to 6 days, then remain in the bloodstream for only minutes before entering the tissues for the remainder of their lives—approximately 12 days. Eosinophils have the capacity to phagocytize microorganisms, but not as efficiently as neutrophils and macrophages. Other immunologic roles of eosinophils include ingesting immune complexes and clearing parasitic organisms from the host.[2,3,6]

Basophils. Basophils make up less than 1% of the total WBC count. They are distinguished by their large, blue-staining, cytoplasmic granules, which contain histamine and other inflammatory mediators. Basophils have on their surface specific receptors that bind IgE antibody molecules secreted

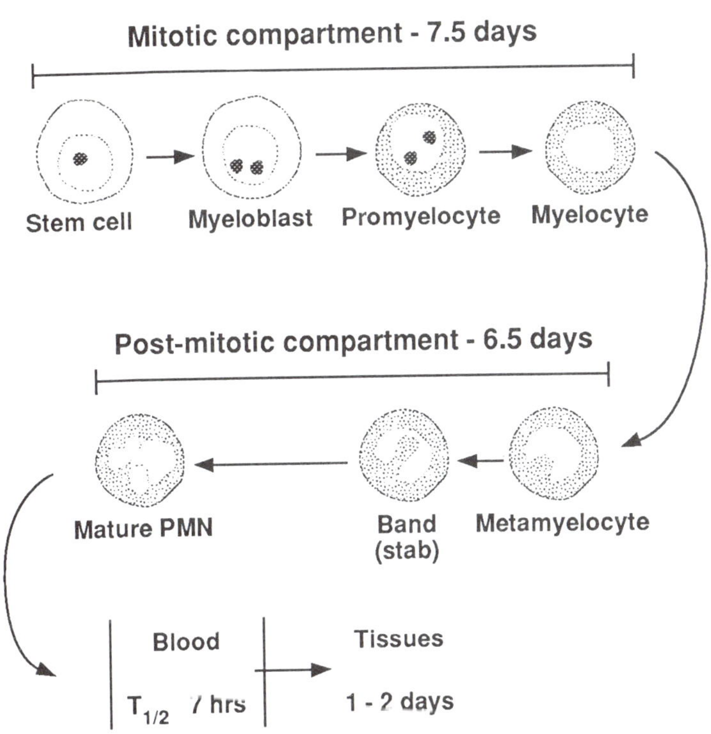

Figure 2-3. Neutrophil development

SOURCE: Reprinted with permission from Chervenick PA. Hematopoiesis. In: Stein JH, ed. Internal medicine. 2nd ed. Boston: Little, Brown;1987:913.

by B lymphocytes. When an antigen molecule interacts with these membrane-bound IgE antibodies, the basophil is triggered to release histamine and other inflammatory mediators. Histamine release increases vascular permeability, allowing deposition of antigen-antibody complexes. Antihistamines block this deposition.[2,6]

Mast Cells. Like basophils, mast cells stain blue, contain histamine and other inflammatory mediators in their granules, and are stimulated when IgE binds to their surface receptors. Mast cells leave the bone marrow more quickly than basophils to enter connective tissue (e.g., the gastrointestinal tract), where they mature. The life span for mast cells is 14 to 18 days. Mature mast cells still have the capacity to differentiate.

Two broad subtypes of mast cells exist. Connective tissue-type mast cells are most commonly found around blood vessels, particularly in the skin, abdominal cavity, and lungs. They contain both heparin and histamine. Most prominent in the gastrointestinal tract are mucosal-type mast cells, which contain histamine but lack heparin.[7]

Platelets

Much like basophils, platelets function as mediator cells. Platelets have a life span of 7 to 9 days. They are cellular fragments from the large megakaryocytes in the bone marrow.[2,6] Platelets are involved primarily in blood clotting. They function immunologically during the inflammatory response by releasing factors that alter permeability and activate complement components to draw other WBCs to the site. The surface of platelets contains receptors for IgG and IgE as well as class I MHC products.

Specific Cellular Components

Lymphocytes

Lymphocytes make up 20% of the circulating white cells. The bone marrow and thymus produce 1 billion lymphocytes per day. The life span of the lymphocyte can be quite long, up to years for memory cells. The lymphoid cells are a very heterogeneous group of cells that can be morphologically described as small lymphocytes or large granular lymphocytes. T lymphocytes, which mature in the thymus, are primarily responsible for cell-mediated immunity; B lymphocytes are responsible for what is historically known as humoral immunity (Figure 2-4), and null cells assist in antibody-dependent cellular cytotoxicity. Physically, these lymphocytes appear quite similar; T and B lymphocytes can be distinguished from one

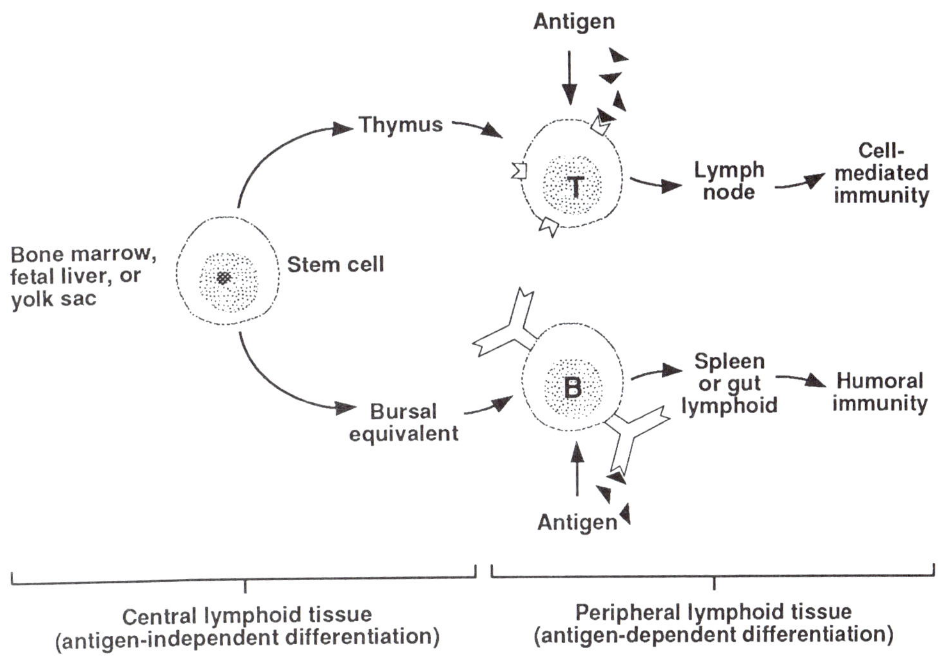

Figure 2-4. Lymphoid system

SOURCE: Reprinted with permission from Bellanti JA, Kadiec JV. General immunobiology. In: Bellanti JA, ed. Immunology III. Philadelphia: W. B. Saunders Company;1985:33.

another by cell surface markers.[10,11] (See Chapter 5 for separation techniques.)

T Lymphocytes (Cell-mediated Immunity)

Function

T lymphocytes develop from stem cells in the bone marrow but differentiate within the thymus. They spend their lives circulating between the bloodstream and the lymphatic system (lymph nodes or spleen). The many T-cell functions include regulating B cells, developing resistance to bacterial or viral invasion, and producing soluble cellular mediators such as the interleukins. T cells are the primary mediators of processes such as graft-versus-host disease, delayed-type hypersensitivity reactions, and allograft rejection. These various aspects of T-cell function are collectively referred to as cell-mediated immunity.

The four classes of T cells are helper (inducer), suppressor, cytotoxic, and memory (delayed hypersensitivity).[1,2,12,13] Helper and suppressor lymphocytes are also known as regulatory cells; cytotoxic lymphocytes are called mediator cells; memory lymphocytes are referred to as effector cells.[1]

Helper T Cells. The primary function of the helper (inducer) cell is to orchestrate communication among the other cell types. This is why helper cells are generically referred to as regulatory cells. When an APC presents an antigen to the helper T cell, the T cell is stimulated to release IL-2, a lymphokine. IL-2 then stimulates other helper T cells, as well as cytotoxic and memory T cells. A second lymphokine secreted by helper T cells, IFN gamma, stimulates natural killer (NK) cells and macrophages. In addition to establishing communication among T lymphocytes, helper T cells produce other lymphokines, such as IL-4, that stimulate the growth and differentiation of B cells.[1,2,12]

Regulatory cells

Suppressor T Cells. Controversy currently exists about whether suppressor cells or a suppressor substance is responsible for the functions ascribed to it. In theory, suppressor T cells function as inhibitors rather than stimulators. Like the helper T cells, suppressor T cells act on other T lymphocytes to inhibit the proliferation and stimulation of these cells. The suppressor cell (or factor) also inhibits plasma cell functions and antibody production. In addition, the suppressor cell (or factor) participates in developing tolerance. Tolerance could be desirable for the host if the antigens are substances used in drug therapy or, as in the case of autoimmune disease, are host cells.[1,2,12]

Cytotoxic T Cells. Cytotoxic cells are the real warriors among the T lymphocytes. They attack cells bearing specific antigens on their membranes. Cytotoxic cells bore holes through the invader's membrane, resulting in cell lysis and death. Cytotoxic cells are thought to be primarily responsible for graft rejection (see Chapter 9). A single cytotoxic T cell can kill more than one target cell, which suggests that cytotoxic T cells are resistant to the lysing substances they contain.[1,2,12]

Because suppressor and cytotoxic T cells bear no surface markers that make it possible to distinguish between them, there has been speculation that they are in fact the same cell type. They do have different functional activities, however, and are generally considered to be two different cell types.

Delayed hypersensitivity

Memory T Cells. These cells are more appropriately called delayed hypersensitivity (DHS) cells because they play a pivotal role in inflammation associated with contact hypersensitivity. T cells that mediate DHS reactions release cytokines that function to activate macrophages and other phagocytic leukocytes for their important role in this inflammatory process. Interferon-gamma secreted by activated T cells plays a central role in the process of macrophage activation. Interferon-gamma enhances the ability of macrophages to migrate to sites of infection, phagocytose particles, and produce microbicidal oxygen metabolites, proteases, and cytokines. Other cytokines, such as IL-4 and GM-CSF, that are produced by T cells also function as macrophage activators. The delayed reaction occurs

24 to 48 hours after initial contact as cells accumulate, causing local tissue damage.[2,12,13]

T-lymphocyte Subpopulation Markers

There are many T-cell surface markers, some more specific than others. The markers are useful for identifying the developmental stage and functional capacity of the T cells. Surface markers also make it possible to isolate T cells from all other cells and isolate specific subtypes of T lymphocytes from one another.[13,14] These markers may appear and disappear during T-cell development.

Sheep Erythrocyte Rosettes. One surface marker found on all T cells is a surface protein (CD2) that naturally serves as an adhesion molecule, allowing T cells to bind to other cells. Sheep erythrocytes (SEs) express CD58, the ligand for CD2, and bind to the T cell at the CD2 surface marker. When combined, the T cells and the SEs form a visible rosette pattern. The T cells can be detected by the fluorescent stain of the nucleus, since the mature SEs are not nucleated. This binding process can also be used to isolate T cells from non-T cells.[2,13,14] (See Chapter 5.)

CD2 binding

Monoclonal Antibodies (MoAbs). MoAbs are immunoglobulins that have been produced by cloning a single cell, resulting in identical antibody molecules (see Chapter 11). The clinical relevance of these lymphocyte markers is that they make it possible to detect quantitative abnormalities of lymphocyte subsets in various disease states. (See Chapter 11 for further information on MoAbs.) On a more sophisticated level than mere separation of broad categories of T versus non-T lymphocytes, monoclonal antibody technology can identify specific lymphocyte subtypes (see Table 2-1). These distinct antigens on the leukocyte surface are categorized as clusters of differentiation (CDs). Some CDs are found on many different cell types; others are very specific to a particular cell type.

Clusters of differentiation

B Lymphocytes (Humoral Immunity)

B lymphocytes are called B cells because they were first identified in the bursa of Fabricius, a specialized organ in chickens. Stimulation of B lymphocyte results in antibody or immunoglobulin production. If serum containing antibodies is given to a host deficient in those antibodies, the host will be protected or may become sensitized to the correlating antigens. Historically, serum was called humor; hence the term humoral immunity.[1,2]

B lymphocytes originate in the bone marrow from a common stem cell, as do the cells described earlier. B-cell maturation in the bone marrow occurs without antigen stimulation. Once B cells have matured, they

Development

Table 2-1 Monoclonal Antibodies to Human T-lymphocyte Surface Antigens

Cluster Designation*	Commercial Monoclonal Antibodies	Molecular Weight of Molecules	Comments
Pan T cell			
CD2	Anti-T11, Leu-5, OKT11	50,000	Erythrocyte rosette-associated protein; adhesion molecule ligand for CD58.
CD3	Anti-T3, Leu-4, OKT3	20,000 22,000 28,000	Modulates antigen-specific T-cell responses; part of the T-cell receptor complex.
CD5	Anti-T1, Leu-1, OKT1	67,000	T- and B-cell marker; ligand for CD72.
T-cell subset			
CD4	Anti-T4, Leu-3a, Leu-3b, OKT4	60,000	CD4+ T cells contain most inducer/helper functions; primarily class II MHC restricted; 50% to 65% of peripheral T cells.
CD8	Anti-T8, Leu-2a, Leu-3b	30,000 32,000	CD8+ peripheral T cells contain most suppressor/cytolytic functions; functions are class I MHC restricted; 25% to 35% of peripheral T cells.
CD25	Anti-tac	55,000	Recognizes low-affinity IL-2 receptor; blocks proliferation and IL-2 binding.

*Designations of clusters of differentiation (CDs) as assigned by the Fourth International Workshop and Conference on Human Lymphocyte Differentiation Antigens.

immediately leave the marrow to reside in peripheral tissues, where they are developed further by antigenic stimulation. After a mature B lymphocyte is

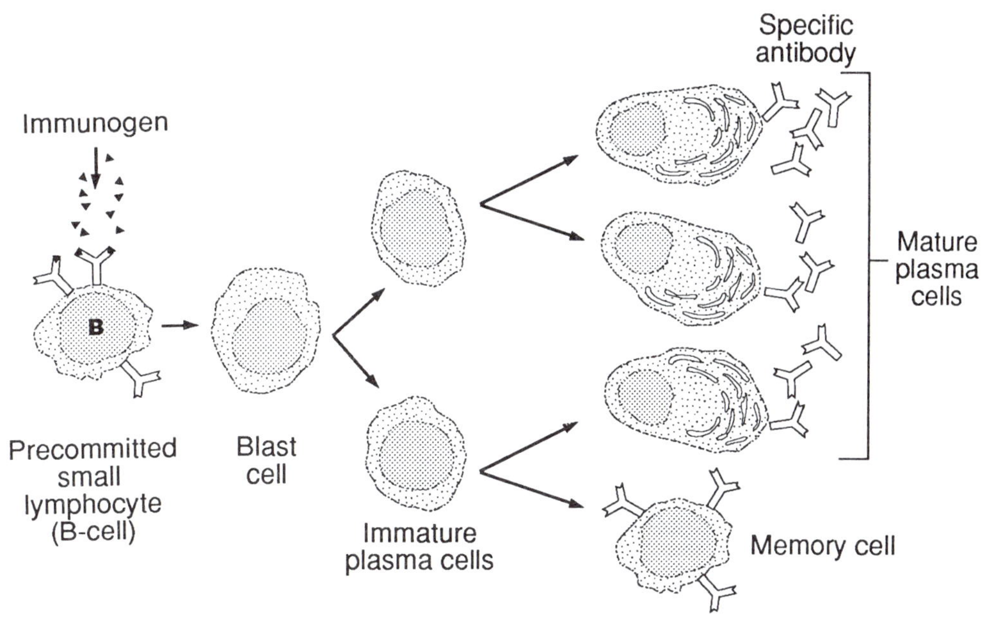

Figure 2-5. Humoral immune responses

SOURCE: Reprinted with permission from Herscowitz HB. Immunophysiology: cell function and cellular interactions in antibody formation. In: Bellanti JA, ed. Immunology III. Philadelphia: W. B. Saunders Company;1985:125.

stimulated by its correlating antigen, it may differentiate into the antibody-producing cell, the plasma cell (Figure 2-5). The B cells that encounter their complementary antigen and are helped by the T lymphocyte may differentiate into memory (effector) cells with a much longer life span.[1,2]

Fc receptors

The membrane of the B cell bears a surface immunoglobulin that is specific for only one antigen. In addition, there are membrane receptors for complement components (C3d and C3b), the Fc portion of the immunoglobulin, IFN, and a B-cell-stimulating factor called BSF-1 (recently renamed IL-4) that is produced by helper T cells and other cells. Activated B cells express other receptors used to modify growth and differentiation. Preliminary work on other B-cell markers has not produced more reliable or specific markers than surface immunoglobulin. Other cells, including T cells, carry Fc receptors, but not all B cells bear them.[2,12,13]

Stimulation

B-lymphocyte stimulation is a complex process that is only partially understood. One known mechanism is the specific antigenic activation of B lymphocytes with the help of T lymphocytes. Another mechanism uses T cells to produce nonspecific activation factors. Mitogens (substances such as lipopolysaccharide or bacterial endotoxin) induce lymphocyte proliferation and may stimulate B cells nonspecifically. B cells may also be simply and directly stimulated by some large polymeric molecules (e.g., antigens such as dextran and polyvinylpyrolidone) without T cell help.[13,15] Once stimulated, B cells can differentiate into plasma cells, which actually produce the antibody.

Antibody. The primary function of the plasma cell is to produce antibodies (immunoglobulins that interact with a specific antigen) against substances potentially harmful to the host. Figure 2-6 shows the basic structure of the IgG class of immunoglobulin.

Structure

Four polypeptide chains make up the basic Y-shaped structure of immunoglobulin. The two smaller ones are identical light chains; the two larger ones are identical heavy chains. The heavy chains are roughly twice as long as the light chains, extending the full length of the Y-shaped molecule, while the light chains are found only along the two arms of the Y. The Fab (fragment of antigen binding) portion of the immunoglobulin contains variable regions of amino acids that allow the Fab molecule to recognize a specific antigen when it binds between the heavy and light chain of the Fab region. The Fc portion of the structure determines the effector function and class (IgG, IgM, IgA, IgD, or IgE) of the

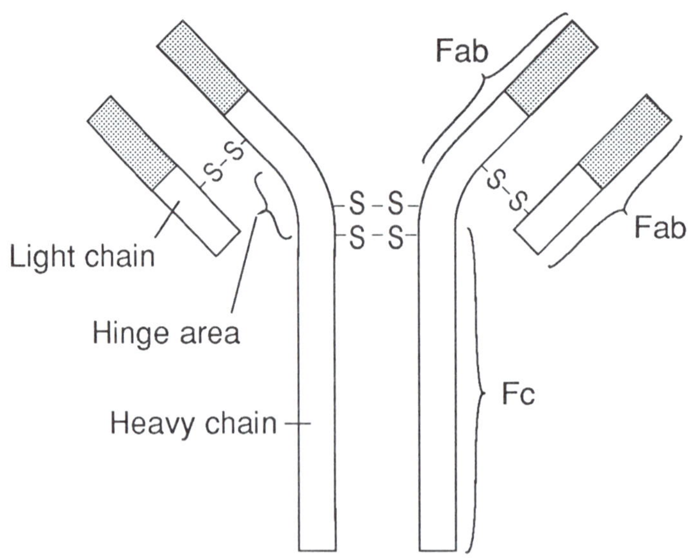

dotted areas = variable regions white areas = constant regions

Figure 2-6. Basic immunoglobulin structure

SOURCE: Adapted with permission from Tami JA, Parr MC, Thompson JS. The immune system. *Am J Hosp Pharm,* 1986;43:2485.

immunoglobulin and is the portion of the antibody that binds to cells bearing Fc receptors.[1,2,15]

Regions

The immunoglobulin molecule can be divided into four regions. The hinge region is a flexible area at the base of the V that allows the two arms of the Y to move closer or further apart. Each arm of the Y is an independent antigen-binding site. The end portion of the V (amino terminal) is known to exhibit variation in amino acid sequence, hence the term variable region. The inner portion of the V (carboxy terminal) remains fairly consistent and is called the constant region. The areas of greater variation within the variable region are referred to as hypervariable regions.[1,2,15]

Classification. Antibodies are glycoproteins that can be classified into five distinct immunoglobulin classes based on the type of heavy chain each contains: IgG, IgA, IgD, IgE, and IgM. The distinguishing letters stand for gamma, alpha, delta, epsilon, and mu, respectively. IgG and IgA can be further subtyped as subclasses IgG1 through IgG4, IgA1, and IgA2. There are only two types of light chains, kappa and lambda. Either may combine with the five different heavy chains, but both light chains within one immunoglobulin will be identical. The four chains are held together by covalent and noncovalent bonds as well as disulfide linkages. IgG, IgD, and IgE all occur as single molecules. IgM occurs as a pentamer in the circulation, but on the surface of the lymphocyte it occurs as a monomer. IgA occurs in monomeric and polymeric forms (Figure 2-7).[2,15]

Properties and Functions. The five immunoglobulin classes or isotypes differ in size, charge, amino acid sequence, and carbohydrate content (Table 2-2). Each class of immunoglobulin is heterogeneous; this can be demonstrated electrophoretically.

Antigen-Antibody Interactions—Binding. Binding occurs between the antigen and the antibody-binding site through multiple noncovalent bonds. These weaker forces, such as hydrogen bonds and Van der Waals forces, are so numerous that they contribute a great deal of binding energy. Close proximity between the antigen and antibody is the primary force creating these noncovalent bonds. In addition, structural characteristics lead to the proper fit between the antigen and antibody, maximizing bond formation and minimizing the development of repulsive forces.[2,15,16]

Binding forces

Affinity. The net result of attractive and repulsive forces between a monovalent antigen and one antibody-binding site is termed affinity. In other words, affinity is an expression of the strength of the interaction between antigen and antibody. The greater the attractive forces, the higher the affinity and probably the better the fit between the antigen and antibody. Conversely, less attractive forces imply less affinity and a poorer fit.[2]

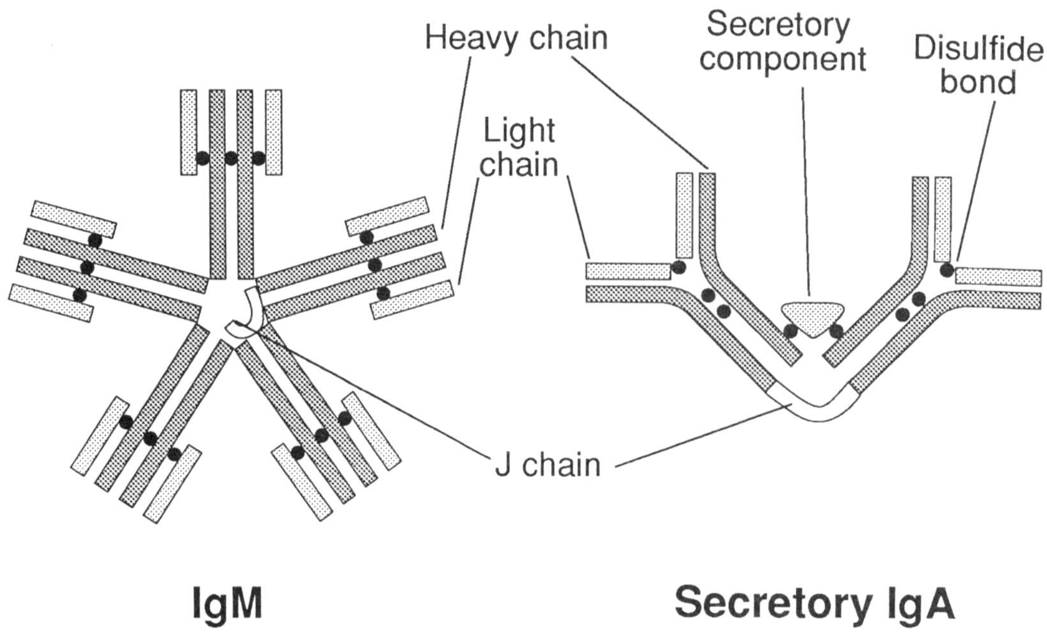

Figure 2-7. The IgM and IgA structure

SOURCE: Reprinted with permission from Bernier GM. Antibody and immunoglobulins: structure and function. In: Bellanti JA, ed. Immunology III. Philadelphia: W. B. Saunders Company;1985:93.

Avidity. Avidity describes the functional combined strength of an antibody to an antigen. Unlike affinity, which can be quantified, avidity is a more general term. In fact, avidity of the antibody for the antigen depends on the affinities at each binding site, but avidity is more than the combined affinities of each binding site. One antigen often has many binding sites, which can give an extra boost to the overall antigen-antibody interaction.

Affinity and avidity are important in biologic reactions such as viral neutralization, enzyme inactivation, and complement fixation. High-affinity reactions are more desirable because high-affinity immune complexes are rapidly cleared from the circulation with little effect on renal function. Low-affinity complexes are cleared more slowly from the circulation and can be deposited on glomerular membranes, causing renal impairment.[2]

Specificity. Specificity is the ability of the antibody to distinguish its own specific antigen from other antigens. The antibody's ability to interact with other related antigens is termed cross-reactivity.[2]

Memory Cells. Both T and B lymphocytes are capable of differentiating into memory (i.e., DHS and effector) cells after initial contact with the

Table 2-2 Immunoglobulin Classification

	Immunoglobulin Class				
Variables	IgG	IgM	IgA	IgE	IgD
Heavy chain	Gamma	Mu	Alpha	Epsilon	Delta
Subclasses	Gamma 1, 2, 3, 4	Mu 1, 2	Alpha 1, 2	None	None
Extra chains	None	Joining	Joining and secretory	None	None
Serum concentration (approximate % of total Ig)	70	20	10	<1	<1
Plasma half-life (days)	IgG 1 = 21 IgG 2 = 20 IgG 3 = 7 IgG 4 = 21	5–10	6	2	3
Molecular weight	150,000 polymer	900,000 polymer	350,000	190,000	100,000
% carbohydrate	3	12	7	12	13
Placental transfer	Yes	No	No	No	No
Major function	Primary or secondary response; fixes complement	Primary response; common antibody to blood group; fixes complement	Secretory response; bodily secretions, such as mucus lining the gastro-intestinal tract	Allergic response	Membrane receptor

SOURCE: Adapted with permission from Tami JA, Parr MC, Thompson JS. The immune system. *Am J Hosp Pharm.* 1986;43:2485.

antigen. After initial contact between the T or B cell and the antigen, lymphocytes are stimulated into proliferation and maturation. Some of the resulting progeny become the plasma cells that develop the antibodies that actually fight the invader. Other lymphocytes are transformed into memory cells that remain in the circulation. Upon future stimulation by the specific antigen, these memory cells can effect a heightened immune response more quickly.[2,13]

Non-B and Non-T Cells (Null Cells)

Killer cells

These lymphoid cells—killer (K) and natural killer (NK) cells—cannot be identified by typical T- or B-cell surface markers and have been called third-population cells or null cells.[2,13] K cells play a role in antibody-dependent cellular cytotoxicity (ADCC). That is, K cells can recognize and kill only target cells that are coated with antibody.

NK cells are another type of lymphocyte (large granular lymphocytes) that do not bear the typical T- or B-cell surface markers. However, by using MoAbs, surface markers have been described for NK cells. The two most useful markers are CD56 and CD16, although not all CD56+ or CD16+ cells are NK cells. The functional capabilities of NK cells are lysing tumor cells, killing virally infected cells, and regulating hematopoiesis. They are found in the bone marrow, peripheral blood, spleen, liver, lung, and intestinal tract.

Development

Although it is accepted that NK cells originate from bone marrow precursors, their exact lineage is unclear. They may represent a third lineage similar to the T- and B-cell families. Little is known about the maturation process of NK cells. Upon escape from the marrow cavity, they are found primarily in the bloodstream or in the spleen and have a life span of days to months. Mature NK cells still retain some capacity to proliferate.

Effects

NK cells are able to kill tumor cells, virally infected cells, and bacterial pathogens through cell lysis without having first been sensitized to the target and without MHC recognition (see Chapter 3). In fact, increased MHC expression probably inhibits NK cell activity. NK cells are also capable of ADCC. NK cells destroy other cells by granules that are released after contact with the target cell.

Inside the granules are perforins, serine esterases, and chondroitin sulfate proteoglycans. Perforins—or, more descriptively, pore-forming proteins—are released as monomers that polymerize when inserted into the target cell, creating transmembrane holes that allow lysis by osmosis. Other factors released by NK cells include TNF, which, by activating endonucleases, breaks DNA into smaller pieces.

The role of NK cells in regulating hematopoiesis is still under investigation; depending on conditions, both hematopoietic stimulation and inhibition have occurred. NK cells play a role in removing malignant cells through lysis and recently have been described in bone marrow transplantation as mediators of the graft-versus-leukemia effect.

Regulation

NK cell regulation is primarily mediated by IL-2 but also by the IFNs. IFNs do not cause an increase in NK cell numbers. However, all IFNs (alfa, beta, and gamma) enhance NK cell-induced lysis, and the effect of IFN alfa is greater than that of IFN beta. The central cytokine that mediates NK cell activity is IL-2. Lymphocytes exposed to IL-2 in culture become lymphokine-activated killer cells capable of destroying tumor cells (see Chapter 10). The effect of IL-2 on NK cells has not been fully elucidated, but it is mediated in part by increases in the quantity and size of the lytic granules.

Communications—Soluble Mediators

The macrophage and helper T cells have pivotal positions in cell-mediated immunity (see Figure 2-8). The activated macrophage is primarily responsible for stimulating the helper T cell, which, in part, activates other lymphocytes. The helper T cell is considered one of the central mediators in the immune response.

Many soluble substances are responsible for stimulating, suppressing, and orchestrating the activities of the immune system, thus maintaining the communication pathways among cells and tissues. These pathways are the sites for the many commercially produced natural or recombinant immunologic agents, such as IFN alfa. In general, these mediators are lymphokines, monokines, CSFs, B-cell growth factors, and other miscellaneous factors such as vasoactive substances and chemotactic factors (Table 2-3).[2,17,18]

Not all the activities of these mediators have been definitively characterized, nor have all the interacting factors been identified. It should also be remembered that the pathways may be affected by more than one mediator and may involve a complex response that subsequently influences other pathways. Chapter 10 gives further details about some of the more well-defined mediators of the immune system.

Tissues of the Immune System

The structural cells of the lymphoid system are found in diffuse collections of tissues and as neatly packaged organs (Figure 2-9). There are two functional types of lymphatic tissue, primary and secondary. Primary lymphatic tissue (thymus and bone marrow) is centrally located within the human body. This is the site of lymphocyte development, beginning with stem cells and resulting in mature, active lymphocytes. Secondary lymphatic tissues (lymph nodes and spleen) provide the stage where lymphocytes communicate among one another as well as with macrophages and antigens.[2,6]

Bone Marrow

Primary lymphatic tissues

Throughout life, the bone marrow is the source of the newly formed cells of the immune system (see Figure 2-1). The location of the active marrow in adults is the proximal ends of the long bones of the body and the sternum.

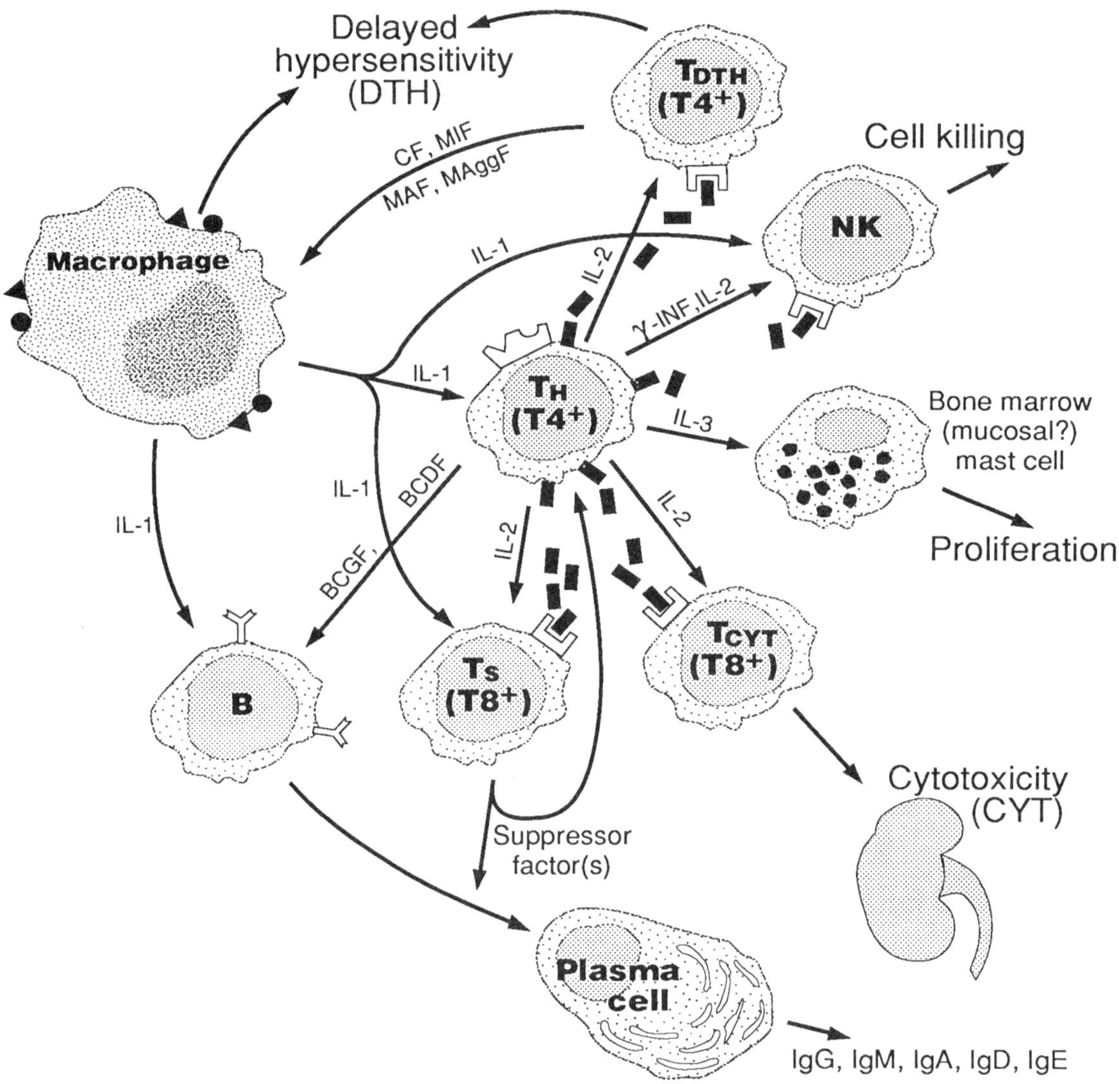

BCDF = B-cell differentiation factor; BCGF = B-cell growth factor; CF = chemotactic factor; γ-INF = interferon gamma; IL-1 = interleukin-1; IL-2 = interleukin-2; IL-3 = interleukin-3; MAF = macrophage activation factor; MAggF = macrophage aggregation factor; MIF = macrophage inhibition factor

Figure 2-8. Cellular events of cell-mediated immunity in humans

SOURCE: Reprinted with permission from Bellanti JA, Rocklin RE. Cell-mediated immune reactions. In: Bellanti JA, ed. Immunology III. Philadelphia: W. B. Saunders Company;1985:181.)

Table 2-3 Sources and Effects of Soluble Mediators[2,6,7,19–24]

Soluble Mediators	Primary Cellular Sources	Principal Effects
Interleukins		
IL-1 (alpha, beta)	Macrophages	Activates lymphocytes, increases WBC adhesion, pyrexia
IL-2	T cells	T-cell growth factor
IL-3	T cells	Multilineage CSF of stem cells
IL-4	T cells	B-cell growth factor
IL-5	T cells	B-cell growth and differentiation
IL-6	Leukocytes	B-cell growth and differentiation, acute phase response
IL-7	Bone marrow, stromal cells	Early lymphocyte proliferation
IL-8	Endothelial cells, monocytes, T lymphocytes	Decrease adhesion of neutrophils to vascular endothelium, attenuate inflammatory events; chemotactic factor for neutrophils
IL-9	Activated T cells	Erythropoiesis
IL-10	Helper T cells	Regulates production of other cytokines
IL-11	Bone marrow, stromal cells	Megakaryocytopoiesis; B-cell development
IL-12	B cells	Activates T lymphocytes, LAK cells
Interferons		
IFN alfa, beta	Leukocytes	MHC class I induction, antiviral IFN effects
IFN gamma	T cells	MHC class I and II induction, macrophage activation, increases lymphocyte adhesion

Table 2-3 (continued)

Soluble Mediators	Primary Cellular Sources	Principal Effects
Colony-stimulating factors		
GM-CSF	Macrophages, T cells	Granulocyte and macrophage growth and differentiation
G-CSF	Macrophages	Granulocyte growth and differentiation
M-CSF	Monocytes	Monocyte and macrophage growth and differentiation
SCF (or MCGF or C-kit ligand)	Bone marrow, stromal cells	Stimulates early hematopoietic progenitor cells
Tumor necrosis factor		
TNF alpha	Monocytes and macrophages	Cachexia; increases activation of lymphocytes, granulocytes, and macrophages; increases cell adhesion
TNF beta (lymphotoxin)	T cells	Cytotoxicity (lymphotoxin)

CSF = colony-stimulating factor; GM-CSF = granulocyte-macrophage colony-stimulating factor; G-CSF = granulocyte colony-stimulating factor; MCGF = mast cell growth factor; M-CSF = monocyte-macrophage colony-stimulating factor; MHC = major histocompatibility complex; LAK = lymphokine-activated killer; SCF = stem cell factor; WBC = white blood cell.

Under the direction of a wide variety of growth factors, the stem cells proliferate and differentiate into mature cells. After release from the bone marrow, each cell has its own life cycle of activity in the secondary lymphatic or other tissues.

Thymus

During the first 3 months of human gestation, the immature T lymphocyte cells leave the bone marrow and travel through the bloodstream to the thymus. Located in the thorax, the thymus overlies the heart and great vessels (see Figure 2-9). This organ is made up of small patches of tissue

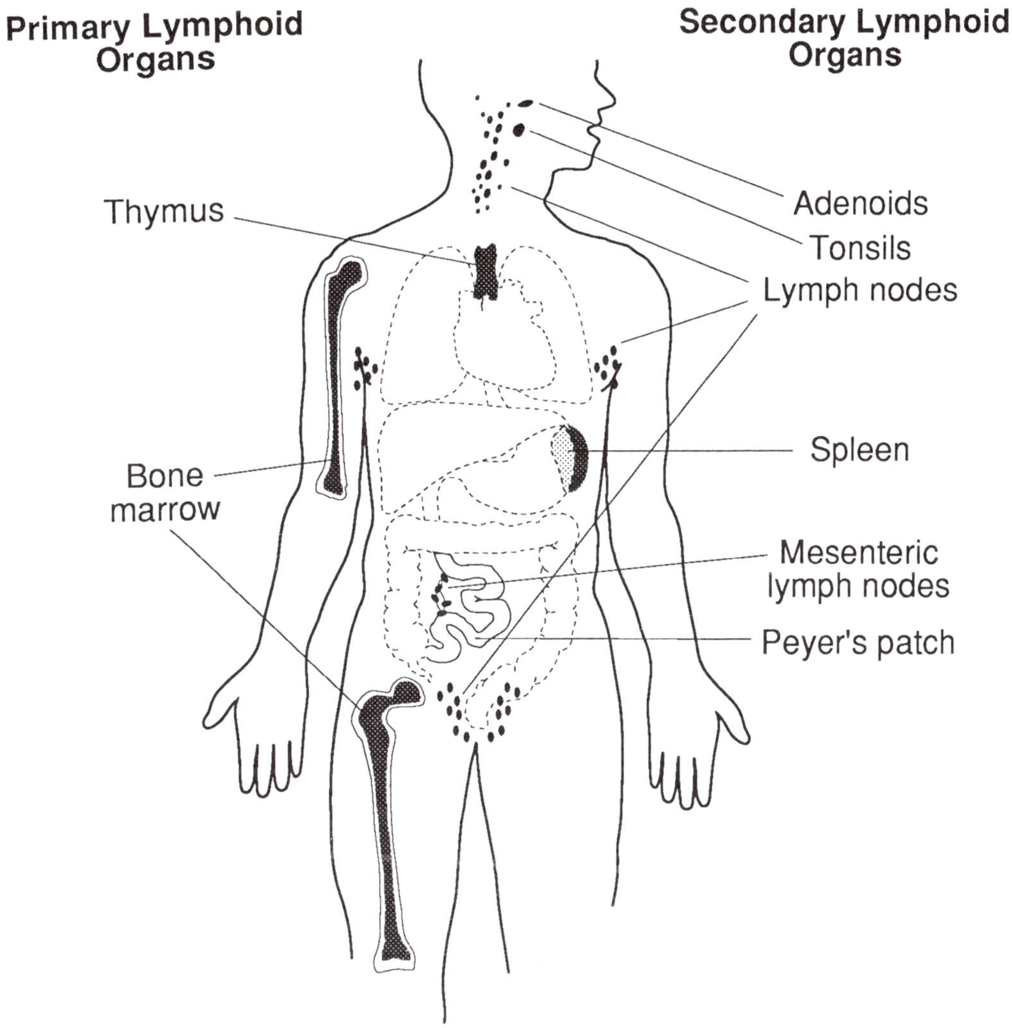

Figure 2-9. General overview of lymphatic tissue

called lobules (Figure 2-10). The lobules have an outer layer of cells (the cortex), where the more immature T lymphocytes proliferate, and an inner layer of cells (the medulla), where the more mature T cells are located. The thymus is made up of epithelial and interdigitating cells that are probably responsible for supporting the lymphocytes through differentiation and by developing the ability to recognize self. Theoretically, the thymus supports the development of the T lymphocyte hormonally.[2,13]

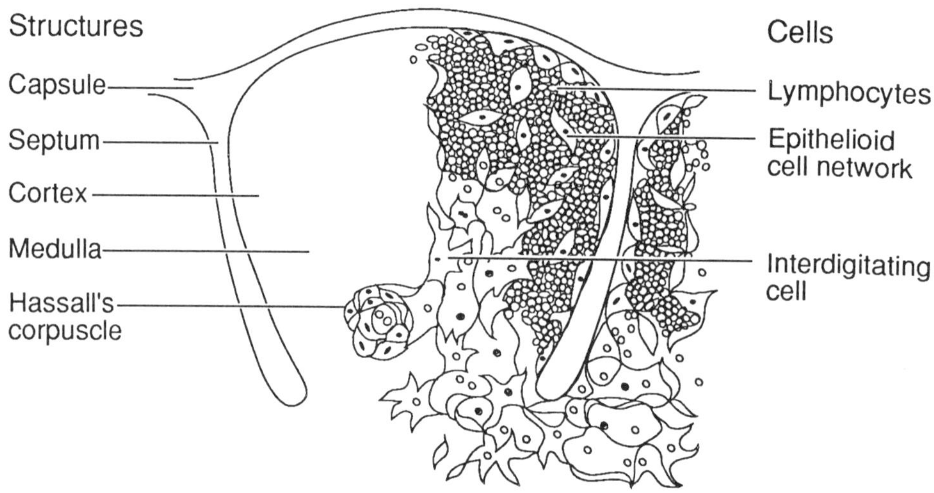

Figure 2-10. The structure of a thymus lobule

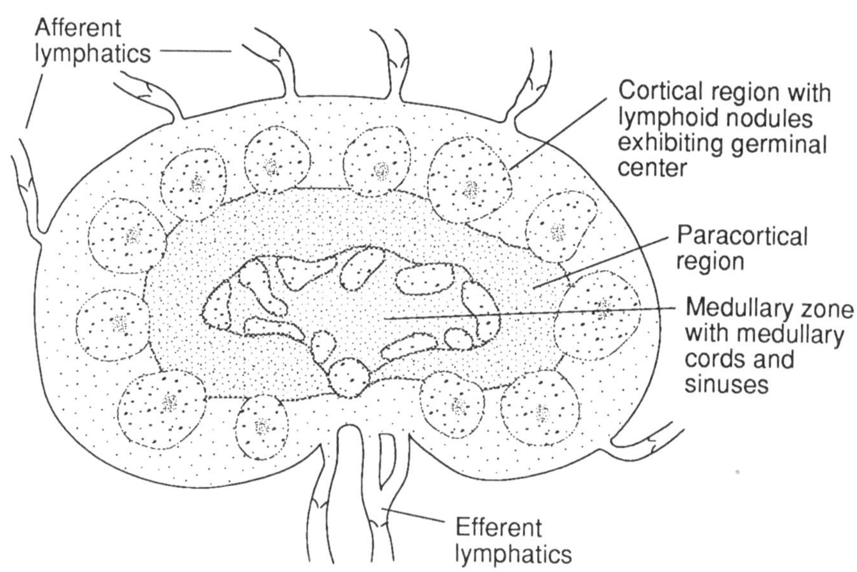

Figure 2-11. Lymph node

SOURCE: Adapted with permission from Mota I. Tissues and cells of the immune system. In: Bier OG, da Silva W, Gotze D et al., eds. Fundamentals of immunology. Heidelberg: Springer-Verlag;1986:23.

Lymph Nodes

Secondary lymphatic tissues

Once the T cell matures, it emigrates out of the thymus to secondary lymphoid tissues. The major network of secondary lymphoid tissue is made up of lymph nodes and lymphatic vessels (Figure 2-11). Lymph nodes are most prominent in the neck, axilla, abdomen (within the mesentery and along the spine), and groin (see Figure 2-9). The lymph nodes filter tissue fluids (lymph) that are eventually returned to the thoracic duct and the bloodstream. Each lymph node is a complex, small (1 to 25 mm), ovoid organ. The outer cortex contains B lymphocytes, and the paracortex houses T lymphocytes and APCs. Some tissue from the outer two layers sends fibrous strands through the inner tissue layer, the medulla, to form sinuses. The sinuses are lined with macrophages, which encounter antigens as the lymph flows through the node. Between these strands are plasma cells. When the node is antigenically stimulated, germinal centers are formed. B cells are the primary focus of the germinal centers; within them are APCs, macrophages, T cells, and NK cells that play crucial roles in the development of the B cells, especially memory B cells.

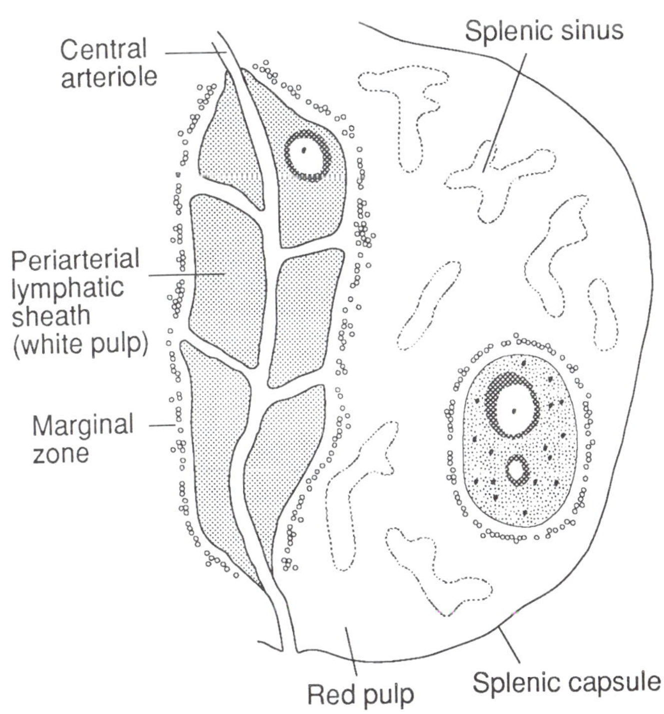

Figure 2-12. Spleen

Spleen

Located in the upper left abdomen behind the stomach, the spleen has two functions: filtering blood and functioning as an organ of immunity. The filtration process removes defective blood cells, sorts cells, and stores some cells. As an organ of the immune system, the spleen is a home base for lymphocytes, monocytes, and macrophages, where they are exposed to immunogenic particles as they patrol.

The spleen also serves as an extramedullary site of hematopoiesis. Red and white pulp are the two major tissue types of the spleen (Figure 2-12). White pulp usually makes up 20% of the spleen, but this percentage varies with the immune status of the host. The lymphoid portion of the spleen is the white pulp, which is positioned around central arterioles. Both T and B cells are found within white pulp, with T cells clustered centrally around the arteriole and the B cells slightly removed from the vessel. As in the lymph nodes, the B cells may be present as unstimulated or stimulated cells in a germinal center. Macrophages and APCs are also part of these centers. The red pulp sinuses are lined with phagocytic cells and lymphocytes that have crossed over from the white pulp.[2,6,12]

Mucosal-associated Lymphoid Tissue (MALT)

Sites

MALT is a generic term for nonencapsulated lymphoid tissues. Mucosal linings of the body are constantly subjected to antigens, pathogens, and toxic substances and hence are the primary portals of entry for invaders. Areas where MALT can be found are the gastrointestinal, respiratory, and urogenital tracts. The nonencapsulated lymphoid tissues found within the gastrointestinal tract are often called gut-associated lymphoid tissue (GALT); a similar system in the lungs is called bronchial-associated lymphoid tissue (BALT). Because these areas are the primary sites of foreign particle invasion, they play a critical role in immunologic defense.

Peyer's patches

MALT, although existing as nonencapsulated cells, may be organized into discrete colonies such as the Peyer's patches of the intestinal tract. The Peyer's patches contain both mature T and B cells and are most numerous in the distal small intestine and the proximal large intestine. There are more than 200 Peyer's patches in the adult. The patch is much like the tissues already discussed, having lymphoid follicles and germinal centers (Figure 2-13). Hosts with minimal antigen stimulation of the intestine have very small Peyer's patches. In addition to the microvilli of the intestinal lumen, the patch is covered by special epithelial cells producing microfolds (hence the name "M cell" in Figure 2-13) over the surface of the patch. The lymphocytes of the patch that are very close to the lumen have ready access to antigens. A large quantity of antigen is present in the intestine, and

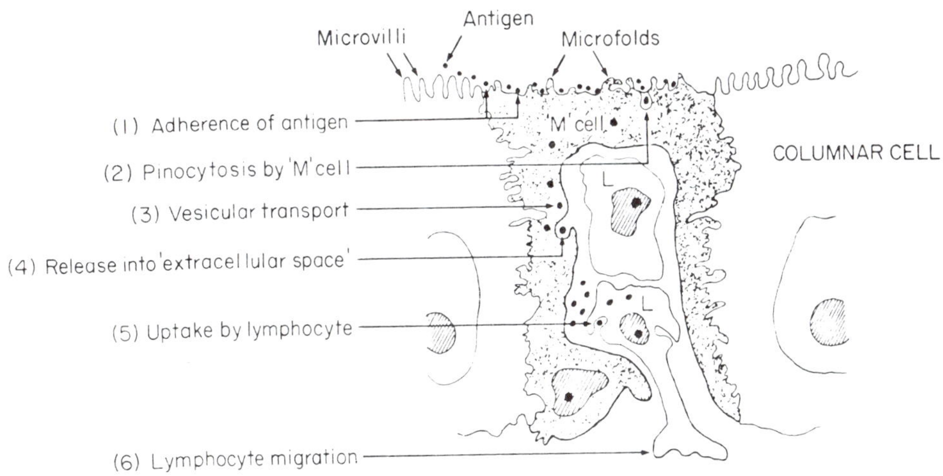

Figure 2-13. Peyer's patch

SOURCE: Reprinted with permission from Chapel H, Haeney M. Essentials of clinical immunology. Oxford: Blackwell Scientific Publications;1984:280.

theoretically the Peyer's patch is responsible for the suppression of the immune response and the development of tolerance; otherwise the system would be overwhelmed. Much remains unknown about Peyer's patches.[2,4,12]

High Endothelial Venule

Migration process

Lymphocytes are able to enter the tissues of the lymphatic system by lymphatic vessels or through the endothelial wall of a blood vessel. The particular region of blood vessels allowing this passage of lymphocytes, called the high endothelial venule (HEV), is made of columnar cells between which the lymphocytes can pass. The HEV, a normal component of lymph nodes and Peyer's patches, can be stimulated by lymphokines (e.g., interferon gamma) and lymphocytes in other tissues involved in an immune reaction. Lymphocytes recognize the HEV with specific receptors. The migration process involves interactions of lymphocytes with various components of the extracellular matrix. Interaction results are varied, but they include enhanced lymphocyte motility, increased lymphocyte adhesion, and T-lymphocyte suppression.[19]

Lymphocyte traffic is the normal circulation of lymphocytes through the secondary lymph tissue and back to the bloodstream (Figure 2-14). Lymphocytes can cross blood vessel walls, moving into specific organs (MALT, spleen, bone marrow, lymph nodes, and thymus), where they may reside in response to antigenic stimuli. They then return to the circulation, making their way through the major vessels of the lymphatic system

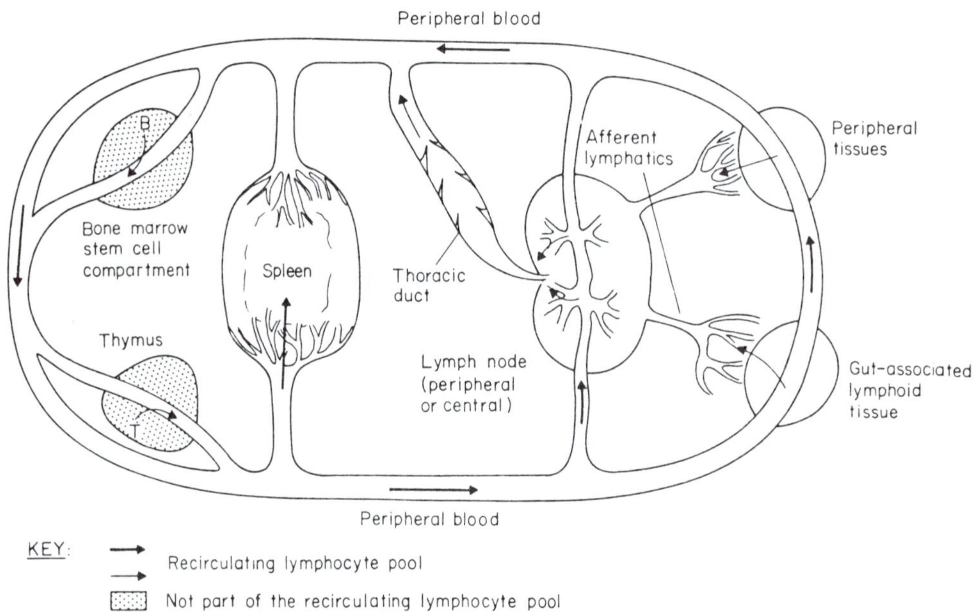

Figure 2-14. Lymphocyte traffic

SOURCE: Reprinted with permission from McConnell I. Lymphocytes and the lymphoid system. In: Lachmann PJ, Peters DK, eds. Clinical aspects of immunology. Boston: Blackwell Scientific Publications;1982:90.

Inductive/latent period

ultimately to the thoracic duct, whence they are emptied into the venous circulation. When an antigen first enters a lymph node, the traffic comes to a halt and areas within the node gear up to respond to the antigen.[2,12]

Immune Regulation and Response

Primary response

The host's first encounter with a specific antigen results in a primary response by the immune system (Figure 2-15). First, the new antigen must be processed and signals sent to the tissues and cells of the immune system to stimulate proliferation and maturation. The time between antigen introduction and host response varies depending on the amount, route, solubility, and immunogenicity of the antigen and the physical status of the host. This length of time is called the inductive or latent period (see upper part of Figure 2-15). The first isotype of antibody produced is IgM, followed by IgG. The rate and amount of antibody production depend on the number of cells that can be activated and on the metabolic rate, or half-life, of each antibody type.[2,13]

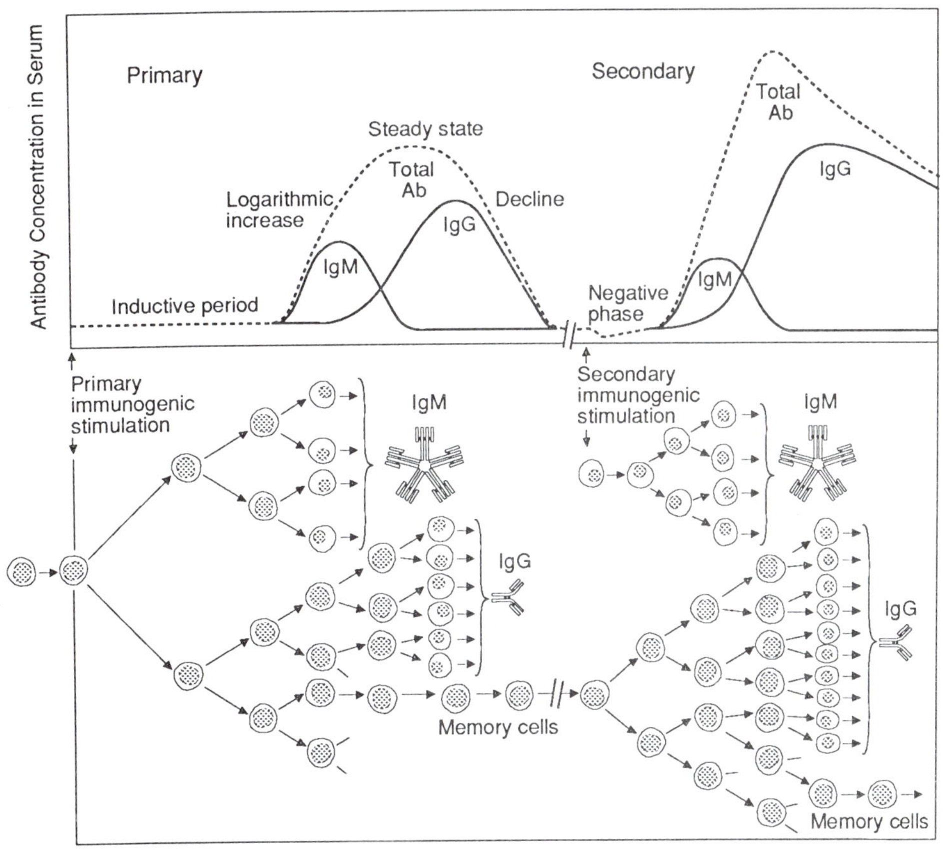

Figure 2-15. Primary and secondary responses of the immune system

SOURCE: Reprinted with permission from Herscowitz HB. Immunophysiology: cell function and cellular interactions in antibody formation. In: Bellanti JA, ed. Immunology III. Philadelphia: W. B. Saunders Company;1985:120.

Memory

Secondary response

As can be seen from Figure 2-15, subsequent encounters between the host and antigen result in a more rapid and enhanced response of the immune system. Memory cells have been produced from both T and B lymphocytes after the first antigenic exposure and can stimulate or generate more antibody-producing (plasma) cells. Antibodies already present react immediately when reexposed to the antigen. A much smaller dose of antigen is needed to evoke a secondary response than to produce the primary response. How much antigen is needed depends on the concentration of preformed antibody and on the length of time between the first and second antigenic stimulations.[2,13]

Immune Tolerance

There are circumstances in which the attenuation or elimination of the immune response is actually beneficial to the host. Tolerance means the selective lack of response to an antigen that has previously been presented to the host. Generally, less mature cells are more likely to become tolerant. For example, a B lymphocyte becomes tolerant more readily than a mature plasma cell. If the host is repeatedly exposed to an antigen early in life, the B-cell response may be lost. T lymphocytes may also become tolerant, but the immature cells are no more susceptible than the mature cells. Overall, T cells become tolerant at much lower doses of antigen than B cells.[2,13]

Other factors in tolerance development are the dose, physical form (monomer versus polymer), and route of entry of the antigen into the host. There are optimal doses of antigens for eliciting an immune response. Exposure to doses at low or high extremes can result in tolerance. For example, intravenous doses of antigen can result in a more concentrated exposure of host to antigen and are therefore more likely to induce tolerance than are doses introduced by other routes. In addition, monomeric forms of antigens are more likely to induce tolerance than are polymers.[2,13]

Summary

The immune system is composed primarily of white blood cells originating in the bone marrow and developing into myeloid or lymphoid cells. Myeloid cells include mononuclear phagocytes and polymorphonuclear granulocytes, some of which are phagocytic while others function as mediator cells. Phagocytosis is the process of attaching to and killing foreign particles or antigens.

Macrophages evolve from monocytes and are capable of cell division. Macrophages (as well as dendritic cells, B lymphocytes, and ciroglial cells) may also function as antigen-presenting cells. Granulocytes have granular nuclei and stain various colors; the granulocytes include neutrophils (polymorphonuclear), eosinophils, basophils, and mast cells.

Platelets are myeloid cells that function as mediator cells and activate complement during the inflammatory process.

Lymphocytes include T, B, and null (K and NK) cells. Subpopulations of T lymphocytes include helper T cells, suppressor T cells, cytotoxic T cells, and memory T cells. T cells are responsible for cell-mediated immunity, while B cells are responsible for humoral immunity. Null cells function in antibody-dependent cellular toxicity. Following activation, B cells may become plasma cells. Plasma cells produce antibodies (immunoglobulin), including IgG, IgA, IgD, IgE, and IgM. Both T and B lymphocytes can become memory cells.

The immune system comprises six tissues: bone marrow, thymus, lymph nodes, spleen, mucosal-associated lymphoid tissue, and high endothelial venule. Bone marrow is the source of immune cells. The thymus is the site where immature T lymphocytes develop. The lymphoid tissues filter foreign particles traveling through the lymph fluid; immune cells in the tissues are responsible for killing the antigens. The spleen filters blood for foreign particles and defective blood cells. Mucosal-associated lymphoid tissues are nonencapsulated tissues found in the gastrointestinal, respiratory, and urogenital tracts and are crucial to first-line immunologic defense. High endothelial venules are blood vessels that allow lymphocytes to pass through the immune tissues.

References

1. Tami JA, Parr MC, Thompson JS: The immune system. *Am J Hosp Pharm.* 1986;43:2483–93.
2. Roitt IM, Brostoff J, Male DK. Immunology. 2nd ed. London: Gower Medical Publishing; 1989.
3. Shevach EM. Macrophages and other accessory cells. In: Paul WE, ed. Fundamental immunology. New York: Raven Press; 1984:71–108.
4. Mota I. Tissues and cells of the immune system. In: Bier OG, da Silva W, Gotze D et al., eds. Fundamentals of immunology. Heidelberg: Springer-Verlag; 1986:1–34.
5. Allison AC. Macrophages and neutrophils. In: Lachmann PJ, Peters DK, eds. Clinical aspects of immunology. Boston: Blackwell Scientific Publications; 1982:101–29.
6. Bellanti JA, Kadlec JV. Introduction to immunology. In: Bellanti JA, ed. Immunology III. Philadelphia: W. B. Saunders Company; 1985:1–15.
7. Kline J. Immunology. Boston: Blackwell Scientific Publications; 1990:26–7.
8. Cline MJ. The white cells. In: Stein JH, ed. Internal medicine. Boston: Little, Brown; 1983:1475–80.
9. Johnston RB. Monocytes and macrophages. *N Engl J Med.* 1988;318:747–52.
10. Barrett JT. Textbook of immunology. St Louis: C. V. Mosby; 1983:50–128.
11. Hutton JJ, Cline MJ. Hematopoieses and the red blood cell. In: Stein JH, ed. Internal medicine. Boston: Little, Brown; 1983:1469–75.

12. McConnell I. Lymphocytes and the lymphoid system. In: Lachmann PJ, Peters DK, eds. Clinical aspects of immunology. Boston: Blackwell Scientific Publications; 1982:72–100.
13. Herscowitz HB. Immunophysiology: cell function and cellular interactions in antibody formation. In: Bellanti JA, ed. Immunology III. Philadelphia: W. B. Saunders Company; 1985:117–59.
14. Royer HD, Reinharz EL. T-lymphocytes: ontogeny, function, and relevance to clinical disorders. *N Engl J Med.* 1987;317:1136–42.
15. Bernier GM. Antibody and immunoglobulins: structure and function. In: Bellanti JA, ed. Immunology II. Philadelphia: W. B. Saunders Company; 1985:89–105.
16. Cooper MD. B-lymphocytes: normal development and function. *N Engl J Med.* 1987;317:1452–56.
17. Bellanti JA, Rocklin RE. Cell-mediated immune reactions. In: Bellanti JA, ed. Immunology III. Philadelphia: W. B. Saunders Company; 1985:176–88.
18. Golde DW, Gasson JC. Hormones that stimulate the growth of blood cells. *Sci Am.* 1988;259:62–70.
19. Gubler U, Chua AO, Schoenhaut DS et al. Coexpression of two distinct genes is required to generate secreted bioactive cytotoxic lymphocyte maturation factor. *Proc Natl Acad Sci USA.* 1991;88:4143–7.

Suggested Reading

For more in-depth information on the cellular and tissue components of the immune system, the reader is strongly encouraged to read the subsequent chapters of this text, especially Chapters 3 and 10.

Self-Study Questions

1. What type of cell is a littoral cell and where does it reside?

   1. A fixed macrophage; in the spleen.

2. What is the function of the microvilli on the outside of a macrophage?

   2. To help the macrophage attach to an antigen.

3. All polymorphonuclear granulocytes function as phagocytes.

   A. True.
   B. False.

   3. B

4. What is the primary immunologic function of platelets?

   A. Attracting other WBCs to the site of inflammation.
   B. Phagocytizing foreign particles.
   C. Clearing parasitic organisms from the host.
   D. Binding to IgE.

   4. A

5. How many days does it take to develop a monocyte cell from a pluripotent stem cell?

   A. 2 days.
   B. 4 days.
   C. 6 days.
   D. 8 days.

   5. C

6. Which cells of the immune system serve as antigen-presenting cells?

   A. Macrophages.
   B. T cells.
   C. Neutrophils.
   D. Lymphokines.

   6. A

7. What is the primary function of the helper T cell?

   7. To orchestrate communication between other cell types.

8. T lymphocytes are responsible for ________________ immunity.

   8. cell-mediated.

Answer	Question
9. A	9. Memory cells may evolve from T or B lymphocytes. A. True. B. False.
10. B	10. Where does a B cell become an antibody-producing cell? A. In the bone marrow. B. In the peripheral tissue. C. In the spleen. D. In the lymph system.
11. D	11. What is the function of the spleen? A. To phagocytize antigens. B. To develop mature B cells. C. To filter tissue fluid. D. To filter blood.
12. To provide communication among lymphocytes, macrophages, and antigens.	12. What is the function of the secondary lymphatic tissue?

CHAPTER 3

The Major Histocompatibility Complex

Kelly A. Scott, Pharm.D.
Oncology Clinical Pharmacist
Pharmacy-IV Department
Good Samaritan Hospital and Medical Center
Portland, OR

Introduction

Advances in the survival of patients undergoing organ transplantation are largely the result of our greater understanding of histocompatibility. The major histocompatibility complex (MHC) is also known as the human leucocyte antigen (HLA). It plays an important role in treating many inpatient and outpatient populations. The MHC significantly affects the success of tissue transplantation and blood transfusions. MHC is also linked to certain disease etiologies, such as some rheumatologic and autoimmune dysfunctions.

Histocompatibility refers to the match between donor and recipient antigens for grafting tissue. A poor match between blood product donor and recipient can result in an MHC rejection, similar to transplant rejection. This same physiologic response is responsible for hemolytic disease of the newborn. It is therefore important that blood typing and MHC crossmatching be conducted for patient populations affected by related therapies and procedures.

Learning objectives

After reading this chapter, the learner will be able to—

- Describe differences among Class I, Class II, and Class III MHC genes.
- Discuss MHC factors influencing the success of organ transplantations.
- Describe the function of the MHC in antigen recognition and response.
- Describe the role played by the MHC in the immunobiology of diseases.
- Describe serologic, cellular, and molecular-biologic MHC typing methods.
- Describe immunogenic determinants of the ABO and Rh blood systems.

Chapter organization

This chapter begins with a review of the structure and function of the MHC and a description of its genetic determination. The major functions of the MHC in the immune system, such as transplantation success, antigen recognition and immune response, complement activation, and disease pathogenesis, are then detailed. The chapter concludes with a discussion of the various methods used for determining a particular individual's genetic makeup or type of blood, the clinical impact of blood nomenclature, and blood typing systems.

Suggested Preparation

A knowledge base of the immune system and its cellular components is necessary to understand fully the important roles of the MHC described in this chapter. Therefore, Chapters 1 and 2 should be read before beginning this chapter.

MHC Genes and Proteins

This section describes the MHC genes, including the history of their discovery and their arrangement and structure. In addition, the genetic determinants of the MHC are detailed, and the functions of the MHC as a part of the human immune system are described.

Human leukocyte antigen

The MHC was first described in 1936 after observations that certain cell antigens were related to transplantation survival. The genes that control graft rejection were soon found to be closely linked to genes of the immune and complement systems.[1] In the late 1950s, scientists discovered that these histocompatibility genes were crucial not only in successful transplantation but also in successful blood transfusions. Since the gene products are located on the surfaces of leukocytes in humans, they are also called human leukocyte antigen (HLA). Based on these observations, it is now known that the MHC or HLA is responsible not only for compatibility of transplants but also for a variety of other functions in the immune system, such as immune response and complement activation. The MHC is a part of the immunoglobulin supergene family, and segments of MHC molecules are similar in composition to immunoglobulins and T-cell receptor molecules, suggesting that all these cells have a common evolutionary ancestry.[2,3]

Arrangement of MHC Genes

The MHC of humans is located on the short arm of chromosome 6. There are currently three known classes of genes in the MHC, class I, class II, and class III (Figure 3-1).

Class I Genes. The three "classical" loci (positions on a chromosome where specific genes are found) that determine the composition of the class I histocompatibility antigens are called HLA-A, HLA-B, and HLA-C. Recently, at least three other MHC class I genes have been described; these

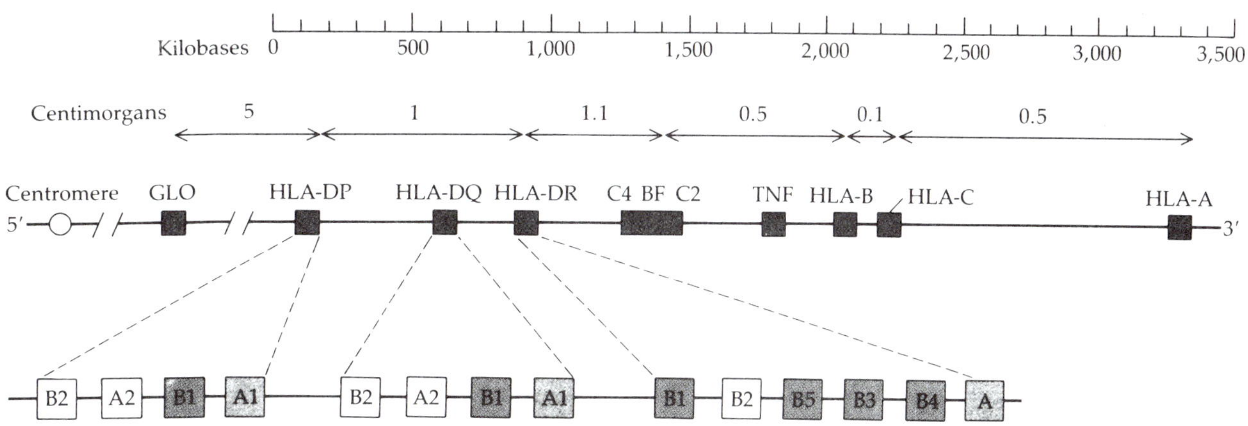

Figure 3-1. Genetic arrangement of the human MHC. An expansion of the class II region is shown in the lower portion of the figure. Distances are shown in recombination units (centimorgans).

SOURCE: Reprinted with permission from Carpenter CB, David J. Histocompatibility antigens and immune response genes. *Scientific American Medicine.* 1991;6(V):1.

"nonclassical" class I genes are different than HLA-A, -B, or -C.[4] The roles or functions of nonclassical class I genes are still unknown, and further discussion of class I genes in this chapter focuses on A, B, and C only. As can be seen in Figure 3-1, the class I genes are separated from the class II genes by the class III genes. Class I molecules have been identified on the surface of nearly all nucleated cells; they are not found on red blood cells (RBCs), which are enucleated.[1,5]

Transplantation antigens

A major role of class I genes is in mediating the immune response to transplantation, and it is these antigens that dominate the graft rejection process. For this reason, class I antigens of the human MHC are also known as the major histocompatibility antigens or transplantation antigens. All types of interferon can increase expression of class I MHC molecules on cell surfaces.[6,7]

Class II Genes. The class II genes are located in a region of chromosome 6 known as the D region; hence, they are also known as the HLA-D genes (see Figure 3-1). The precise number of genes in the D region is currently unknown. However, it is widely accepted that there are at least three specific genes, designated DR, DP, and DQ. Class II molecules have a more limited expression than class I molecules; they are located primarily on the cell surfaces of immunocompetent cells, such as B lymphocytes, macrophages, and monocytes, and on activated T lymphocytes.[3,6,8]

Intercellular communication

Class II genes encode for molecules that regulate immune response via cell-cell interactions; that is, they participate in communication among cells during the immune response.[9] The main role of class II genes is in regulating this immune response by a proliferative response of lymphocytes to foreign antigens.

Class III Genes. Class III genes are located between class I and class II genes on chromosome 6 (see Figure 3-1). There are at least four loci in the class III gene region, namely, C2, C4-A (also called C4-1), C4-B (also called C4-2), and Bf. Many of the class III genes are associated with the complement system and are the structural genes for production of the C2, C4, and factor B1 proteins of the complement system (see Chapter 1 for a review of the complement system).

Complement cascade

The role of class III genes in relation to the MHC and antigen recognition and response is less well understood than the roles of class I and II genes,[8] but it is known that the complement proteins produced from class III genes are important components of the complement cascade.[1] The genes for tumor necrosis factor (TNF), TNF alpha and TNF beta (or lymphotoxin), are also found in the class III region.[2]

In addition, a new cluster of eight genes has recently been isolated within the human MHC and has been termed HLA-B-associated transcripts (BATs).[10] At this time, the structure and function of BATs are unknown. Since the roles of class III genes and BATs in the MHC are unclear, they are not discussed further in this chapter.

Structure of the MHC Molecules

The structures of the human MHC molecules are very similar to those found in mice. Each MHC molecule is composed of polypeptide chains of various sizes in specific configurations.

Class I. Each class I molecule consists of two proteins: a large protein and a noncovalently associated smaller beta$_2$ microglobulin (Figure 3-2). The larger protein is made up of 354 amino acids and is divided into five segments including three globular (alpha$_1$, alpha$_2$, and alpha$_3$) domains. The alpha$_1$ and alpha$_2$ domains, being most exterior, are responsible for most of the antigenic specificity of the class I antigens. The three other segments have fairly constant amino acid sequences in all individuals and do not contribute greatly to antigenic specificity.[6]

The second protein in the class I gene structure is a beta$_2$ microglobulin that is encoded for by chromosome 15 and not by the HLA complex.[6,8] This protein is noncovalently bound to the larger protein. The beta$_2$ portion is an

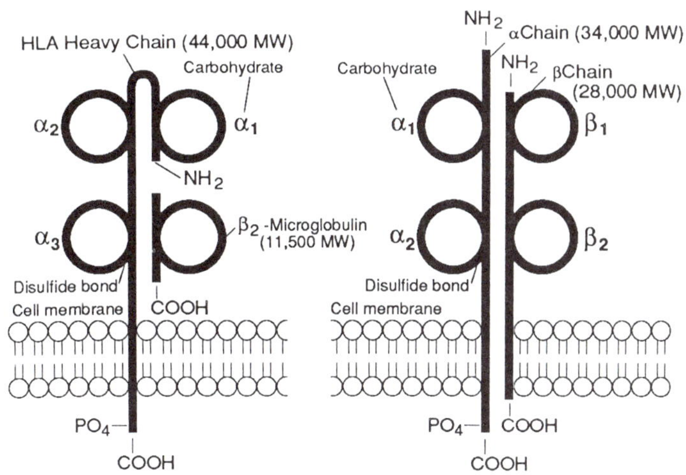

Figure 3-2. Structure of class I (left) and class II (right) histocompatibility antigens

SOURCE: Reprinted with permission from Carpenter CB, David J. Histocompatibility antigens and immune response genes. *Scientific American Medicine.* 1991;6(V):2.

identical protein in all class I genes, and it does not contribute greatly to the antigenic specificity of the class I antigens.[1] A three-dimensional representation of an MHC class I molecule (HLA-A2) is now possible using X-ray crystallography techniques.[11] This technique has also advanced knowledge of the structure-function relationship of the MHC (see the discussion on antigen recognition in this chapter). Figure 3-3 shows a side view of an MHC class I molecule, depicting the three alpha domains as well as the $beta_2$ microglobulin.

Class II. The structure of the class II (HLA-D) molecules differs from that of the class I molecules. As can be seen in Figure 3-2, each class II molecule consists of two polypeptide chains, the larger alpha chain (molecular weight 34,000 consisting of 229 amino acids) and the smaller beta chain (molecular weight 29,000 consisting of 237 amino acids). The alpha and beta chains are ionically bound and are subdivided into four smaller units ($alpha_1$, $alpha_2$, $beta_1$, $beta_2$).

The $alpha_1$ and $beta_1$ domains appear to be responsible for most of the antigen specificity of the HLA-D molecules, whereas the $alpha_2$ and $beta_2$ regions appear to be fairly constant in all class II gene products. In contrast to class I molecules, there is no $beta_2$ microglobulin associated with class II molecules.[1]

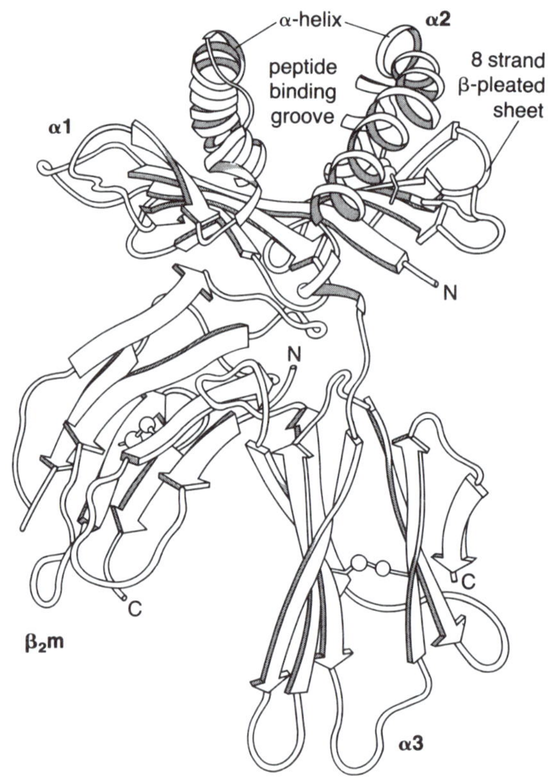

Figure 3-3. The diagrammatic crystalline structure of a class I MHC molecule (side view)

SOURCE: Reprinted with permission from Stites DP, Terr AI. Basic and clinical immunology. 7th ed., copyright Appleton & Lange 1991.

In summary, each HLA gene encodes for an immunologically distinct protein. These proteins, found on the surfaces of body cells, assist the immune system in a variety of functions. Table 3-1 summarizes the major characteristics of the three classes of HLAs.

Genetic Determinants of the MHC

A brief review of some basic genetic nomenclature is necessary before beginning this discussion of genetic determination of the MHC.

Haplotype

The human genome comprises 23 pairs of chromosomes, one of which is the pair of sex chromosomes. Within each pair, one chromosome is inherited from each parent. Each chromosome has a variety of loci where specific genes are found. An allele is one variation or alternate form of a given gene, and alleles vary widely among individuals. The term *haplotype*

Table 3-1 Summary of Main Characteristics of HLA Antigen Classes

Characteristic	Class I	Class II	Class III
Synonyms	Histocompatibility or transplant antigens	Immune response (Ir) genes	Complement activators
Loci	HLA-A, HLA-B, HLA-C	HLA-DP, HLA-DQ, HLA-DR	HLA-C2, HLA-C4A (C41), HLA-C4B (C42), HLA-Bf
Location	Nearly all nucleated cells	B lymphocytes, macrophages and monocytes, activated T lymphocytes	Serum, red blood cell membranes
Components	Large protein with five segments associated with a beta$_2$ microglobulin	Alpha and beta chains	

describes the combination of alleles at each locus on a single chromosome; the haplotype is usually inherited as a unit. Each person has two haplotypes at each MHC locus, one inherited from each parent. Thus, the genetic composition of an individual is determined by the paternal haplotype and the maternal haplotype. The term *genotype,* which describes all the alleles detected in a given individual, can be thought of as one's genetic portrait.

Genotype

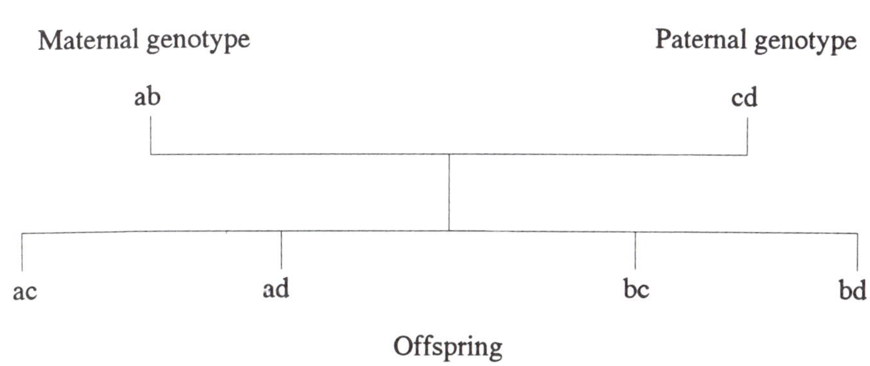

Figure 3-4. Inheritance of HLA haplotypes (depicted as a, b, c, d)

Let us now turn specifically to the genetic determinants of the HLA region on chromosome 6 in humans. Figure 3-4 illustrates this discussion. Each person has two HLA haplotypes. In Figure 3-4, a, b, c, and d denote parental haplotypes; ab denotes the maternal genotype and cd denotes the paternal genotype. When these parents produce offspring, four genetic combinations or genotypes are possible in the children: ac, ad, bc, and bd. By simple Mendelian inheritance patterns, it is known that 25% of siblings will have HLA-identical haplotypes (ac, ac); 50% of siblings will have HLA-semi-identical haplotypes—that is, they will share one haplotype (ac and ad, or ad and bd); and 25% of siblings will be HLA-nonidentical—that is, they will share no common haplotypes (ac and bd).

Codominance

Thus, despite the complexity and diversity of the HLA system, within offspring of a given couple there are only four possible genotypes based on inheritance patterns.[3] In the case of class I genes (HLA-A, HLA-B, HLA-C), each human has six alleles, three from each parent. Another important fact in HLA genetics is that HLA genes are codominant; that is, the alleles inherited from each parent are expressed equally. This genetic trait contrasts with many others, in which one allele is either dominant or recessive.

The reason for reviewing the genetic determinants of MHC and the haplotype-phenotype patterns of individuals is that these factors are very important in the association of MHC with successful transplantation, disease predisposition, and a variety of other immune functions. These functions will now be addressed.

Functions of the MHC

The first work on the MHC and its name were derived from work with engrafted animals. Subsequent investigations recognized the role of the MHC in successful transplantation. However, the question soon arose, Why would the human body develop such an elaborate system to regulate transplantation, which is an unnatural, artificial phenomenon? Research thus moved toward finding other functions of the MHC in the human immune system. It soon became apparent that the HLA and MHC were closely related, if not one and the same.

It is now known that each of the three portions of the MHC plays a different role in the immune system: class I genes are primarily associated with transplantation; class II genes are associated with eliciting an immune response; and class III genes are associated with the complement system. Thus, the MHC plays a major role in body defense as well as in histocompatibility.

Transplantation. Work by scientists in the mid-1900s described the important role of the class I genes in determining acceptance or rejection of transplanted tissues, or allografts (tissues or organs grafted between two genetically dissimilar members of the same species).[3] Antigens on transplant tissue stimulate the transplant recipient's immune system to either accept or reject the graft. The recipient recognizes the graft as either self or foreign on the basis of its antigens and responds accordingly. Many proteins in graft tissue may be viewed as alloantigens (antigens present on the cells of some individuals of a given species)[3] by the recipient. However, only the antigens of the HLA system and the antigens of the ABO blood group system appear to affect graft survival significantly.

Alloantigens

In the HLA system, the class I antigens (HLA-A, -B, and -C) play the largest role in transplantation; hence, they are also known as the major histocompatibility or transplantation antigens. Class II antigens (HLA-D) also play a role in transplantation. However, it appears that HLA-DR matching of donor and recipient is more important for successful bone marrow transplantation than for successful kidney transplantation.[9] Other minor non-HLA histocompatibility antigens may also contribute to graft rejection. However, the use of immunosuppressive drugs usually abates the immune response to these minor incompatibilities.

Syngeneic/ congenic grafts

On the basis of our understanding of the immune system, it appears obvious that tissue transplanted between two genetically identical people (identical phenotypes) would not be rejected. This is known as *syngeneic* or *congenic* transplantation—a transplant between identical twins. Because the body does not recognize the graft as foreign, the transplant is generally quite successful.[1] (The mechanism of graft acceptance and rejection is covered in Chapter 9.)

Unfortunately, most individuals do not have an identical twin and must therefore receive graft tissue from a sibling, another relative, or an unrelated donor. Because each class I gene has many different alleles, which are determined by inheritance of maternal and paternal haplotypes, it follows that tissue for transplantation is preferably harvested from a matched sibling or related donor. Kidney transplants are much more successful from living related donors than from unrelated cadaver donors.[12] In fact, the greatest success is found with HLA-identical sibling donor grafts (85% to 90% long-term survival in kidney transplants), followed by transplants from relatives with one common haplotype (semi-identical). Relatives who are HLA nonidentical have a lower success rate.[1] The process of histocompatibility testing, or HLA typing, is the ideal method for identifying suitable tissue donors.

Effect on Antigen Recognition. Early in the study of MHC, investigators realized that there must be roles for MHC in the human immune system other than transplantation. In the early 1970s it was discovered that the ability to respond to a specific antigen by mounting an immune response is genetically controlled and that the genes involved in this control are located in the MHC.[9] Thus, it was established that these immune response (Ir) genes reside in the MHC.

However, at that time the exact mechanism of the cell-cell interactions of the immune cells and the MHC was still unclear. A theory evolved that MHC genes on the surface of B lymphocytes, macrophages, and other cells formed a complex with an antigen. T lymphocytes that bore the appropriate receptors would then recognize this MHC-antigen complex and would initiate an immune response.[5,8,13] Figure 3-5 represents the crystalline structure of a class II HLA molecule as it might appear to a T-cell receptor (the crystalline structure for class II MHC molecules is extrapolated from research done on the structure of a class I molecule, HLA-A2).[11] A "peptide groove," formed by the $alpha_1$ and $beta_1$ domains, is the antigen peptide-binding site. The variable regions of the molecule are located primarily along this groove, which is also found in class I MHC molecules. Thus, the antigen-binding site varies between different molecules, and a given MHC molecule can bind only a limited number of antigenic peptide fragments.[3]

Antigen binding sites

Superantigens

One exciting area of research in immunology relates to the role of superantigens. These superantigens, such as staphylococcal enterotoxin, do

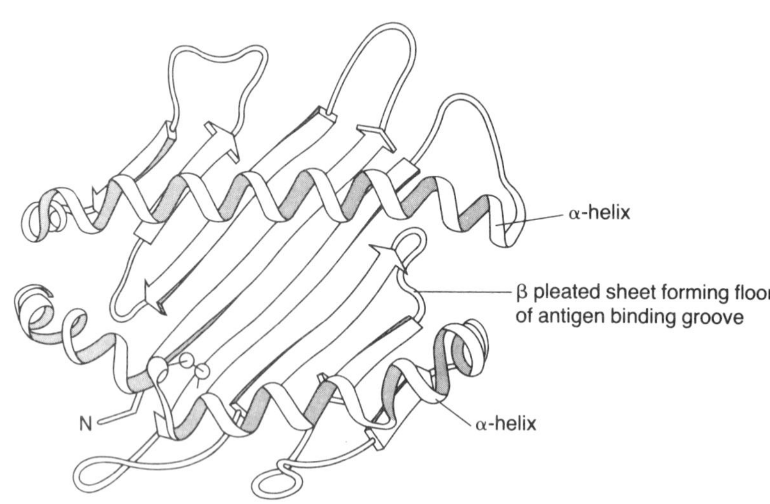

Figure 3-5. Structure of a class II HLA molecule (top view) as it might appear to a T-cell receptor

SOURCE: Reprinted with permission from Stites DP, Terr AI. Basic and clinical immunology. 7th ed., copyright Appleton & Lange 1991.

not bind to MHC molecules the way most antigens do (by wedging into the peptide groove). Rather, preliminary evidence suggests that superantigens have the ability to bind to MHC molecules outside the peptide groove. By binding on the edge of the groove, they may act like vices, cementing the antigen-presenting cell to the T cell and leading to T-cell activation.[14,15]

Another unique aspect of superantigens is that they can directly activate subsets of T cells. As we have seen, normal antigens bind to T cells at an antigen receptor, and less than 1% of all T cells proliferate in response.[14] In contrast, superantigens can bind to a particular part of the T-cell receptor named the V beta chain. Superantigens can engage the V beta on many T cells, quickly stimulating the activation of a large number of T cells. In the mouse model, superantigens can activate as many as 10% of all T cells.[14,15]

Known superantigens include staphylococcal enterotoxin as well as a group of proteins produced by streptococcal species. The proteins produced may lead to toxic shock, septic shock, or food poisoning in the human host. The clinical symptoms of these illnesses are probably due to the overstimulation of T cells, with a subsequent, paradoxical, profound immunosuppression. Bacteria, such as staphylococci and streptococci, probably developed superantigens as an evolutionary survival mechanism: the superantigens cause such chaos in the host's immune response that the bacteria can slip by, unnoticed by the host's immune surveillance. The exact roles of these and other superantigens in humans are still being investigated.[15]

Antigen complex

With the exception of superantigens, the receptors on the T cells recognize a foreign antigen only when the antigen is part of a complex with a cell surface molecule encoded by the MHC. This observation helped to confirm that the immune response to antigen was MHC dependent. The isolation of the molecules that make up the T-cell antigen receptor molecule and the genes that encode it have recently been made possible via monoclonal antibodies (MoAbs) and recombinant DNA technology.[16,17] Recent studies strongly suggest that two distinct T-cell receptors may be involved.[17] Figure 3-6 provides a schematic representation of the association among the HLA molecule, antigen, and T cell.

MHC restriction

Another way of expressing this concept is that it takes a self component (an HLA molecule) and an antigenic component (often called X) to be recognized as nonself by the immune system. The T cells then proliferate and differentiate and can then recognize and attack the nonself complex via the T-dependent immune response.[6] Thus, the effector phase of the immune response depends on the receptor on T cells recognizing self structure plus antigen.[5,6,13,16] The term *MHC restriction* refers to the concept that there must be a self component and an antigen component to elicit a T-cell-mediated immune response. This process has also been called the altered self theory and the self plus X theory.

The case of infection by an influenza virus illustrates these concepts. When a cell is infected by influenza virus (acting as a foreign antigen, or X), fragments of proteins encoded by the viral genome form an external complex with an HLA molecule (acting as self). Then, T-cell receptors on cytotoxic T cells recognize this complex as nonself and kill the virally infected cells.

Tumor surveillance

While cytotoxic T cells must recognize self + X, natural killer (NK) cells may recognize antigen via a different process. This theory suggests that NK cells kill antigenic targets because they express low levels of MHC class I genes (self). In other words, this "missing self" theory proposes that NK cells recognize and kill cells, such as tumor cells, that fail to express self class I genes.[18]

It has also been recognized that both class I molecules (A, B, C) and class II molecules (D region) participate in the cell-cell interactions between the MHC and T lymphocytes. Receptors on helper T cells must recognize class II molecules before eliciting an immune response. This is why class II genes have also been called the Ir genes; specifically, the HLA-DR region in humans is believed to contain these Ir genes. In contrast, cytotoxic T cells have receptors that recognize class I molecules. Both classes of molecules must be in a complex with an antigen before the helper or cytotoxic T cell receptors can recognize the antigen (see Figures 3-5 and 3-6).

Maternal-fetal histocompatibility

The phenomenon of MHC restriction is a vital control mechanism in enabling the human immune system to differentiate between self and nonself. That is, it helps the T cells recognize which cells to destroy (virally infected cells). In addition, the MHC plays a role in immune surveillance against other foreign or altered cells, such as cancer cells that may develop over a life span.[3] MHC restriction also prevents T cells from destroying certain desirable nonself cells, such as the cells of a fetus in a pregnant woman. The MHC plays a vital role in the maternal-fetal relationship by ensuring histocompatibility between the mother and fetus, although the exact mechanism of this compatibility is not well understood. It is now recognized that MHC restriction in the efferent immune response is important in other areas, such as autoimmune disease, cancer, and organ transplantation.[12]

Disease Association. As we have seen, the HLA complex plays many helpful roles in the immune system, such as successful transplantation, promotion of antibody response to antigen, tumor surveillance, and

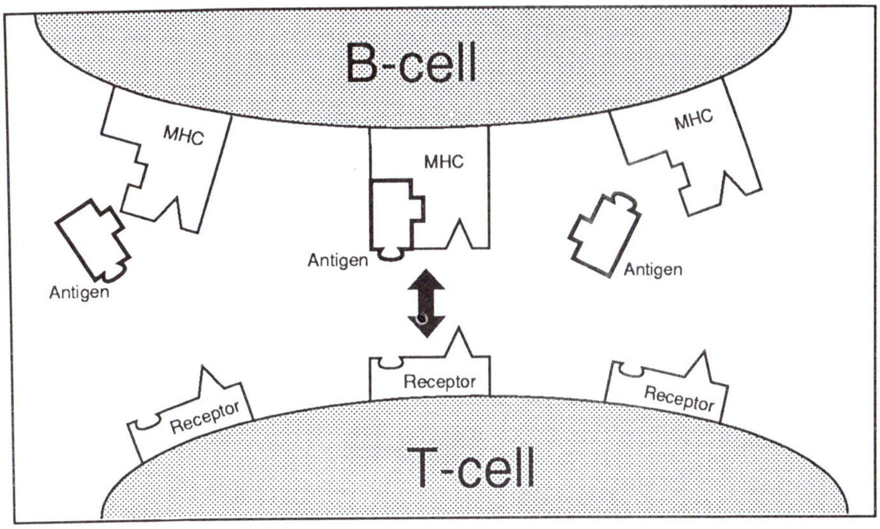

Figure 3-6. T-cell receptor binding with MHC-antigen complex

maternal-fetal histocompatibility. However, the HLA complex also has a striking role in the immunobiology of certain diseases. It has been found in recent years that certain HLA alleles may predispose individuals to specific disease processes. Genes of the HLA complex have been associated with more than 100 diseases,[5,6] many of which are listed in Table 3-2.

Table 3-2 Diseases Showing Positive HLA Associations

Disease	HLA Antigen	Relative Risk[a]
Rheumatic		
Ankylosing spondylitis	B27	69.1
Reiter's syndrome	B27	37.0
Acute anterior uveitis	B27	8.2
Reactive arthritis (*Yersinia, Salmonella,* gonococcus)	B27	18.0
Psoriatic arthritis, central	B27	10.7
	B38	9.1
Psoriatic arthritis, peripheral	B27	2.0
	B38	6.5
Juvenile rheumatoid arthritis	B27	3.9

Table 3-2 (continued)

Disease	HLA Antigen	Relative Risk[a]
Juvenile rheumatoid arthritis (pauciarticular)	DR5	3.3
Rheumatoid arthritis	Dw4/DR4	3.8
Sjögren's syndrome	Dw3	5.7
Systemic lupus erythematosus	DR3	2.6
Gastrointestinal		
Gluten-sensitive enteropathy	DR3	11.6
Chronic active hepatitis	DR3	6.8
Ulcerative colitis	B5	3.8
Hematologic		
Idiopathic hemochromatosis	A3	6.7
	B14	26.7
	A13, B14	90.0
Pernicious anemia	DR5	5.4
Skin		
Dermatitis herpetiformis	DR3	17.3
Psoriasis vulgaris	Cw6	7.5
Psoriasis vulgaris (Japanese)	Cw6	8.5
Pemphigus vulgaris (Jews)	DR4	14.6
	A26	4.8
Behcet's anemia	B5	3.8
Endocrine		
Insulin-dependent diabetes mellitus (juvenile diabetes mellitus)	DR4	3.6
	DR3	4.8
	DR2	0.2
	BfF1[b]	15.0
Graves' disease	B8	2.5
	DR3	3.7
Graves' disease (Japanese)	B35	4.4
Addison's disease	Dw3	10.5
Subacute thyroiditis (de Quervain)	B35	13.7

Table 3-2 (continued)

Disease	HLA Antigen	Relative Risk[a]
Hashimoto's thyroiditis	DR5	3.2
Congenital adrenal hyperplasia	Bw47	15.4
Neurologic		
Myasthenia gravis (without thymoma)	B8	3.3
Multiple sclerosis	D/DR2	2.7
Manic-depressive disorder	B16	2.3
Narcolepsy	DR2	130.0
Schizophrenia	A28	2.3
Renal		
Idiopathic membranous glomerulonephritis	DR3	5.7
Goodpasture's syndrome (anti-GBM)	DR2	15.9
Minimal change disease (steroid responsive)	DR7	4.2
IgA nephropathy (French, Japanese)	DR4	3.1
Gold/penicillamine nephropathy	DR3	14.0
Polycystic kidney disease	B5	2.6
Infectious		
Tuberculoid leprosy (Asians)	B8	6.8
Paralytic polio	B16	4.3
Low vs. high response to vaccinia virus	Cw3	12.7

SOURCE: Reprinted with permission from Carpenter CB. The major histocompatibility gene complex. In: Wilson JD, Braunwald E, Isselbacher KJ, et al, eds. Harrison's principles of internal medicine. 12th ed. New York: McGraw-Hill; 1991:91.

[a]Relative risk $= \dfrac{(\text{\% antigen-positive patients}) \times (\text{\% antigen-negative controls})}{(\text{\% antigen-negative patients}) \times (\text{\% antigen-positive controls})}$

[b]BfF1 is an allele of the complement system that is HLA linked, but it is not antigen.

Predisposing factors

The most striking association between HLA and disease is the one found with the HLA-B27 allele and an increased frequency of some rheumatic diseases, such as ankylosing spondylitis.[5,6,8,19] In fact, the B27 allele is found in 80% to 90% of patients with ankylosing spondylitis, whereas only 7% of the healthy control population has the B27 allele.[5] Thus, individuals with the B27 allele have a risk of developing ankylosing spondylitis about 87 times greater than that of the general population.[5]

Aside from the B27 haplotype, most HLA disease associations are found in the D region (i.e., associated primarily with class II molecules). Most HLA-associated diseases share some other common characteristics: inheritance patterns do not follow simple Mendelian genetics; they are associated with immunologic abnormalities (especially autoimmunity); and they follow chronic courses.[6] The most profound HLA-D-associated disease is narcolepsy, a disease characterized by constant excessive sleepiness. The association of narcolepsy with the DR2 allele is virtually 100%.[2,6,20]

Another example of D-related disease association is that of HLA-DR3, which carries a 21 times greater risk than normal toward development of gluten-sensitive enteropathy. DR3 is found in 63% to 96% of patients with this gastrointestinal disorder, versus only 22% to 27% of the general population. Type I (insulin-dependent) juvenile-onset diabetes mellitus has also been associated with DR3 and DR4.

Many of the other D3- and DR3-associated diseases are of an autoimmune or hyperimmune pathogenesis, such as Graves' Disease (see Chapter 6). This tendency toward autoimmunity makes sense when one considers that class II antigens are responsible for immune response.

Diagnostic value

Currently, the only clinically valuable tool in the diagnosis of disease is the relationship of HLA-B27 in ankylosing spondylitis, and MoAbs are available to assist in the typing of B27.[8]

The exact causative role of these HLA haplotypes in disease predisposition is unclear. Three possible explanations are as follows.

Possible causes

First, some HLA phenotypes respond poorly to pathogen elimination because of difficulties in T-cell interactions with class I and II molecules on immune cells and their targets (i.e., problems with MHC restriction).[3,9] These difficulties in interaction may include failure to generate antigenic peptides, failure of generated peptides to associate with the MHC antigen-binding groove, and failure of T cells to recognize a peptide associated within the MHC molecule.

Second, specific DR genes (Ir genes) may not act appropriately in eliciting an immune response. Therefore, individuals become more prone to autoimmune disease (because of excessive immune response) or infection (because of inadequate immune response).[3,9]

Third, HLAs may act as inappropriate receptors for a pathogen (such as a virus), which infects the cell and causes changes in cellular function and subsequent disease expression.[3,5]

Susceptibility alleles

Certainly, the predisposition to these diseases may be multifactorial, since not everyone with a given allele contracts the disease. In fact, only

20% of B27 individuals actually develop ankylosing spondylitis.[5,8] Seventy percent of multiple sclerosis patients carry the DR2 allele.[21] Because of this tendency toward predisposition to a disease, these alleles such as B27 and DR2 are also termed susceptibility alleles. It is probable that other cofactors, such as environmental influences or other genetic influences, ultimately cause onset of the disease.[6,8,12]

It has also been postulated that normal controls who carry a susceptibility gene may also have a protective gene that is dominant and therefore prevents disease onset. Insulin-dependent diabetes mellitus has been extensively studied in this regard; data reveal that most people have haplotypes that confer either an increased susceptibility or a dominant protective effect.[21] New techniques developed to rapidly characterize DNA sequences in the MHC (such as the polymerase chain reaction [PCR], described in the next section) provide improved data on allele sequencing and have furthered our understanding of HLA disease susceptibility on a molecular level.

Since HLA diseases often run in families (based on the relevant inherited haplotype), knowledge of a certain HLA phenotype may prove helpful in genetic counseling of people who are at risk for certain diseases but who wish to have children. In addition, HLA typing can be performed on cells obtained from amniotic fluid, and thus the degree of risk for disease development in the unborn fetus can be assessed.

Further study is needed on the role of the HLA system in disease association. Better understanding of the pathogenesis may someday lead to the possibility of therapeutic interventions in HLA-associated diseases.

MHC Typing

HLA matching of donor and recipient results in a higher degree of success in organ transplantation, and HLA matching is the ideal method for donor selection. This section discusses the various methods of HLA typing and describes the application of HLA typing in clinical practice.

There is a great deal of polymorphism in the HLA system; each allele determines a product. The products of class I and II genes are molecules on the cell surface that bear specific antigenic determinants. These molecules provide the targets for HLA typing. There are two older, classic methods of HLA typing, serologic typing (antibody screening tests of serum and lymphocytes) and cellular typing (evaluations of reactions between sets of lymphocytes). A newer form of HLA typing using molecular biology and DNA technology is also described.

Serologic Typing

Serologic typing is one of the simplest and fastest techniques for HLA testing and is one of the most widespread and standard typing methods. The process of serologic typing is based on the fact that antibodies in the serum of immunized individuals react with lymphocytes being tested only if differing HLA haplotypes are present. Sera from individuals with identical phenotypes do not react. Therefore, if the lymphocytes of the individual to be tested are run against a battery of sera containing antibodies to known HLAs, the HLA profile of the tested individual can be established by examining the subsequent reactions.

Antisera

The sera used for testing are of a human source, obtained primarily from multiparous women,[3,6] and they have lymphocytotoxic antibodies directed at certain HLA haplotypes. These sera, known as antisera, contain high titers of cytotoxic antibodies directed against a limited number of HLA antigenic determinants.

Many attempts have been made to develop MoAbs (see Chapter 11) with enough specificity for use as typing reagents. Although some MoAbs are currently available to type particular HLA antigens (such as HLA-DP), the majority cannot "fix" complement, a vital component of most serologic assays. Therefore, MoAbs are not widely used in serologic HLA typing.[3,6] The tests used for serologic typing are the lymphocytotoxicity assay and the crossmatch test.

Lymphocytotoxicity Assay. Serologic testing using this assay is useful primarily to identify class I antigens (A, B, C), but it can also identify DR and DQ antigens from class II. Lymphocytotoxicity assays, such as the complement-dependent lymphocytotoxicity assay, are the most widely applied tests in determining histocompatibility. The test is performed as shown in Figure 3-7.

Procedures

Lymphocytes from the donor are purified and added to antisera targeted against specific HLAs. Complement is added and the lymphocyte-antisera mixture is incubated. Antigens present on donor lymphocytes react with the targeted antisera specific for certain HLA products, and the lymphocytes are killed by the antibodies and complement. When a dye (such as eosin) is added, dead lymphocytes absorb the dye and appear red, whereas living lymphocytes do not absorb the dye.

By examining the percentage of cells killed by each antiserum (patterns of reactivity), one can identify which antisera were specific for the donor lymphocytes and thus assign an HLA type. When this test is performed with a battery of antisera, the HLA types of both donor and recipient can be established on the basis of their reaction patterns. A determination can then

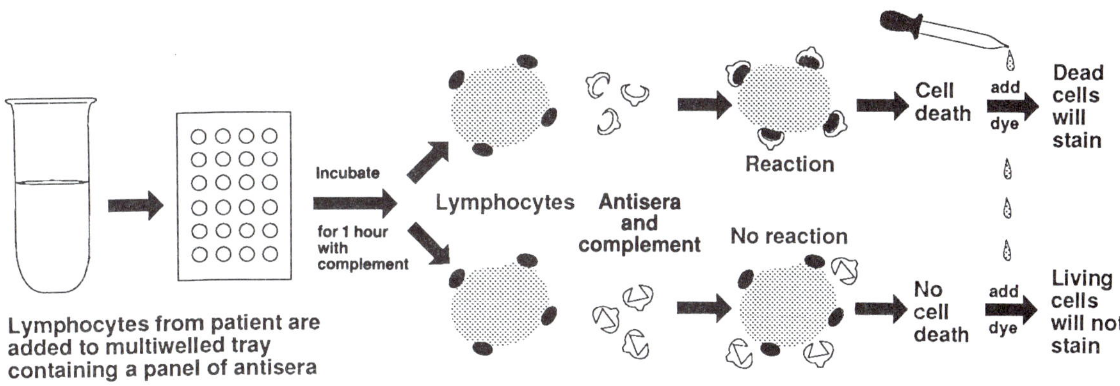

Figure 3-7. Complement-dependent lymphocytotoxicity assay for HLA antigens

be made as to whether the donor and recipient have identical HLA haplotypes, semi-identical haplotypes, or nonidentical haplotypes. If donor and recipient are compatible, a crossmatch test is performed.

Serologic Crossmatch. In the crossmatch test, serum from the recipient is incubated with lymphocytes from the potential donor for 30 minutes, then the same process of the lymphocytotoxicity assay is followed (i.e., addition of complement, 1 hour's incubation, then addition of dye).

If the two individuals were found to be HLA identical from the initial lymphocytotoxicity test, one would expect no cytotoxic antibodies to be present in the recipient, and the crossmatch results would be negative. However, in the case of HLA semi-identical patients, the recipient may have antibodies directed against the donor lymphocytes, which would lead to graft rejection, and the two individuals would be judged incompatible. The recipient may have developed these antibodies from previous exposure to the mismatched haplotype, such as through a blood transfusion. Thus, for HLA semi-identical patients, the crossmatch is either positive or negative, depending on whether the recipient has been previously exposed. Like lymphocytotoxicity assay results, results from the crossmatch test are obtained fairly quickly.

Cellular Typing

Antagonistic reactions

Cellular typing does not use antisera containing cytotoxic antibodies. Instead, this method is based on the fact that when lymphocytes from one individual are mixed with lymphocytes from another individual, the cells mount an immune response and are stimulated to divide or proliferate. Thus, in cellular typing, donor and recipient lymphocytes are mixed together and observed for antagonistic reactions that denote incompatibility. Cellular typing does not necessarily determine an individual's HLA type (as is possible with the serologic typing methods), but, rather, it assesses the compatibilities of mixtures of lymphocytes.

Mixed lymphocyte reactions and cultures

Cellular typing is often preferred over serologic typing because it more closely mimics the natural course of events when tissues are transplanted. By actually testing the interactions of donor and recipient lymphocytes, one can assess not only HLA histocompatibilities but also other minor non-HLA histocompatibilities that may contribute to graft rejection.[9] The proliferation seen when different sets of lymphocytes are mixed together in vitro is caused by the incompatibility of genes in the D region of the MHC, especially the DR region.[9] This proliferation is known as the mixed lymphocyte reaction (MLR). However, if lymphocytes with identical haplotypes are mixed, stimulation and proliferation do not occur and no MLR takes place. The mixed lymphocyte culture (MLC) technique uses the MLR to assess compatibility.

MLC measures the amount of proliferation and reflects the response of T cells to antigens present on other lymphocytes. When HLAs A, B, and C are identical between the two sources of lymphocytes (identical class I phenotypes as assessed by serologic typing), then any proliferation that occurs is due solely to incompatibilities in the D region.

One-way MLC

To identify which lymphocytes (donor or recipient) are actually proliferating, a test known as the one-way MLC is used (Figure 3-8). In this technique, the donor lymphocytes are poisoned with either radiation or mitomycin C before they are mixed with the recipient's lymphocytes. Then the donor lymphocytes can act only as antigen bearers but cannot confuse the MLC results by proliferating. In this way, one can be sure that any proliferation (called a positive MLC) is due solely to a response of the recipient's lymphocytes directed against the donor's antigens.

The degree of proliferation in the one-way MLC is determined by using radiolabeled thymidine. The DNA of cells that are actively proliferating takes up (incorporates) this labeled thymidine. The amount of incorporated radiolabeled thymidine indicates the amount of cell proliferation and the lack of compatibility of the donor and recipient's lymphocytes.

The disadvantage of MLC is that 5 to 7 days of culturing may be necessary before results are obtained. MLC is used in transplantation typing, as in the case of HLA-identical donor and recipient (as judged by serologic typing). Thus, cellular typing is used to confirm patient/donor "identicalness," and it also assesses non-HLA incompatibilities between the two individuals. In the case of transplant typing, if MLC is positive, the donor and recipient are incompatible, and prospects for a graft are poor.

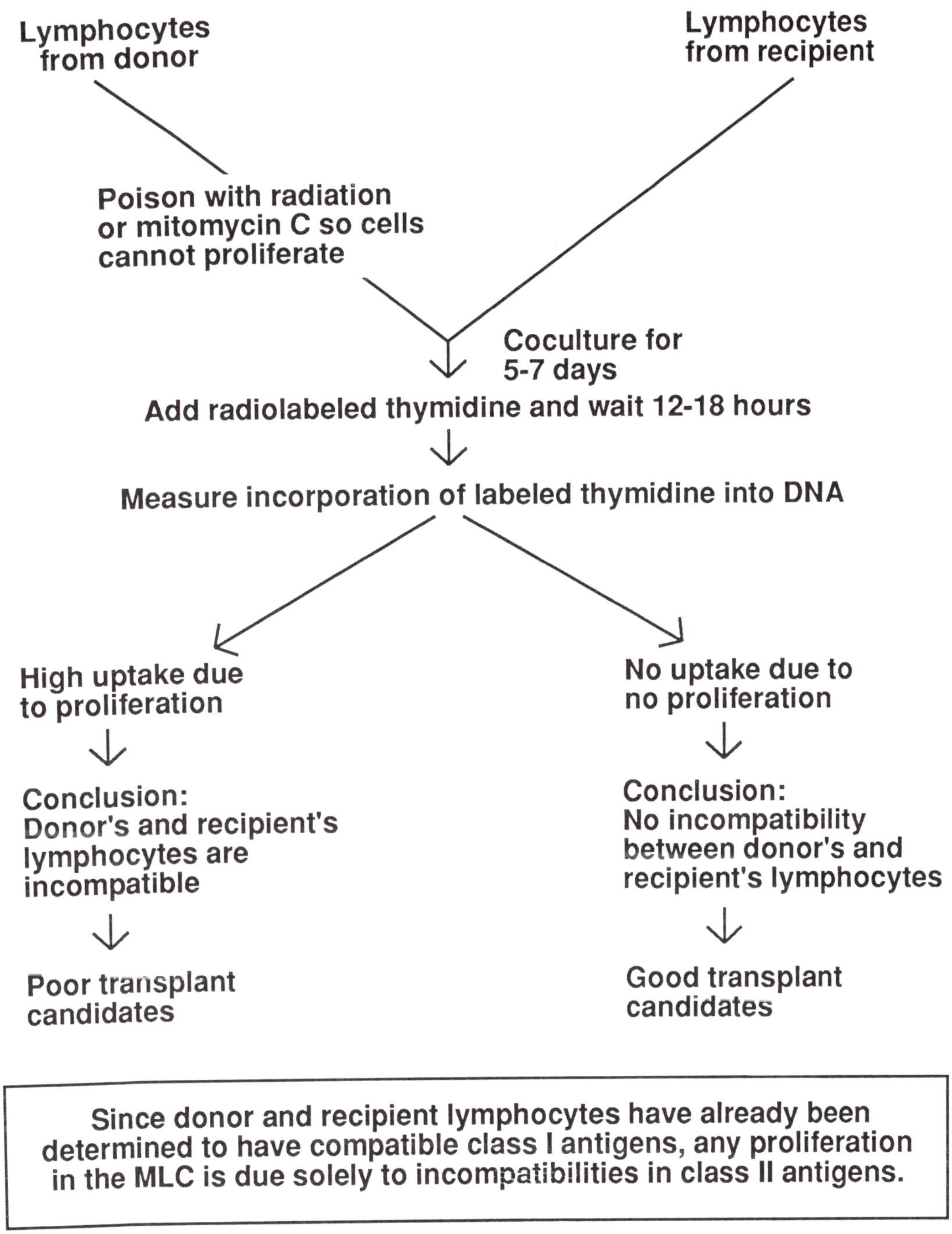

Figure 3-8. One-way MLC test to determine HLA-D compatibility

Cell-mediated lympholysis assay

Another cellular method of typing is the cell-mediated lympholysis assay. During MLC, the recipient cells may have generated cytotoxic T lymphocytes directed against the donor's lymphocytes (antidonor T cells).

In the cell-mediated lympholysis assay, the cells from the MLC are mixed with fresh living donor cells, and the lysis of donor cells reflects the presence of antidonor cytotoxic T lymphocytes.

In summary, even though cellular typing may detect some antigens not detected by antisera, as well as assess non-HLA incompatibilities, its clinical utility is limited to use in typing of living related donors for transplant. Table 3-3 summarizes the main assays used in serologic and cellular HLA typing.

Molecular-biologic Typing

Until recently, HLA haplotypes were determined primarily by using serologic typing analysis. In the 1990s, however, many HLA alleles can be identified by using biochemical and DNA sequencing techniques. These developments in the field of molecular biology reveal the structure and amino acid sequence of many specific HLA antigens. In fact, HLA alleles are now officially recognized by their DNA sequences rather than by their

Table 3-3 Serologic and Cellular Methods Used in Histocompatibility Testing

Test	Test Components	Time	Applications
Serologic lymphocytotoxicity	HLA antisera; complement; test cells	3 hours	Identification of class I and II HLA antigens
Serologic crossmatch	Recipient serum; donor cells; complement	3 hours	Detection of preformed antidonor antibodies in recipient's serum
Cellular			
Mixed lymphocyte culture (MLC)	Donor and recipient cells combined in tissue culture	6 days	Class II HLA compatibility
Cell-mediated lympholysis	Recipient cells from MLC; donor cells as targets	4 hours	Detection of anti-donor cytotoxic T lymphocytes

SOURCE: Reprinted with permission from Stites DP, Terr AI. Basic and clinical immunology. 7th ed. Copyright Appleton & Lange 1991.

serologic patterns. Three molecular biology methods for HLA typing are described in this section: (1) restriction fragment length polymorphism (RFLP), (2) oligonucleotide probes (ONPs), and (3) PCR.

Restriction Fragment Length Polymorphism. The RFLP test is based on the finding that a high degree of homology exists in the DNA sequences of class I and II genes. Variations in these common DNA sequences appear at predictable sites on the molecule, and these unique sequences define specific HLA alleles. The points of variation are thus made targets for cleavage by enzymes called restriction endonucleases, each of which recognizes a specific cleavage site of a unique DNA sequence.

DNA cleavage

Therefore, in RFLP typing the HLA haplotype is cleaved into DNA fragments of different lengths (restriction fragment lengths). These DNA fragments can then be generated and visualized by means of further methods, including blotting and electrophoresis. In this way, a specific HLA antigen can be assigned.[3] RFLP analysis may be especially useful in identifying antigens in the HLA-DR and -DQ regions.[22]

Limitations of the RFLP include the fact that not all HLA antigens have corresponding restriction endonucleases available and that the procedure can take several weeks.[3] Because of these limitations, it would be desirable to have specific DNA "probes" for each unique sequence of an HLA antigen. Two recent molecular biology developments, ONPs and PCR, provide solutions to the RFLP's shortcomings.

Oligonucleotide Probes. ONPs are small DNA segments consisting of 20 to 25 nucleotides. This length is short enough that each segment is likely to be unique to a particular individual. Even differences in a single nucleotide can imply a different HLA antigen, so the specificity of these probes is necessary for accurate HLA typing.

HLA specificity

The ONP assay is illustrated in Figure 3-9. Samples of DNA (denoted as A, B, C, or D) are dotted onto a support membrane in a column on a slot template. This membrane is then cut into strips, and each strip is exposed to sequence-specific ONPs, such as probes for DR1 or DR2. The membrane is then reassembled, and a band appears on film to indicate a match between the DNA sample and the sequence-specific ONP used. Thus, a patient's HLA type can be assigned.[3]

The Polymerase Chain Reaction. The PCR process amplifies one DNA fragment or a single gene into many copies in a short time, thus allowing greater expression of DNA sequences. PCR technology can be applied to HLA genes.[3,23] A segment of DNA containing the HLA gene of interest is sequenced, and oligonucleotide primers are synthesized to complement each end of the DNA segment. The gene of interest is then amplified

DNA amplification

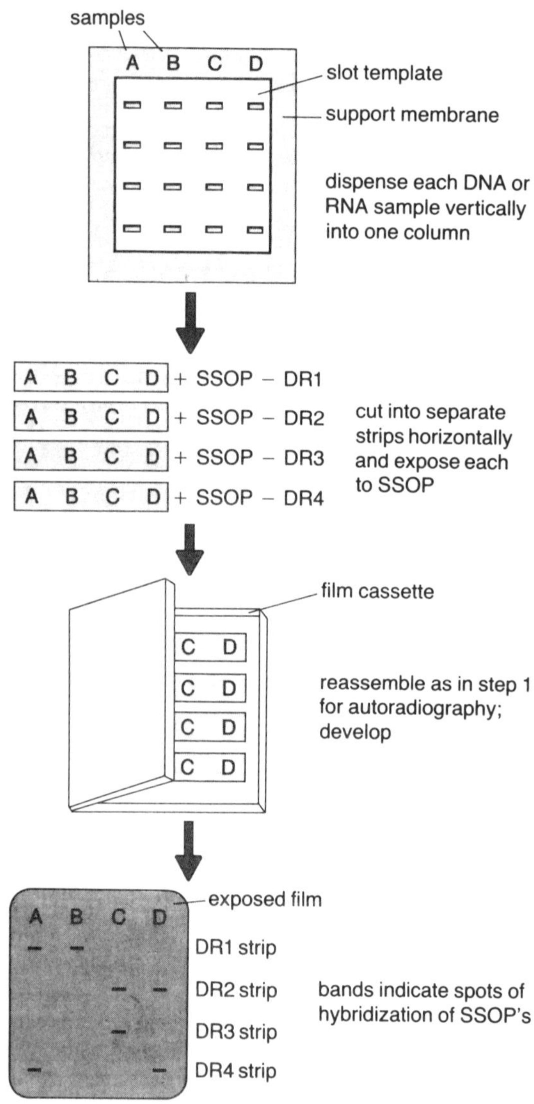

sample	results
A	DR1, DR4
B	DR1 only
C	DR2, DR3
D	DR2, DR4

Figure 3-9. Oligonucleotide probes

SOURCE: Reprinted with permission from Stites DP, Terr AI. Basic and clinical immunology. 7th ed., copyright Appleton & Lange 1991.

through a series of reactions in a chain reaction (reaction products become the templates for the next cycle of the process). Over a few hours, this repetition of amplification (approximately 25 to 30 cycles) generates more than 1 million copies of the chosen DNA sequence.

The PCR thus enables very minute quantities of DNA to be amplified into quantities sufficient for HLA typing and testing for donor-recipient compatibility. The PCR is an accurate, convenient method of typing HLA alleles, and it provides results as quickly as standard serologic methods.[23] Although histocompatibility testing by PCR techniques is available today in only a few laboratories, its applications will surely grow in the coming years.

In summary, the uses of molecular-biologic HLA typing include confirming the serologic results of compatibilities between transplant donors and recipients. In addition, these new technologies can help select the best nonrelated potential donor for a transplant patient. These tests also may be used in combination for typing (e.g., use of PCR for DNA amplification, followed by use of RFLP).[24] With further refinement and wider availability, molecular-biologic typing will probably become the standard HLA typing method.

Uses of MHC Typing. MHC typing is a valuable tool used primarily for predicting success of organ transplantation and choosing appropriate donors.

Use of MLC as a means of cellular typing has been shown to provide better graft outcomes than serologic typing alone for both living related donors and cadaveric donors in kidney transplant.[5] It has been shown repeatedly that the results of cellular typing, focusing on the D region, are better predictors of graft outcome than serologic typing methods alone.[19] Fortunately, the results of MLC usually agree fairly closely with those of the lymphocytotoxicity assays for the major HLAs.

Predicting graft outcomes

Most labs continue to use serologic testing of HLA-A, -B, -C, -DQ, and -DR with lymphocytotoxicity assays and crossmatching if HLA typing is needed immediately (as in the case of a cadaveric kidney transplant). The cell-mediated lympholysis assay can also quickly detect antidonor T lymphocytes in the patient. In other situations, as in the case of using a living related donor for kidney or bone marrow transplant, there may be no need for immediate HLA typing. In these cases, one often has the luxury of enough time to perform cellular typing using the one-way MLC. Table 3-4 lists the sequence of compatibility tests used in renal transplantation (including ABO and Rh typing, which is discussed in the next section).

Table 3-4 Sequence of Histocompatibility Testing for Renal Transplant Patients

A. Perform preliminary immunologic evaluation

1. Patient

   HLA typing

   ABO/Rh typing

   Screening of serum for antibodies reactive with HLA antigens

   Testing of serum for autoantibodies

2. Living related donors

   HLA typing

   ABO/Rh typing

   Crossmatch with serum of patient to detect anti-donor antibodies

   MLC test with patient

B. Select living related donor

This is based on:

ABO compatibility

Best match for HLA antigens

Low stimulation of patient's cells in MLC test

Negative preliminary crossmatch

If there is no appropriate living related donor, then

C. Place patient on waiting list for cadaver kidney

Register patient with UNOS

Screen serum sample monthly for antibodies reactive to HLA antigens

D. Select appropriate recipient for cadaver kidney

HLA and ABO type cadaver donor

Crossmatch cadaver with ABO-compatible recipients

Select candidates having no antibodies to donor's HLA antigens

Table 3-4 (continued)

E. Transplant: living-related and cadaver donors
Crossmatch with most recent patient sample drawn immediately pretransplant

SOURCE: Reprinted with permission from Stites DP, Terr AI, eds. Basic and clinical immunology. 7th ed. Copyright Appleton & Lange 1991.

MLC = mixed lymphocyte culture; UNOS = United Network for Organ Sharing.

There is now a nationwide computer bank that can help match possible donors with waiting recipients across the country. The United Network for Organ Sharing, established in 1987, links local and regional transplant centers with a national registry of waiting recipients.

Platelet matching

However, there are also several other uses of MHC typing. Typing is useful in certain patients who require platelet transfusions. If these patients have received multiple blood and platelet transfusions, they may have high titers of cytotoxic antibodies directed against many of the blood component antigens to which they have been exposed. These sensitized patients often react against subsequent platelet transfusions by destroying the platelets, thus gaining no therapeutic benefit. However, since platelets express only class I HLA molecules and not class II molecules, serologic typing can be done via the lymphocytotoxicity assay. This assay identifies platelets that are histocompatible (HLA-matched platelets) and that will not be destroyed in sensitized patients.[5]

Paternity testing

In addition, the genetic polymorphism of the HLA system proves useful in other applications. Because so many variations of alleles exist in humans, the chance of having a phenotype in common with another individual who is unrelated is approximately one in 20 million. This high degree of polymorphism provides the basis for HLA typing in paternity testing and other medical and legal applications. The distribution of HLAs is also specific for certain races, and typing can thus serve as a helpful tool for anthropologists studying migration patterns and evolution.[5] HLA typing is also useful in establishing HLA-disease associations, such as the one seen between HLA-B27 and ankylosing spondylitis.

Blood Group Detection

This section provides a brief history of the development of blood grouping systems and discusses their application in clinical practice.

The history of blood transfusions dates back to the late 17th century. Initial attempts at blood transfusion for humans used sheep's blood, which led to many deaths and the subsequent outlawing of transfusion therapy in England. By the 1800s it was determined that blood could be transfused only between individuals of the same species.[12] Blood transfusion can be thought of as a form of tissue transplantation, and it is actually the safest form of allotransplantation.

Immunohematology

There are many applications of immunohematology, not only in the medical field but also in law, genetics, and anthropology. The use of blood transfusions is one of the most important lifesaving measures known in medicine. However, because severe hemolytic reactions can occur if incompatible blood is transfused, nomenclature and typing systems are essential.

Many systems are used to classify blood groups. Currently, there are at least 22 different blood grouping systems that describe approximately 400 blood group antigens in humans. The two most widely used are the ABO system and the Rh system.

The ABO System

At the turn of the 20th century, a relatively simple RBC antigen-grouping system was designed. This system was based on the fact that there are two main immunogenic antigens associated with RBCs, A and B. A person may have one, both, or neither of these two antigens. A third RBC antigen was then described and was denoted as *H*. H is a precursor of both A and B antigens. People who have neither A nor B antigens have high titers of the H antigen.

Blood group

The nomenclature of this ABO system is based on which antigen or antigens are present on an individual's RBCs. People with the A antigen are blood group A, those with B antigens are blood group B, those with both A and B are blood group AB, and those who have neither A nor B antigens but have high levels of H antigen are blood group O.[9] The ABO nomenclature system is summarized in Table 3-5.

Antibody designates

It was also found that the serum of many people contains antibodies that are directed against whichever antigen or antigens are not expressed on their RBCs. That is, the antibodies do not react against and destroy the person's own RBCs, which would be incompatible with life. Therefore, A individuals have anti-B antibodies, B individuals have anti-A antibodies, AB individuals have no antibodies, and O individuals have both anti-A and anti-B antibodies. Table 3-5 summarizes the antibody distribution in the ABO blood grouping system.

Table 3-5 ABO(H) Blood Group System

Blood Group Phenotype	Possible Genotypes	Antigen on Red Blood Cells*	Antibody in Serum	Incidence in U.S. Population (%)
A	AA, AO	A	Anti-B	42
B	BB, BO	B	Anti-A	10
O(H)	OO	Neither A nor B	Both anti-A and anti-B	45
AB	AB	Both A and B	Neither anti-A nor anti-B	3

*Cells of all blood groups contain the H substance.

SOURCE: Reprinted with permission from Barrett J. Textbook of immunology. 5th ed. St. Louis: C.V. Mosby; 1988:233.

Blood grouping was first used as a prerequisite to blood transfusion in the early 1900s, and in 1949 the actual structure of the three ABO antigens was described. The presence of antigens on RBCs is genetically controlled; the inheritance of these ABO antigens follows simple Mendelian patterns. Each individual possesses two alleles at the ABO locus (located on chromosome 9 in humans), one derived from each parent. There are six possible ABO genotypes based on the three available antigens: AA, AO, BB, BO, AB, and OO. The genotypes determine people's blood types. For instance, people with genotype AA and AO have blood type A; those with BB or BO have blood type B; those with AB have blood type AB, and those with genotype OO have blood type O (see Table 3-5).

Genotypes

The ABO antigens are present on virtually all cells and tissues of the body, with the exception of lymphocytes and cells of the spinal cord and brain. The matching of blood groups in medicine is useful primarily in transfusions, allografts, and hemolytic disease of the newborn (HDN).

Before blood is transfused, compatibility between the donor and recipient must be established by typing the blood of both individuals. In addition to determining the blood type, tests must verify the absence of cytotoxic antibodies in the recipient that may be targeted against the donor's RBCs. In fact, most severe hemolytic reactions that occur after transfusion are due to ABO mismatches.

Procedure

Blood Typing. In determining a patient's blood type, both the cells and the serum are tested. When the cells are typed, they are mixed with serum containing known antibodies, and agglutination reactions are assessed. This method of RBC antigen typing is also referred to as forward grouping. In testing a patient's serum, the serum is mixed with RBCs containing known antigens, and agglutination reactions are assessed. This method is also known as reverse grouping.[9] Because correct typing of ABO antigens is vital, both forward and reverse grouping are routinely done. Table 3-6 summarizes the agglutination reactions found in ABO blood typing.

Type and cross

Crossmatching. The crossmatch test is a very important pretransfusion test, second only to typing in importance. A physician ordering a *type and cross* would receive results of both of these testing methods. In crossmatching, the recipient's serum is incubated with the donor's RBCs to assess the presence of antibodies that could cause hemolysis. If the cells agglutinate after this procedure, antibodies are present and the donor and recipient are judged incompatible.

Type and screen

For situations in which the transfusion will probably not be needed within the ensuing 48 hours, a *type and screen* may be performed. In this case, the patient's blood type is determined and then the blood is screened for the presence of antibodies by being mixed with a variety of common RBC antigens. When the patient is actually ready to receive the transfusion, a crossmatch must be done between the recipient and the actual donor's blood.[16] The crossmatch must be performed within 24 hours of the proposed transfusion, because the antibody status of the recipient can change rapidly and unexpectedly.[12]

When available, only ABO- and Rh-matched blood should be transfused. It was previously believed that type O blood (containing "no" antigens) could safely be given to any patient, and type O patients were referred to as universal donors. Conversely, it was thought that AB patients (having "no" antibodies) could receive any blood and were referred to as universal recipients. This concept has now been abandoned, because patients who receive repeated transfusions can develop high titers of antibodies directed

Table 3-6 Results of ABO Typing

Blood Type	RBCs plus Anti-A Serum	RBCs plus Anti-B Serum
A	+	0
B	0	+
AB	+	+
O	0	0

+ = agglutination; 0 = no agglutination.

against antigens of various blood groups. Also, prior pregnancy or organ transplant can prompt a patient to develop high titers. Thus, "universal" donor whole blood should be used only in emergency situations when typing and crossmatching are not possible. However, administering packed RBCs (from which the serum containing most of the antibodies is removed) is safer than administering whole blood in emergency situations.[5]

The Rh System

The Rh system is antigenically separate from the ABO system and is the most complex of all the RBC antigen systems. The nomenclature most widely used for the Rh system was developed by Fisher and Race. The Fisher-Race nomenclature system is approved by the World Health Organization and is the simplest and easiest to understand.

Nomenclature

The Rh gene complex, located on chromosome 1 in humans, consists of three closely linked loci containing three pairs of allelic genes. The alleles are denoted as C, c, D, d, E, and e. (In reality, the d allele has never been isolated, and the notation *d* simply means that D is not present.) Since the gene loci of the Rh system are so closely linked, they are generally inherited as a gene complex. In contrast to the ABO system, no naturally occurring antibodies are directed against Rh antigens. The only way such antibodies can develop is from sensitization via blood transfusions, organ transplants, or pregnancy.[16]

Agglutination techniques

Methods of Rh Blood Group Detection. The assignment of an Rh type is based on the use of antisera, which are obtained from sensitized humans. To determine an Rh type, the antisera are mixed with the patient's RBCs and agglutination is assessed. The presence or absence of the D antigen determines whether an individual is Rh positive (Rh+) or Rh negative (Rh-). In fact, the terms Rh+ and D+ are synonymous, as are the terms Rh- and D-.[12]

The D antigen is often called the Rh antigen, because it is the most clinically important and the most immunogenic of the Rh antigens. This D antigen often induces antibody production after blood transfusions, and it is also responsible for the maternal-fetal incompatibilities seen in HDN. The D antigen is the only Rh antigen that is crossmatched between donor and recipient, since the C, c, E, and e antigens are much less immunogenic.[5] Patients whose blood agglutinates with anti-D serum are termed Rh+, while those exhibiting no agglutination are termed Rh-.

In addition to the importance of Rh matching before blood transfusions, the Rh system also plays a critical role in the development of HDN, also known as Rh disease. A brief review of the pathogenesis of this disease illustrates the importance of the Rh system.

Hemolytic Disease of the Newborn. This condition was first described in 1936, when it was found that mothers of some infants had antibodies in their serum directed against the newborn's RBCs. These destructive antibodies are primarily anti-D antibodies, accounting for 95% of cases of HDN. The development mechanism of the anti-D antibodies and HDN is as follows.

During normal pregnancy, fetal RBCs do not enter the maternal circulation. However, during the placental trauma that occurs at delivery or miscarriage, fetal RBCs may cross the placenta and enter the mother's bloodstream. If the mother is Rh- and the infant is Rh+, the fetal RBCs stimulate the mother to produce cytotoxic antibodies after birth. The firstborn child is spared any problems with HDN. However, during subsequent pregnancies, a strong secondary response occurs and maternal antibodies could cross the placenta and destroy the fetal Rh+ RBCs.

Anemia and jaundice

Erythroblastosis fetalis

The clinical features of HDN include anemia and jaundice developing within 24 hours after birth. The high concentrations of bilirubin can cause permanent damage to the central nervous system. High circulating levels of erythroblasts (RBC precursors) are also seen. Consequently, this clinical syndrome is also known as erythroblastosis fetalis.

The best treatment for HDN is prevention. As a rule, all premenopausal women who are Rh- should only receive Rh- blood to avoid sensitization. If the father of the child is Rh+, the likelihood of HDN increases. Therefore, all pregnant women should undergo prenatal screening for this disease with ABO and Rh blood grouping and testing of the mother's serum against paternal RBCs, as well as possible testing of the amniotic fluid.

Treatment

In the first pregnancy, treatment is not necessary before delivery. The preferred treatment is administration of exogenous anti-D antibody (Rh immunoglobulin). Administered within 72 hours after the birth of the first child, it reacts with the Rh+ fetal RBCs (neutralizes them), thus preventing the production of maternal anti-D antibodies and avoiding sensitization. If the mother has already been sensitized to Rh+ RBCs through a previous pregnancy or an Rh+ blood transfusion, the prenatal screening may show increased titers of anti-D antibodies, and treatment with Rh immunoglobulin would need to be started before the baby is delivered. Figure 3-10 illustrates the sequence of events in the development and prevention of HDN.

Thus, the pathogenesis of HDN graphically illustrates the importance of knowing the patient's Rh status. Fortunately, the use of Rh immunoglobulin has drastically reduced the incidence of HDN and has a success rate of 98% to 99%.[9]

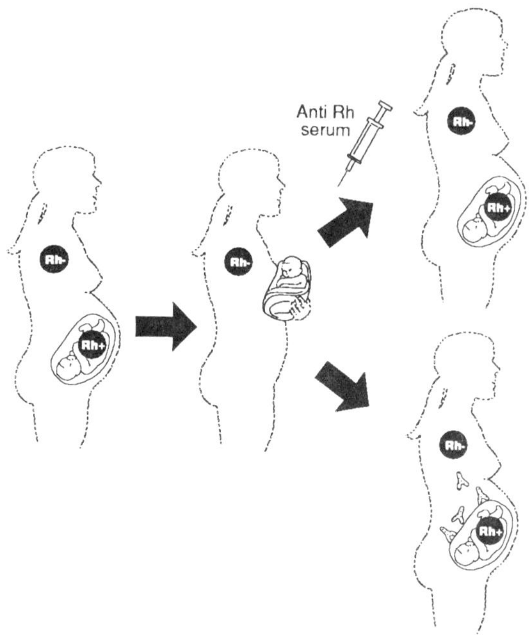

Figure 3-10. Development and prevention of hemolytic disease of the newborn

The Rh-mother is exposed to Rh+ antigens during the birth of her Rh+ child. If passively immunized with anti-Rh sera immediately after delivery, the maternal anti-Rh immune response is suppressed. A subsequent Rh+ fetus is uncomplicated by HDN (upper right). When passive immunization is not practiced, erythrocytes of an Rh+ fetus are subject to destruction by maternal antibodies and complement (lower right).

SOURCE: Reprinted with permission from Barrett J. Textbook of immunology. 5th ed. St. Louis: C.V. Mosby; 1988:339.

In summary, the use of the ABO and Rh blood systems is very important in determining the antigenicity of blood products and the compatibility of donor and recipient before blood transfusion and organ transplant and in maternal-fetal relationships. There are also nonmedical uses for the blood group systems. The use of ABO and Rh phenotypes can help solve crimes involving blood traces. Furthermore, the genetic determination of these phenotypes can be used in solving cases of disputed parentage and baby mix-ups occurring in nurseries.[5] The extensive polymorphism seen, especially in the Rh and HLA antigens, can also prove valuable to anthropologists studying relationships among human populations, including migration and breeding patterns.

Summary

The MHC plays a vital role in many aspects of the human immune system. The human MHC, or HLA, is a structurally complex and genetically polymorphic entity. The function of the MHC is significant for the acceptance or rejection of transplanted tissue and in cell-cell interactions involving antigen recognition and response. Unfortunately, certain HLA haplotypes are also etiologically associated with a number of diverse diseases, such as ankylosing spondylitis.

The typing methods of the MHC (serologic, cellular, and molecular-biologic typing), as well as the ABO and Rh blood groups, prove to be important tools for transplantation and blood transfusion procedures as well as in certain areas of law, genetics, and anthropology.

References

1. Barrett J. Textbook of immunology. 5th ed. St Louis: C.V. Mosby; 1988:76-83, 232-42, 272-98.
2. Carpenter CB, David J. Histocompatibility antigens and immune response genes. *Scientific American Medicine.* 1991;6(V):1-10.
3. Stites DP, Terr AI, eds. Basic and clinical immunology. 7th ed. Los Altos, CA: Lange Medical Publications; 1991.
4. Holmes N. New HLA class I molecules. *Immunology Today.* 1989;10(2):52-53.
5. Wilson JD, Braunwald E, Isselbacher KJ et al, eds. Harrison's principles of internal medicine. 12th ed. New York: McGraw-Hill; 1991.
6. Schwartz BD. The major histocompatibility complex and disease susceptibility. In: Wyngaarden JB, Smith LH, eds. Cecil's textbook of medicine. 18th ed. Philadelphia: W. B. Saunders Company; 1988:1962-8.
7. David-Watine B, Israel A, Kourilsky P. The regulation and expression of MHC class I genes. *Immunology Today.* 1990;11(8):286-92.
8. Statsny P, Ball EJ, Dry PJ et al. The human immune response region (HLA-D) and disease susceptibility. *Immunological Reviews.* 1983;70:113-53.
9. Virella G, Goust JM, Fudenberg HH, eds. Introduction to medical immunology. New York: Marcel Dekker, Inc.; 1986.
10. Spies T, Blanck G, Bresnahan M et al. A new cluster of genes within the human MHC. *Science.* 1989;243(4888):214-7.
11. Bjorkman PJ, Saper MA, Samraoui B et al. Structure of the human class I histocompatibility antigen, HLA-A2. *Nature.* 1987;329:506-13.

12. Myrvik QN, Weiser RS. Fundamentals of immunology. 2nd ed. Philadelphia: Lea and Febiger; 1984.
13. deVries RR, vanRood JJ, eds. Immunobiology of HLA class I and class II molecules. *Progress in Allergy.* 1985;36:1-189.
14. Hoffman M. "Superantigens" may shed light on immune puzzle. *Science.* 1990;243(4956):685-6.
15. Marrack P, Kappler J. The staphylococcal enterotoxins and their relatives. *Science.* 1990;248(4956):705-11.
16. Davis M. Molecular genetics of T-cell antigen receptors. *Hospital Practice.* 1988;23(5):115-28.
17. Existence of second type of T-cell receptor confirmed. *Scientific American Medicine Bulletin.* 1990;13(12):1-2.
18. Ljunggren H, Karre K. In search of the "missing self": MHC molecules and NK cell recognition. *Immunology Today.* 1990;11(7):237-44.
19. Roitt IM. Essential immunology. 6th ed. Oxford: Blackwell Scientific Publications; 1988:220-30.
20. Tiwari JL, Terasaki PI. HLA and disease association. New York: Springer-Verlag; 1985:33, 184.
21. Bell JI, Todd JA. HLA class II sequences infer mechanisms for MHC-associated disease susceptibility. *Molecular Biology and Medicine.* 1989;6(1):43-53.
22. Bidwell J. DNA-RFLP analysis and genotyping of HLA-DR and -DQ antigens. *Immunology Today.* 1988;9(1):18-23.
23. Anon. PCR technique now being used to type HLA alleles. *Scientific American Medicine Bulletin.* 1991;14(3):9.
24. Uryu N, Maeda M, Ota M et al. A simple and reproducible method for HLA-DRB and -DQB typing by digestion of PCR-amplified DNA with allele specific restriction endonucleases. *Tissue Antigens.* 1990;35:20-31.

Suggested Reading

Completing Chapter 9 of this text will give the reader additional information on the clinical utility of HLA typing in transplantation.

Self-Study Questions

1. A

1. Which MHC gene class mediates the immune response to transplantation?

   A. Classical class I genes.
   B. Nonclassical class I genes.
   C. Class II genes.
   D. Class III genes.

2. C

2. Which MHC gene class communicates among cells during the immune response?

   A. Classical class I genes.
   B. Nonclassical class I genes.
   C. Class II genes.
   D. Class III genes.

3. C

3. Which type of donor would be the ideal candidate for a transplantation procedure?

   A. Mother.
   B. Father.
   C. Identical twin.
   D. Sibling (not twin).

4. B

4. Many proteins in graft tissue can be alloantigens to a recipient, all of which significantly affect graft survival.

   A. True.
   B. False.

5. Alpha I, Beta I.

5. The peptide groove is formed by the _______________ and the _________________ domains.

6. Because superantigens bind to MHC molecules outside the peptide groove.

6. Why do superantigens cause a greater T-cell response than normal antigens?

7. Which MHC class is associated with a risk of rheumatic diseases such as ankylosing spondylitis? — 7. A

A. Classical class I.
B. Nonclassical class I.
C. Class II.
D. Class III.

8. What allele would be associated with a predisposition to developing juvenile-onset diabetes mellitus? — 8. B

A. DR2.
B. DR3.
C. B27.
D. D3.

9. Which MHC typing method permits rapid duplication of one DNA fragment or a single gene? — 9. B

A. Restriction fragment length polymorphism test.
B. Polymerase chain reaction.
C. Oligonucleotide probes.
D. One-way MLC.

10. Which MHC typing method is conducted before a serologic crossmatch is performed? — 10. D

A. Oligonucleotide probes.
B. Cell-mediated lympholysis.
C. One-way MLC.
D. Lymphocytotoxicity assay.

11. The crossmatch test given prior to transplantation is used to detect antibodies in which of the following? — 11. D

A. Donor's RBCs.
B. Donor's serum.
C. Recipient's RBCs.
D. Recipient's serum.

12. B

12. Which sequence of events best describes the development of hemolytic disease of the newborn?

    A. Fetal Rh+ serum stimulates maternal RBC production.
    B. Fetal Rh+ RBCs stimulate maternal antibody production.
    C. Maternal Rh+ RBCs stimulate fetal antibody production.
    D. Maternal Rh+ serum stimulates fetal antibody production.

CHAPTER 4

Hypersensitivity Reactions

Jeffrey C. Delafuente, M.S.
Associate Professor and Associate Chairman
Department of Pharmacy Practice, College of Pharmacy,
and Associate Professor
Division of Clinical Immunology, Rheumatology, and Allergy
Department of Medicine, College of Medicine
University of Florida
Gainesville, FL

Introduction

Hypersensitivity to drugs and other antigenic substances results in both drug-related problems and indications for the use of pharmacologic agents to modulate inflammatory responses. The role of the pharmacist in preventing, identifying, and managing these drug-related problems necessitates an understanding of the pathogenesis of hypersensitivity reactions. Many acute and chronic pathologic states, including allergies, drug reactions, serum sickness, and organ transplant rejection, are caused by hypersensitivity reactions that are immunologically mediated.

Learning objectives

After reading this chapter, the learner will be able to—

- Discuss the prevalence and severity of Type I hypersensitivity reactions.
- Describe the mechanisms of action of the four types of hypersensitivity reactions.
- Match examples of hypersensitivity reactions to one of four types.
- Describe the mediators of immediate hypersensitivity reactions.
- Describe diagnostic techniques for immediate hypersensitivity reactions.
- Describe therapy options for immediate hypersensitivity reactions.

Chapter organization

This chapter discusses four types of hypersensitivity reactions, their mechanisms, diagnosis, and treatment: anaphylactic reactions, cytotoxic reactions, immune complex-mediated reactions, and cell-mediated reactions. Each type of hypersensitivity is described in the context of its symptoms, causes, immune mechanism, prevalence and incidence, methods of diagnosis, and therapies.

Suggested Preparation

To maximize learning, it is recommended that the user read Chapters 1 through 3 of this text to prepare for this chapter.

Classification of Hypersensitivity Reactions

The immunologic mechanisms involved in hypersensitivity reactions are often categorized in four types: type I, anaphylactic; type II, cytotoxic; type III, immune complex-mediated; and type IV, cell-mediated. This classification scheme, originally developed by Coombs and Gell more than two decades ago, is illustrated in Figure 4-1.

Immunologic mechanisms

Type I reactions involve IgE and are responsible for many common allergies. Type II reactions, which involve IgG or IgM, are causes for many drug reactions involving destruction of blood cells. Immune complexes are responsible for type III hypersensitivity reactions, which contribute to many of the rheumatic diseases. Type IV reactions are primarily mediated by sensitized T lymphocytes, with participation by other cell types such as monocytes and macrophages. These reactions are responsible for delayed cutaneous hypersensitivity reactions, organ transplantation rejection, and other immunologic phenomena.

Since the Coombs and Gell[1] system was developed, numerous other immunologic mechanisms have been described that do not precisely follow this classification scheme, and the original classification has been modified to include newer findings.[2] It has become evident from recent research that in many immunologically mediated disease states more than one type of hypersensitivity reaction is responsible for tissue damage. For example, mononuclear cell-derived factors and inflammatory cells (type IV reaction) may have roles in some type I reactions.[3,4] Also, type I mediators may have a role in diseases that are generally thought to be type III reactions.[5]

Anaphylactic Reactions

Immediate hypersensitivity

Type I (anaphylactic) reactions are immediate hypersensitivity reactions that are usually mediated by the interaction of mast cell-bound antigen-specific IgE and a specific antigen. These reactions develop within minutes of an IgE-antigen interaction. Clinically, the reaction may be systemic, resulting in a shocklike state, or local, involving only one target site, such as the skin or nasal mucosa. Systemic reactions, known as anaphylaxis, can be life threatening. Within seconds to minutes after antigen exposure the anaphylactic reaction begins. It can be manifested as

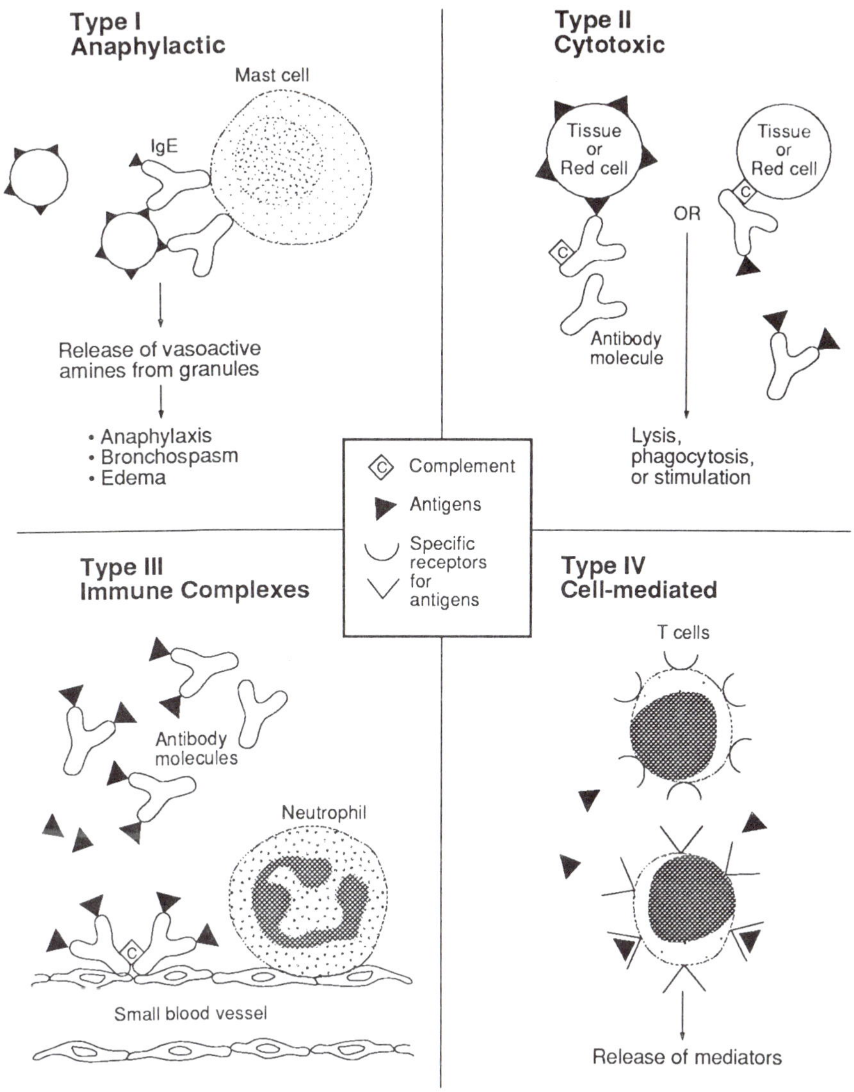

Figure 4-1. Hypersensitivity reactions

SOURCE: Reprinted with permission from Stites DP, Stobo JD, Fudenberg HH, et al. Basic and clinical immunology. 4th ed. Los Altos, CA: Lange Medical Publications; 1982:137.

respiratory distress, laryngeal edema, and vascular collapse. This state of shock is often fatal if not immediately treated. Other anaphylactic manifestations include pruritus, urticaria, and angioedema.

Mechanism

The manifestation of a type I hypersensitivity reaction is preceded by a precise sequence of events. Numerous factors play roles in this development.

Allergens. The term *allergen* usually refers to an antigen that elicits an allergic immune reaction. A few examples of allergens that cause type I hypersensitivity reactions are plant pollens, house dust mite, fungi spores, animal dander, foods, drugs, and insect venoms. The route of entry into the body can be inhalation (e.g., pollen, mold spores), ingestion (e.g., food, drugs), or injection (drugs, bee stings). Most allergens must have large molecular weights to bridge adjacent IgE molecules on mast cells. Substances of smaller molecular weight, such as drugs, become allergenic by covalently binding to protein molecules.[6]

Sensitization

Role of IgE. An individual must be sensitized for an immediate hypersensitivity reaction to occur. This sensitization process occurs after the individual has been exposed to a particular antigen. Antigen-specific IgE antibodies are produced after the first exposure to the antigen. An immediate reaction does not occur at this point. After antigen-specific IgE antibodies are produced, they attach to Fc receptors on mast cells and basophils.[7] Upon subsequent exposure to the antigen, antigen-specific IgE on mast cells or basophils combines with the antigen to activate the cells, which then release inflammatory mediators. A clinical example of this phenomenon is a type I reaction to penicillin. Exposure to penicillin must have occurred at least once before to produce penicillin-specific IgE. The previous exposure allows mast cells to become sensitized, that is, coated with penicillin-specific IgE. Upon subsequent exposure to penicillin, the sensitized cells combine with penicillin to release mast cell mediators. Immediate reactions to penicillin range from local reactions, such as urticaria and pruritus, to fatal systemic anaphylaxis. The type of reaction depends on the location of the sensitized mast cells interacting with the allergen.

Mast Cell and Basophil Mediators. Mediators derived from mast cells and basophils are responsible for type I reactions. Human mast cells are found in skin, synovium, and mesentery; around large and small blood vessels; in the mucosa of the respiratory tract; and in the subserosal and submucosal layers of the gastrointestinal tract.[8] Basophils make up 0.5% to 2% of circulating white blood cells. Both mast cells and basophils have surface receptors for the Fc portion of IgE. These receptors have a high affinity for the Fc portion of IgE; when an individual produces IgE, a large percentage of it is bound to the mast cell membrane. There are between 100,000 and 500,000 IgE Fc receptors per mast cell, about 10% of which are occupied with IgE in vivo.[8] Basophils have approximately 40,000 to 100,000 IgE Fc receptors per cell.[7] Both mast cells and basophils contain mediators of inflammation. Antigen must bridge two adjacent antigen-specific IgE molecules for mediators to be released from these cells.[9] After this step, cellular granules are secreted through the outer cell membrane. These granules contain preformed mediators as well as precursors for the generation of other mediators.[10,11] For example, arachidonic acid, which is

Fc receptors

liberated upon activation of mast cells, is used to synthesize prostaglandins and leukotrienes. Secretion of lipid mediators allows mast cells to regenerate their membranes, thereby allowing cells to participate in subsequent reactions. Table 4-1 lists mediators that are released or rapidly generated after mast cell activation.

Early events occurring after mast cell mediator release include increased vascular permeability, contraction of smooth muscle, and mucus secretion in the tissue where mediator release occurred. Increased vascular permeability allows for the leakage of intravascular fluid (thereby causing edema) as well as serum proteins, such as antibodies and complement. Mast cell mediators also promote chemotaxis through the release of chemotactic mediators, which attract a variety of inflammatory cells into the area. These cells may continue the inflammatory process hours after the initial release of mast cell constituents. Mast cell mediators involved in the pathogenesis of asthma have been well characterized.[12] Their roles in this disease are shown in Table 4-2. Some of the more important mediators of type I reactions are described in the following paragraphs.

Mediator effects

Histamine. The best-known mast cell mediator is histamine. Histamine is stored in the granules of mast cells and basophils and is released after the granules have been released from the cells. Histamine is responsible for reactions such as smooth muscle contraction of bronchioles and small blood vessels, increased permeability of capillaries, and increased mucus secretion.

Eosinophil Chemotactic Factor. Eosinophil chemotactic factor (ECF) is another preformed mediator. After release from mast cells, this mediator attracts eosinophils into the area of allergic inflammation. Eosinophils are now thought to have a major role in the tissue damage seen in some allergic reactions.[13]

Table 4-1 Human Mast Cell Inflammatory Mediators

Preformed Mediators	Newly Generated Mediators
Histamine	Leukotrienes (SRS-A)
Eosinophil chemotactic factor	Prostaglandins
Neutrophil chemotactic factor	Thromboxanes
Kininogenase	Platelet-activating factor
Arylsulfatase A	Monohydroxyeicosatetraenoic acids (HETE)
Exoglycosides	Hydroperoxyeicosatetraenoic acids (HPETE)

Table 4-2 Roles of Mast Cell Mediators in Asthma

Mediators	Physiologic Response
Histamine	Bronchospasm
Prostaglandins	
Leukotrienes	
Bradykinin	
Platelet activating-factor	
Histamine	Mucus secretion
Prostaglandins	
Leukotrienes	
Monohydroxyeicosatetranoic acids (HETE)	
Histamine	Mucosal edema
Prostaglandins	
Leukotrienes	
Bradykinin	
Neutrophil chemotactic factor	Airway inflammation
Eosinophil chemotactic factor	
Platelet activating-factor	
Leukotriene B_4	

Neutrophil Chemotactic Factor. A high-molecular-weight neutrophil chemotactic factor (HMW-NCF) is released after mast cell activation.[14] This mediator has not been identified in human mast cell granules, and its site of synthesis is not certain. However, HMW-NCF is readily found in serum of patients undergoing allergic reactions, and its presence in serum parallels that of histamine.[15] This mediator is a potent stimulus for attracting polymorphonuclear leukocytes (neutrophils). Although neutrophils contain numerous enzymes that can be destructive to normal host tissue, whether they participate in IgE-mediated allergic inflammation is still a matter for speculation. Neutrophils as well as other leukocytes produce factors capable of causing additional histamine release from mast cells that are perpetuating the allergic response.[16]

Leukotrienes. Leukotrienes (LTs) are lipoxygenase metabolites of arachidonic acid that have potent bronchoconstricting and vasodilatory properties.[11] In allergic asthma, LTC_4, LTD_4, and LTE_4 have been identified as mediators of disease activity.[12] Before leukotrienes were discovered, this mixture of leukotrienes identified in asthma was known as slow-reacting substance of anaphylaxis.

Prostaglandins. Prostaglandins (PGs) are cyclo-oxygenase metabolites of arachidonic acid that are generated after mast cell release. PGD_2 is formed from human lung mast cells and is a potent vasodilator.[17] The inflammatory cells attracted to the area of allergic inflammation, such as neutrophils and macrophages, produce additional bronchoconstricting and vasodilatory prostaglandins that further exacerbate the inflammatory reaction.

Platelet Activating-factor (PAF). PAF is a low-molecular-weight substance released during certain type I reactions. It is the most potent bronchoconstrictor identified, and its effect on human airways is long-lived.[18] PAF stimulates the accumulation of eosinophils in the area of inflammation. Numerous inflammatory cells produce PAF, including platelets, macrophages, eosinophils, neutrophils, and perhaps mast cells.[10,17]

Prevalence and Incidence

Atopics

Individuals with a predisposition for IgE-mediated allergic reactions are known as atopics. There are more than 35 million atopic persons in the United States, 8.9 million with asthma, 14.7 million with hay fever, and 11.8 million with other allergic manifestations.[19] Some of the IgE-mediated allergic disorders are hay fever (allergic rhinitis), allergic asthma, urticaria, insect venom allergy, anaphylaxis, food and drug allergies, and atopic dermatitis (eczema).

The onset of common allergies is usually in childhood, although an allergy can develop at any age. The prevalence of atopy increases with age during the first two decades of life and then gradually declines.[20] The symptoms vary depending on the target organ involved in the type I reaction. For example, rhinitis may be the symptom when only the upper respiratory tract is exposed to an allergen. If the allergen gets into the circulation, as with a bee sting, then anaphylaxis may occur. Symptoms may be seasonal (grass pollen allergy) or perennial (house dust mite hypersensitivity). Many patients with multiple allergies have perennial symptoms with exacerbations during pollen season. There is a genetic predisposition for developing allergies. If both parents are atopic there is a 75% chance that an offspring will also be atopic, whereas if only one parent is atopic there is a 50% chance that a child will be atopic.[17]

Diagnosis of Atopy

History and exam

Allergies may be diagnosed in a variety of ways. None of the tests available supplant a good medical history and physical examination. The symptoms elicited during the medical history may be sufficient to diagnose an allergy. Variations in symptoms with the time of day, season, or environment give important information toward an accurate diagnosis. An occupational allergen may be suspected as a cause of an allergy if an individual has symptoms only in the workplace; an allergy to cat dander may be suspected when symptoms consistently occur after exposure to cats. When a particular allergen cannot be identified by history, skin testing or in vitro testing may be carried out to aid in the diagnosis and treatment strategy.

Wheal-and-flare

Skin Testing. The mainstay for immediate hypersensitivity diagnosis is the skin test. Extracts of allergens are placed in the skin, and within minutes a reaction occurs. The reaction is caused by mast cell-bound allergen-specific IgE combining with the test allergen. Mast cells become activated and release histamine and other mediators. These mediators cause local vasodilation and increased capillary permeability, resulting in a wheal-and-flare reaction usually within 15 minutes. The most common method of introducing the allergen into the skin is by scratch testing.[19] In this procedure a drop of the allergen is placed on the skin, and a needle is inserted through the solution, penetrating the external surface of the skin. Another method is the use of intradermal allergen injection. Antihistamine drugs decrease or block the development of the wheal-and-flare response; therefore, these drugs must be discontinued before skin testing.

Skin testing is the preferred procedure for most patients because there has been extensive experience with it, it is inexpensive and easy to administer, and the results are immediately available. However, skin testing is not without risk. Since the antigen is being injected, there is a possibility of a systemic anaphylactic reaction occurring; resuscitation equipment and epinephrine should be readily available.

RAST and ELISA tests

In Vitro Testing. Although in vitro tests for measuring total serum IgE and antigen-specific IgE are often useful in diagnosing allergy, their true place in allergy diagnosis is not well established.[21] For determining total IgE levels a radioallergosorbent test (RAST) or paper radioimmunosorbent test is commonly used.[19] These are radioimmunoassays that are highly specific and sensitive for detecting serum IgE. Enzyme-linked immunosorbent assay (ELISA) is now being used in some laboratories to measure IgE antibodies. Allergen-specific IgE can be semiquantitatively measured by using RAST or ELISA, provided the antigen can be coupled to an insoluble matrix (e.g., plastic ELISA plate, filter paper, dextran beads).

In vitro testing has some advantages over skin testing. There is no risk to the patient. Numerous in vitro allergen-specific assays can be done with a single venipuncture, whereas with skin testing multiple sites are needed. Antihistamine drugs do not interfere with in vitro tests and do not have to be discontinued before testing. In vitro tests are useful in infants and in patients with skin disorders such as eczema, in whom it may be difficult to find an unaffected area for skin testing.

Advantages and drawbacks

There are also disadvantages to in vitro testing. The tests are considerably more expensive and less sensitive than skin testing, and they may produce false-negative results.[21] There is a lag in getting the results back from the laboratory. Because only a limited number of in vitro tests are available, commercial laboratories cannot test for all antigens that may be suspected of causing a patient's symptoms. The presence of antigen-specific IgE in serum does not give direct information about its pathogenetic role.[21] Whereas a wheal-and-flare reaction from skin testing provides direct evidence of allergen hypersensitivity, a positive in vitro test detects only serum IgE, which may not be synonymous with hypersensitivity.

Treatment of Type I Reactions

Treatment of immediate hypersensitivity reactions varies depending on the clinical manifestations. The simplest treatment is avoidance of the offending antigen. In the case of pollen allergy, total avoidance may be impractical; however, exposure to other allergens such as animal danders can be avoided. When eliminating the offending antigens is impossible, pharmacologic and immunologic therapies are alternatives.

Avoidance

Pharmacologic Therapies. Type I reactions can be blocked at various stages with antihistamines, sympathomimetic agents, and antiallergic agents.

Antihistamines. Antihistamine agents are helpful in treating the symptoms of type I reactions. Unfortunately, because histamine is only one mediator involved in the pathogenesis of these reactions, blocking histamine receptors only partially alleviates symptoms. The H_1 histamine receptor is predominantly involved in allergic reactions, and H_1 antagonists are therefore used for these conditions. The newer generation H_1 antagonists, such as astemizole and terfenadine, do not produce much sedation—a major advantage compared with many older antihistamines (e.g., diphenhydramine).[22] H_2 receptor antagonists, such as cimetidine, have no effect by themselves on attenuating type I reactions. However, for patients refractory to standard H_1 antihistamines, the addition of an H_2

Sedation

antihistamine may be beneficial.[23] H_2 receptors are present in cutaneous vasculature, and the combination of H_1 and H_2 antihistamines has been most effective in certain urticarial syndromes.

Sympathomimetic Agents. Sympathetic nervous stimulation is useful to counteract some of the manifestations of mast cell degranulation. For example, stimulation of beta$_2$ receptors leads to bronchodilatation and may reverse some or all of the bronchoconstricting effects from allergen-induced asthma. Alpha$_1$ agonists such as phenylpropanolamine and phenylephrine constrict mucosal vasculature and are used predominantly as nasal decongestants. For systemic anaphylaxis, epinephrine is the preferred sympathomimetic agent because of its potent alpha- and beta-stimulating effects.

Antiallergy Agents. Antiallergy drugs are classified as noncorticosteroidal agents that can modify the acute and chronic tissue responses associated with type I reactions. The prototype drug in this class is cromolyn sodium. This agent can inhibit mast cell degranulation and prevent the clinical symptoms that follow antigen exposure.[24] Cromolyn sodium also modulates the effector functions of neutrophils and eosinophils,[25] both of which may have active roles in many allergic reactions. Other antiallergic drugs that may be clinically useful are nedocromil sodium, azelastine, and ketotifen.[26-29]

Corticosteroids. In many allergic conditions, such as asthma and allergic rhinitis, chronic inflammation is present. Corticosteroids do not help to relieve the acute allergic symptoms that follow allergen exposure, but they help suppress the inflammatory response seen in late-phase and chronic allergic reactions.

The mechanisms of action of corticosteroids are still unclear. Steroids do not prevent mediator release from mast cells. Among their many actions, they are effective at inhibiting the actions of leukocytes that are involved in chronic inflammation, reduce vascular leakage thereby decreasing edema, and prevent the influx of inflammatory cells into the area of mast cell degranulation. Corticosteroids can also up-regulate beta receptors, enhancing the efficacy of beta agonists.

Corticosteroids can be given systemically or topically. Topical corticosteroids have proven to be effective for diseases such as asthma and hay fever. The use of inhaled and intranasal corticosteroids has circumvented many of the side effects of systemic administration.

Desensitization

Immunotherapy. Immunotherapy, also known as hyposensitization or desensitization, is an effective adjunct therapy for patients with seasonal allergic rhinitis, allergic asthma, or insect venom hypersensitivity.[30,31]

Immunotherapy consists of injecting allergens subcutaneously in increasing doses over a prolonged period. Many controlled trials using immunotherapy have been carried out in patients with allergic rhinitis or asthma. Most studies demonstrate clinical improvement in 60% to 90% of patients.[31] Allergy immunotherapy results in reduction, not complete elimination, of symptoms. The selection of allergens for injection is based on positive skin test results, clinical history, and sometimes RAST when the other methods of diagnosis are inconclusive.

Regimen

Immunotherapy is used mainly in patients whose symptoms are not adequately controlled by pharmacologic means and avoidance of the offending antigens. Immunotherapy usually begins with weekly injections of low concentrations of appropriate allergens. The dose of allergen administered is increased weekly until a maintenance dose is achieved. Under certain circumstances, rush immunotherapy has been used to achieve maintenance dose within a few days.[32] This form of therapy has been shown to result in a quicker IgG response.[33] Therapy then continues with monthly injections. Duration of treatment varies for each patient. Therapy should be discontinued if symptoms do not improve after 2 or 3 years of treatment.[31] The usual recommended length of treatment is 3 to 5 years, although some patients may require longer treatment periods.[31] There is always a risk of inducing an anaphylactic reaction with each injection. Because of this potentially severe risk, for a disease such as allergic rhinitis a combination of a new-generation antihistamine plus a topical corticosteroid may be preferred therapy.[34] Immunotherapy should be used only after appropriate pharmacotherapy fails to improve symptoms satisfactorily.

Mechanisms

The mechanisms by which hyposensitization reduces allergic symptoms are not clearly established. Skin test reactivity to the offending antigens decreases after a successful course of immunotherapy. Antigen-specific serum IgE levels diminish with a concomitant rise in antigen-specific serum IgG levels.[29,35] This IgG is thought to be a "blocking antibody" competing with mast cell-bound IgE for binding to the allergen. Immunotherapy has also been shown to induce T-suppressor lymphocytes, which suppress the production of antigen-specific IgE.[36]

Cytotoxic Reactions

Type II hypersensitivity reactions are antibody-mediated cytotoxic reactions. Both IgG and IgM antibodies are involved in type II reactions. Cytotoxicity occurs when these antibodies are directed against intrinsic cell surface antigens or against antigens that have been absorbed on a cell surface. Some examples of clinically relevant type II reactions are drug reactions, erythroblastosis fetalis, Graves' disease, hemolytic anemia, idiopathic thrombocytopenic purpura, myasthenia gravis, and transfusion reactions.

Mechanisms

Several different mechanisms are involved in type II reactions. Antigen bound to IgG or IgM activates the complement cascade. Activation of complement at or near a cell membrane results in cell lysis and cell death.[2] Another mechanism of cytotoxicity involves phagocytic cells such as neutrophils, monocytes, and macrophages. These cells have Fc receptors for IgG. Once antigen-specific IgG has attached to cell surface antigens via its Fab region, the Fc region of IgG becomes available to bind phagocytic cell Fc receptors. The IgG-coated cell is then phagocytized and destroyed. Phagocytic cells also have receptors for various components of activated complement proteins. After IgG or IgM attaches to cell surface antigens, complement is activated and deposited at the site of this antibody-antigen reaction (see Chapter 1). Complement on a cell surface also leads to phagocytosis and destruction of the cell. The process of enhanced phagocytosis by IgG and complement is known as opsonization. IgG is also involved in cytotoxicity mediated by subpopulations of lymphocytes. Some T lymphocytes and natural killer cells have IgG Fc receptors.[2] IgG that is bound to cell surface antigens can also bind to these lymphoid cells, which lyse the IgG-bound cell. This process is referred to as antibody-dependent cellular toxicity. Some tumor cells are destroyed by this mechanism.[37] (See Chapter 10.)

Although type II reactions were originally described by Coombs and Gell as cytotoxic reactions, other nonlytic antibody-mediated pathologic processes are now classified as type II reactions. For example, in some autoimmune diseases, antibodies are produced that are directed against various receptors.[38] These antibodies may stimulate a receptor to mimic a natural hormone, as in Graves' disease, or they may block receptor stimulation, as in myasthenia gravis, in which antibodies block acetylcholine from binding to its receptor. Noncytolytic antibodies may also protect a cell with foreign cell surface antigens from being destroyed by normal immunologic cytotoxic mechanisms. Antibodies can mask these foreign antigens, thereby preventing them from being recognized by the immune system. This process has been described for some tumor-associated antigens.[37]

Drug-induced reactions

Numerous medications can cause type II reactions. The predominant feature is destruction of the formed elements of blood: red blood cells, white blood cells, and platelets. The drug molecule or its metabolites may become antigenic by covalently binding to cell surface proteins and ultimately causing cell destruction by the mechanisms that have been described. The penicillins and cephalosporins are examples of drugs that cause this type of reaction. Other drugs cause type II reactions by first forming antigen-antibody complexes in plasma; these complexes then become nonspecifically absorbed to cell membranes. Complement may then be activated, and cell lysis soon follows. This mechanism, which is referred to as the innocent bystander reaction, is usually the reason some drugs cause hemolytic anemia.[39] Other drugs such as methyldopa induce autoantibodies against red blood cells. These autoantibodies destroy cells in the absence of the drug. Altered suppressor cell function caused by methyldopa has been implicated in the production of these autoantibodies.[40] Drug-induced type II reactions are usually reversible after the implicated drug is discontinued.

Treatment

The treatment for a type II immune reaction varies depending on the causes of the reaction and the clinical manifestations. If a medication is the cause, stopping the offending agent may be all that is necessary. For a disease such as idiopathic thrombocytopenic purpura (ITP), in which IgG antiplatelet antibodies lead to the destruction of platelets, treatment may involve corticosteroids or immunosuppressive drugs. Splenectomy is frequently performed, because the spleen is the primary location for platelet destruction in this disease. Intravenous immunoglobulin is also useful in therapy for ITP. Immunosuppressive therapy is being tested for many autoimmune diseases characterized by type II mechanisms, such as diabetes mellitus.

Immune Complex-mediated Reactions

Type III hypersensitivity reactions are immune complex mediated (antigen-antibody complexes). These reactions result when circulating immune complexes (usually IgG or IgM) are deposited on endothelial surfaces or when the immunoglobulin is directed toward a tissue antigen. Immune complexes activate complement, which is chemotactic for polymorphonuclear leukocytes (neutrophils). As the neutrophils phagocytize the immune complexes, they release their intracellular array of lysosomal enzymes. These enzymes, which are destructive to normal host tissue, cause inflammation. Blood vessels are a frequent target for immune complex deposition; the resultant clinical manifestation is vasculitis. Immune complexes have pathogenic roles in many disease states, such as rheumatoid arthritis, systemic lupus erythematosus, poststreptococcal glomerulonephritis, hypersensitivity pneumonitis, and the serum sickness prodrome of hepatitis B infection.[41]

Inflammation

Serum sickness

Serum sickness is the classic example of a type III reaction. Before the advent of antibiotics, heterologous antiserum (usually from horses) was used to treat certain infectious diseases, and serum sickness reactions would ensue. Serum sickness reactions have been a useful model for increasing our understanding of type III hypersensitivity reactions. Circulating immune complexes form, are deposited systemically in various tissue target sites, and cause an inflammatory reaction. Signs and symptoms of serum sickness, which usually begin 1 to 2 weeks after exposure to the offending antigen, include fever, arthritis, arthralgias, rashes, vasculitis, lymphadenopathy, and splenomegaly. These symptoms are common to many multisystem, immune complex-mediated diseases.

Drugs can combine with drug-specific antibodies to form circulating immune complexes and cause serum-sickness-like reactions. The penicillins and sulfonamides are common causes of these reactions.[39] Symptoms usually begin 7 to 10 days after therapy begins and may include the symptoms just listed for serum sickness. Symptoms may occur earlier if the patient has been previously exposed to the causative drug. Symptoms abate within a few days after discontinuing the drug.

Treatment

Clinical signs and symptoms determine the treatment for type III reactions. Therapy may range from a simple analgesic to treat pain associated with rheumatoid arthritis, to potent immunosuppressive therapy for lupus nephritis. In general, drugs that suppress the inflammatory response caused by immune complex deposition are used. These drugs include corticosteroids, nonsteroidal anti-inflammatory agents, and immunosuppressive drugs such as azathioprine, cyclophosphamide, cyclosporine, gold compounds, and methotrexate. Plasmapheresis is occasionally used to remove circulating immune complexes.

Cell-mediated Reactions

Delayed hypersensitivity

T lymphocytes are primarily responsible for type IV hypersensitivity reactions, also known as delayed hypersensitivity reactions. These reactions generally occur days after antigen exposure and are independent of antibodies and complement. The classic example of this type of reaction is the delayed cutaneous hypersensitivity reaction used to identify individuals exposed to *Mycobacterium tuberculosis.* Purified protein derivative is injected intradermally and a positive reaction (induration) slowly develops, reaching its maximum size 48 to 72 hours after the injection. In addition to delayed-type skin testing, other clinical examples of type IV reactions include contact dermatitis, organ transplant rejection, and the killing of viruses, fungi, and tumor cells by antibody-independent cellular-mediated reactions.

Mechanisms

T lymphocytes possess antigen-specific receptors and undergo a state of activation when antigen is presented to them by macrophages (see Chapter 3). Resting T lymphocytes produce interleukin-2 (IL-2) receptors within hours after appropriate antigen stimulation.[42] Cellular activation also leads to the generation of IL-2. DNA synthesis and cell mitosis occur once a sufficient number of IL-2 receptors have been bound with IL-2. IL-2 secreted by antigen-activated T cells also stimulates non-antigen-specific T lymphocytes to become activated and participate in the type IV reaction. In addition to secreting IL-2, activated T lymphocytes also produce many other lymphokines that are pathogenically involved in type IV hypersensitivity reactions. For example, macrophage-activating factor increases the phagocytic and cytodestructive properties of macrophages. Activated T cells also produce the antiviral protein interferon, which also regulates cell-mediated cytotoxicity.[43] Table 4-3 lists some of the cytokines that are responsible for the cellular infiltration and effector functions seen in type IV reactions. (See Chapter 2 for additional information.)

In addition to the tuberculin skin test, delayed cutaneous hypersensitivity (DCH) testing using multiple ubiquitous antigens is commonly used to evaluate a patient's cellular immunity, especially when an immunodeficiency syndrome is suspected.[44] (See Chapter 6 for more details.) Although DCH testing is a simple and useful procedure, there are

Table 4-3 Selected Cytokines and Their Effects

Cytokine	Effects
Interleukin-1	Activates resting T and B cells
Interleukin-2	Growth factor for activated T cells
Interleukin-3	Mast cell growth factor; stimulates pluripotent stem cells
Interleukin-4	Growth factor for activated B cells, resting T cells, and mast cells
Interleukin-5	Promotes B-cell differentiation; induces differentiation of eosinophils
Interleukin-6	Promotes B-cell differentiation
Colony-stimulating factors	Promotes neutrophilic, eosinophilic, and macrophagic bone marrow colonies
Interferon gamma	Antiviral activity; enhances cellular cytotoxicity; activates macrophages
Tumor necrosis factor	Cytotoxic for some tumor cells; pyrogenic; endotoxic shock
Migration inhibition factor	Inhibits macrophage migration away from inflammatory site
Macrophage activation factor	Activates macrophages

problems associated with it. For example, a negative purified protein derivative test cannot be properly interpreted without a positive control to indicate the presence of an intact immune system. Control antigens commonly used include *Candida albicans* and mumps; however, these two antigens may not be sufficient for all patients.

Anergy

The lack of DCH response, known as anergy, indicates a defective cellular immune response. However, anergy can often be misdiagnosed because skin tests are interpreted improperly. False-negative results can occur if too few antigens are used. To avoid this problem, four to six antigens should be used,[45,46] particularly in elderly patients.[47] If only one or two antigens are used, there is a possibility of getting negative test results, not because of anergy but, rather, because of a lack of recent antigen exposure.[44] Several investigators have shown that almost half of all negative DCH reactions to a variety of antigens convert to positive on repeat testing.[48,49] It is believed that the first test injection serves as a booster that enhances the sensitivity that had waned below the level of detection.[44] Therefore, serial testing may be useful to prevent a false diagnosis of anergy.

Treatment

As with the other types of hypersensitivity reactions, treatment of type IV reactions is dictated by the clinical situation. The goal of therapy is to suppress the activities of inflammatory cells at the pathologic site. Treatment may range from prednisone for contact dermatitis to combination potent immunosuppressive drugs to prevent organ transplant rejection. (See Chapters 6 and 9 for more thorough discussions of immunosuppressive drug therapy.)

Summary

Hypersensitivity reactions can be categorized as type I (anaphylactic), type II (cytotoxic), type III (immune complex-mediated), and type IV (cell-mediated) reactions.

The mechanism of type I reactions is an interaction among allergens, IgE, and mast cell and basophil mediators, such as histamine, eosinophil chemotactic factor, neutrophil chemotactic factor, leukotrienes, prostaglandins, and platelet activating factor. Type I hypersensitivity can be detected with skin or in vitro testing and may be treated with antihistamines, sympathomimetic agents, antiallergy agents, corticosteroids, or immunotherapy.

Type II reactions involve IgG and IgM antibodies and may be treated by administering corticosteroids or immunosuppressive drugs and sometimes by a splenectomy. Medications may cause type II reactions.

Type III reactions involve circulating immune complexes. Their therapies differ depending on the clinical signs and symptoms but generally utilize anti-inflammatory agents.

Type IV hypersensitivity is a delayed reaction involving T lymphocytes and may range from contact dermatitis to organ transplant rejection. Causes and therapies vary, as with type III reactions, but continue to stress inflammation suppression.

References

1. Coombs RRA, Gell PGH. The classification of allergic reactions underlying disease. In: Gell PGH, Coombs RRA, eds. Clinical Aspects of Immunology. Philadelphia: F.A. Davis Company; 1963:317-37.
2. Rodnan GP, Schumacher R, eds. Primer on the rheumatic diseases. 8th ed. Atlanta: Arthritis Foundation; 1983:25-8.
3. Younger RE, Henry HG, Lieberman PL et al. Characterization of mononuclear cell-derived histamine release enhancing factor. *J Allergy Clin Immunol.* 1987;80:547-57.
4. Frew AJ, Kay AB. Eosinophils and T-lymphocytes in late-phase reactions. *J Allergy Clin Immunol.* 1990;85:533-9.
5. Godfrey HP, Ilardi C, Engber W et al. Quantitation of human synovial mast cells in rheumatoid arthritis and other rheumatic diseases. *Arthritis Rheum.* 1984;27:852-6.
6. DeSwarte RD. Drug allergy—problems and strategies. *J Allergy Clin Immunol.* 1984;74:209-21.
7. Kulczycki A. Role of immunoglobulin E and immunoglobulin receptors in bronchial asthma. *J Allergy Clin Immunol.* 1981;68:5-14.
8. Marom Z, Casale TB. Mast cells and their mediators. *Ann Allergy.* 1983;50:367-70.
9. Ishizaka T. Analysis of triggering events in mast cells for immunoglobulin E-mediated histamine release. *J Allergy Clin Immunol.* 1981;67:90-6.
10. Peters SP, Schleimer RP, Naclerio RM et al. The pathophysiology of human mast cells: in vitro and in vivo function. *Respir Dis.* 1987;135:1196-200.
11. Schleimer RP, MacGlashan DW, Peters SP et al. Inflammatory mediators and mechanisms of release from purified human basophils and mast cells. *J Allergy Clin Immunol.* 1984;74:473-80.
12. Friedman MM, Kaliner MA. Human mast cells and asthma. *Respir Dis.* 1987;135:1157-64.
13. Frigas E, Gliech GJ. The eosinophil and the pathophysiology of asthma. *J Allergy Clin Immunol.* 1986;77:527-37.

14. Lee TH, Nagy L, Nagakura T et al. Identification and partial characterization of an exercise-induced neutrophil chemotactic factor in bronchial asthma. *J Clin Invest.* 1982;69:889–99.
15. Belcher NG, Murdoch R, Dalton N et al. Circulating concentrations of histamine, neutrophil chemotactic activity, and catecholamines during the refractory period in exercise-induced asthma. *J Allergy Clin Immunol.* 1988;81:100–10.
16. White MV, Phillips RL, Kaliner MA. Neutrophils and mast cells: nedocromil sodium inhibits the generation of neutrophil-derived histamine-releasing activity (HRA-N). *J Allergy Clin Immunol.* 1991;87:812–20.
17. Frick OL. Immediate hypersensitivity. In: Stites DP, Stobo JD, Wells JV, eds. Basic clinical immunology. 6th ed. Norwalk, CT: Appleton & Lange; 1987:197–227.
18. Barnes PJ, Chung KF, Page CP. Platelet-activating factor as a mediator of allergic disease. *J Allergy Clin Immunol.* 1988;81:919–34.
19. Slavin RG. Diagnostic tests in clinical allergy. *Postgrad Med.* 1980;67:72–81.
20. Marsh DG, Meyers DA, Bias WB. The epidemiology and genetics of atopic allergy. *N Engl J Med.* 1981;305:1551–8.
21. Terr AI. In vitro tests for immediate hypersensitivity. *Annu Rev Med.* 1988;39:135–45.
22. Delafuente JC, Davis TA, Davis JA. Pharmacotherapy of allergic rhinitis. *Clinical Pharmacy.* 1989;8:474–85.
23. Delafuente JC. Use of H_2 histamine antagonists in allergic disorders. *Clinical Pharmacy.* 1988;7:422.
24. Godfrey S. The relative merits of cromolyn sodium and high dose theophylline therapy in childhood asthma. *J Allergy Clin Immunol.* 1980;65:97–104.
25. Kay AB, Walsh GM, Mogbel R et al. Disodium cromoglycate inhibits activation of human inflammatory cells in vitro. *J Allergy Clin Immunol.* 1987;80:1–8.
26. Ruhno J, Denberg J, Dolovich J. Intranasal nedocromil sodium in the treatment of ragweed-allergic rhinitis. *J Allergy Clin Immunol.* 1988;81:570–4.
27. Spector SL, Perhach JL, Rohr AS et al. Pharmacodynamic evaluation of azelastine in subjects with asthma. *J Allergy Clin Immunol.* 1987;80:75–80.
28. Kakuta Y, Kato T, Sasaki H et al. Effect of ketotifen on human alveolar macrophages. *J Allergy Clin Immunol.* 1988;81:469–74.
29. Volovitz B, Varsano I, Cumella JC. Efficacy and safety of ketotifen in young children with asthma. *J Allergy Clin Immunol.* 1988;81:526–30.
30. Patterson R. Clinical efficacy of allergen immunotherapy. *J Allergy Clin Immunol.* 1979;64:155–8.

31. Rocklin RE. Clinical and immunologic aspects of allergen-specific immunotherapy in patients with seasonal allergic rhinitis and/or asthma. *J Allergy Clin Immunol.* 1983;72:323–34.
32. Horst M, Hejjaoui A, Horst V et al. Double-blind, placebo-controlled rush immunotherapy with a standardized alternaria extract. *J Allergy Clin Immunol.* 1990;85:460–72.
33. Weber RW. Allergen immunotherapy and standardization and stability of allergen extracts. *J Allergy Clin Immunol.* 1989;84:1093–6.
34. Bousquet J, Hejjaoui A, Michel FB. Specific immunotherapy in asthma. *J Allergy Clin Immunol.* 1990;86:292–305.
35. Patterson R. Allergen immunotherapy with modified allergens. *J Allergy Clin Immunol.* 1981;68:85–90.
36. Tamir R, Castracane JM, Rocklin RE. Generation of suppressor cells in atopic patients during immunotherapy that modulate IgE synthesis. *J Allergy Clin Immunol.* 1987;79:591–8.
37. Greenberg PD. Tumor immunology. In: Stites DP, Stobo JD, Wells JV, eds. Basic and clinical immunology. Norwalk, CT: Appleton & Lange; 1987:192–3.
38. Wilkin TJ. Receptor autoimmunity in endocrine disorders. *N Engl J Med.* 1990;323:1318–24.
39. Witte KW, West DP. Immunology of adverse drug reactions. *Pharmacotherapy.* 1982;2:54–65.
40. Kirtland HH, Mohler DN, Horwitz DA. Methyldopa inhibition of suppressor-lymphocyte function. *N Engl J Med.* 1980;302:825–32.
41. Panush RS, Brestel EP, Delafuente JC et al. Diagnostic studies for the rheumatic diseases. In: Panush RS, ed. Principles of rheumatic diseases. New York: John Wiley & Sons; 1981:47.
42. Royer HD, Reinherz EL. T lymphocytes: ontogeny, function, and relevance to clinical disorders. *N Engl J Med.* 1987;317:1136–42.
43. Dinarello CA, Mier JW. Lymphokines. *N Engl J Med.* 1987;317:940–5.
44. Delafuente JC, Eisenberg JD, Hoelzer DR et al. Tetanus toxoid as an antigen for delayed cutaneous hypersensitivity. *JAMA.* 1983;249:3209–11.
45. Spitler LE. Delayed hypersensitivity skin testing. In: Rose NR, Friedman H, eds. Manual of clinical immunology. Washington, DC: American Society for Microbiology; 1976:53–63.
46. Decker EL. Skin testing for anergy: a review with proposed guidelines. *Hospital Formulary.* 1980;15:369–74.
47. Delafuente JC, Meuleman JR, Nelson RC. Anergy testing in nursing home residents. *Journal of the American Geriatrics Society.* 1988;36:733–5.
48. Fereebee SH, Mount FW. Evidence of booster effect in serial tuberculin testing. *Am Rev Respir Dis.* 1963;88:118–9.

49. Keystone EL, Demerieux P, Gladman D et al. Enhance delayed hypersensitivity skin test reactivity with serial testing in healthy volunteers. *Clinical and Experimental Immunology.* 1980;40:202–5.

Self-Study Questions

1. Which is the most common atopic disease? — 1. D

   A. Urticaria.
   B. Eczema.
   C. Asthma.
   D. Hay fever.

2. How quickly do type I hypersensitivity reactions develop? — 2. A

   A. Within minutes.
   B. Within hours.
   C. Within days.
   D. Within weeks.

3. Type I hypersensitivity reactions occur after the first exposure to the antigen. — 3. B

   A. True.
   B. False.

4. Which type of hypersensitivity reaction is independent of antibodies and complement? — 4. D

   A. Type I.
   B. Type II.
   C. Type III.
   D. Type IV.

5. Which of the following is an example of a type IV hypersensitivity reaction? — 5. C

   A. Erythroblastosis fetalis.
   B. Eczema.
   C. Contact dermatitis.
   D. Systemic lupus erythematosus.

6. Which of the following is an example of a type I hypersensitivity reaction? — 6. B

   A. Post-streptococcal glomerulonephritis.
   B. Insect venom allergy.
   C. Graves' disease.
   D. Transfusion reactions.

7. C

7. Which of the following mediators is responsible for increased permeability of capillaries during an immediate hypersensitivity reaction?

   A. Eosinophil chemotactic factor.
   B. Leukotrienes.
   C. Histamine.
   D. Neutrophil chemotactic factor.

8. A

8. Which of the following is the most potent bronchoconstrictor?

   A. Platelet activating-factor.
   B. Histamine.
   C. Neutrophil.
   D. Prostaglandins.

9. B

9. Which of the following is an advantage of in vitro testing over skin testing? It...

   A. is quicker.
   B. is safer.
   C. is more accurate.
   D. provides direct evidence of allergen hypersensitivity.

10. A

10. A radioallergosorbent test is used to detect what type of hypersensitivity?

   A. Type I.
   B. Type II.
   C. Type III.
   D. Type IV.

11. A

11. Immunosuppressive drugs such as cyclosporine and methotrexate may be used to treat types III and IV hypersensitivity reactions.

   A. True.
   B. False.

12. B, D, A, C

12. Match the pharmacologic therapy in the left column with its descriptor in the right column. Write in the letter of the descriptor next to the therapy.

___ Antihistamine	A. Cromolyn sodium
___ Sympathomimetic agents	B. Terfenadine
___ Antiallergy agents	C. Inhibit action of leukocytes
___ Corticosteroids	D. Alpha and beta stimulator

CHAPTER 5

Immunologic Tests and Separation Techniques

Karl Kwok, Pharm.D.
Clinical Pharmacist in Oncology
Pharmacy Services, University of Washington Medical Center, and
Clinical Associate Professor
Department of Pharmacy Practice, School of Pharmacy
University of Washington
Seattle, WA

Introduction

Pharmacists who engage in clinical activity are routinely called upon to integrate the results of laboratory tests into drug regimen decisions. Many laboratory tests today employ principles of immunology because of the sensitivity and specificity of these methods. The immunologic techniques incorporated into these tests have made some procedures less expensive, easier, quicker to perform, and often more accurate than traditional tests. These techniques are being refined continuously, and many of them are being incorporated into products used daily by the general public, such as early pregnancy tests.

The cornerstone of these immunologic tests is the union of antibody and antigen, which results in formation of an antibody-antigen complex. Reading this chapter will help the practicing pharmacist understand this principle. Methods that detect these antibody-antigen complexes are the basis for immunologic tests.

After reading this chapter, the learner will be able to—

Learning objectives

- Match acronyms and abbreviations to the names of their corresponding immunologic tests.
- Match the acronym or abbreviation of the immunologic test to one of the four testing classifications: precipitation test, agglutination test, complement fixation, or immunoassay.
- Describe mechanisms of common immunologic tests.
- Discuss the advantages and drawbacks of common immunologic tests.
- State typical applications of immunologic tests.
- Describe typical immunologic applications of separation techniques.

Chapter organization

The first section of this chapter presents information about various immunoprecipitation, agglutination, and labeled antibody or antigen methods used in some of the immunologic tests. Included is a discussion of the applications, advantages, and drawbacks of these immunologic tests. The chapter then describes many of the separation techniques that use immunologic principles to separate the immunologic components. For information about the specific step-by-step methods of the immunologic tests and separation techniques the reader is referred to standard laboratory manuals.

Immunologic Tests

Immunologic tests are often used to measure and identify, or localize, antibody-antigen reactions. This section examines some of the qualitative and quantitative methods for detecting and measuring antibody and antigen reactions as they are applied in diagnostic and screening assays. These immunologic tests include precipitation tests, agglutination tests, a complement fixation test, and some of the currently applied immunoassays.

Precipitation

The type of antibody-antigen complex depends on the nature of the antigens and antibodies and on the relative amounts of each. Antigens that are soluble proteins react with antibodies to produce an antibody-antigen complex that precipitates; antigens that are insoluble (i.e., particulate antigens), such as red blood cells (RBCs), form agglutinates. Not all antibody-antigen reactions, however, cause precipitation or agglutination. The precipitin reaction (Figure 5-1) depends on the relative amounts of antibody and antigen. There is an equivalence zone where the optimal proportion of components is present and maximum lattice formation of complexes occurs. Many of the immunologic tests depend on identifying the precipitin reaction.

Immunodiffusion

Many qualitative and quantitative immunochemical methods are carried out in a gel-like semisolid medium such as agar or agarose, through which antibody and antigen can diffuse and form a precipitin complex. Immunodiffusion in a semisolid medium has the advantages of decreasing unwanted mixing caused by vibration and allowing visualization of precipitin bands. One approach uses passive diffusion. Passive diffusion methods include the double immunodiffusion technique known as the Ouchterlony test and the single immunodiffusion technique incorporated into radial immunodiffusion (RID). Another approach, which uses electrophoretic separation diffusion, is called immunoelectrophoresis (IEP).

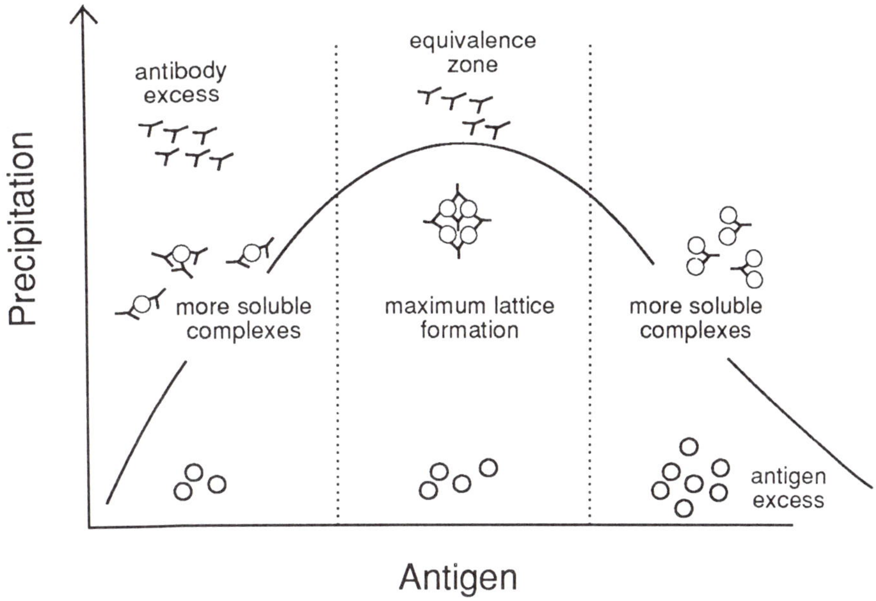

Figure 5-1. Precipitin reaction

SOURCE: Adapted with permission from Buffone GJ. Principles of immunochemical techniques. In: Tietz NW, ed. Fundamentals of clinical chemistry. 3rd ed. Philadelphia: W.B. Saunders Company;1987:147-8.

Radial Immunodiffusion. RID is a single immunodiffusion technique in which either the antibody or the antigen remains fixed and the other reactant is allowed to move and complex with it. The method is used for quantitative determination of antigen or antibody. RID is based on the principle that a quantitative relationship exists between the amount of antigen placed in a well that is cut into an agar plate containing antibody and the resulting ring of precipitation. The antigen is allowed to equilibrate for 24 hours. The antigen diffuses outward, forming soluble complexes with the antibody until the equivalence point is reached and the complexes precipitate in a ring (Figure 5-2).

Quantitative test

The applications of RID include routine quantitation of many serum proteins. The immunoglobulins that are typically quantitated by this method are IgG, IgA, and IgM. RID is less useful for quantitating IgD and IgE because of the relatively low levels of these immunoglobulins in human serum. RID can also be used to measure complement components. The RID method may be used to quantitate a specific antibody by uniformly dispersing the antigen instead of the antibody into the agar.

RID applications are limited; newer techniques are faster and more sensitive. RID can quantitate any antigenic protein that exists in

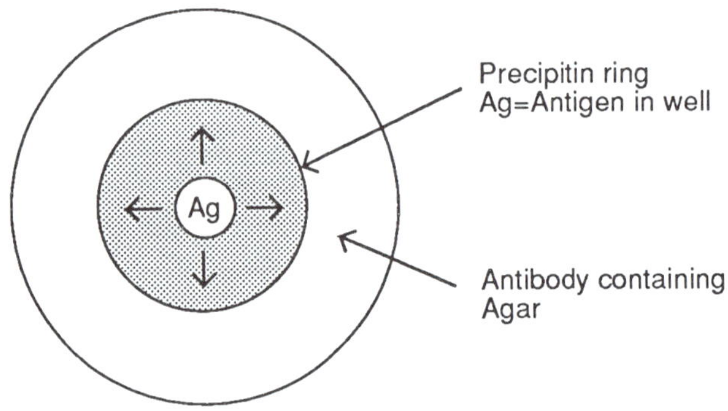

Figure 5-2. Radial immunodiffusion

concentrations higher than 5 μg/mL. In general, excellent technical skills, especially in the tedious process of preparation and execution, are required to identify and quantitate antigens or antibodies by means of any gel-based methodology. For this reason most laboratories today use RID only for qualitative studies or as a reference method.

Double Immunodiffusion (Ouchterlony Technique). Double immunodiffusion is a passive diffusion technique in which a concentration gradient is established for both the antibody and the antigen.[1] Antigen and antibody are placed in wells in a support matrix and are allowed to diffuse toward each other; a precipitin line forms at the point of antibody-antigen equivalence. This method is useful for determining the presence or absence of a given antigen by using a defined antibody or for determining antibody presence or absence if a purified antigen is available. Double immunodiffusion allows comparison between two or more test specimens to determine whether the antigens or antibodies in the specimens are identical, nonidentical, or partially identical. Semiquantitative analysis of antigen and antibody may be performed by double immunodiffusion. Three basic patterns of reactions may occur as the antibody and antigen are allowed to diffuse toward each other and precipitin lines form (Figure 5-3).

Semiquantitative analysis

A continuous precipitin arc indicates that the antibody is precipitating identical antigens in each preparation. Crossing precipitin arcs and multiple arcs indicate the presence of different antigens. A spur from a precipitin arc indicates partial identity between the antigen preparations.

Disadvantages

The usefulness of the double diffusion method is limited by its relative insensitivity compared with newer techniques. Time is also a limiting factor, because full development of precipitin patterns requires 18 to 96 hours. The double immunodiffusion method is rarely used today, but it is more sensitive than the IEP method. A negative reaction does not

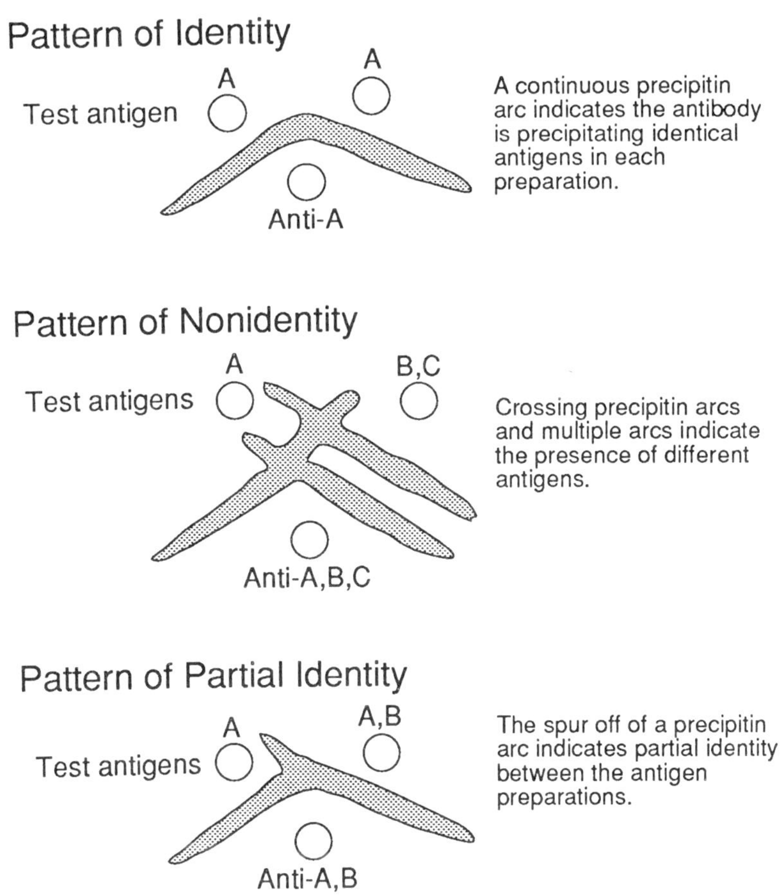

Figure 5-3. Three basic patterns of double immunodiffusion

SOURCE: Adapted with permission from Roitt IM, Brostoff J, Male DK, eds. Immunology. 2nd ed. London: Gower Medical Publishing, 1989:25.1.

necessarily imply absence of antibody or antigen but may be the result of using amounts too small for the sensitivity of the method or the presence of a nonprecipitating antibody.

Immunoelectrophoresis. IEP is a technique in which mixtures of antigen may be separated and identified in a two-step procedure.[2,3] The sample is applied to a well cut into thin, semisolid agarose poured onto a glass slide. The sample is then separated by electrophoresis for 30 to 60 minutes (Figure 5-4). After the electrophoretic step, specific antisera are added to a trough that is cut into the agarose parallel to the electrophoretic separation of the sample antigens. The separated antigens and the antisera diffuse toward one another, and at the equivalency zone of the antibody-antigen a precipitin pattern forms that is characteristic of the antigens in the sample.

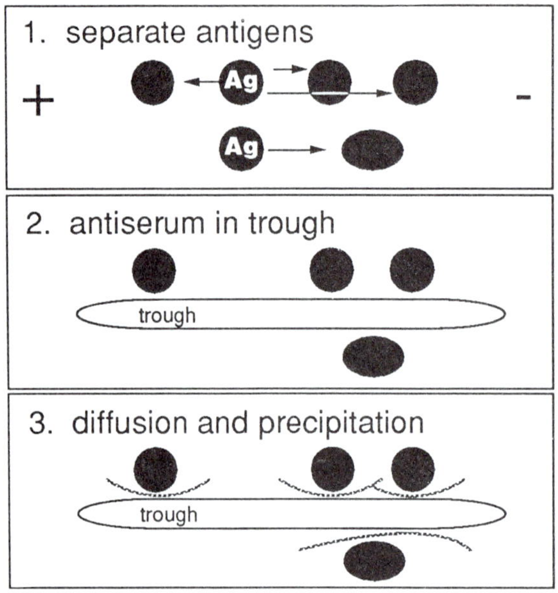

1. Antigens are separated in an agar gel by placing an electric charge across the gel. The pH is chosen so that positively charged proteins move to the negative electrode and negatively charged proteins to the positive.
2. A trough is then cut between the wells, filled with the antibody and the plate is left to diffuse.
3. The antigens and antibody form precipitin arcs.

Figure 5-4. Immunoelectrophoresis

SOURCE: Reprinted with permission from Roitt IM, Brostoff J, Male DK, eds. Immunology. 2nd ed. London: Gower Medical Publishing, 1989:25.2.

The precipitin patterns are then interpreted by comparison with known controls. IEP is used to identify and characterize serum proteins, particularly immunoglobulin abnormalities found in serum and urine. IEP tests are the least sensitive of the gel and agar tests.

Agglutination

Qualitative or quantitative

Antibody-antigen ratio

When the antigen is a particle or is coated on cells, the resulting antibody-antigen reaction leads to clumping or agglutination of the particles or cells. Agglutination assays have been used for qualitative and quantitative measurements of antigens and antibodies. Agglutination reactions require the availability of a stable cell or uniform particle, the presence of pure antigens or antigens close to the surface of the cell or particle, and a specific antibody. The type of antibody is important; IgM antibodies may produce more complete agglutination than IgG antibodies because of the size and valence of the IgM molecule. As with precipitation reactions, the ratio of antibody to antigen is important. Extremes in either antigen or antibody concentration result in false-negative results with no agglutination.

Agglutination reactions may be classified as either direct or indirect (passive). The direct reaction involves the antibody directly agglutinated to the cell or insoluble particulate antigen. Indirect agglutination is the agglutination of antigen-coated cells or inert particles that are passive carriers of otherwise soluble antigens. Agglutination methods have many clinical applications that include using RBCs, microorganisms, or inert particles (e.g., latex, bentonite) coated with antigen. Hemagglutination is one of many techniques for detecting antibodies on the basis of agglutination of RBCs. Three classes of hemagglutination are used in many tests: direct hemagglutination, indirect (passive) hemagglutination, and a variation known as hemagglutination inhibition. Types of hemagglutination tests and their most common applications are shown in Table 5-1.

Clinical applications

In direct hemagglutination, the antigens to which the antibodies are directed are antigenic determinates native to the surface of the RBC. Direct hemagglutination is useful for direct testing of the erythrocytes for ABO, Rh, and other blood groups. A qualitative agglutination test may be conducted either on a slide or in a test tube.

In indirect or passive hemagglutination, the erythrocytes are used as particulate carriers of foreign antigen. Many soluble antigens can be passively adsorbed or chemically coupled to RBCs. Antigens that can spontaneously couple with RBCs to form stable reagents for antibody detection are listed in Table 5-2. Chemical coupling of antigens with the surface of RBCs can involve many different types of coupling reactions (e.g., adsorption, cross-linking, covalent coupling of the antigen to the RBC surface).

Table 5-1 Major Types of Hemagglutination Tests

Type	Applications
Direct	Blood groups: ABO, Rh Paul-Bunnell test: diagnosis of infectious mononucleosis
Indirect	Rose-Waaler test: diagnosis of rheumatoid arthritis Antithyroid antibody test Infectious disease diagnosis: diphtheria, tetanus, leptospirosis, toxoplasmosis, treponematosis Coomb's test
Inhibition	Hemophilia test for factor VIII antigen Hepatitis B surface antigen Viruses: influenza, rubella, mumps, measles

Table 5-2 Substrates Adsorbed Spontaneously to RBCs for Hemagglutination

Drugs	Antibiotics (e.g., penicillin)
Proteins	Bovine serum albumin Ovalbumin Purified protein derivative
Infectious organisms	*Escherichia coli* antigens Yersinia antigens Toxoplasma antigens Lipopolysaccharide from *Neisseria meningitides* Endotoxin of *Mycoplasma species* Viruses
Others	DNA Haptens

SOURCE: Adapted with permission from Stites DP, Rodgers RP. Clinical laboratory methods for detection of cellular antigens and antibodies. In: Stites DP, Terr AI, eds. Basic and clinical immunology. 7th ed. Norwalk, CT: Appleton and Lange; 1991:252.

Hemagglutination inhibition allows the presence of a soluble antigen to be detected in body fluids. In this test the suspected soluble antigen is detected by its ability to reduce the agglutinating activity of a known antiserum. The hemagglutination inhibition method is useful in detecting factor VIII antigen in hemophilia and related clotting disorders and hepatitis B surface antigen (HBSAg) in patients with hepatitis.

A modification of the hemagglutination inhibition method is used to determine the presence of antibodies to viruses. Some RBCs of given species may be directly agglutinated by viruses. This agglutination is inhibited if the virus is first exposed to serum containing an antibody for that virus. The principle of viral hemagglutination inhibition is used to test for antibodies to influenza, rubella, mumps, and measles viruses.

Coombs' test

The Coombs' (or antiglobulin) test is a hemagglutination test used to detect the presence of antibodies that coat the surface of RBCs but cannot form the necessary lattice for agglutination. The presence of subagglutinating or nonagglutinating antibodies may be detected by adding a second antibody or antiglobulin directed against the specific serum proteins. The addition of the secondary antibody or antiglobulin results in hemagglutination if the antibody of interest is on the RBCs.

The Coombs' test is useful for determining the presence of antibodies against RBCs that may cause hemolysis. There are two types of Coombs' test, direct and indirect (Figure 5-5).

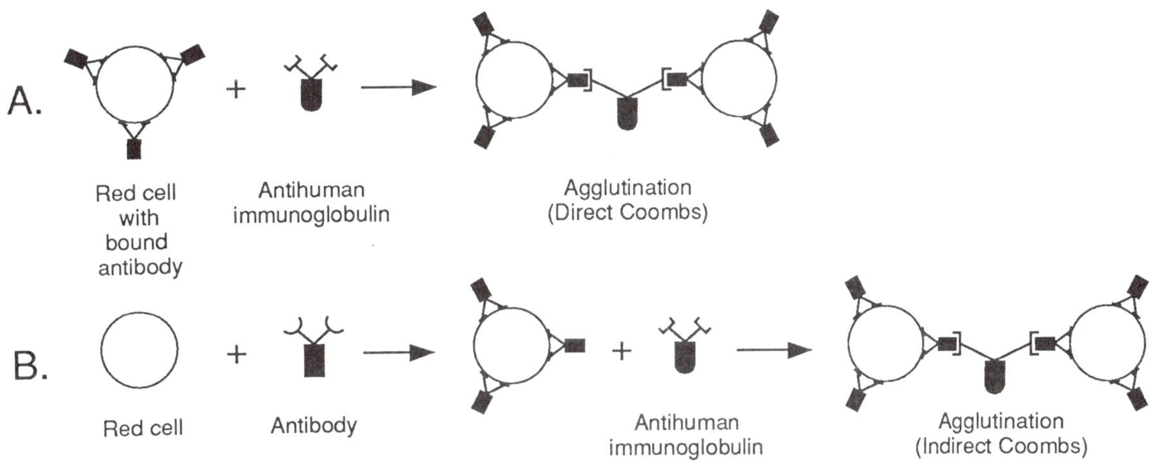

Figure 5-5. Antiglobulin (Coombs') technique, the direct (A) and indirect (B) methods of hemagglutination

SOURCE: Reprinted with permission from Nichols WS, Nakamura RM. Agglutination and agglutination inhibition assays. In: Rose NR, Friedman H, Fahely JL, eds. Manual of clinical laboratory immunology. Washington, DC: American Society for Microbiology; 1986:52.

The direct Coombs' test detects the presence of antibody-antigen complexes on the RBC membrane. The addition of rabbit antihuman gamma globulin to the RBC mixture induces agglutination if immunoglobulins are bound to the cell surface. Nongamma Coombs' reagents (i.e., anticomplement) directed against complement components such as C3 or C4 are also available. The addition of anti-C3 to the RBC mixture can produce hemagglutination in the case of autoimmune hemolytic anemia in which complement has bound to the RBC surface. Applications of the direct Coombs' test include the diagnosis of hemolytic disease of the newborn, acquired hemolytic anemia, transfusion reaction, and RBC sensitization caused by drugs.[4]

The indirect Coombs' test is a two-part test to determine the presence of antibody in serum against normal RBCs. The test is performed by incubating the serum containing the antibody in question with RBCs, then performing the direct Coombs' test on the mixture by adding the antiglobulin. A positive agglutination reaction reflects the presence of specific antibody present in the serum against the RBC. This test is important for determining major crossmatch and is used by blood banks for blood typing.

In general, agglutination methods are more sensitive than precipitation methods. Antibody concentrations as low as 0.01 μg/mL have been detected with modified passive hemagglutination. Agglutination reactions, however, are not as quantitative as the newer immunoassay techniques that are slowly replacing the agglutination methods.

Complement Fixation Test

Complement is a substance in the serum that causes lysis when it combines with antibody-antigen complexes involving antibodies of the IgG or IgM classes. Complement fixation reactions are sensitive serologic tests for detecting antibody or antigen. The method involves two main steps. The first step is to incubate the antibody-containing serum with antigen and a small amount of complement. If the antibody directed at the antigen is present, complexes form and complement is fixed to the complex; if no antibody is present, active complement remains. The second step, which allows the results of the first step to be visualized, involves using an indicator made of RBCs coated with antibodies to the RBC antigens. These sensitized RBCs are added to the first mixture. If active complement is still present, the sensitized RBCs lyse and the test reaction is considered negative; if the sensitized RBCs do not lyse, the test reaction is positive for the presence of the antibody, since active complement was fixed to the antibody-antigen complex during the test reaction. The steps for the complement fixation test are shown in Figure 5-6.

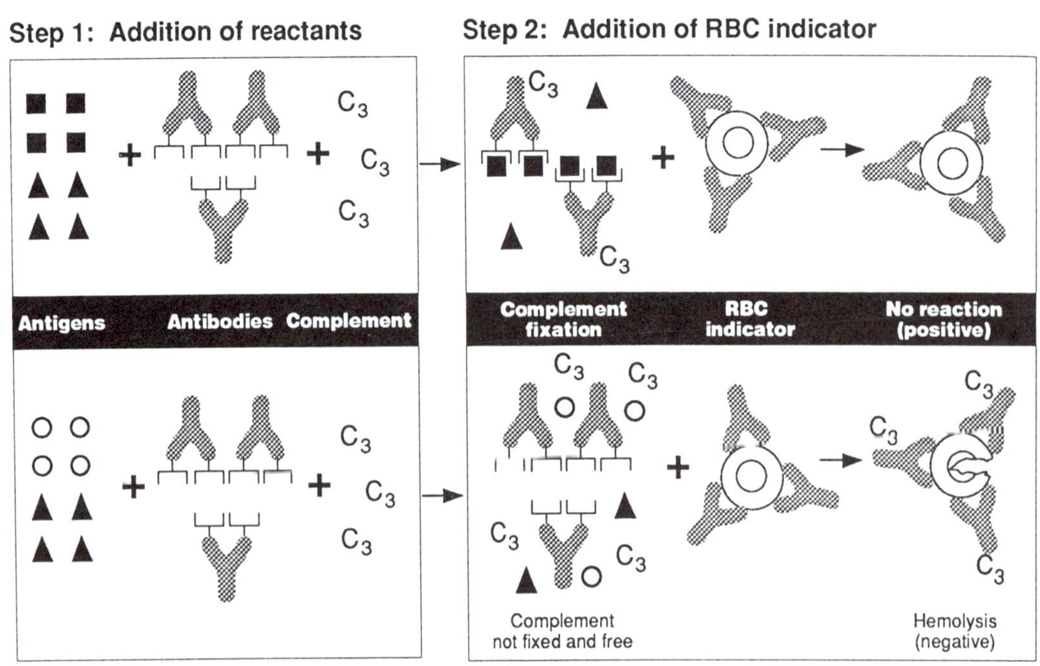

Figure 5-6. Complement fixation test

Applications

The complement fixation method can be used to detect antibodies to *Mycoplasma pneumoniae, Bordetella pertussis, Coccidioides immitis* antigen, *Cryptococcus, Histoplasma,* hepatitis-associated antigen, viruses, and other diseases. Complement fixation is also the basis of the Wassermann test for syphilis.

Immunoassays

The previously discussed precipitin, agglutination, and complement fixation techniques rely on detecting the immune complex formation as the index of the antibody-antigen reaction. The primary reaction between antibody and antigen can also be measured by other immunoassay techniques. Many of these immunoassays have been modified for various diagnostic or quantitative applications such as measuring the concentration of drugs. The two major immunoassay methods used for measuring initial antigen and antibody reactions are the competitive and noncompetitive immunoassays.

General Methods. Competitive immunoassays have a labeled and an unlabeled antigen competing for a limited number of antibodies or protein binding sites. The label on the labeled antigen varies depending on the manner of measuring the label. In a competitive immunoassay, the number of labeled antigens must be greater than the number of protein binding sites or antibodies, while the concentrations of the labeled antigen and antibody are kept constant. The concentration of unlabeled antigen varies depending on the sample. As the concentration of unlabeled antigen increases, labeled antigen bound to the binding protein decreases because of displacement by the nonlabeled antigen, and the amount of free labeled antigen increases. Some immunoassays that employ competitive methodology include classic radioimmunoassay (RIA), enzyme-multiplied immunoassay, and fluorescence immunoassay (FIA).

Noncompetitive versus competitive assays

Sandwich assay

Noncompetitive immunoassays measure the reaction between antibody and antigen. The major difference between these methods and the competitive binding immunoassays is the lack of competitive binding between the labeled protein and the antigen for the antibody. Most of the noncompetitive immunoassay techniques use a general assay method known as the sandwich assay, which has the advantage of two distinct antigenic sites. In its most basic form, the sandwich assay involves the use of an antibody (binder) that has been immobilized on a solid surface. The antigen (ligand) is added and binds to the antibody. A second labeled antibody (binder) is added, causing a reaction with the antigen at a different site, thus forming the antibody-antigen-antibody sandwich while labeling the complex. Noncompetitive immunoassay techniques are used in radioimmunosorbent tests, immunoradiometric assays, enzyme-linked immunosorbent assay (ELISA), and some FIAs. The majority of immunoassays used today are noncompetitive.

Specific Types of Immunoassays. Although immunoprecipitation and agglutination provide a visual detection of the antibody-antigen reaction, not all antibody-antigen reactions are detectable with the unaided eye. Many of the immunoassays have incorporated labels (e.g., radioactive isotopes, enzymes, fluorescence) to facilitate detection of the antibody-antigen reaction. These methods have improved the overall sensitivity, specificity, and turnaround time of the assays, thus making them more clinically applicable. Furthermore, they have decreased the need for the large sample volumes seen with the older methods. Some of the commonly used immunoassay methods are presented in the following paragraphs.

Radioimmunoassay. RIA includes a variety of techniques that use a radioisotope label to detect antigens or antibodies. Most of the RIAs used today are noncompetitive. Figure 5-7 shows a noncompetitive RIA technique, the immunoradiometric assay (IRMA). In the IRMA technique the radioisotope is on an antibody instead of on the antigen. Antibodies with affinity for the antigen of interest are first attached to a solid phase by passive absorption or by covalent binding. The antigen of interest is then added and allowed to react with the antibody attached to the solid phase. Other proteins are washed away, and the radioisotope-labeled antibody is added; it then reacts with the bound antigen through a second and distinct epitope. After a second washing, the remaining antibody-antigen radiolabeled antibody complex is measured with a gamma counter or by scintillation. The amount of radiation measured is directly proportional to the concentration of antigen. IRMA is a common approach for protein antigen measurement. The IRMA methodology has been applied in an assay to detect the ovarian carcinoma tumor marker CA 125 in the serum, as well as to detect growth factors such as granulocyte-macrophage colony-stimulating factor.[5]

IRMA

Classic RIA

Classic RIA is one of the oldest competitive binding immunoassay techniques. This assay was developed originally by Berson and Yalow, who used human anti-insulin antibodies to detect human insulin.[6] In this assay, the antigen is labeled with a radioactive isotope (usually iodine 125) and a fixed amount of the labeled antigen is added to a fixed quantity of antibody and the unlabeled antigen. The reactants are mixed together simultaneously as the labeled and unlabeled antigens compete for binding to the antibody (Figure 5-8). The antibody binds both the labeled and unlabeled antigens, and some excess labeled and unlabeled antigens are left unbound in the supernatant. The amount of free (unbound) labeled antigen is proportional to the quantity of unlabeled antigen added. A standard curve may be constructed by plotting the percentage of antibody-bound labeled antigen against known concentrations of standard unlabeled antigen.

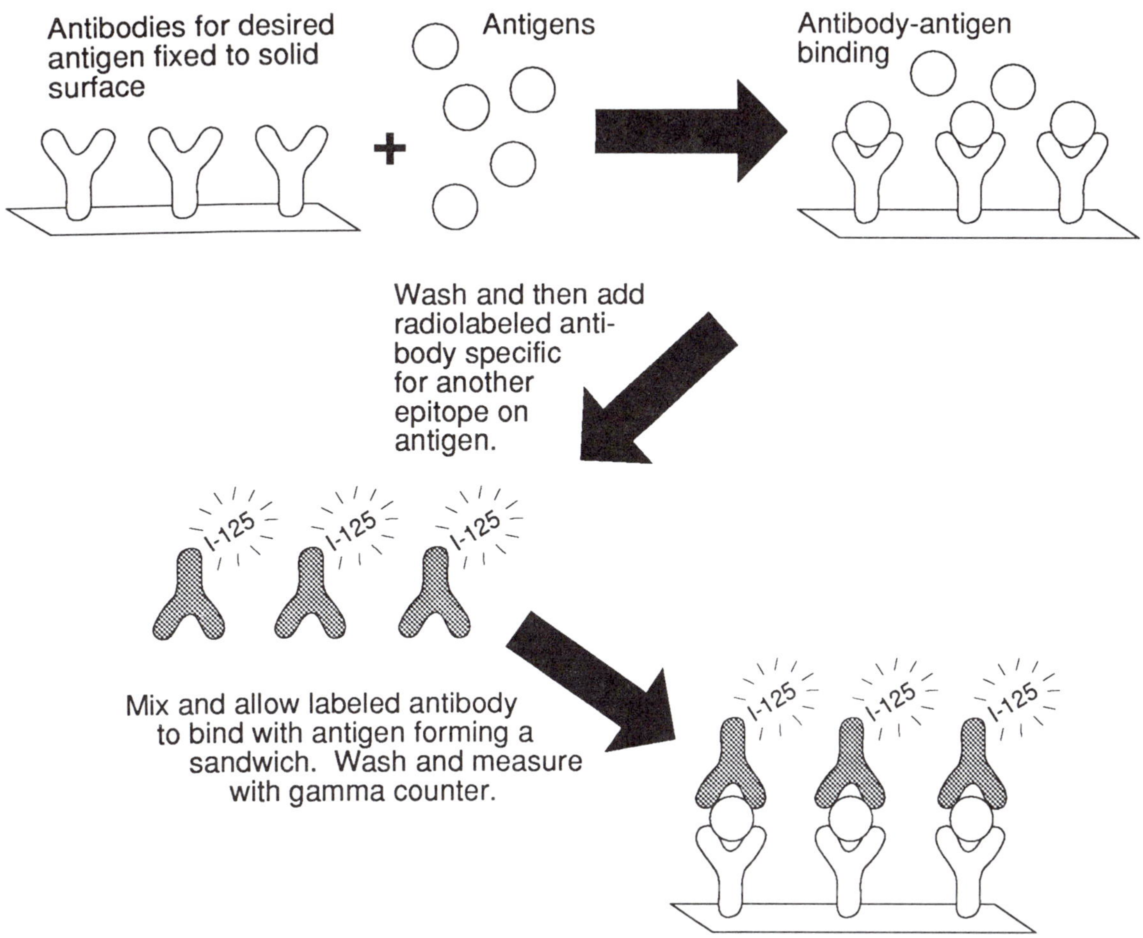

Figure 5-7. Immunoradiometric assay, a noncompetitive RIA technique

Technique

The classic RIA technique requires a method of separating free labeled antigen and antibody-bound labeled antigen so that the radiolabeled immune complexes may be quantitated with either a liquid scintillation counter or a gamma counter. Among the partitioning and separation techniques are salting out (or precipitating out) the proteins, adsorption, electrophoresis, and gel filtration. The easiest method includes use of a solid-phase RIA, in which the antibody is attached to an inert particle (e.g., cellulose, Sephadex®, glass beads) that can be centrifuged. The supernatant can be separated from the solid phase and both samples can be measured for labeled antigen content. Standard solutions are run in parallel with patient's samples for use in preparing the standard curve. RIA can be used to measure protein antigens. It has been used primarily to quantitate hormones and drugs. Good RIAs have been developed to detect such hormones as insulin, aldosterone, human follicle-stimulating hormone,

Applications

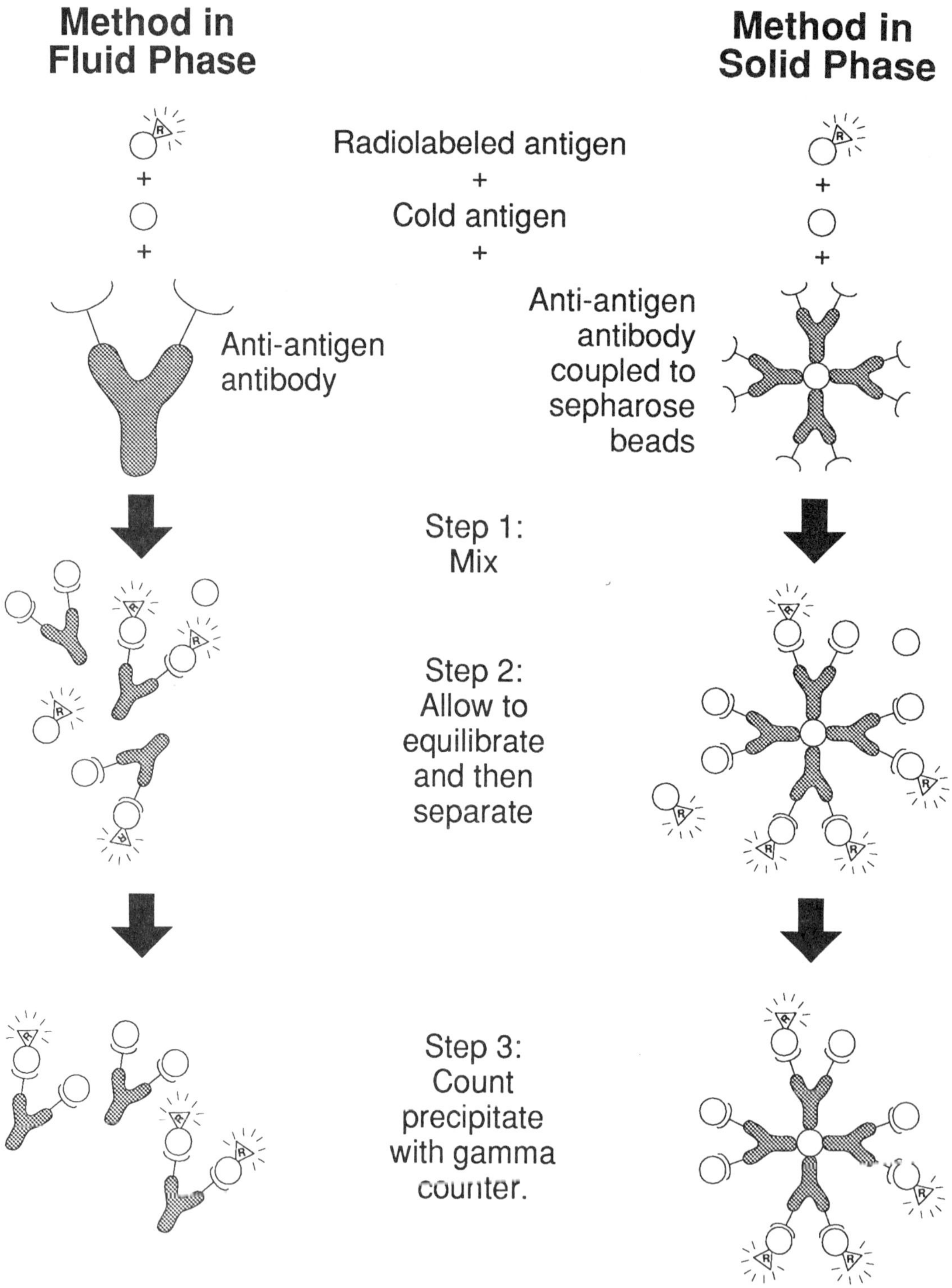

Figure 5-8. Radioimmunoassay competitive binding technique

SOURCE: Adapted from Virella G, Goust JM, Fundenber HH, et al., eds. Introduction to medical immunology. New York: Marcel Dekker; 1986:241, 242. Reprinted with permission.

progesterone, testosterone, thyroxin, and vasopressin. They have also been used to detect such proteins as alpha-fetoprotein, carcinoembryonic antigen, and IgE; vitamins; enzymes (e.g., pepsin); antibodies to DNA; HBSAg; and such drugs as digoxin, lysergic acid diethylamide, theophylline, aminoglycosides, and barbiturates.[7,8] The major limitations to RIA are the cost of detection equipment, the short stability of the reagents, and the need to handle and eliminate radioactive materials.

Enzyme-multiplied Immunoassay Technique (EMIT). Another competitive binding immunoassay is the EMIT, which uses an enzyme detection system.[9,10] In EMIT, the antigen is coupled to an enzyme that remains active when unbound, but its activity is altered when the antigen binds to the antibody. This enzyme-labeled antigen competes for antibody binding with the unlabeled antigen. The bound labeled antigens may be separated from the free labeled antigen by the same methods described in RIA. The detection system depends on the enzyme used, but it usually catalyzes a colored chemical reaction that can be quantitated. A standard curve must be prepared to interpolate the measured concentration of antigen. The EMIT method does not enhance the sensitivity or the precision of the immunoassay as significantly as the name implies. Enzyme immunoassays are more sensitive than agglutination reactions but not as sensitive as RIA. Advantages of enzyme immunoassay techniques include the safety of a nonradioactive test, the stability of the reagents, and the ability to use colored substances in the detection system. The EMIT method has been most widely used for therapeutic monitoring of drugs such as the anticonvulsants,[11] aminoglycosides, theophylline,[12] antiarrhythmics, digoxin,[13] and others.[14] The EMIT method is also available for toxicologic detection in the urine of a variety of drugs such as amphetamines, barbiturates, benzodiazepines, opiates, phencyclidine, cannabinoids, and others.[15] Inherent to drug screening programs, use of an immunoassay like EMIT imparts some degree of nonspecificity due to cross-reactivity of the antibodies.[16] Some prescription drugs and over-the-counter medications can give a false-positive result for another agent. Fenoprofen can give a false-positive test for tetrahydrocannabinol (THC), and cold medications containing pseudoephedrine or phenylpropanolamine can give a false-positive test for amphetamines. In addition, cough preparations containing dextromethorphan can give a false-positive test for opiates. Until newer, more specific antibodies are developed and incorporated into these drug-screening assays, it is important to confirm these tests by other methods such as gas chromatography-mass spectrometry.

Technique

Advantages

Applications

Fluorescence Immunoassay. FIA includes a group of immunoassays that use fluorescein-labeled antigens or antibodies and an emitted-light monitoring system.[17] FIA procedures are widely used in clinical laboratories for detecting and quantitating drugs, hormones, proteins, and peptides in biologic fluids. The various FIAs may be classified as

Applications

homogeneous or heterogeneous; antigen or antibody labeled; competitive or noncompetitive; and solid or nonsolid phase. The element common to all FIA techniques is the fluorescein labeling and detection method. Two types of FIAs are shown in Figure 5-9.

Technique

In FIAs, the antigen or antibody is labeled with a fluorophore or fluorescent compound. These compounds contain a chemical ring structure that can absorb light of a short wavelength and emit light of a longer wavelength. The very short time interval from absorption to emission of the light is measured in nanoseconds. The development of special instrumentation and the use of a time-resolved fluorometer have increased the sensitivity of the method and minimized the interference of background fluorescence caused by serum and other biologic fluids. The FIA method involves a fast light pulse that excites the label; the fluorescence is measured after a certain time has elapsed. Depending on the type of FIA, the amount of measured fluorescence correlates with the presence of the antigen or antibody of interest. FIA techniques have been incorporated into many systems and are providing alternatives to RIAs and enzyme immunoassays. FIAs can be developed to have sensitivities in the range of the RIAs.

Advantages

Advantages of FIAs include stability of reagents, rapid sensitivity, adaptability to automation, and the development of homogeneous FIA methods that do not require a separation step. Disadvantages include the expensive instrumentation necessary to achieve adequate sensitivity and the need for purified antibody reagents and special fluorophore labels.

Technique

Enzyme-linked Immunosorbent Assay. The ELISA is a noncompetitive immunoassay used to detect the presence of antibody (Figure 5-10).[18] The technique is similar to IRMA except that the labeled antibody has an enzyme linked to it instead of a radionuclide. The general approach to performing an ELISA test involves adding a sample or standard containing the antibody to be quantitated to antigen, which is adsorbed to a solid phase such as a plastic plate. The reaction is allowed to equilibrate so that the antibody may bind to the antigen adsorbed to the solid phase. After the solid phase is washed, an enzyme-labeled antibody (either polyclonal or monoclonal) directed toward the antibody of interest is added. It can form an antigen-antibody-antibody complex. Excessive enzyme-labeled antibody is washed away and an enzyme substrate is added that can be hydrolyzed by the enzyme on the antigen-antibody-antibody complex, causing a color formation proportional to the amount of antibody in the sample.

The choice of ELISA enzyme label depends on the application. Labels include alkaline phosphatase, b-glucuronidase, glucose-6-phosphate dehydrogenase, and horseradish peroxidase. Various detection systems ranging from visual to photometric have aided the expansion and use of the ELISA procedure.[19] Newer ELISAs have sensitivities similar to or higher

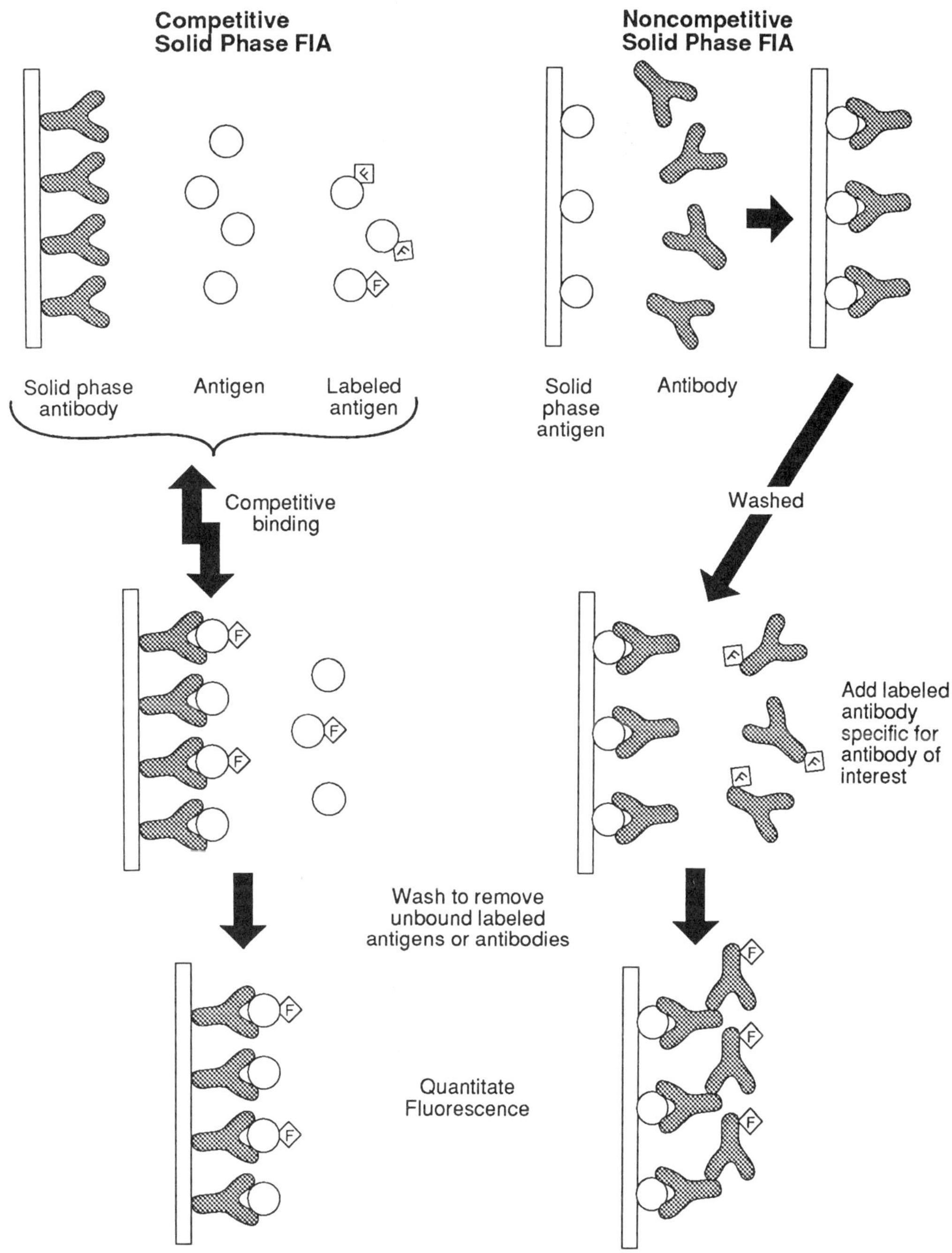

Figure 5-9. Competitive and noncompetitive immunoassays

SOURCE: Adapted from Nakamura RM, Robbins BA. Analytical fluid-phase fluorescence immunoassay. In: Rose NR, Friedman H, Fahely JL, eds. Manual of clinical laboratory immunology. 3rd ed. Washington, DC: American Society of Microbiology; 1986:118.

than RIAs. These improvements in sensitivities are achieved by increasing the number of available enzyme labels per analyte molecule or amplifying substrate or both.[20] The technique has been applied recently for determining serum erythropoietin levels. A labeled complex consisting of a tetrameric

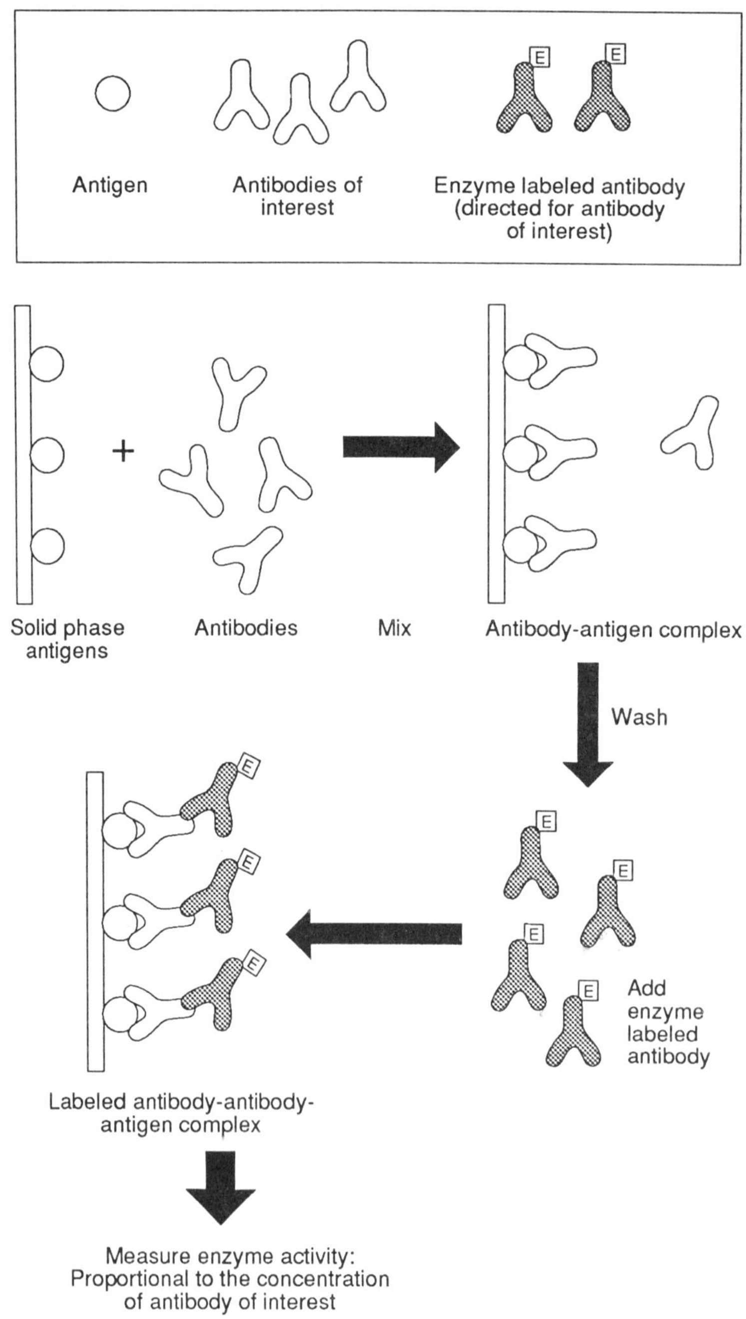

Figure 5-10. Enzyme-linked immunoassay, a noncompetitive binding immunoassay

antialkaline phosphatase-antierythropoietin complex together with substrate amplification improved sensitivity tenfold.[21]

Applications

ELISA methods have been applied to the detection of circulating antibodies in candidiasis, aspergillosis, toxoplasmosis, and rheumatoid arthritis and have been used to diagnose rubella and hepatitis. The greatest explosion of ELISA-based assays has been in detecting in serum the presence of antibodies against human immunodeficiency virus (HIV).[22-24]

Radioimmunosorbent Test (RIST). The RIST is an immunoassay technique used to detect IgE in the serum. This highly sensitive technique can detect an IgE content of 100 ng/mL or less and is useful in determining allergic conditions. Both competitive binding (indirect) and noncompetitive binding (direct) RIST methods are available. The direct RIST method is the more commonly used method of the two, because of the relatively easy use of and commercial availability of reagents.

Applications

TDx. The TDx system is the current standard for monitoring therapeutic drug and hormone levels using fluorescence polarized immunoassay (FPIA) technology and competitive binding immunoassay methodology.[25] In the TDx system, fluorescein-labeled antigen and patient antigen compete for binding sites on the antibody. The relative binding of the fluorescein-labeled antigen and the patient antigen to the antibody depends on the relative concentrations of antigen and antibody. As more of the fluorescein-labeled antigen binds to the antibody, less of the fluorescein-labeled antigen remains in the solution. The mixture is allowed to reach a steady state. The amount of fluorescein-labeled antigen in solution and the amount bound to the antibody can be determined by a simple procedure. The mixture is exposed to a polarized blue light of 485 nm, which raises the fluorescein molecule on the antigen to an excited state. When it returns to a steady state, a green light (of a wavelength of 525 to 550 nm) is emitted. If the fluorescein-labeled antigen is bound to the antibody, it cannot rotate freely; the emitted green light is in the same plane as the blue light and polarization is retained. Free labeled antigen is allowed to rotate freely and the emitted green light does not maintain its polarization. The principles of FPIA as used in the TDx system may be seen in Figure 5-11.

Technique

The solution has a polarization value based on the concentration of the unlabeled drug or hormone in the specimen. This value can establish the concentration of the drug or hormone in the sample by being compared with known standards. The TDx system can determine the concentrations of thyroid hormones in the serum as well as most of the typical therapeutically monitored drugs.[26-28]

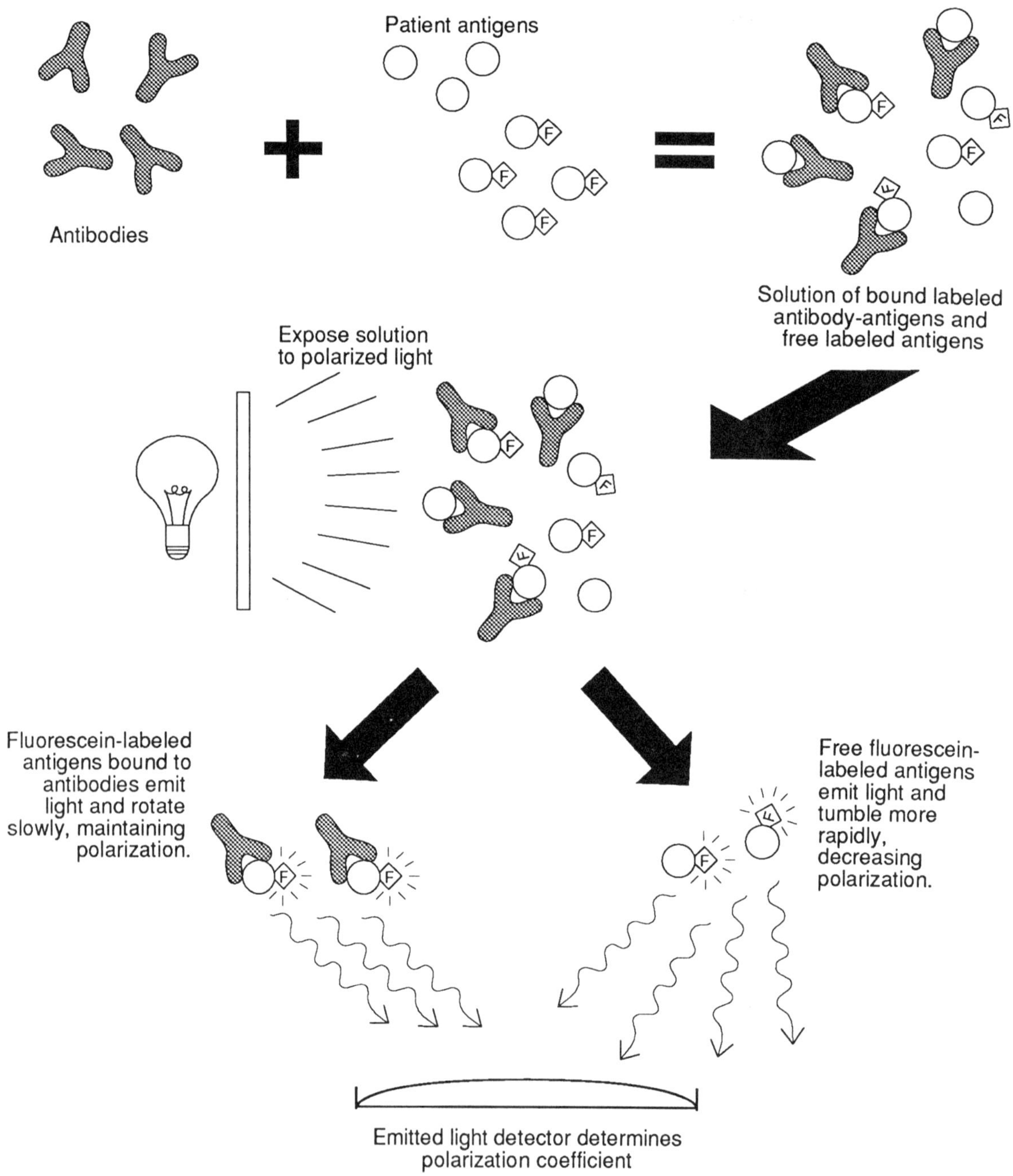

Figure 5-11. Fluorescence polarized immunoassays

Many other modifications of the basic immunologic tests are used to localize and quantitate desired antigens or antibodies. The major differences among the immunologic tests are their practical applications and their relative sensitivities. The sensitivity limits of all these tests vary with the affinity of the antibody and antigen tested, their concentration, variations among the lots of antisera, temperature, length of reaction, preparation of reagents, and individual laboratory differences. The relative sensitivity of immunologic assays for antigen and antibodies is listed in Table 5-3. One of the oldest immunoassay techniques, RIA, is still one of the most sensitive tests available; IEP is one of the least sensitive of the immunologic tests discussed.

Separation Techniques

This section examines three major separation techniques that use immunologic methods: affinity chromatography, purification of lymphocyte populations, and Western blot techniques.

Table 5-3 Relative Sensitivity of Immunologic Tests

Techniques	Minimum detectable antibody (µg/mL)
Precipitation in liquid	20
Precipitation in gel	
Immunoelectrophoresis	50–200
Double diffusion	3–20
Radial diffusion	3–20
Agglutination	
Qualitative	0.05
Quantitative	0.02–0.1
Hemagglutination	0.001–0.01
Coombs' test	0.01
Complement fixation	0.01–0.05
Immunoassays	
Enzyme immunoassay	0.01
Fluorescence immunoassay	0.001
Radioimmunoassay	0.001

SOURCE: Reprinted with permission from Friedman H, Fahely JL, eds. *Manual of clinical laboratory immunology*. 3rd ed. Washington, DC: American Society for Microbiology; 1986:50. In: Stites DP, Terr AI, eds. Basic and clinical immunology. 7th ed. Norwalk, CT: Appleton and Lange; 1991.

Affinity Chromatography

Technique

Affinity chromatography is a purification technique used to remove particular protein from a complex protein mixture. The basis of this technique involves an immobilized ligand that interacts specifically with the desired protein. The desired protein in the mixture can interact strongly with the ligand and bind while the unwanted proteins are washed through. The desired protein is then eluted from the immobilized ligand.

Immunologists have developed the use of affinity chromatography to isolate pure antibodies or pure antigens. The availability of monoclonal antibodies (MoAbs) (see Chapter 11) has made it possible to construct high-capacity, specific immunoadsorbents to almost any antigen.

The preparation of an affinity column requires the covalent coupling of the MoAbs to gels in a column. The desired antigen is then isolated by running the mixture containing the antigen through the column.

MoAb applications

A MoAb affinity column can purify a membrane molecule up to several hundredfold, giving a good yield. The columns may also be used for bulk purification of molecules. Affinity columns prepared with MoAbs are important in enzyme purification, especially when purification by conventional procedures is difficult. An example of commercial application of MoAb affinity chromatography is the bulk purification of interferon.[29] Another clinically significant application of MoAb affinity chromatography is the MoAB purification of factor VIII for use with hemophiliacs.[30] This process is useful in reducing contamination by viruses, especially HIV, and other extraneous proteins in the final, purified factor VIII concentrate.

Limitations

However, MoAb affinity columns have some limitations. The type of antibody is important because, although most of the columns prepared with IgG MoAbs function well, IgM MoAbs usually do not function as well as immunoadsorbents. Desired antigens may also pass unretarded through a column because either the antibody has too low an affinity for the antigens or the antibody was denatured by the coupling procedure. Antigens may also pass through if not enough specific antibodies are coupled. Other limitations include inability to elute the antigen from the column because of too high an antibody affinity or because the antigen was in a denatured form.

Purification of Lymphocyte Populations

The cellular system primarily responsible for immunity is composed of lymphocytes located in tissue or circulating in blood or lymph. There are a number of functional classes and subclasses of lymphocytes (see Chapters 1 and 2). The two major functional classes are the T lymphocytes and the B lymphocytes. When observed through a microscope the lymphocytes have a homogeneous appearance, making it difficult to distinguish the two major lymphocytes from each other.

Lymphocytes and their subpopulations may be separated from other cell populations and purified for study. The lymphocytes can be separated from other cells by their physical characteristics (e.g., density, size) or by their cell surface properties (e.g., differential adherence to such substrates as glass or specific ligands). The subpopulations of lymphocytes may be determined by the presence or absence of receptors located on the cell surface. The receptors that permit identification of lymphocytes include surface immunoglobulins, B-cell- and T-cell-specific antigens, and receptors for complement components. This section reviews the methods used to separate and purify lymphocytes.

Techniques

Ficoll-Hypaque. Lymphocytes must first be separated from other blood plasma cells. Lymphocytes may be separated by density-gradient centrifugation—for example, with the Ficoll-Hypaque technique. This method depends on the specific gravity of a gradient solution. The blood is diluted in tissue culture medium and layered on top of a tube partially full of Ficoll (Figure 5-12). (Ficoll is denser than lymphocytes, but less dense than RBCs and granulocytes.) After centrifugation, the RBCs and granulocytes settle to the bottom of the Ficoll layer and the lymphocytes are located at the interface between the plasma and Ficoll.

Rosetting. Rosetting is another method of isolating lymphocytes by allowing them to associate with RBCs.[31] Human T lymphocytes may be identified by their binding reactions with sheep erythrocytes (this reaction involves the CD2 receptor on the T cells); B lymphocytes may be identified by their reactions with antibody- and complement-treated erythrocytes. Once the lymphocytes have become surrounded by RBCs through a rosetting technique, the cells may then be isolated by sedimentation through Ficoll gradients. There are three basic types of rosetting: erythrocyte rosette formation, erythrocyte-antibody rosette formation, and erythrocyte-antibody-complement rosette formation.

Panning. Panning is another technique used to separate lymphocyte subpopulations. The panning technique involves differential adherence of lymphocytes to various solid surfaces coated with antibodies or antigens. Plastic plates sensitized with antibodies or antigens are incubated with the mixture of cells. The cells bind to the sensitizing agents if they have the appropriate receptors; thus, they are separated on the basis of their cell surface properties. MoAbs are often used to separate B lymphocytes and T lymphocytes. A plate coated with anti-Ig or anti-B cell antibodies has B lymphocytes adhering to the plate and T lymphocytes in suspension. A plate coated with anti-T-cell antibodies has T lymphocytes on the plate and B lymphocytes in suspension. The desired subpopulation of lymphocytes

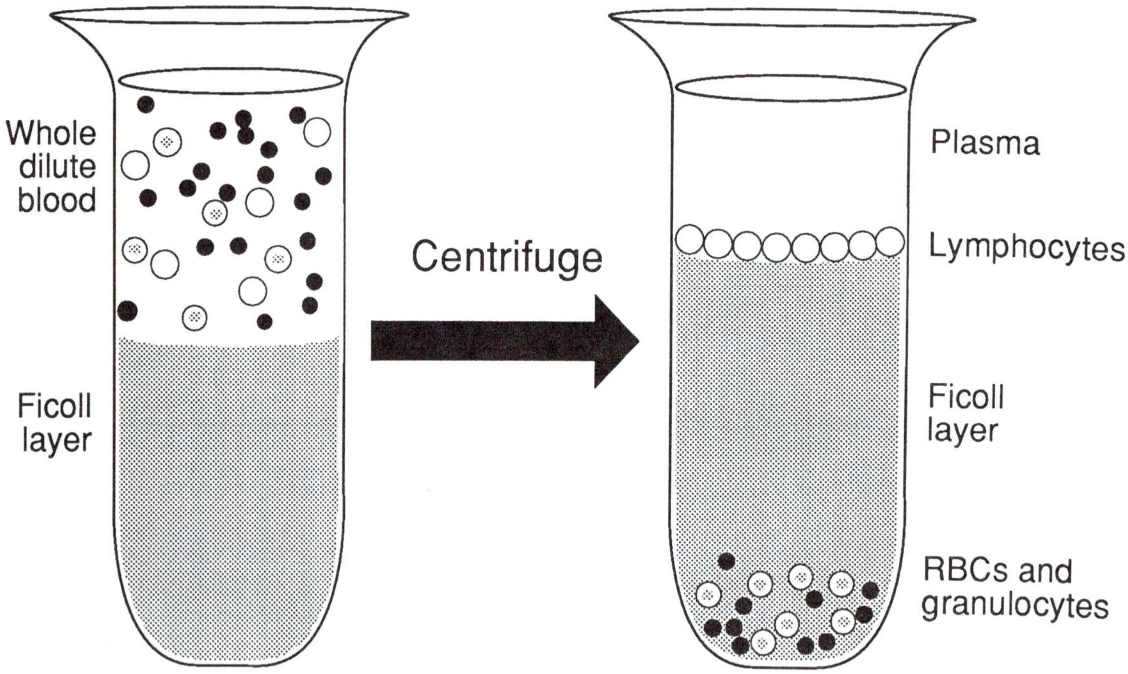

Figure 5-12. Ficoll-Hypaque technique

SOURCE: Adapted from Roitt IM, Brostoff J, Male DK, eds. Immunology. 2nd ed. London: Gower Medical Publishing; 1989:25.10.

may be recovered from the plates by collecting the suspension or by pouring off the suspension and releasing the desired bound lymphocytes by enzymatic treatment.

Flow Cytometer. The flow cytometer or flow microfluorimeter (FMF) is an instrument for analyzing the size, cytoplasmic granularity, and fluorescence intensity of single cells stained with fluorescent dyes or bound by specific fluorescent antibodies.[32] This instrument uses laser and MoAb technology to separate subpopulations of cells. The FMF has many applications in immunologic research and is now being introduced into clinical laboratory immunology for analyzing T lymphocytes, B lymphocytes, and other subsets of lymphocytes. The system by which the FMF isolates, sorts, and counts lymphocytes is illustrated in Figure 5-13.

A single-cell suspension is isolated from blood or other tissue and labeled with either fluorescent antibodies or other fluorochrome dyes. The cells are forced under pressure through a nozzle in a liquid jet surrounded by a sheath of saline or water. The stream of liquid is broken up into a series of droplets by vibration at the tip of the nozzle assembly. The size of the droplets may be regulated so that each droplet contains only one cell.

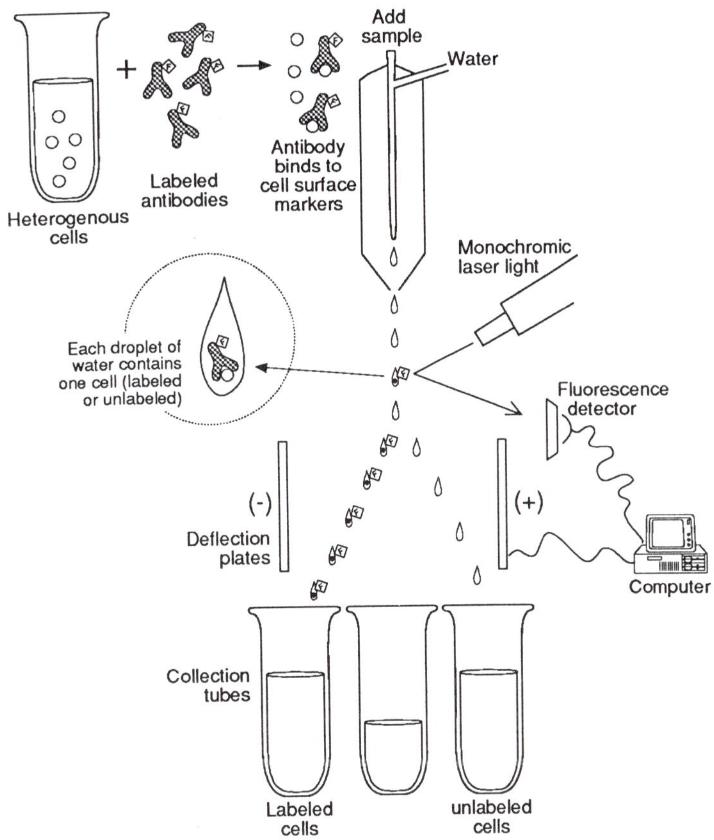

Figure 5-13. Flow cytometer or flow microfluorimeter

SOURCE: Adapted from Golub ES. Immunology: a synthesis. Sunderland, MA; 1987:135.

The droplets are illuminated by the monochromic laser beam and electronically monitored by fluorescence detectors. Droplets with cells that emit appropriate fluorescence signals are electrically charged in a high-voltage field between two deflector plates and may then be sorted into collection tubes. The FMF separates cells rapidly and accurately while preserving their sterility and viability. Once separated, the cells can then be analyzed, cultured, and assayed. The FMF can rapidly process thousands of cells per minute, and measurements can be made by the instrument and stored and analyzed by computer.

Applications

MoAbs conjugated to fluorescent dyes can be prepared for certain receptors on subpopulations of cells; these subpopulations can then be separated and analyzed with the aid of an FMF. In clinical medicine, the

FMF is useful for typing leukemias and lymphomas,[33] looking at T-cell distribution in multiple sclerosis, and studying other diseases that can disturb immunoregulation (e.g., HIV infection). FMF methods may detect alterations in subpopulations of lymphocytes in some diseases that may not be detected by examining the total white blood cells or lymphocytes. Monitoring these slight changes may provide diagnostic or prognostic information or may be useful in determining the effects of pharmacologic treatment.

Many other applications of flow cytometry exist with slight modifications of the basic principles. A newer application of flow cytometry includes analyzing DNA content of cells to quantitiate tumor pathology.[34] Rapidly growing tumors generally contain many cells that are doubling their DNA content. These cells often have abnormal chromosome numbers known as aneuploidy, which can be detected by flow cytometry and often indicate a poor prognosis. Investigators and clinicians are now applying DNA flow cytometry to help determine the prognosis for breast cancer patients.[35] These procedures may be further expanded with labeled MoAbs for tumor surface markers on cells to select and sort these cells for additional investigational studies.

Western Blots

Applications

The Western blot is an immunoblotting method used for identifying specific proteins recognized by antibodies. The Western blot, in contrast to Northern and Southern blotting methods for identifying nucleic acids (RNA and DNA, respectively), is used primarily to identify proteins, but it may also be used to identify carbohydrates. Protein immunoblotting is a powerful tool for analyzing both the antigens of infectious agents and the host's immune response. The method can directly determine which proteins are being recognized by an antibody and may help in the development of vaccines and diagnostic tests. Western blotting is particularly useful in diagnosing HIV-1 infection. Other applications of Western blotting include tests for antibodies against such viruses as herpes and HIV-2, and for analyzing serologic response in systemic candidiasis.[36,37]

Procedure

The procedure for Western blotting was originally described by Towbin[38] and modified by Burnett.[39] It includes the fractionation of proteins based on molecular weight in sodium dodecyl sulfate-polyacrylamide gel electrophoresis (SDS-PAGE), and the electrophoretic transfer of the protein from the SDS polyacrylamide gels to membrane sheets such as unmodified nitrocellulose, which act as an immunoblotting matrix. These immobilized proteins are allowed to react with specific antibodies; then, secondary radiolabeled antibody or radioiodinated staphylococcal protein A binds to the immune complexes. The membrane is then air dried, and autoradiography with X-ray film is performed to visualize the denatured antigen protein.

HIV testing

Currently, the Western blot technique finds greatest commercial use as a confirmation test for diagnosing or validating HIV-1 infections.[40] This application of the technique has been compared with other retrovirus serologic tests including ELISA and immunofluorescence assay.[41,42] The Western blot has demonstrated greater than 99% sensitivity and specificity for HIV-1 proteins, but the technique is time-consuming and labor-intensive, and it relies on subjective interpretation of the banding patterns of the viral proteins. The Western blot is a useful tool to confirm the diagnosis of the deadly HIV-1 virus. False positives are possible, and careful interpretation of band patterns is critical to avoid distressing the patient with an incorrect diagnosis.[43]

The immunoblotting technique is being used to advance the understanding of autoimmune diseases and allergies. Nuclear antigens such as Sm and ribonucleoprotein (RNP) are being investigated by immunoblotting.[44] Anti-RNP antibodies are associated with mixed connective tissue diseases, while Sm antibodies are associated with systemic lupus erythematosus. Immunoblotting has also facilitated the identification and quantitation of IgE and other immunoglobulins against specific allergens. These applications and others, along with modifications to amplify the sensitivity of immunoblotting, have increased the use of the technique in both immunology research and clinical medicine.[45]

Summary

Immunologic tests for detecting antibodies or antigens include precipitation tests, agglutination tests, a complement fixation test, and applied immunoassays. They may be used to obtain quantitative or qualitative results.

Precipitation test methods include immunoelectrophoresis (IEP), radial immunodiffusion, and double immunodiffusion. Agglutination test methods, which may be classified as either direct or indirect, are generally more sensitive than precipitation methods.

Immunoassays may be competitive or noncompetitive. The classic radioimmunoassay (RIA) and enzyme-multiplied immunoassay technique (EMIT) are examples of competitive immunoassays. The immunoradiometric assay (IRMA) and enzyme-linked immunosorbent assay (ELISA) are examples of noncompetitive immunoassays. The fluorescence immunoassay (FIA) may be competitive or noncompetitive, homogeneous or heterogeneous, and solid or nonsolid. The radioimmunosorbent test (RIST) may be noncompetitive, even though the competitive method is more commonly used. TDx is a type of competitive immunoassay used to monitor drug and hormone levels using a fluorescence-polarized immunoassay (FPIA).

Immunologic separation techniques include affinity chromatography, purification of lymphocyte populations, and Western blot tests. Affinity chromatography is a purification technique that may use monoclonal antibody columns. Lymphocyte purification techniques include Ficoll-Hypaque, rosetting, panning, and the use of the flow cytometer. The Western blot may be used to identify proteins and carbohydrates.

Factors to consider when using these tests are the time required to obtain results, the quantity of sample required, and the relative sensitivity of each test. Immunologic testing and separation techniques are being applied with increasing frequency in clinical medicine.

References

1. Check IJ, Piper M. Quantitation of immunoglobulins. In: Rose NR, Friedman H, Fahely JL, eds. Manual of clinical laboratory immunology. Washington, DC: American Society for Microbiology; 1986:138–51.
2. Ouchterlony O, Nilsson LA. Immunodiffusion and immunoelectrophoresis. In: Weir DM, ed. Handbook of experimental immunology. Oxford, England: Blackwell Scientific Publications; 1978:19.1–19.44.
3. Johnson AM. Immunoprecipitation in gels. In: Rose NR, Friedman H, Fahely JL, eds. Manual of clinical laboratory immunology. Washington, DC: American Society for Microbiology; 1986:14–24.
4. Petz LD, Branch DR. Serological tests for the diagnosis of immune hemolytic anemias. In: McMillan R, ed. Methods in hematology: immune cytopenias. New York: Churchill Livingstone; 1983:9–48.
5. Bast RC, Klug TL, Schaetz LE et al. Monitoring human ovarian carcinoma with a combination CA 125, CA 19-9, and carcinoembrogenic antigen. *Am J Obstet Gyneco.* 1984;149:553–9.
6. Yalow RS, Berson SA. Immunological specificity of human insulin: application to immunoassay of insulin. *J Clin Invest.* 1961;40:2190–8.
7. Neese AL, Soyka LF. Development of a radioimmunoassay for theophylline: applications to studies in premature infants. *Clin Pharmacol Ther.* 1977;21:633–41.
8. Sun L, Spiehler V. Radioimmunoassay and enzyme immunoassay compared for determination of digoxin. *Clinical Chemistry.* 1976;22:2029–31.

9. Sharpe SL, Gorman WM, Blomme WJ et al. Quantitative enzyme immunoassay: current status. *Clinical Chemistry.* 1976;22:733–8.
10. Rubenstein KE. Homogenous enzyme immunoassay today. *Scandinavian Journal of Immunology.* 1987;8:57–62.
11. Schottelius DD. Homogenous immunoassay system (EMIT) for quantitation of antiepileptic drugs in biological fluids. In: Pippenger CE, Penry JK, Kutt H, eds. Quantitative analysis and interpretation. New York: Raven Press; 1978:95–108.
12. Koup JR, Brodsky B. Comparison of homogenous enzyme immunoassay and high pressure liquid chromatography for the determination of theophylline concentrations in serum. *Am Rev Respir Dis.* 1978;117:1135–8.
13. Rosenthal AF, Vargas MG, Klass CS. Evaluation of enzyme-multiplied immunoassay technique (EMIT) for determination of serum digoxin. *Clinical Chemistry.* 1976;22:1899–1902.
14. Atkinson AJ Jr, Ambre JJ. Kalman and Clark's drug assay, the strategy of therapeutic drug monitoring. 2nd ed. New York: Masson Publishing USA; 1984:169–71.
15. Allan LV, Stiles ML. Specificity of the EMIT drug abuse urine assay methods. *Clin Toxicol.* 1981;18:1043–65.
16. McBay AJ. Drug analysis technology pitfalls and problems of drug testing. *Clinical Chemistry.* 1987;32:33B–40B.
17. Nakamura RM, Robbins BA. Analytical fluid-phase fluorescence immunoassay. In: Rose NR, Friedman H, Fahely JL, eds. Manual of clinical laboratory immunology. Washington, DC: American Society for Microbiology; 1986:116–23.
18. Engvall E. Enzyme immunoassay: ELISA and EMIT. *Methods in Enzymology.* 1980;70:419–38.
19. Voller A, Bidwell DE. Enzyme-linked immunosorbent assay. In: Rose NR, Friedman H, Fahely JL, eds. Manual of clinical laboratory immunology. Washington, DC: American Society for Microbiology; 1986:99–109.
20. Nilsson B. A general reaction for amplifying ELISAs. *Journal of Immunological Methods.* 1988;114:89–93.
21. Wognum AW, Lansdorp PM, Eaves AC et al. An enzyme-linked immunosorbent assay for erythropoietin using monoclonal antibodies, tetrameric immune complexes, and substrate amplification. *Blood.* 1989;74:622–8.
22. Weiss SH, Goedert JJ, Sarngadharan MG et al. Screening test for HTLV III (AIDS agent) antibodies. *JAMA.* 1985;253:221–5.
23. Carlson JR, Hinrichs SH, Yee J et al. Evaluation of three commercial screening tests for AIDS virus antibodies. *Am J Clin Pathol.* 1986;86:357–9.

24. Smith KO, Ludwig MJ, Stigall BW et al. Enzyme-linked immunosorbent assay (ELISA) for HIV antibody by a glass slide technique. *Journal of Immunological Methods.* 1991; 136:239–46.
25. Jolley ME. Fluorescence polarization immunoassay for the determination of therapeutic drug levels in human plasma. *Journal of Analytical Toxicology.* 1981;5:236–40.
26. Jolley ME, Stroupe SD, Wang CJ et al. Fluorescence polarization immunoassay I: monitoring aminoglycoside antibiotics in serum and plasma. *Clinical Chemistry.* 1981;27:1190–7.
27. Lu-Sleffes M, Pittluck GW, Jolley ME et al. Fluorescence polarization immunoassay IV: determination of phenytoin and phenobarbital in human serum and plasma. *Clinical Chemistry.* 1982;28:2278–82.
28. Hill HD, Jolley ME, Wang CJ et al. Fluorescence polarization immunoassay (FPIA) for theophylline: clinical correlation and reagent stability. *Clinical Chemistry.* 1981;27:1086. Abstract.
29. Secher DS, Burke DC. A monoclonal antibody for large-scale purification of human leukocyte interferon. *Nature.* 1980;285:446–50.
30. Brettler DB, Fosber AD, Levine PH et al. Factor VIII: C concentration purified from plasma using monoclonal antibodies: human studies. *Blood.* 1989;73:1859–63.
31. Rowlands DT, Whiteside TL, Daniele RP. Cells of the immune system. In: Henry JB, ed. Todd, Stanford, Davison: clinical diagnosis and management by laboratory methods. 17th ed. Philadelphia: W.B. Saunders Company; 1984:835–7.
32. Jackson AL, Warner NW. Preparation, staining, and analysis by flow cytometry of peripheral blood leukocytes. In: Rose NR, Friedman H, Fahely JL, eds. Manual of clinical laboratory immunology. Washington, DC: American Society for Microbiology; 1986:226–35.
33. Carey L. Flow cytometric immunoassays of leukemia and lymphoma. *Journal of Clinical Immunoassay.* 1989;12:21–8.
34. Gansler T. Applications of flow cytometric DNA quantitation in tumor pathology. *Journal of Clinical Immunoassay.* 1989;12:30–5.
35. Clark GM, Dressler LG, Owens MA et al. Prediction of relapse or survival in patients with node-negative breast cancer by DNA flow cytometry. *N Eng J Med.* 1989;320:627–33.
36. Towbin H, Gordon J. Immunoblotting and dot immunobinding: current status and outlook. *Journal of Immunological Methods.* 1984;72:313–40.
37. Matthews RC, Burnie JB, Tabaqchali S. Immunoblot analysis of serologic response in systemic candidiasis. *Lancet.* 1984;2:1415–8.
38. Towbin H, Staehelin T, Gordon J. Electrophoretic transfer of proteins from polyacrylamide gels to nitrocellulose sheets: procedures and some applications. *Proc Natl Acad Sci USA.* 1979;76:4350–4.

39. Burnett NW. "Western blotting": electrophoretic transfer of proteins from sodium dodecyl sulfate-polyacrylamide gels to unmodified nitrocellulose and radiographic detection with antibody and radioiodinated protein A. *Analytical Biochemistry.* 1981;112:195–203.
40. Sever JL, Madden DL. Serologic tests for AIDS. *Clinical Immunology Newsletter.* 1986;7:137–40.
41. Gallo D, Diggs JL, Sheil GR et al. Comparison of detection of antibody to the acquired immune deficiency syndrome virus by enzyme immunoassay, immunofluorescence, and Western blot methods. *Journal of Clinical Microbiology.* 1986;23:1049–51.
42. Ward JW, Grindona J, Feorino PM et al. Laboratory and epidemiology evaluation of an enzyme immunoassay for antibodies to HTLV-III. *JAMA.* 1986;256:351–61.
43. Zolla-Pazner S, Gornay NK, Honnen WJ et al. Reinterpretation of human immunodeficiency virus western blot patterns. *N Eng J Med.* 1989;320:1280–1.
44. Combe B, Rucheton M, Graffland H et al. Clinical significance of anti-RNP and anti-Sm autoantibodies as determined by immunoblotting and immunoprecipitation in sera from patients with connective tissue diseases. *Clinical Experimental Immunology.* 1989;75:18–24.
45. Stott DI. Immunoblotting and dot blotting. *Journal of Immunological Methods.* 1989;119:153–87.

Suggested Reading

Buffone GJ. Principles of immunochemical techniques. In: Tietz NW, ed. Fundamentals of clinical chemistry. 3rd ed. Philadelphia: W. B. Saunders Company; 1987:144–59.

Dalchau R, Fabre JW. Monoclonal antibodies and immunochemistry. In: Beverly PCL, ed. Methods in hematology: monoclonal antibodies. New York: Churchill Livingstone; 1986:34–59.

Melamed MR, Lindmo T, Mendelson ML, eds. Flow cytometry and sorting. 2nd ed. New York: Wiley-Liss; 1990:660–802.

Miller LE, Ludke HR, Peacock JE, eds. Manual of laboratory immunology. 2nd ed. Philadelphia: Lea and Febiger; 1991.

Rose NR, Friedman H, Fahely JL, eds. Manual of clinical laboratory immunology. 3rd ed. Washington, DC: American Society of Microbiology; 1986.

Stites DP, Rodgers RPC. Clinical laboratory methods for detection of antigens and antibodies. In: Stites DP, Terri AI, eds. Basic and clinical immunology. 7th ed. Norwalk, CT: Appleton and Lange; 1991:217–62.

Tietz NW, ed. Clinical guide to laboratory tests. 2nd ed. Philadelphia: W. B. Saunders Company; 1990.

Virella G. Immunoserology and diagnostic immunochemistry. In: Virella G, Goust JM, Fundenber HA, eds. Introduction to medical immunology. New York: Marcel Dekker; 1986:225–45.

Self-Study Questions

1. What does IEP stand for?

   1. Immuno-electrophoresis.

2. What does RIA stand for?

   2. Radioimmunoassay.

3. What type of immunologic test is the Coombs?

   A. Precipitation test.
   B. Agglutination test.
   C. Complement fixation.
   D. Immunoassay.

   3. B

4. What type of immunologic test is the Wasserman?

   A. Precipitation test.
   B. Agglutination test.
   C. Complement fixation.
   D. Immunoassay.

   4. C

5. Which of the following immunologic tests detects antibody-antigen complexes photometrically?

   A. ELISA.
   B. FIA.
   C. IEP.
   D. IRMA.

   5. B

6. Which of the following immunologic tests gives results by a color formation proportional to the amount of antibody in the sample?

   A. ELISA.
   B. FIA.
   C. RIST.
   D. IEP.

   6. A

7. Which immunologic test is seldom used by laboratories due to the need for excellent technical skills?

   A. RIST.
   B. FIA.
   C. ELISA.
   D. RID.

   7. D

8. C

8. Which immunologic test is the least sensitive of the gel and agar tests?

A. RIST.
B. IRMA.
C. IEP.
D. RID.

9. D

9. Which immunologic testing method or test should be used for initially detecting antibodies against the human immunodeficiency virus?

A. Complement fixation.
B. Direct hemagglutination.
C. Indirect hemagglutination.
D. Enzyme-linked immunosorbent assay.

10. D

10. Which immunologic test should be used to detect the ovarian carcinoma tumor marker CA 125 in the serum?

A. ELISA.
B. RIA.
C. FIA.
D. IRMA.

11. A

11. A Western blot is an immunoblotting method used primarily to identify which of the following?

A. Proteins.
B. DNA.
C. RNA.
D. Toxic substances.

12. A

12. Which separation technique is being used to help determine the prognosis of breast cancer?

A. Flow cytometer.
B. Ficoll-Hypaque.
C. Rosetting.
D. Panning.

CHAPTER 6

Autoimmune and Immunodeficiency Disease

Jeffrey C. Delafuente, M.S.
Associate Professor and Associate Chairman
Department of Pharmacy Practice, College of Pharmacy, and
Associate Professor
Division of Clinical Immunology, Rheumatology, and Allergy
Department of Medicine, College of Medicine
University of Florida
Gainesville, FL

Introduction

The immune system is designed to provide a complex response to an antigenic challenge. When it functions as it should, the immune system prevents and fights disease. However, sometimes the immune response does not function properly and mistakes self for nonself tissue. Autoimmune disease is a disorder caused by an immune response directed at self antigens, causing the immune system to attack the patient's tissues. Immunodeficiency diseases are characterized by abnormally low immune responses, resulting in chronic opportunistic infections.

Autoimmune diseases are common, and the pharmacist needs to understand the pathophysiology involved with these diseases in order to select appropriate drug therapies. There are many new immunotherapies on the horizon that will make rational therapeutic interventions more complex in treating these disorders.

Learning Objectives

After reading this chapter, the learner will be able to—

- Describe pathogenic mechanisms involved in autoimmunity.
- Describe therapeutic agents for autoimmune diseases.
- Describe treatment modalities for antibody and cellular deficiencies.
- List physical conditions that can impair the immune function.

Chapter Organization

This chapter presents an introductory description of autoimmunity and its possible causes. A discussion of the immunopathologic mechanisms and treatment of autoimmune diseases follows. Immunodeficiency diseases are introduced next with a discussion of antibody and cellular deficiency diseases and their therapies. Last, the chapter provides information about risk factors associated with secondary immunodeficiency diseases.

Suggested Preparation

To maximize learning, it is recommended that the user read Chapters 1 through 4 of this text before beginning this chapter.

Autoimmunity

Autoimmune diseases are caused by immunopathologic mechanisms that are destructive to host tissue. There are many autoimmune diseases; some affect a single organ or tissue site, whereas others have multisystem effects. Treatment for these diseases varies depending on clinical manifestations and may range from simple nonsteroidal anti-inflammatory agents to potent immunosuppressive drugs.

Mechanism

Autoimmunity is the process of developing an immune response to self antigens (autoantigens). In the past two decades numerous investigators have repeatedly shown that the generation of sensitized T lymphocytes and immunoglobulins (antibodies) that are reactive to autoantigens is a normal process. This type of autoreactivity is necessary for T-lymphocyte receptors to recognize host major histocompatibility complex (MHC) antigens on macrophages to initiate both humoral and cellular immune responses to foreign antigens (see Chapter 3). Other cell-cell interactions also require recognition of self antigens to produce a proper immune response. Idiotypic and anti-idiotypic antibodies are required for immunoregulation and maintenance of homeostasis. Anti-idiotypes are antibodies reactive to the antigen-binding Fab portion of an immunoglobulin; in other words, antibodies against antibodies. Autoreactive sensitized cells to host MHC antigens and anti-idiotypic antibodies are beneficial forms of autoimmunity. Autoimmune diseases occur when there is uncontrolled production of autoantibodies or development of excessive autoreactive T lymphocytes resulting in tissue injury.

There are numerous autoimmune diseases and a wide spectrum of clinical manifestations. An autoimmune disease may be organ specific, affecting only one tissue or organ site (as in myasthenia gravis) or non-organ specific, causing systemic manifestations (as in systemic lupus erythematosus [SLE]). The autoantigens and pathogenetics involved in these myriad diseases may vary among different disease processes. Table 6-1 lists some of the autoimmune diseases and associated autoantigens. No attempt is made in this chapter to describe each of these diseases in detail. Where applicable, selected diseases are used as examples to discuss research findings.

Table 6-1 Autoantigens Associated with Diseases

Autoimmune Diseases	Autoantigen
	Intracellular
SLE, chronic active hepatitis, Sjögren's syndrome	DNA
SLE, Sjögren's syndrome	RNA
SLE, PSS, polymyositis	Nucleolus
SLE, PSS, polymyositis, mixed connective tissue disease	Sm-RNA
	Membrane receptors
Graves' disease (stimulates), autoimmune thyroiditis (blocks)	Thyrotropin
Myasthenia gravis (blocks)	Acetylcholine receptor
IDDM (blocks)	Insulin receptor
	Cell membranes
Autoimmune hemolytic anemia, SLE	Red blood cells
SLE	Lymphocytes
Autoimmune neutropenia, SLE	Neutrophils
ITP, SLE	Platelets
Polymyositis, RA, SLE	Muscle
IDDM	Islet cells
	Plasma Proteins
RA, SLE, Sjögren's syndrome	Immunoglobulins
SLE, RA	Complement
SLE	Clotting factors
	Hormones
IDDM	Insulin
Autoimmune thyroiditis	Thyroid hormones
IDDM	Glucagon
Pernicious anemia	Intrinsic factor

SOURCE: Adapted from Smith HR, Steinberg AD. Autoimmunity—a perspective. *Annual Review of Immunology*. 1983;1:175–210.

IDDM = insulin-dependent diabetes mellitus; ITP = idiopathic thrombocytopenia purpura; PSS = progressive systemic sclerosis; RA = rheumatoid arthritis; SLE = systemic lupus erythematosus.

Causes

There is no single concept to explain the causes and pathogenesis of the autoimmune diseases. Numerous theories have been generated and tested for many decades, and it is clear that the development of autoimmune diseases involves genetic, hormonal, infectious, immunologic, environmental, and other factors acting singly or in combination.[1] Some of the more substantiated theories are discussed in this chapter.

Genetic Factors. Data from inbred strains of animals unequivocally show that there is a genetic predisposition to the development of certain autoimmune diseases. In humans the data are not as convincing. That some families have a greater incidence of autoimmune disease than others suggests a genetic relationship to disease development.[2] In humans, there are correlations to certain autoimmune diseases and specific human leukocyte antigens (HLAs), particularly the D gene locus, which is closely linked to immune response (Ir) genes (see Chapter 3). Since Ir genes determine how an individual reacts to a foreign antigen, it is quite conceivable that they also determine how an individual reacts to autoantigens and, hence, disease susceptibility.[3] Table 6-2 lists HLA antigens associated with selected autoimmune diseases. The association of a particular HLA gene and an autoimmune disease does not necessarily mean that the gene is responsible for the disease. Many people have an associated HLA antigen and never develop the disease, and some people with a particular disease may not have the associated HLA antigen. However, possessing an associated HLA gene may predispose an individual to a disease, although perhaps only in combination with other etiologic factors. For example, in insulin-dependent diabetes mellitus (IDDM), with which HLA antigens are associated, a surprising discordance rate is found in identical twins, strongly suggesting that contributing environmental factors may also have a role in disease susceptibility.[4] (See Chapter 3.)

Ir genes

Estrogen risk

Hormonal Factors. Sex hormones may play a role in the development of some autoimmune diseases. Many autoimmune diseases such as rheumatoid arthritis, Graves' disease, and SLE are much more prevalent in females. In animal models of SLE, estrogens have been shown to enhance disease development, whereas androgens inhibit the expression of autoimmunity.[5] The exact role of sex hormones in human autoimmune diseases still needs to be determined.

Infectious Factors. Viral infections have been implicated in certain autoimmune diseases. Viruses may alter normal cell surface antigens, making them immunogenic. MHC antigens are likely targets in virus-infected cells, forming viral complexes that may serve as autoantigens.[2] Viruses may also induce expression of antigens normally repressed in host cells.[2] Infectious causes have been suggested in IDDM,

Table 6-2 Selected Autoimmune Diseases and Associated HLA Antigens

Disease	Associated HLA
Rheumatoid arthritis	Dw4, DR4
Systemic lupus erythematosus	DR2, DR3
Polymositis	DR3, DRw6
Sjögren's syndrome	DR2, DR3
Insulin-dependent diabetes mellitus	DR3, DR4
Hashimoto's thyroiditis	DR3, DR5
Graves' disease	DR3
Multiple sclerosis	DR2
Ankylosing spondylitis	B27

multiple sclerosis (MS), rheumatoid arthritis, SLE, and other autoimmune diseases.[4,6–8]

Epstein-Barr virus

The Epstein-Barr virus (EBV) has been associated with diseases such as rheumatoid arthritis. This virus may be important in autoimmunity because it is ubiquitous and persistent and it can modulate the immune system.[8] EBV is a polyclonal activator of B lymphocytes, capable of inducing DNA synthesis, mitosis, and immunoglobulin secretion in B cells, including synthesis of autoantibodies.[7] Although evidence suggests that EBV may be involved in the pathogenesis of autoimmune diseases, no direct connection has been proved.

That people have EBV infections such as mononucleosis yet never develop rheumatoid arthritis or other autoimmune diseases suggests that the virus is not the only factor involved in development of autoimmune disease. Other viruses have also been implicated as causative agents in human autoimmunity: myxoviruses, hepatitis viruses, cytomegaloviruses, coxsackieviruses, retroviruses, and others.[8]

Immune Factors. Host immunologic factors have a major role in autoimmune diseases. Many theories have been proposed to explain the role of the immune system in autoimmunity pathogenesis. A few of the more feasible theories are discussed here.

Sequestered Antigens. An immune response to most autoantigens does not occur under normal conditions because of tolerance to those antigens. Tolerance to autoantigens occurs during embryonic development of the immune system, when autoantigens are in contact with developing immunoregulating mechanisms. However, some autoantigens do not normally come in contact with the immune system; when they do, these sequestered antigens may be seen as foreign. Autoantibodies are found in instances of tissue injury in which sequestered antigens become exposed to circulating T and B lymphocytes. For example, antibodies to sperm are detected after vasectomy. Also, antibodies to proteins of the crystalline lens have been found after eye injury, and antibodies to heart muscle antigens may occur after a myocardial infarction.[8] In all of these examples, the antigens eliciting an antibody response do not normally come in contact with immunocompetent cells. The autoantibody response usually subsides after tissue repair, and no sustained autoimmune pathology occurs.

Defective cells

Immunoregulatory T Cells. Numerous investigations have been conducted into the role of defective suppressor or helper T cells. Although defects in immunoregulation have been demonstrated in human autoimmune diseases, their role in autoimmunity is controversial. It seems likely that uncontrolled helper T-cell activity could result in the excessive generation of autoantibodies. Some animal models have demonstrated that helper T cells are the primary mediators of autoimmunity.[9] Likewise, diminished suppressor T-cell function could also account for disease activity. There is a correlation between suppressor T-cell activity and disease exacerbation in multiple sclerosis, suggesting that immunoregulation contributes to the pathogenesis. During periods of disease activity there are decreases in the number of suppressor T cells and suppressor function.[6,10] Similar correlations between suppressor T-cell function and active disease have also been identified in SLE and rheumatoid arthritis.[11,12] The loss of suppressor cell function in SLE may be due to an IgG antisuppressor T-cell antibody.[13]

Cross-reacting Antigens. Another reason for autoimmunity may involve cross-reactivity between exogenous and autologous antigens. The possibility exists that complex foreign antigens may share an epitope (antigenic determinant) with the host tissue, resulting in cross-reactivity. A clinical example is rheumatic fever, a disease occurring after group A streptococcal pharyngitis. Patients with acute rheumatic fever may develop serum antibodies against group A streptococcal antigens that cross-react with antigens on organs affected by rheumatic fever (e.g., myocardium, heart valves, joint capsules).[3] In vitro experiments have shown that T lymphocytes sensitized to streptococcal antigens are cytotoxic for cardiac cells, lending further evidence that cross-reacting antigens are a cause of an autoimmune disease.[3] More than 90% of individuals with ankylosing spondylitis have the HLA-B27 gene. In ankylosing spondylitis, homology between amino acid sequences on the HLA-B27 molecule and various bacterial proteins has been identified, suggesting a possible cross-reacting link in this disease process.[14] When a microorganism elicits an immune response that cross-reacts with host constituents the process is known as molecular mimicry.

Immunopathologic Mechanisms

The immunopathologic mechanisms of tissue injury in autoimmune disease are described by Coombs and Gell.[15] Most autoimmune diseases involve IgG or IgM autoantibodies and elicit either type II or type III hypersensitivity reactions (see Chapter 4).

Type I

Type I hypersensitivity reactions probably do not have a significant role in autoimmunity. However, IgE and mast cells have been implicated in some autoimmune diseases. Mast cells are believed to be involved in the pathogenesis of progressive systemic sclerosis, an autoimmune disease characterized by serum antinuclear antibodies and often seen in association with other autoimmune diseases.[16] Mast cells may also have a role in joint inflammation of rheumatoid arthritis.[17] IgE rheumatoid factor (IgE anti-IgG) has been isolated from synovial fluid in patients with rheumatoid arthritis and can cause in vitro mast cell degranulation when binding to IgG.[18]

Type II

Cytotoxic antibodies mediating type II reactions are commonly found in autoimmune diseases. These reactions are responsible for clinical entities such as autoimmune hemolytic anemia, thrombocytopenia, neutropenia, and destruction of other formed elements of the blood. The endocrine system is particularly susceptible to autoimmune phenomena.[19] Autoantibodies to pancreatic beta cells are believed to be responsible for beta cell destruction resulting in diabetes mellitus. Autoantibodies can also bind to cell receptors to cause other disease. For example, Graves' disease is manifested by autoantibodies to thyroid-stimulating hormone (TSH) receptors. These antibodies mimic the actions of TSH, activating the receptors to produce symptoms of hyperthyroidism.[20] In myasthenia gravis, antibodies are produced to nicotinic acetylcholine receptors. Antibodies binding to these receptors block the actions of acetylcholine and result in muscle weakness.[20]

Type III

Immune complexes, which are responsible for type III hypersensitivity reactions, are common to many autoimmune diseases. For example, DNA-anti-DNA complexes are frequently found in sera of patients with SLE, and immune complexes containing anti-IgG antibodies are prevalent in rheumatoid arthritis sera.[21] The multisystem involvement of these diseases reflects deposition of circulating immune complexes into various tissues as well as local production of immune complexes at the site of tissue injury.[22]

Type IV

Type IV hypersensitivity reactions may account for some pathology in autoimmunity. Animal models have shown that sensitizing T cells to autoantigens results in autoimmune diseases.[23] In Hashimoto's thyroiditis, intradermal injection of thyroglobulin causes a type IV reaction, suggesting a lymphocyte-mediated pathogenesis.[23] Circulating activated T lymphocytes are found in IDDM, Graves' disease, and MS.[24,25] Activated T cells are also present in the lesions of affected target areas, such as the synovium in rheumatoid arthritis and the pancreas in diabetes mellitus. Because autoantibodies are often found in conjunction with sensitized T cells, it is difficult to know which pathologic mechanism predominates in disease activity; however, both are probably important.

Treatment of Autoimmune Diseases

Anti-inflammatory and immuno-suppressive drugs

The treatment of autoimmune diseases varies depending on the disease and clinical manifestations. Therapy may range from simple analgesics in rheumatoid arthritis to high-dose corticosteroids or cytotoxic drugs for life-threatening manifestations of SLE. In general, anti-inflammatory and immunosuppressive drugs are the cornerstone to pharmacologic management of autoimmune diseases. Commonly used agents include nonsteroidal anti-inflammatory drugs, corticosteroids, gold compounds, hydroxychloroquine, and cytotoxic drugs such as cyclophosphamide, azathioprine, and methotrexate. Immunosuppressive agents such as cyclosporine look promising for these diseases. All these drugs interfere with the inflammatory response, some affecting predominately humoral immunity and some affecting cellular immunity. Immunosuppressive therapy has induced remission in IDDM, SLE, rheumatoid arthritis, MS, and other autoimmune diseases.[25-29]

A better understanding of the mechanisms involved in immune responses has led to new types of therapy for autoimmune diseases. Recent advances in biotechnology have identified and cloned numerous cytokines as well as determined cellular receptors involved in immune responses. These discoveries will greatly influence the way autoimmune diseases are treated in the 21st century.

New therapies

An example of new therapies being studied is the use of an anti-CD4 antibody in the treatment of rheumatoid arthritis. Preliminary data showed that injection of these monoclonal anti-CD4 antibodies improved clinical symptoms and laboratory parameters of inflammation in patients with severe disease not responsive to conventional drug therapy.[30] Other possible new modes of therapy may include (1) monoclonal antibodies against a particular T-cell clone (a unique T-cell subset) involved in the autoimmune process and (2) antibodies to cytokines or their receptors.[31] Designing therapy that suppresses only the aberrant immune response involved in the autoimmune pathogenesis appears to be on the horizon. This type of therapy would be extremely advantageous over current pharmacotherapy, which nonspecifically suppresses all immune responses, leading to infection and other complications.

Primary Immunodeficiency Diseases

The causes of immunodeficiency diseases may be either primary, (i.e., intrinsic) or secondary (i.e., resulting from an external source). The primary immunodeficiencies are rare and may involve only humoral immunity, cellular immunity, or both.

Classification

Immunodeficiencies are a diverse group of diseases with varying pathogeneses, causes, and clinical manifestations. More than 20 different forms of primary immunodeficiencies have been recognized since the first human immunodeficiency disease was described in 1952.[32] The World Health Organization has classified the primary immunodeficiency diseases into three major categories: predominantly antibody deficiencies, combined immunodeficiency, and immunodeficiencies associated with other major defects.[33] Tables 6-3, 6-4, and 6-5 list some diseases in these categories. The pathogenesis for most of these diseases remains unknown, although the functional and cellular abnormalities of the various immunodeficiencies are well characterized. None of these diseases has been associated with any HLA antigen, although many of the immunodeficiency diseases are associated with the X chromosome and therefore occur mostly in males.[34]

An exact incidence for the various immunodeficiency diseases is not known. Fortunately, these serious and often fatal diseases are rare. A few of the more common immunodeficiencies are discussed in this chapter, but even these diseases are quite rare.

Antibody Deficiency Diseases

Antibody deficiency diseases may be either congenital or acquired disorders, with deficiencies of all immunoglobulin classes or in just one class or subclass of immunoglobulin. The inability to form an antibody against a specific antigen or the absence of a subclass of immunoglobulin may be seen in patients with normal total serum immunoglobulin concentrations. Clinical attributes may range from severe recurrent pyogenic bacterial infections, as seen in X-linked agammaglobulinemia, to asymptomatic, as in many patients with selective IgA deficiency.

Table 6-3 Predominantly Antibody Deficiencies

Disorder	Functional Deficiencies	Presumed Pathogenesis	Inheritance
X-linked agammaglobulinemia	↓ all Ig isotypes	Defect in pre-B cell to B-cell differentiation	
IgA deficiency	↓ IgA	Failure of terminal differentiation	AR, unknown
Selective IgM deficiency	↓ IgM	Abnormal helper T cells	Unknown
Ig deficiency with ↑ IgM	↑ IgM, ↓ all other isotypes	Isotype switch defect	X-linked, AR, unknown
Immunodeficiency with thymoma	↓ all Ig isotypes	↑ suppressor T cells, B-cell defects	Unknown
Transient hypogammaglobulinemia of infancy	↓ IgG, ↓ IgA	Cellular maturation defect, ↓ helper T cells in some	Unknown

SOURCE: Adapted from the following: (1) Anon. Primary immunodeficiency diseases: report of a World Health Organization Scientific Group. *Clinical Immunology and Immunopathology.* 1986;40:161–96. (2) Buckley RH. Immunodeficiency diseases. *JAMA.* 1987;258:2841–50.

AR = autosomal recessive; ↓ = decreased; ↑ = increased.

Table 6-4 Combined Immunodeficiencies

Disorder	Functional Deficiencies	Presumed Pathogenesis	Inheritance
Common variable immunodeficiency	↓ various Ig isotypes, ↓ T cells	B-cell defect, ↓ helper T cell ↑ suppressor T-cell function, ↓ T-cell numbers	AR, AD, unknown AR, unknown
Severe combined immunodeficiency	↓ Ig, ↓ B cells, ↓ T cells	Defective T- and B-cell differentiation	AR
Nezelof's syndrome	↓ T cells	Abnormal thymus architecture	AR, X-linked

SOURCE: Adapted from the following: (1) Anon. Primary immunodeficiency diseases: report of a World Health Organization Scientific Group. *Clinical Immunology and Immunopathology.* 1986;40:161–96. (2) Buckley RH. Immunodeficiency diseases. *JAMA.* 1987;258:2841–50.

AD = autosomal dominant; AR = autosomal recessive; ↓ = decreased; ↑ = increased.

Clinical features

Common clinical features of antibody deficiencies are recurrent pyogenic infections with encapsulated bacteria, chronic sinopulmonary problems, enteroviral infections, and low or absent antibodies in serum and secretions. B cells may be present in circulation.

Table 6-5 Immunodeficiencies Associated with Other Major Defects

Disorder	Functional Deficiencies	Presumed Pathogenesis	Inheritance	Major Defects
Wiskott-Aldrich syndrome	↓ IgM, ↓ T cells	Cell membrane defect affecting stem cell derivatives	X-linked	Thrombocytopenia, eczema
Ataxia telangiectasia	↓ IgA, ↓ IgE, ↓ IgG, ↑ IgM	Unknown	AR	Cerebellar ataxia, ovarian dysgenesis, chromosomal instability
DiGeorge's syndrome	↓T cells, some ↓Ig	Abnormal thymus	Unknown	Hypoparathyroidism, cardiac malformation, abnormal facies

SOURCE: Adapted from the following: (1) Anon. Primary immunodeficiency diseases: report of a World Health Organization Scientific Group. *Clinical Immunology and Immunopathology.* 1986;40:161–96; (2) Buckley RH. Immunodeficiency diseases. *JAMA.* 1987;258:2841–50.

AR = autosomal recessive; ↓ = decreased; ↑ = increased.

X-linked Agammaglobulinemia. This disease is also known as Bruton's disease and congenital, infantile, or sex-linked agammaglobulinemia. The term *agammaglobulinemia* is a misnomer, because small amounts of serum immunoglobulins are usually detectable. Affected infants usually do well during the first 6 to 9 months of life, because maternal antibodies are still present. Recurrent pyogenic infections begin to appear during infancy and early childhood as maternal antibody levels decrease. Common infectious bacteria include pneumococci, streptococci, and Haemophilus.[34,35] Sinusitis, pneumonia, otitis, furunculosis, meningitis, and septicemia are common types of infections. Chronic viral and fungal infections are not usually a problem, since cellular immunity remains functional.[35] These patients are at risk for developing vaccine-associated poliomyelitis and infections from certain enteric pathogens, such as echoviruses and *Giardia lamblia.*[36] X-linked agammaglobulinemia occurs only in males. The diagnosis is suspected if serum IgA, IgG, and IgM are less than the 95% confidence limits for age- and race-matched controls.[35] A block in the maturation of pre-B cells to B cells appears to be the pathogenetic defect.[36] Normal numbers of pre-B cells are found in bone marrow, but there are few B cells in peripheral circulation.[35] Prognosis is good if immunoglobulin replacement therapy is initiated early.

Common Variable Agammaglobulinemia. This deficiency is also known as agammaglobulinemia with immunoglobulin-bearing B lymphocytes, idiopathic late-onset immunoglobulin deficiency, and common variable immunodeficiency. This immunodeficiency can occur at any age in both males and females.[36] Its clinical presentation may be similar to that of X-linked agammaglobulinemia. In common variable immunodeficiency there is a high incidence of gastrointestinal abnormalities often due to *G. lamblia* and gastrointestinal tumors. Recurrent bacterial infections of the sinuses and respiratory tract are common; frequently involved organisms include *Haemophilus influenzae, Pneumococcus pneumoniae, Streptococcus pyogenes,* and *Staphylococcus aureus.*[37] Pernicious anemia is a common feature, and bronchiectasis and lymphoreticular malignancies may also be concomitant diseases.

Normal numbers of circulating B lymphocytes are usually seen in common variable agammaglobulinemia, although some patients may have decreased B-cell numbers. As implied in the name of the disease, variable pathogenetic mechanisms are responsible for this immunodeficiency. The major defect is in the differentiation of mature B lymphocytes into antibody-secreting plasma cells.[35] Abnormal regulatory T lymphocyte function may be a factor in some patients, with either an abnormality in helper T cells or overactive suppressor T cells.[36,38,39] Autoantibodies to lymphocytes may also be involved with this disease.[37]

Selective IgA Deficiency. The most common immunodeficiency in humans is selective IgA deficiency; the frequency is approximately 1 in 300 to 1 in 3,040 people.[37] Many people are unaware that they have abnormally low serum IgA concentrations because they never develop any signs or symptoms of this disorder. Infections of the respiratory, gastrointestinal, and genitourinary tracts predominate in symptomatic patients. Encapsulated bacteria are usually responsible for recurrent infections; IgA may prevent bacteria from attaching to mucosal surfaces. There is no evidence for increased susceptibility to viral infections. IgA deficiency may be associated with certain autoimmune diseases, such as rheumatoid arthritis, SLE, pernicious anemia, and thyroiditis.[40] It is not known why some individuals with this deficiency remain healthy while others become seriously ill.

Blood product risk

There is no specific therapy for IgA deficiency other than appropriate treatment for concomitant infections. Replacing serum IgA is not useful, because it is not transported into secretions. Many of these patients have antibodies directed against IgA.[41] These patients should not receive any blood products containing IgA, because fatal anaphylactic reactions can occur. Selective IgA deficiency may involve both subclasses of IgA: IgA1 and IgA2. Abnormalities in both subclasses are sometimes accompanied by decreases in the IgG subclasses IgG2, IgG3, or IgG4. In addition, IgA deficiency may occur, with only a single subclass of IgA being markedly decreased or absent.

Therapy for Antibody Deficiencies

Goal

The primary goal of therapy for immunoglobulin deficiencies is to control the frequency and severity of acute infections. Prophylactic long-term antibiotics may be needed for selected patients. The mainstay of treatment for most antibody deficiency diseases is replacement therapy with immunoglobulin administered either intramuscularly or intravenously. A large multicenter crossover study showed no differences between these two routes of administration in preventing acute and chronic infections.[42] The intravenous route allows for administering the larger doses that are often needed in immunodeficiency diseases.

IM therapy

Problems associated with intramuscular therapy for primary antibody deficiencies include (1) experiencing acute pain at the injection site; (2) experiencing pain for several days because of prolonged distribution of the bolus from the injection site; (3) being required by small muscle mass (in infants and children) to limit the dose; (4) immunoglobulin being degraded by proteolytic enzymes at the injection site before absorption takes place; (5) not achieving high serum IgG concentrations; and (6) needing 1 to 2 weeks to reach peak serum concentrations.

IV therapy

Intravenous immunoglobulin has eliminated many of the problems associated with intramuscular administration and is now the preferred route for most patients. Agreement is not unanimous on the optimal dose of intravenous immunoglobulin. An initial dose of 150 to 300 mg/kg as a monthly infusion may be tried, but some patients require higher doses (400 to 600 mg/kg) and shorter administration intervals. There is large interpatient variability in the pharmacokinetics of intravenous immunoglobulin, but little intrapatient variability. It is therefore necessary to establish a time-dose relationship for each patient. Sequential serum IgG levels obtained every 7 days throughout two cycles of therapy have been recommended.[43] The goals of treatment are to maintain trough IgG concentrations above 350 to 500 mg/dL and prevent infections.

Selective IgA deficiency patients should never receive any immunoglobulin preparation containing IgA because of the risk of a life-threatening allergic reaction. Many of these reactions are due to IgG anti-IgA antibodies. Patients with IgA deficiency with IgG subclass deficiencies and the inability to produce antigen-specific IgG may benefit from intravenous immunoglobulin replacement. However, the immunoglobulin preparation that contains the least amount of IgA should be selected for these patients. Also, patients with common variable hypogammaglobulinemia and undetectable IgA in their serum can develop IgE anti-IgA antibodies and experience an anaphylactic reaction.[44]

Combined Immunodeficiency Diseases

Combined immunodeficiency diseases have both a cellular and a humoral defect. The pathogenesis of combined immunodeficiencies is highly variable among affected individuals. Some patients may exhibit severe loss of both T-cell and B-cell function, whereas other patients may have only slightly impaired function of either cellular or humoral immunity.

Clinical features

The general clinical features of cellular immunodeficiency diseases are recurrent infections with opportunistic organisms such as fungi, viruses, and *Pneumocystis carinii*; lack of delayed cutaneous hypersensitivity; high incidence of malignancy; and major developmental defects.

Combined Immunodeficiency with Predominant T-Cell Defect. This immunodeficiency, also known as Nezelof's syndrome, is characterized by lymphopenia. Patients have normal serum immunoglobulin concentrations, although they often fail to make specific antibody in response to a foreign antigen. Patients with Nezelof's syndrome often present with recurrent or chronic infections of the lung, skin, genitourinary tract, and blood, and failure to thrive.[34] Patients are anergic and long-term prognosis is poor.

Severe Combined Immunodeficiency Disease (SCID). This disorder, which presents as a heterogeneous clinical entity, is the most severe form of immunodeficiency. The most common clinical symptoms are failure to thrive and severe illness in the first few months of life.[45] Persistent oral and perianal candidiasis, intractable diarrhea, and malabsorption are common.[45] Pneumonia from *P. carinii* is often seen.[36]

SCID is inherited as an autosomal recessive or X-linked recessive trait; about 75% of cases occur in males.[36,45] Both cellular and humoral immunity are affected. Patients are anergic and specific antibodies do not form in response to vaccinations.

The pathogenesis of this disease is very heterogeneous. In some patients there is a total absence of B lymphocytes, while others have markedly elevated numbers of circulating B cells.[46] Lymphocyte dysfunction is the result of defects in cellular differentiation.[47] In about 40% of SCID patients the immunologic defect is due to an absence of adenosine deaminase (ADA). In addition, increased suppressor T-cell activity or decreased helper T-cell function may have a role in the pathogenesis of SCID.[46]

Therapy for Cellular Deficiencies

The only useful treatment is immunologic reconstitution. Bone marrow transplantation can restore both cellular and humoral abnormalities in SCID.[48,49] If bone marrow transplantation is unsuccessful, death is almost certain in the first year of life. For patients with SCID due to ADA deficiency an enzyme replacement product, polyethylene glycol ADA, can be used. Only limited data are available for this product, but immunologic improvement can be seen from weekly intramuscular injections. Gene transfer therapy using the ADA gene has been performed experimentally in one SCID patient with ADA deficiency. Long-term follow-up on this patient is not available at the time of this writing, but short-term data are encouraging.

Secondary Immunodeficiency Diseases

Etiology

The immunodeficiencies that have been discussed are primary immunodeficiencies, all presumed to be due to intrinsic defects of the immune system.[33] Secondary immunodeficiencies can be caused by infectious agents, malignancies, malnutrition, aging, drugs, and a variety of disease processes. Both primary and secondary immunodeficiencies may present with similar clinical signs and symptoms. This section deals with some of the causes of secondary immune deficiencies.

Infectious Agents

An acute viral infection may cause a transient immunodeficiency, with lymphopenia, decreased cellular immunity, and reversed ratio of helper T cells to suppressor T cells. In congenital rubella infection, cellular immunity may be depressed and hypogammaglobulinemia may be present. Measles infection causes a transient suppression of cellular immunity with normal humoral function.[50] These temporary conditions do not have any lasting detrimental effects. Persistent immunodeficiency can be caused by the human immunodeficiency virus. (See Chapter 8.)

Malignancy

A number of malignant neoplastic diseases are associated with secondary immunodeficiencies. In Hodgkin's disease, cellular immunity is suppressed and humoral immunity may also be impaired. Both acute and chronic leukemia may be associated with decreased cellular immunity, and variable immunoglobulin levels are seen in patients with these diseases. In myeloma there is an impairment in antibody responses. In addition to the effects of a malignancy on immune function, therapy for these diseases (such as chemotherapy and radiation therapy) can cause immune dysfunction by killing immunocompetent cells.

Malnutrition

Malnutrition can markedly impair immunologic function. Children with protein-calorie malnutrition show a high incidence of death from infections due to immunodeficiency states.[51] Common communicable diseases such as mumps can be fatal in these children. Replenishment with nutrients improves immunologic functions and decreases mortality. The effects of protein-calorie malnutrition on the immune system include thymic atrophy, decreased spleen weight, decreased circulating T cells, increased circulating non-T and non-B cells, impaired lymphokine production, anergy, decreased thymic hormone production, and impaired antibody formation.

Single-nutrient deficiencies can also impair immune function.[52,53] This phenomenon has been studied mostly in animals because it is possible to deprive an animal of a single nutrient. Data from animal and human studies on nutrient deficiencies are summarized in Table 6-6.

Aging

Immunosenescence

Aging is associated with a decline in immune function. This abnormality, referred to as immunosenescence, contributes to the high incidence of autoantibodies and neoplastic and infectious diseases seen in the elderly population.[54] Both cellular and humoral immunity may be affected. It is common to find decreased numbers of circulating T lymphocytes in elderly people. They often are anergic, and in vitro studies demonstrate depressed lymphocyte function. The ability to make specific antibody after an

Table 6-6 Effects of Single-nutrient Deficiencies on Immune Function

	Primary cells affected			
Nutrient	T cells	B cells	Macrophages	Neutrophils
Vitamin A	+	+		
Thiamine		+		+
Vitamin B_6	+	+		
Vitamin B_{12}	+	+		+
Riboflavin		+		
Biotin		+		
Pantothenic acid		+		
Folic acid	+	+		

Table 6-6 (continued)

	Primary cells affected			
Nutrient	T cells	B cells	Macrophages	Neutrophils
Vitamin C	+		+	+
Vitamin D		+		
Vitamin E	+	+	+	
Niacin		+		
Iron	+	+	+	+
Magnesium		+		+
Zinc	+		+	+
Selenium	+			

SOURCE: Adapted from the following: (1) Beisel WR, Edelman R, Nauss K et al. Single-nutrient effects on immunologic functions. *JAMA.* 1981;245:53–8. (2) Delafuente JC. Nutrients and immune responses. *Rheumatic Disease Clinics of North America* 1991;17:1–10.

immunization may also be depressed, although enough antibody is usually made to offer some protection. Because immunosenescence abates immunologic responses, it is extremely important that elderly people receive proper immunizations to enhance their immunity to common infectious pathogens. Recommended are a yearly influenza immunization and a pneumococcal immunization, which should be given only once.[55]

Drugs

A number of drugs used clinically can cause a secondary immunodeficiency. In some cases this is a desired effect, for example, when a cytotoxic agent is used to suppress an autoimmune pathologic process. In other cases, such as cancer chemotherapy, it is an undesired effect. The effects of corticosteroids and cytotoxic agents on the immune system can easily be explained on the basis of their pharmacology.[56] Table 6-7 lists the effects of corticosteroids on various immune functions. The cytotoxic drugs impair immune function by destroying or blocking the proliferation of immunocompetent cells. In addition, phenytoin and penicillamine have been reported to decrease serum IgA concentration.[57,58] Apparently, phenytoin can induce suppressor cells, causing hypogammaglobulinemia.[57] This drug-induced effect resolves after the drugs are discontinued.

Table 6-7 Immunologic Effects of Corticosteroids

Lymphocytes	
↓	Cellular proliferation
↓	Lymphokine production or release or both
↓	Delayed cutaneous hypersensitivity reactions
	Selective depletion from blood (T cells more than B cells)
Neutrophils	
	Blood neutrophilia
↓	Egress from circulation
↑	Release from bone marrow
↑	Circulating half-life
	Blocked migration into inflammatory areas
Monocytes-macrophages	
	Depletion from blood
	Inhibition of mediator production or release or both
	Blocked migration in response to cytokines
Eosinophils	
	Depletion from blood
Other Effects	
↓	Specific antibody formation
↓	Synthesis of prostaglandins

↓ = decreased; ↑ = increased.

Summary

Autoantibodies and sensitized lymphocytes to self antigens are necessary for maintaining normal homeostasis. Autoimmune diseases occur when this process becomes excessive and uncontrolled. There are numerous autoimmune diseases with a wide spectrum of clinical manifestations. The etiologies for these diseases remain unknown, but there are probably many factors involved, including genetic predisposition, environmental factors, and host immune responses. Tissue damage is mediated through sensitized cells or autoantibodies; both may play a role in some diseases. Generally, the treatment goal is to suppress the disease activity with anti-inflammatory and immunosuppressive drugs.

Clinical manifestations of the primary immunodeficiency diseases range from asymptomatic in some cases of IgA deficiency to chronic, severe infections. In many cases, the immunodeficiency is fatal. Fortunately, the primary immunodeficiency diseases are rare. Treatment strategies usually focus on replacing the deficiency by administering immunoglobulin for antibody deficiency diseases or transplanting bone marrow for cellular deficiencies. Secondary immunodeficiencies may be iatrogenically caused by drugs or may result from a variety of disease states, including malignancies, malnutrition, viral infections, and some autoimmune diseases. Aging is also known to blunt the immune response.

References

1. Smith HR, Steinberg AD. Autoimmunity—perspective. *Annual Review of Immunology.* 1983;1:175–210.
2. Cruse JM, Lewis RE. Contemporary concepts of autoimmunity. In: Cruse JM, Lewis RE, eds. Autoimmunity: basic concepts; systemic and selected organ-specific diseases. Basel: Karger; 1985:1–31.
3. Rodnan GP, Schumacher HR, eds. Primer on the rheumatic diseases. 8th ed. Atlanta: Arthritis Foundation; 1983.
4. Cahill GF, McDevitt HO. Insulin-dependent diabetes mellitus: the initial lesion. *N Engl J Med.* 1981;304:1454–65.
5. Steinberg AD, Raveche ES, Laskin CA et al. Systemic lupus erythematosus: insights from animal models. *Ann Intern Med.* 1984;100:714–27.
6. McFarlin DE, McFarland HF. Multiple sclerosis, parts 1 and 2. *N Engl J Med.* 1982;307:1183–8, 1246–51.
7. Tosato G, Steinberg AD, Blaese RM. Defective EBV-specific suppressor T-cell function in rheumatoid arthritis. *N Engl J Med.* 1981;305:1238–43.
8. Theofilopoulos AN. Autoimmunity. In: Stites DP, Stobo JD, Wells JV, eds. Basic and clinical immunology. 6th ed. Norwalk, CT: Appleton & Lange; 1987:128–58.
9. Kumar V, Kono DH, Urban JL et al. The T-cell receptor repertoire and autoimmune diseases. *Annual Review of Immunology.* 1989;7:657–82.
10. Reinherz EL, Weiner HL, Hauser SL et al. Loss of suppressor T cells in active multiple sclerosis: analysis with monoclonal antibodies. *N Engl J Med.* 1980;303:125–9.
11. Sakane T, Steinberg AD, Green I. Studies of immune functions of patients with systemic lupus erythematosus. V. T cell suppressor function and autologous mixed lymphocyte reaction during active and inactive phase of disease. *Arthritis Rheum.* 1980;23:225–31.

12. Lau C, Budz-Tymkewycz S, Ramsden M et al. Impaired release of a T-cell specific suppressor factor in rheumatoid arthritis. *Clinical and Experimental Immunology.* 1985;61:489–95.
13. Sagawa A, Abdou NI. Suppressor-cell antibody in systemic lupus erythematosus: possible mechanism for suppressor-cell dysfunction. *J Clin Invest.* 1979;63:536–9.
14. Tsuchiya N, Husby G, Williams RC et al. Autoantibodies to the HLA-B27 sequence cross-react with the hypothetical peptide from the arthritis-associated Shigella plasmid. *J Clin Invest.* 1990;86:1193–203.
15. Coombs RRA, Gell PGH. The classification of allergic reactions underlying disease. In: Gell PGH, Coombs RRA, eds. Clinical aspects of immunology. Philadelphia: FA Davis Company; 1963:317–37.
16. Hawkins RA, Claman HN, Clark RAF et al. Increased dermal mast cell populations in progressive systemic sclerosis: a link in chronic fibrosis. *Ann Inter Med.* 1985;102:182–6.
17. Godfrey HP, Ilardi C, Engber W et al. Quantitation of human synovial mast cells in rheumatoid arthritis and other rheumatic diseases. *Arthritis Rheum.* 1984;27:852–6.
18. Gruber B, Ballan D, Gorevic PD. IgE rheumatoid factors: quantification in synovial fluid and ability to induce synovial mast cell histamine release. *Clinical and Experimental Immunology.* 1988;71:289–94.
19. Wilkin TJ. Receptor autoimmunity in endocrine disorders. *N Engl J Med.* 1990;323:1318–24.
20. Fraser CM, Venter JC. Anti-receptor antibodies in human diseases. *J Allergy Clin Immunol.* 1984;74:661–73.
21. Barnett EV, Knutson DW, Abrass CK et al. Circulating immune complexes: their immunochemistry, detection, and importance. *Ann Intern Med.* 1979;91:430–40.
22. Halla JT, Schrohenloher RE, Volanakis JE. Immune complexes and other laboratory features of pleural effusions: a comparison of rheumatoid arthritis, systemic lupus erythematosus, and other diseases. *Ann Intern Med.* 1980;92:748–52.
23. Barrett JT. Autoimmunity. In: Barrett JT. Textbook of immunology: an introduction to immunochemistry and immunobiology. 4th ed. St. Louis: C.V. Mosby; 1983:402–31.
24. Jackson RA, Morris MA, Haynes BF et al. Increased circulating Ia-antigen-bearing T cells in type I diabetes mellitus. *N Engl J Med.* 1982;306:785–8.
25. Hafler DA, Fox DA, Manning E et al. In vivo activated T-lymphocytes in peripheral blood and cerebrospinal fluid of patients with multiple sclerosis. *N Engl J Med.* 1985;312:1405–11.

26. Stiller CR, Dupre J, Gent M et al. Effects of cyclosporine immunosuppression in insulin-dependent diabetes mellitus of recent onset. *Science.* 1984;223:1362–7.
27. Harrison LC, Colman PG, Dean B et al. Increase in remission rate in newly diagnosed type I diabetic subjects treated with azathioprine. *Diabetes.* 1985;34:1306–8.
28. Burlingame MB, Delafuente JC. Treatment of system lupus erythematosus. *Drug Intelligence and Clinical Pharmacy.* 1988;22:283–9.
29. Pugh MC, Pugh CB. Current concepts in clinical therapeutics: disease-modifying drugs for rheumatoid arthritis. *Clinical Pharmacy.* 1987;6:475–91.
30. Horneff G, Burmester GR, Emmrich F et al. Treatment of rheumatoid arthritis with an anti-CD4 monoclonal antibody. *Arthritis Rheum.* 1991;34:129–40.
31. Wofsy D. Regulation of immunity by anti-T-cell antibodies. *West J Med.* 1990;153:265–8.
32. Bruton OC. Agammaglobulinemia. *Pediatrics.* 1952;9:722–7.
33. World Health Organization Scientific Group. Primary immunodeficiency diseases: report of a World Health Organization Scientific Group. *Clinical Immunology and Immunopathology.* 1986;40:161–96.
34. Buckley RH. Immunodeficiency. *J Allergy Clin Immunol.* 1983;72:627–41.
35. Buckley RH. Immunodeficiency diseases. *JAMA.* 1987;258:2841–50.
36. Rosen FS, Cooper MD, Wedgwood RJP. The primary immunodeficiencies, parts 1 and 2. *N Engl J Med.* 1984;311:235–42, 300–10.
37. Huston DP, Kavanaugh AF, Rohane PW et al. Immunoglobulin deficiency syndromes and therapy. *J Allergy Clin Immunol.* 1991;87:1–17.
38. Geha RS, Schneeberger E, Merler E et al. Heterogeneity of "acquired" or common variable agammaglobulinemia. *N Engl J Med.* 1974;291:1–6.
39. Waldmann TA. Disorders of suppressor cells with common variable hypogammaglobulinemia and selective IgA deficiency. In: Waldmann TA, moderator. Disorders of suppressor immunoregulatory cells in the pathogenesis of immunodeficiency and autoimmunity. *Ann Intern Med.* 1978;88:226–38.
40. Ammann AJ, Hong R. Selective IgA deficiency: presentation of 30 cases and a review of the literature. *Medicine.* 1971;50:223–36.
41. Koistinen J, Heikkila M, Leikola J. Gammaglobulin treatment and anti-IgA antibodies in IgA-deficient patients. *Br Med J.* 1978;2:923–4.
42. Ammann AJ, Ashman RF, Buckley RH et al. Use of intravenous gamma globulin in antibody immunodeficiency: results of a

multicenter controlled trial. *Clinical Immunology and Immunopathology.* 1982;22:60–7.

43. Pirofsky B. Intravenous immune globulin therapy in hypogammaglobulinemia. *Am J Med.* 1984;76(3A):53–60.
44. Burks AW, Sampson HA, Buckley RH. Anaphylactic reactions after gamma globulin administration in patients with hypogammaglobulinemia. Detection of IgE antibodies to IgA. *N Engl J Med.* 1986;314:560–4.
45. Gelfand EW, Dosch HM. Diagnosis and classification of severe combined immunodeficiency disease. *Birth Defects.* 1983;19(3):65–72.
46. Pahwa SG, Pahwa RN, Good RA. Heterogeneity of B lymphocyte differentiation in severe combined immunodeficiency disease. *J Clin Invest.* 1980;66:543–50.
47. Pahwa RN, Pahwa SG, Good RA. T-lymphocyte differentiation in vitro in severe combined immunodeficiency. *J Clin Invest.* 1979;64:1632–41.
48. Reinherz EL, Geha R, Rappeport JM et al. Reconstitution after transplantation with T-lymphocyte-depleted HLA haplotype-mismatched bone marrow for severe combined immunodeficiency. *Proc Nat Acad Sci USA.* 1982;79:6047–51.
49. Reisner Y, Kapoor N, Kirkpatrick D et al. Transplantation for severe combined immunodeficiency with HLA-A, B, C, D, DR incompatible parental marrow cells fractionated by soybean agglutinin and sheep red blood cells. *Blood.* 1983;61:341–8.
50. Ammann AJ. Immunodeficiency Diseases. In: Stites DP, Stobo JD, Wells JV, eds. Basic and clinical immunology. Norwalk, CT: Appleton & Lange; 1987:347–50.
51. Worthington BS. Effect of nutritional status on immune phenomena. *Journal of the American Dietetic Association.* 1974;65:123–29.
52. Delafuente JC. Nutrients and immune responses. *Rheumatic Disease Clinics of North America.* 1991;17:1–10.
53. Beisel WR, Edelman R, Nauss K et al. Single-nutrient effects on immunologic functions. *JAMA.* 1981;245:53–8.
54. Delafuente JC. Senescence of the immune system: nutritional and pharmacologic modulation. *Journal of Geriatric Drug Therapy.* 1990;4:7–27.
55. Immunization Practices Advisory Committee, Centers for Disease Control. General recommendations on immunization. *Ann Intern Med.* 1989;11:133–42.
56. Katz P. Immunosuppressant therapy. *Advances in Internal Medicine.* 1984;29:167–92.
57. Cooper MD, Buckley RH. Developmental immunology and the immunodeficiency diseases. *JAMA.* 1982;248:2658–69.

58. Dosch HM, Jason J, Gelfand EW. Transient antibody deficiency and abnormal T suppressor cells induced by phenytoin. *N Engl J Med.* 1982;306:406–9.

Self-Study Questions

1. A
2. A
3. B
4. A
5. 350 to 500; infections
6. A
7. D

1. Systemic lupus erythematosus, progressive systemic sclerosis, and polymyositis are all associated with antigens from the nucleus of cells.

   A. True.
   B. False.

2. Insulin-dependent diabetes mellitus is associated with autoantigens for glucagon and islet cells.

   A. True.
   B. False.

3. Anti-CD4 monoclonal antibodies are the cornerstone to pharmacologic management of autoimmune diseases.

   A. True.
   B. False.

4. Multiple sclerosis may be brought into remission with the use of immunosuppressive therapy.

   A. True.
   B. False.

5. The therapy goals for treating antibody deficiencies are to maintain trough IgG concentrations above _________mg/dL and to prevent_____________.

6. Intravenous immunoglobulin is the preferred route for most patients with antibody deficiencies.

   A. True.
   B. False.

7. Which of the following infectious agents has lasting detrimental effects on the immune system?

   A. Measles.
   B. Varicella zoster.
   C. Mumps.
   D. Human immunodeficiency virus.

8. The use of corticosteroids increases the formation of specific antibodies.

   A. True.
   B. False.

8. B

CHAPTER 7

Immunization

Karen I. Plaisance, Pharm.D.
Associate Professor
Department of Clinical Pharmacy
University of Maryland
School of Pharmacy
Baltimore, MD

Kelly A. Scott, Pharm.D.
Oncology Clinical Pharmacist
Pharmacy IV Department
Good Samaritan Hospital and Medical Center
Portland, OR

Introduction

Even centuries ago, it was noted that people exposed to certain diseases acquired a tolerance to developing those diseases a second time. This basic observation led scientists to investigate ways of artificially producing immunity against disease. Today, the widespread use of vaccines has led to the global eradication of smallpox, the near elimination of polio and diphtheria from the United States, and dramatic reductions in the incidence rates of other infectious diseases.

The pharmacist can play a major role in the field of immunization. A knowledge of vaccine sources provides needed information related to product selection and storage. In addition, the selection of patients requiring either prophylaxis or treatment of disease using passive or active immunization techniques, or both, can be facilitated by the pharmacist, as can the timing of vaccine administration. Because of the toxicities related to certain vaccines, the pharmacist must also realize the clinical and legal risks of vaccine use and provide appropriate patient counseling while serving as a patient advocate. The use of passive immunization and therapeutic intervention with intramuscular and intravenous immunoglobulins is an expanding field in medicine. The pharmacist can use the information in this chapter to make recommendations regarding product selection, appropriate route of administration, and monitoring endpoints of these new immunoglobulin therapies.

After reading this chapter, the learner will be able to—

Learning objectives

- Describe risk factors associated with active immunization.
- Describe the development of traditional vaccines.
- Describe the development of biotechnological vaccines.
- Discuss the therapeutic applications of intramuscular immunoglobulins.
- Discuss considerations in the use of intravenous immunoglobulins.

Chapter organization

This chapter highlights the results of early investigations into active immunization followed by a discussion of modern vaccine development —both traditional and biotechnological approaches. Similarities and differences between active and passive immunization are next described. Finally, the principles of serotherapy are presented with a focus on the use of immunoglobulins for imparting passive immunity.

Suggested Preparation

This chapter is designed for pharmacists who want to gain a basic understanding of the history, theory, method, and utility of immunizations. The reader should have a knowledge base in the immune system, including the cellular and tissue components. Thus, Chapters 1 and 2 of this text should be reviewed before beginning this chapter. In addition, the following sources may be helpful:

- Plotkin SA, Mortimer EA Jr. Vaccines. Philadelphia: W. B. Saunders Company; 1988.
- Roitt IM. Immune intervention: new trends in vaccines. New York: Academic Press; 1984.

Active Immunization (Vaccination)

This section provides a brief history of active immunization, including a review of some of the milestones in early vaccine development. The different types of vaccines and their methods of development are also discussed. Included is a summary of the risk factors associated with vaccines. The next two sections address traditional and biotechnologic approaches to vaccine development. Finally, methods of stimulating the immune response to vaccines are addressed.

Brief History of Vaccines

Specific active immunity may be acquired naturally through exposure to infectious agents, or it may be induced by means of immunization with killed or attenuated organisms or toxoids.

As described in Chapters 1 and 2, the body's first contact with an organism (i.e., antigen) imprints some specific information into a memory bank so that the body may effectively repel any later invasion by that same organism. This process explains why we rarely suffer twice from certain diseases such as mumps, chicken pox, and measles, but instead develop a complete and long-lasting immunity to those infections. The process of active immunization uses this basic principle by exposing the body to a relatively harmless form of the antigen to imprint memory and stimulate the body's defenses against any subsequent exposure.

Risk Factors of Vaccines

Goal

Although the goal of active immunization (vaccination) is to establish adequate levels of memory cells and thus provide immunity upon renewed contact with the antigen, the first contact with the antigen during vaccination should not be deleterious to the patient. The goal is to modify the pathogenic effect of the organism without losing the antigenicity.

The first written record of vaccination was by a Chinese Buddhist nun around A.D. 1000. Her crude vaccination attempts involved obtaining live smallpox organisms from the scabs of patients with the disease and introducing them into the nostrils of infants or children to induce a mild form of the disease.[1] Although this method of vaccination was dangerous, a similar approach is used for some modern vaccines, such as those for diphtheria and tetanus, and these specific vaccines are associated with few significant side effects. However, even in today's era of technologic advancement, certain other vaccines still carry real, if relatively rare, risks to the recipient. For example, vaccines for measles and rabies have been associated with postvaccination complications such as encephalitis.[2] This complication can cause permanent brain damage and mental retardation. The rate of postvaccination encephalitis with the measles vaccine is approximately one case per million vaccinations. This small incidence rate is approximately one fifth to one tenth the rate of encephalitis after natural measles. Since the introduction of the measles vaccine, the rate of postmeasles encephalitis has dropped tenfold.[2,3] Therefore, the potential benefit from measles vaccination far outweighs the small risk of postvaccination encephalitis.

Another risk is the potential for the vaccine to elicit an allergic response. This allergenicity usually results from the method of production, such as the use of chicken embryo culture media. When such cultures are used in the production of a vaccine, complete purification may not be possible, and trace contaminants (such as egg protein) may persist in the final product. The use of human diploid cell lines as viral hosts, a method developed in the 1980s, has limited the risk of both allergenicity and oncogenicity.[4]

Viral DNA might be incorporated into the human genome with the use of live viral vaccines, potentially resulting in the disease the vaccine was intended to prevent.

Benefit-risk assessment

The risk of complication from the vaccine must be balanced against the risk of contracting the disease. For diseases with low occurrence rates, such as smallpox, the risk of untoward effects from vaccination outweighs the possible benefits. In contrast, the documented benefits of vaccines against other diseases, such as measles, far outweigh the small percentage of postvaccination complications. Factors to consider when assessing risks and benefits of vaccination include the risk of infection, the consequences of natural unmodified illness, the availability of a safe and effective vaccine, and the duration of vaccine effect.

It is clear that immunization is a vital component of pediatric and adult health care. Unfortunately, immunization is quite underused, even though it is one of the most cost-effective measures available for preserving and protecting health. The incidence rates of vaccine-preventable diseases in the United States have decreased dramatically since the mid-1950s, primarily because of the widespread public acceptance and availability of effective vaccines. For example, before the vaccine for measles became available in

Measles

1963, 400,000 cases of measles were reported each year. In the era after the introduction of this vaccine, a 99% reduction in reported measles cases has been documented.[3] Unfortunately, in recent years outbreaks of measles in unvaccinated school-aged children have been noted by the Centers for Disease Control (CDC). An outbreak of measles in 1989 affected a substantial number of people on college campuses. It has been estimated that approximately 88% of inner-city youth are unvaccinated and thus unprotected against measles.[3] The pharmacist, like all health care providers, should encourage parents to comply with vaccination recommendations from the CDC.

However, it is also the pharmacist's or physician's responsibility to educate the patient or patient's parent about the risks of immunization, and it is the responsibility of all health care providers to use (i.e., store, dose, administer) the vaccines in an appropriate manner. Pharmacists should ensure compliance with, and advocate, patient safety measures.

It is also apparent that companies involved in vaccine development and production must carefully weigh all known risks involved in vaccination to minimize adverse effects to the patient. However, some adverse events occur in such a small percentage of patients that the incidence and severity of the effect may not be known until mass production and vaccination are under way.

The 1976 nationwide swine flu immunization program provides a classic example of this problem.[2] A careful monitoring program revealed a fivefold increase in the development of Guillain-Barré syndrome in vaccinated people versus unvaccinated controls.[5] The rarity of this complication made it impossible to predict or detect during initial trials, illustrating the difficulty in predicting all risks of immunization.

VAERS

Because of the untoward complications arising from this immunization program and the increasing concern regarding the possible impact of lawsuits for vaccine-related complications, the Vaccine Adverse Event Reporting System (VAERS), an ongoing nationwide surveillance program, was instituted.[6] VAERS was established in late 1990 by the Department of Health and Human Services to centralize reports of adverse reactions to vaccines. Under this system, health care providers administering vaccines and vaccine manufacturers as well are required by law to report all suspected adverse events following any vaccination.[6] Adverse events that must be reported under VAERS include specific events following vaccination with diphtheria, measles, mumps, pertussis, polio, rubella, and tetanus vaccines. "Reportable events" as delineated in information available from VAERS, as well as any other suspected vaccine adverse event, should be reported. A sample VAERS reporting form is shown in Figure 7-1. All pharmacists should also report adverse reactions to vaccines according to their own institution's procedures for reporting adverse drug reactions or other quality assurance programs within their departments, as well as to VAERS.

Government bodies such as the Food and Drug Administration (FDA) carefully review the sale and use of all vaccine products.[2,7] A decision by the U.S. Supreme Court in 1988 holds the federal government financially liable if government officials are negligent in enforcing strict vaccine safety guidelines.

Manufacturer liability

In general, manufacturers of vaccines are held legally and financially accountable for failure to comply with known safety standards in vaccine production methods. However, the threat of legal action based on unpredictable side effects could force private industry to abandon research and development to ensure financial survival. To address this concern, Congress has passed laws to facilitate the settlement of lawsuits brought against vaccine manufacturers and to protect them from financial ruin. In this system, pharmaceutical companies put money into a central fund that is used to settle lawsuits brought against companies for adverse vaccine reactions that were not due to substandard manufacturing processes. In this way the continued incentive to pursue research and production efforts of these lifesaving therapeutic agents has been preserved. Other nations, such as the United Kingdom and Japan, have their own national compensatory mechanisms to cover costs of vaccine-related complications.[2]

VAERS

VACCINE ADVERSE EVENT REPORTING SYSTEM
24 Hour Toll-free information line 1-800-822-7967
Patient identity kept confidential

For CDC/FDA Use Only
VAERS Number ______
Date Received ______

Patient Name: ______
Last First M.I.
Address ______
City State Zip
Telephone no. (____)______

Vaccine administered by (Name): ______
Responsible Physician ______
Facility Name/Address ______
City State Zip
Telephone no. (____)______

Form completed by (Name): ______
Relation to Patient ☐ Vaccine Provider ☐ Patient/Parent ☐ Manufacturer ☐ Other
Address *(if different from patient or provider)* ______
City State Zip
Telephone no. (____)______

1. State
2. County where administered
3. Date of birth __/__/__ mm dd yy
4. Patient age
5. Sex ☐M ☐F
6. Date form completed __/__/__ mm dd yy

7. Describe adverse event(s) (symptoms, signs, time course) and treatment, if any

8. Check all appropriate:
☐ Patient died (date __/__/__) mm dd yy
☐ Life threatening illness
☐ Required emergency room/doctor visit
☐ Required hospitalization (____days)
☐ Resulted in prolongation of hospitalization
☐ Resulted in permanent disability
☐ None of the above

9. Patient recovered ☐ YES ☐ NO ☐ UNKNOWN

10. Date of vaccination __/__/__ mm dd yy Time ______ AM PM

11. Adverse event onset __/__/__ mm dd yy Time ______ AM PM

12. Relevant diagnostic tests/laboratory data

13. Enter all vaccines given on date listed in no. 10

	Vaccine (type)	Manufacturer	Lot number	Route/Site	No. Previous doses
a.					
b.					
c.					
d.					

14. Any other vaccinations within 4 weeks of date listed in no. 10

	Vaccine (type)	Manufacturer	Lot number	Route/Site	No. Previous doses	Date given
a.						
b.						

15. Vaccinated at:
☐ Private doctor's office/hospital ☐ Military clinic/hospital
☐ Public health clinic/hospital ☐ Other/unknown

16. Vaccine purchased with:
☐ Private funds ☐ Military funds
☐ Public funds ☐ Other /unknown

17. Other medications

18. Illness at time of vaccination (specify)

19. Pre-existing physician-diagnosed allergies, birth defects, medical conditions (specify)

20. Have you reported this adverse event previously? ☐ No ☐ To health department ☐ To doctor ☐ To manufacturer

Only for children 5 and under
22. Birth weight ____ lb. ____ oz.
23. No. of brothers and sisters

21. Adverse event following prior vaccination (check all applicable, specify)

	Adverse Event	Onset Age	Type Vaccine	Dose no. in series
☐ In patient				
☐ In brother or sister				

Only for reports submitted by manufacturer/immunization project
24. Mfr. / imm. proj. report no.
25. Date received by mfr. / imm. proj.
26. 15 day report? ☐ Yes ☐ No
27. Report type ☐ Initial ☐ Follow-Up

Health care providers and manufacturers are required by law (42 USC 300aa-25) to report reactions to vaccines listed in the Vaccine Injury Table. Reports for reactions to other vaccines are voluntary except when required as a condition of immunization grant awards.

Form VAERS-1

Figure 7-1. Vaccine Adverse Event Reporting System report form (copyright Williams & Wilkins.)

Traditional Approaches to Vaccine Development

Active immunization traditionally uses either live, attenuated microorganisms or inactive microbial products. For some diseases, such as poliomyelitis, both approaches have gained acceptance. Vaccines used in the United States are summarized in Table 7-1.

Live vaccines

Generally, live vaccines induce an immunologic response closely resembling natural infection. The organisms in a live, attenuated vaccine replicate logarithmically in the host until halted by the immunologic response to the vaccine. This multiplication of organisms produces a cumulatively greater antigenic load with live vaccines even though the amount of antigen initially administered with inactive vaccines is usually greater. In addition, following vaccination with an attenuated strain, primary and secondary responses are merged during amplification. Thus, vaccines containing live, attenuated viruses (e.g., oral polio vaccine) often generate lifelong immunity with a single dose or a primary series of doses, and subsequent booster doses are not usually required.[8-10]

Inactivated vaccines

An inactivated vaccine may contain killed whole organisms (e.g., pertussis), inactivated bacterial toxins (toxoids), or extracts of capsular material (e.g., *Haemophilus influenzae* type b) or other component (e.g., hepatitis B surface antigen). In contrast to attenuated vaccines, inactive vaccines usually do not provide permanent protection with a single dose, and repeated vaccinations are generally necessary to maintain protective levels of antibody and generate long-lasting immunity. Table 7-2 summarizes the characteristics of attenuated and inactive vaccines.[8,10]

The relative merits of attenuated, inactive vaccines have been debated. The controversy focuses on relative immunogenicity, safety, ease of production, distribution, administration, stability, and cost. This section discusses the various classic approaches to vaccine development.

Live, Attenuated Vaccines. The pathogenicity of an organism must be reduced substantially to produce a safe vaccine, yet, for the vaccine to be effective, the organism must retain enough pathogenicity to infect the host. After administration, an ideally attenuated organism should produce infection that mimics the immune response to the natural infection as closely as possible while producing little or no illness. The live virus should be free of latency, teratogenic, abortogenic, and oncogenic properties. The organism's ability to disseminate throughout a population should be minimal. Finally, the attenuated organism must be genetically stable and incapable of reverting to a pathogenic form.[10]

Genetic stability

The genetic stability of attenuated strains is of utmost concern. Even a minimal level of reversion that produces only one case of disease per

Table 7-1 Recommended Immunizations in the United States

Patients	DPT	Td	MMR	OPV	Hib	Flu	PnV	HBV	Other
General Use									
Infants	a		a	a	a			b	
Adolescents		a	c						
Adults									
18-64		a	c	d					
≥ 65		a				a	a		
Special Groups									
Pregnant women			e					b	
Health care workers		a				a		f	
Day care									
Attendees	a		a	a	a				
Workers		a				a			
Veterinarians									Rabies
Homosexual males								a	
Parenteral drug users								a	

SOURCE: Adapted from American College of Physicians Task Force on Adult Immunization and Infectious Diseases Society of America. Guide for adult immunization. 2nd ed. American College of Physicians. Tables 1 and 2; pp xii–xiv.

DPT = diphtheria-tetanus-pertussis; Td = tetanus/diphtheria; MMR = measles-mumps-rubella; OPV = oral polio; Hib = *Haemophilus influenzae* type b; Flu = influenza; PnV = *Streptococcus pneumoniae*; HBV = hepatitis B.

[a]Routine immunization.

[b]If mother is a chronic carrier of hepatitis B surface antigen (HBsAg), newborns should receive active and passive immunization.

[c]All persons born after 1956 should have evidence of immunity to measles.

[d]Inactivated polio vaccine may be given to nonimmune parents of children scheduled for OPV.

[e]MMR is contraindicated in pregnancy.

[f]If anticipated exposure to blood or blood products of patients who are likely to be positive for HBsAg.

Table 7-2 Characteristics of Vaccines

Live, attenuated vaccines
Diminished pathogenicity
Both cell-mediated and humoral immunity
Longer lasting antibody protection
Ability to revert to pathogenic variant
Killed, inactive vaccines
Nonreplicating and noninfectious
Need for multiple, booster administrations

100,000 vaccinated subjects would be unacceptable if that case provided a focus of outbreak. The use of attenuated oral polio vaccine is an example of genetic reversion.[10] The frequency of vaccine-associated poliomyelitis has been estimated at 2.5 cases per 1 million live-born infants.[11] Oral polio vaccine was associated with 76% of the 138 cases of paralytic poliomyelitis reported in the United States from 1973 through 1984.[12]

Techniques

The various approaches to the attenuation of organisms are summarized in Table 7-3. These methods, based largely on trial and error, were developed in the 1950s and 1960s and focused on producing organisms that grew optimally under different conditions than those found in their natural hosts. Although the organism would be unable to reproduce in numbers adequate to cause disease, this subclinical infection would be sufficient to stimulate both cellular and humoral responses.[10] The general methods for attenuation on which this section focuses include adaptation to a foreign host (either species or tissue) and modification of optimal growth conditions.

The use of cowpox virus (vaccinia) to prevent smallpox (variola virus) is an example of a relatively nonpathogenic virus used to stimulate immunity

Table 7-3 Traditional Approaches to Developing Attenuated Vaccines

Method	Example
Passage in cell culture (tissue adaptation)	Measles-mumps-rubella
Species adaptation	Smallpox
Temperature-selected mutants	Influenza

to a closely related pathogen. More commonly, however, live, attenuated vaccines have been produced by adapting virulent viruses to unnatural host cells. This process is illustrated by the attenuation of the Sabin poliovirus strain through growth in monkey kidney cells. Live attenuated measles, mumps, and rubella vaccines have been produced in a similar manner. The success of attenuation through adaptation depends on the characteristics of the organisms involved, the type of culture media and conditions, and the number of passages through laboratory culture. Although these procedures may be successfully applied to some viruses, problems may still arise with application even to closely related viruses (e.g., poliovirus and foot-and-mouth disease virus). Mutations occurring during passage in culture are probably the cause of the problem, but the precise molecular effects of these mutations are not yet understood.[10]

Another classic approach to attenuation involves adaptation by growth at suboptimal temperatures. This approach is illustrated with poliovirus. When adapted to growth at 23°C in monkey kidney cell cultures, poliovirus had diminished neurovirulence and was unable to replicate at temperatures of 39°C to 40°C. Procedures for attenuation by growth under suboptimal conditions vary dramatically depending on the organisms involved.[10]

Multiple doses

Inactive, Killed Vaccines. Because inactive vaccines do not replicate and are generally less efficient in inducing an immune response than attenuated vaccines, two or three doses of inactive vaccine must usually be given to stimulate the primary and secondary responses necessary to produce long-lasting immunity. With a live, attenuated vaccine, the primary and secondary responses are merged during amplification. Therefore, a single dose of a live, attenuated vaccine is often sufficient.

The antigenic mass required for an inactive vaccine to generate a protective immune response is often many times greater than the antigenic mass required for live, attenuated vaccines. In terms of vaccine production procedures, cost, and administration, this difference in dose size may be considerable. In addition, inactivated vaccines are often prepared from infected cell cultures or the tissues of infected animals or eggs. Given the large doses required, inactivated vaccines often contain large amounts of extraneous material, increasing the possibility of adverse reactions.

Because inactive vaccines are noninfectious and incapable of replicating in the host, they are unable to revert to a pathogenic variant and cause clinical disease. However, outbreaks of polio have been attributed to incomplete inactivation of the virus.[13] Several approaches have been used to produce inactive, or killed, vaccines. These strategies and examples of vaccines produced through these methods are listed in Table 7-4. The classic approaches to producing inactivated vaccines employ techniques of biochemical purification and biophysical inactivation, such as physical inactivation of whole viruses or bacteria, use of inactivated toxoids produced by bacteria, purification of surface components of viruses or bacteria, and conjugation of purified surface components to other immunogens. This last approach, illustrated by the conjugated vaccines for *H. influenzae,* is particularly attractive for poorly immunogenic antigens.

Techniques

Hib

H. influenzae type b (Hib) is the leading cause of pediatric bacterial meningitis in the United States and is the cause of other serious infections including bacteremia, epiglottitis, pneumonia, septic arthritis, osteomyelitis, pericarditis, and cellulitis.[14] Most Hib disease occurs in children younger than 2 years.[15] The cumulative risk of contracting Hib (estimated at 1 in every 200 children during the first 5 years of life) approximates that of paralytic poliomyelitis during the peak epidemic years in the early 1950s.[14] Type b capsular polysaccharide (polyribosylribitol phosphate [PRP]) vaccine, licensed in 1985, became the first vaccine available for preventing Hib disease. Because polysaccharide vaccines are generally T-cell independent, children younger than 24 months respond poorly, antibody levels wane rapidly, and repeated doses of PRP vaccine fail to induce booster responses.[16,17] In children aged 12 to 24 months, antibody responses to PRP vaccine are marginal; better responses are seen in children older than 24 months. The best responses are seen in older children and adults, but there is considerable variability in immunogenicity. The results of protective efficacy studies reflect the poor immunogenicity of the purified PRP. Even in children older than 24 months, the vaccine was not completely protective. The protective efficacy of this vaccine was 80% with a 95% confidence interval of 7% to 96%.[18,19] In case-controlled studies, the protective efficacy of this vaccine ranged from 45% to 88%.[19]

When the poorly immunogenic PRP is combined with a protein carrier, the immunologic response to PRP is enhanced. Conjugate vaccines employ a highly immunogenic protein carrier that is covalently linked to the PRP antigen. The antigenicity of the protein is incorporated in the immune response to the protein-PRP conjugate. PRP has been conjugated to a

Table 7-4 Traditional Strategies for Developing Inactive Vaccines

Method	Example
Inactivate whole pathogens	Pertussis
Inactivate toxins (toxoids) from pathogens	Diphtheria, tetanus
Purify surface components	Hepatitis B
Conjugate surface components	*Haemophilus influenzae* type b

diphtheria toxoid (PRP-D), a nontoxic mutant diphtheria toxin (HbOC), tetanus toxoid (PRP-T), and the outer membrane protein of *Neisseria meningitidis* (PRP-OMP). These conjugate vaccines have three advantages. First, they produce a T-cell-dependent immune response that is quantitatively enhanced, particularly in younger children. Second, repeat administrations of conjugate vaccines elicit booster responses. Third, a greater proportion of anti-PRP antibodies produced through vaccination are of the IgG class. The conjugate vaccines currently available in the United States are listed in Table 7-5. Although the purposes of these vaccines are the same, important differences in immunologic response exist among them. These differences are reflected in their respective immunization schedules.

Conjugate vaccines

Figure 7-2 shows the responses in children aged 15 to 24 months who were immunized with PRP vaccine or PRP-D vaccine. Antibody responses are at least 10 times greater to PRP-D than to PRP, and they are less dependent on age. Young infants respond to PRP-D, although multiple doses are required. Furthermore, conjugate vaccines such as PRP-D induce booster responses.[14] An evaluation of the clinical efficacy of PRP-D was conducted in Finland. This open trial enrolled 60,000 newborn children who were vaccinated at 3, 4, 6, and 14 months of age. After an average follow-up time of 9 months, there were three cases of invasive Hib infection among those who had received three doses of PRP-D and 20 cases among the controls, indicating 87% protective efficacy. Only minor adverse effects were reported.[20] However, limited efficacy (35%) with PRP-D in young infants of Native Alaskan heritage has been observed.[21] The difference in age distribution of Hib infection between the Finnish children and the Native Alaskan children may have contributed to this apparent difference in efficacy between the two populations. Although most reported Hib disease in Native Alaskan children occurs before 1 year of age, this age group accounts for only 28% of the reported illness in Finland.[22] PRP-D is currently not approved for use in infants younger than 15 months.

Table 7-5 *Haemophilus influenzae* Conjugate Vaccines Licensed in the United States

Vaccine	Carrier	Age (months)
HibTITER®	Mutant diphtheria toxin	2, 4, 6, and 15
ProHIBit®	Diphtheria toxoid	≥15
PedvaxHIB®	Outer membrane protein of *Neisseria meningitidis*	2, 4, and 12

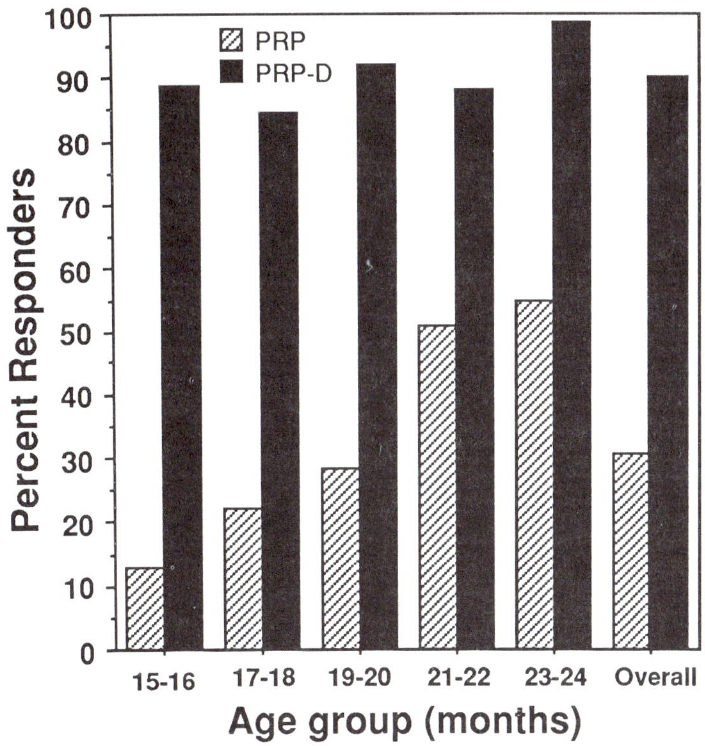

Figure 7-2. Immune responses to polyribosylribitol phosphate (PRP) and PRP diphtheria toxoid by age

SOURCE: Reprinted with permission from Ward J. Newer *Haemophilus influenzae* type b vaccines and passive prophylaxis. *Pediatric Infectious Diseases Journal.* 1987;6:799-803. (copyright by AAAS.)

Vaccine efficacy

Both the HbOC and the PRP-OMP conjugates are immunogenic in infants aged 2 months.[23,24] Comparing the immunogenicity of these vaccines is problematic because of the lack of standardized assays for antibody to PRP. It appears that the antibody response is more brisk to PRP-OMP than to HbOC. However, the antibody response to HbOC appears more prolonged than with PRP-OMP.[22] In a large study conducted in the United States, the protective efficacy of three doses of HbOC was 100% (0 cases in 20,800 children). There were 22 cases of *H. influenzae* disease in the 30,680 unvaccinated children and 3 cases in the 4,919 children who received only one dose of the vaccine.[23] Finally, a randomized trial vaccinated Navajo infants with PRP-OMP at 2 and 4 months of age. Efficacy in this trial was estimated at 93%; 1 case of invasive disease occurred in the children who completed the two-dose series, and 14 cases occurred in placebo recipients.[22] These trials suggest the greater promise of conjugated vaccines for the prevention of *H. influenzae* illness.

Biotechnologic Approaches to Vaccine Development

Safer, more efficient methods of vaccine production are attainable through biotechnology. An understanding of molecular genetics enables attenuated vaccines to be developed with well-defined mutations instead of an accumulation of random mutations. In addition, recombinant DNA techniques allow the cloning and efficient expression of proteins for use in vaccines that contain a few precisely defined antigens. These strategies offer the promise of vaccines without the potential to revert to pathogenic variants, as well as vaccines with fewer contaminants and, therefore, fewer side effects. These techniques also make possible the development of vaccines against organisms such as *Treponema pallidum,* which are difficult to grow. Finally, biotechnologic methods for creating cancer vaccines (see Chapter 10) and vaccines against the human immunodeficiency virus (HIV) (see Chapter 8) are under evaluation.

This section addresses various biotechnologic methods used in vaccine development, including subunit approaches (both cloned proteins and synthetic peptides), attenuation approaches, and approaches using carrier organisms. These methods are summarized in Table 7-6.

Subunit Vaccines. There are two types of subunit vaccines: those made with cloned proteins and those made with synthetic peptides.

Cloned Proteins. Genes that encode for a specific antigen can be cloned and expressed in a variety of vectors. An example of an approach using cloned proteins is the genetically engineered vaccine for hepatitis B.

Table 7-6 Biotechnological Methods of Developing Vaccines

Method	Vaccine Example
Subunit approaches	
Cloned proteins	Hepatitis B, malaria
Synthetic peptides	Hepatitis B, malaria
Attenuated organisms	
Eliminate virulence factor	Cholera
Delete metabolic factor	Typhoid fever
Vaccinia carriers	Herpes simplex, rabies
Anti-idiotypic vaccines	Hepatitis B, rabies

HBV vaccine

The incidence of reported hepatitis B virus (HBV) infection has increased steadily in the past decade, even after the effective plasma-derived vaccine became available. Globally, this disease is associated with acute and chronic hepatitis and primary liver cancer. The incidence of HBV infection in the United States is now estimated at more than 300,000 cases per year.[25]

The crucial immunogen in the HBV vaccine is the surface polypeptide antigen HBsAg. The gene encoding this peptide has been cloned and expressed in yeast, *Escherichia coli,* and mammalian cells. The first licensed recombinant vaccine for HBV was approved by the FDA in July 1986. Currently, there are two recombinant HBV vaccines licensed in the United States.

Technique

These vaccines are produced by inserting the gene containing the HBsAg subtype adw into a plasmid and inserting the plasmid into the yeast *Saccharomyces cerevisiae.* The recombinant antigen forms spherical aggregate particles 17 to 25 nm in diameter, similar to the purified antigen from the plasma-derived HBV vaccine. Although as much as 25% of the plasma-derived antigen is glycosylated, the antigen expressed in yeast is not. This lack of glycosylation has not had any effect on either antigenicity or ability to stimulate neutralizing antibodies. In addition, up to 5% of this final product may consist of yeast-derived proteins, although no yeast DNA is detectable.[25,26] No adverse consequences related to the development of antibody to these yeast proteins were observed during clinical trials.[25] Mammalian cells—Chinese hamster ovary (CHO) cells—have also been used as vectors for production of recombinant HBV vaccine.[27] Both yeast and CHO-derived vaccines confer excellent antibody response with minimal adverse reactions.

Efficacy

The immunogenicity of the recombinant HBV vaccine is comparable to that of the plasma-derived product. More than 90% of healthy adults demonstrate protective antibodies to HBsAg (more than 10 mIU/mL) after a series of three 10-μg doses of the recombinant vaccine; equal rates of seroconversion have been demonstrated after three doses of either the plasma-derived vaccine (20 μg per dose) or recombinant vaccine (10 μg per dose).[28-30] Older adults demonstrate a lower antibody response than younger adults to either vaccine. In studies using three 5-μg doses of recombinant vaccine for children younger than 12 years, more than 99% of the recipients developed protective levels of antibodies.[25] Field trials conducted in the United States suggest that recombinant vaccines are 80% to 95% effective in preventing infection and clinical disease in susceptible individuals.[25,26] In studies of infants born to HBsAg- and HBeAg(envelope)- positive mothers, the combination of hepatitis B immunoglobulin (HBIg) (0.5 mL at birth) and recombinant HBV vaccine (5 μg in each of three doses) was shown to protect 95% of these infants from developing the chronic carrier state; this efficacy equals that of HBIg plus plasma-derived vaccine.[31] However, hemodialysis patients develop a poorer response to the recombinant vaccine than do healthy adults, as shown by one study in which only 64% of hemodialysis patients developed protective levels of antibodies after receiving three 40 μg doses of recombinant HBV vaccine.

Because the surface coat of the virus is the only part of the HBV genome present in the yeast vector, no infectious viral DNA can be produced. Adverse reactions to recombinant HBV vaccine during prelicensure trials were similar in extent and variety to those observed with the plasma-derived vaccine.[25]

Malaria vaccine

The development of malaria vaccines is a second example of a potentially useful application of the subunit approach. Malaria is a major public health problem, particularly in Third World countries, affecting 300 million people per year and causing 1 million to 2 million deaths. Developing a vaccine against this disease is more difficult than developing an HBV vaccine because, in the life cycle of the causative agent, *Plasmodium falciparum,* different antigens are expressed at different stages (Figure 7-3). Because of this difficulty, recombinant DNA methods are being used to develop an effective vaccine, which may serve as a prototype for vaccines against other diseases.

The life cycle of *P. falciparum* begins in the human host when the sporozoite form of the parasite is injected into the host's bloodstream by a mosquito bite. Within minutes the sporozoites invade the hepatocytes, where they are protected from the body's defenses. Once inside the liver cells, the sporozoites reproduce until the hepatocytes burst, releasing thousands of merozoites. These merozoites invade red blood cells (RBCs), where they undergo repeated cycles of intracellular asexual multiplication, resulting in RBC lysis, release of more merozoites, and infection of other RBCs. A few merozoites differentiate into sexual forms called gametocytes, which are then ingested by a mosquito feeding on the host's blood. The cycle begins again as the gametocytes are released from RBCs in the mosquito's stomach, eventually resulting in the production of thousands of sporozoites.

Developing a vaccine against malaria is complicated by the expression of different antigens at each stage in the Plasmodium life cycle. The first attempts at developing a vaccine were directed against the sporozoite stage; however, the time from sporozoite injection to invasion of the hepatocyte is very short. Clinical disease could result if even one sporozoite escapes the antibodies engendered by a vaccine. On the other hand, merozoite vaccines may ameliorate clinical illness, but they cannot prevent infection.

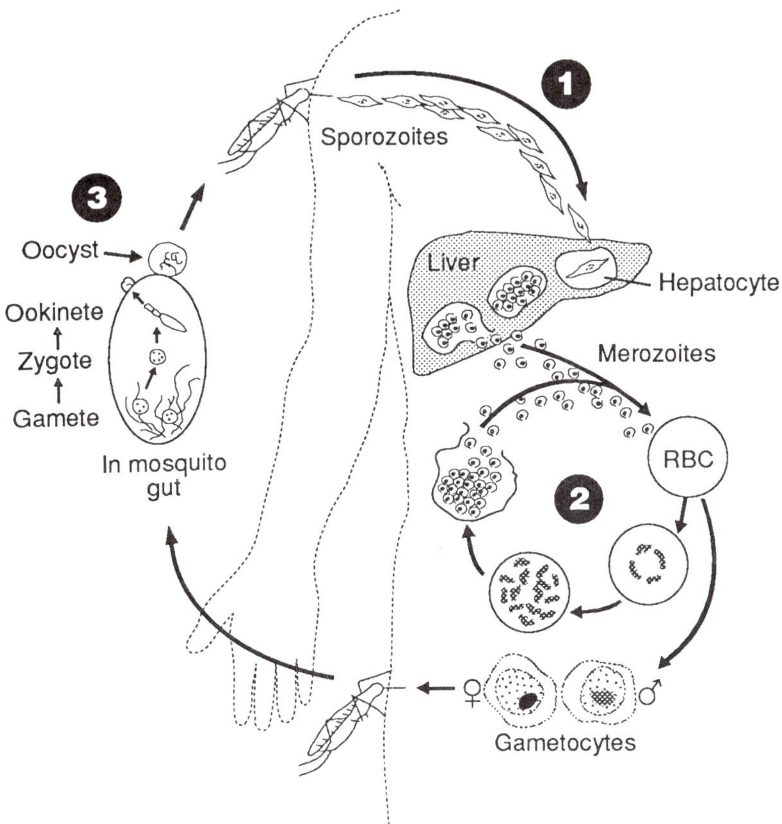

1. Sporozoites; one sporozoite develops into 20,000 merozoites within a hepatic cell. 2. Merozoites rupture from hepatic cells and invade erythrocytes. 3. Cycle in mosquito.

Figure 7-3. Life cycle of malaria

SOURCE: Reprinted with permission from Miller LH, Howard RJ, Carter R, et al. Research toward malaria vaccines. *Science.* 1986;234:1349–56. 1

Efficacy

A recombinant vaccine expressed in *E. coli* and composed of the dominant epitope of the circumsporozoite (CS) protein, which coats the sporozoite, has been developed.[32] Volunteers who were immunized with this vaccine developed antibodies that reacted with *P. falciparum* sporozoite antigen. The efficacy of the vaccine was tested by exposing volunteers to mosquitoes infected with virulent *P. falciparum.* Only one subject was completely protected from parasitemia, two others were partially protected, and no protection was conferred to the remaining three subjects.[33] Such results are far from optimal, but they do suggest that higher doses of this sporozoite vaccine, perhaps in combination with merozoite antigens, may be a useful strategy.

Synthetic Peptides. Synthesizing peptide antigens suitable for vaccination is an alternative to purifying antigens cloned in *E. coli,* yeast, or mammalian cells. The DNA sequence of the gene that encodes the critical immunogen forms the basis for the chemical synthesis of these peptides. An advantage of this approach is that multiple related peptides may be synthesized incorporating variations found between strains. Peptide synthesis may also be directed at conserved, rather than variable, regions of the genome.

Influenza

In one study, investigators working with epitopes of influenza virus synthesized 20 peptides corresponding to 75% of the influenza hemagglutinin. Antibodies directed at 85% of these peptides bound to influenza virus, suggesting that a peptide may stimulate an antibody response capable of binding the virus. In addition, a peptide synthesized from a region conserved in both influenza types A and B produced neutralizing antibodies for the different viral subtypes, indicating that synthetic peptide vaccines may provide protection against organisms with antigenic variability.[34]

Malaria

As an alternative to the cloned protein approach, synthetic peptides have been used as antigens in a vaccine for preventing malaria. This sporozoite vaccine contains the major epitope of the CS protein consisting of a four-amino-acid sequence (asparagine-alanine-asparagine-proline) tandemly repeated 37 times. Nussenzweig and associates developed a synthetic vaccine consisting of three of these four-amino-acid sequences.[35] This 12-amino-acid peptide was conjugated to tetanus toxoid with aluminum hydroxide as an adjuvant and administered to volunteers. The vaccinated subjects were challenged by mosquitoes harboring virulent *P. falciparum.* The results were similar to those seen with the cloned CS vaccine: one volunteer was completely protected from parasitemia and two others showed a significant delay in parasitemia.[36] This synthetic vaccine appears to be immunogenic, stimulating the production of biologically active antibody. Nevertheless, in the doses evaluated thus far, the vaccine did not protect against parasitemia. It may be necessary to combine peptides from both sporozoite and merozoite epitopes to develop an effective synthetic vaccine for malaria.

The studies discussed in this section indicate that it is possible to elicit protective antibody responses in humans with subunit vaccines. These results with both cloned proteins and synthetic peptides are important not only for the development of malaria and HBV vaccines but also for the general approach to vaccine design.

Attenuated Vaccines. Recombinant DNA techniques allow a more defined approach to the rational design of attenuated organisms. DNA sequence analysis and viral genetics may be used to identify regions of the viral genome where alteration reduces the pathogenicity of the organism. In vitro site-directed mutagenesis allows point mutations into, or deletions from, any piece of cloned DNA in a selected, predefined position. The approach to genetically engineered live, attenuated vaccines contrasts with the approach taken with subunit vaccines, in which recombinant technology is used to produce large amounts of a critical antigen isolated from the organism. Site-directed mutagenesis alters genes that encode a critical virulence or growth factor, retaining the organism as a vaccine.[10,37] Cholera and typhoid fever vaccines are examples of two different approaches to live, attenuated vaccines. In the first approach, the gene that encodes for a critical virulence factor (e.g., cholera toxin) may be altered so that the organism survives and multiplies but does not produce disease.[38] In the second approach, a metabolic factor is modified so that the organism does not survive long enough to result in disease. This second approach has been used in the development of a vaccine for *Salmonella typhimurium,* which has additional growth requirements because of the deletion of two genes.[39] Because the vaccines are produced by eliminating a key region in the genome, the vaccine strains are incapable of reverting to pathogenic variants.

Selective mutations/ deletions

Carrier Organisms: The Vaccinia Model. In 1980, following global eradication of smallpox, the World Health Organization (WHO) suspended the use of the wild-type vaccinia virus vaccine. Vaccines may be produced by using vaccinia or other DNA viruses as carriers for one or more foreign antigens.[37] The vaccinia genome may be modified to incorporate foreign genetic material, thus producing a vaccine directed against a wide variety of dissimilar infectious agents. There are a number of examples in which foreign genes encoding pertinent antigens have been expressed by vaccinia virus. Animals inoculated with these recombinant viruses responded with serologic evidence of successful immunization, and, in some cases, protection of these vaccinated animals against subsequent challenge with the infectious agent has been demonstrated.[40] Figure 7-4 outlines the basic strategy for creating recombinant vaccinia carriers through the introduction of foreign DNA sequences into infectious vaccinia virus.

Technique

Foreign genetic material is isolated and inserted into a cloned fragment of the vaccinia genome at a region that is nonessential to vaccinia replication (e.g., thymidine kinase [TK] activity). It is crucial that the flow of genetic information essential for virus replication not be interrupted by insertion of this plasmid. Next, this donor DNA is introduced into tissue culture that has been coinfected with vaccinia virus. In vivo recombination occurs between the vaccinia DNA sequences flanking the foreign DNA and the homologous DNA sequences on the wild-type replicating vaccinia, resulting in recombinant progeny virus.[40] Genes encoding for rabies glycoprotein, HBsAg, HIV envelope glycoprotein, influenza hemagglutinin, herpes simplex glycoprotein D, and Plasmodium CS protein have all been cloned into the TK gene under transcriptional control of the vaccinia promotor.[37]

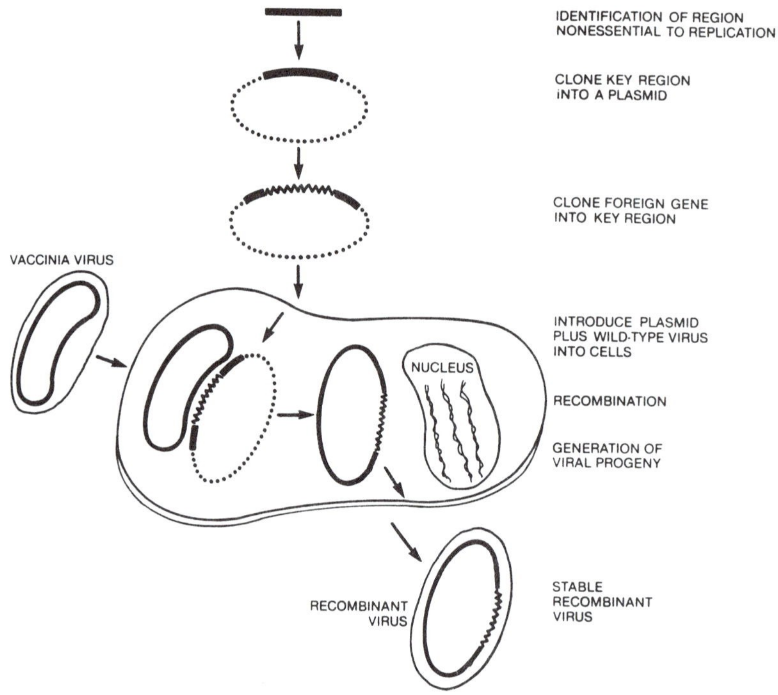

Figure 7-4. Strategy for creating recombinant vaccinia carriers

SOURCE: Reprinted with permission from Ellis RW. New technologies for making vaccines. In: Plotkin SA, Mortimer EA Jr, eds. Vaccines. Philadelphia: W. B. Saunders Company; 1988:570.

Vaccinia advantage

The vaccinia virus is attractive as a vector because, unlike the DNA from other animal viruses, the naked DNA of vaccinia is noninfectious and does not integrate into the host chromosome. In addition, a large amount of foreign DNA can be stably integrated into vaccinia. Thus, a number of foreign genes can be expressed in a single recombinant vaccinia virus, providing a live polyvalent vaccine that may be capable of eliciting immunity against a number of unrelated pathogens. The ability of the human immune system to respond adequately to such an antigenic intrusion, however, remains to be established, as do the relative immunogenicity of, and potential interferences among the various antigens.[40]

Whether a recombinant vaccinia vaccine will be able to induce an immunologic response in an individual previously immunized against smallpox is a critical question. Vaccination usually involves administration of an antigen with the immune response being modulated by homologous controls. With a vaccinia vector, however, the ability to generate an effective antigenic response may depend on the antibody status of the individual to vaccinia as well as on the ability of vaccinia antibody to modulate the multiplication of the recombinant. Since smallpox immunization was discontinued, the populations of vaccinia-naive children and adults with waning immunogenicity have been increasing. Infants with variable transplacental antibodies to vaccinia may be candidates to receive polyvalent vaccinia recombinant vaccines. Given the complexity of this epidemiologic setting, assessing the efficacy of recombinant vaccinia vaccines may be difficult.[41] Nevertheless, encouraging results have been observed in studies of previously vaccinated animals. These animals, already vaccinated with recombinant vaccinia virus, were revaccinated with a second vaccinia recombinant expressing a new foreign antigen. The second vaccination resulted in antibodies to both the new antigen and to the vaccinia itself; however, no increase was observed in antibody response to the initial foreign antigen expressed by the first vaccinia recombinant.[40]

Polyvalent vaccinia vaccines

The manipulation of vaccinia virus illustrates the potential of carrier organisms to generate immunity against a broad spectrum of viral, parasitic, and bacterial pathogens. Multiple antigens may be cloned into vaccinia, as demonstrated by antibody response to three distinct antigens in animals vaccinated with a trivalent vaccinia recombinant.[42] Polyvalent vaccinia vaccines may make possible fewer immunizations, perhaps allowing a combination of vaccines against the childhood diseases in a single vaccination.

Although the benefits of such vaccines appear to outweigh the risks, the safety of these vaccines must be addressed. Wild-type vaccinia has been associated with severe, although infrequent, reactions. Vaccinia recombinant vaccines must be evaluated for the propensity for such reactions. The pathogenesis of vaccinia encephalitis (caused by vaccinia that is tropic for neural tissue) is poorly understood. The impact, if any, that the introduction of foreign antigens may have on tissue tropism is of concern. The safety of these vaccines in immunosuppressed patients must be evaluated.[37]

Approaches to Increasing Immunogenicity

Adjuvants. Adjuvants such as aluminum salts have been useful in enhancing the immune response to some vaccines or toxoids. Although the mechanism of potentiating antigenicity needs further clarification, it is known that a soluble antigen may become particulate when combined with an adjuvant. This property may be essential for synthetic vaccines, which tend to be water soluble and less immunogenic.[43] In addition, adjuvants prolong the release of antigen and mobilize phagocytes at the site of antigen deposition.[8]

FCA

Many of the structural components of microorganisms are themselves antigenic and may be suitable for use as adjuvants. For example, Freund's complete adjuvant (FCA) contains killed mycobacteria dispersed in a water-and-oil emulsion. Though this adjuvant usually stimulates high-level, prolonged immunity, local reactions preclude its use in humans.

MDP

The minimal structure that can replace the adjuvant activity of mycobacteria in FCA is synthetic N-acetyl-muramyl-L-alanyl-D-isoglutamine, called muramyl dipeptide (MDP). Unlike other mycobacterial components, the adjuvant properties of MDP are present when administered either parenterally or orally in an aqueous medium. MDP exerts activity on several cell lines, including T cells, macrophages, and B cells. The essential mediators of this adjuvant effect appear to be T lymphocytes, as shown in transfer experiments and by stimulation of helper cell function in various carrier-hapten systems.[40] Depletion and even removal of macrophages do not reduce the adjuvant effect of MDP. B lymphocytes reconstituted with a monokine and interleukins can be stimulated by MDP, perhaps through enhancing differentiation of B cells into antibody-producing cells.[44]

Adjuvants may also be capable of suppressing the immune response. Immunosuppression has been described with BCG and lipopolysaccharide adjuvants and may occur with large doses of MDP. The antibody response to both particulate and soluble antigens is depressed in mice pretreated with high doses of MDP. T lymphocytes may mediate the suppressive effect of MDP. The capacity of MDP to inhibit the production of interleukin-2 and to increase the secretion of prostaglandins and oxygen metabolites may also play a role in its immunosuppressive effect. Because cell-mediated immunity is regulated by MDP, treatment of mice with a water-and-oil emulsion of MDP may induce nonspecific suppressor T cells.[44]

Mechanism

Anti-idiotypes. Idiotypes are unique epitopes either within the variable regions of immunoglobulin molecules produced by each individual B-cell clone or within T-cell receptors on each individual T-cell clone. Antibodies bear a structural image of their primary antigen at the antigen-binding site (idiotype). Therefore, antibodies directed at these antibodies (anti-idiotypes) must have antigen-binding sites similar to the antigen. Administration of an anti-idiotypic antibody would stimulate an anti-anti-idiotypic antibody, which should be identical to the primary antibody (Figure 7-5). This strategy is analogous to making a negative from a photographic negative to produce a positive image.

In vaccination experiments, anti-idiotypic antibodies have been used increasingly, either alone or in combination with vaccinating antigens. In one study, pretreatment of mice with anti-idiotypic antibodies 2 weeks before vaccination enhanced the immune response to HBsAg. These

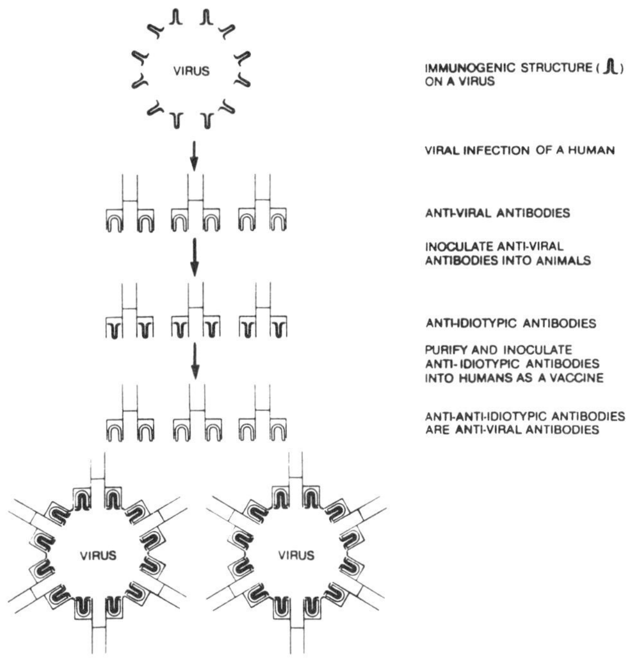

Figure 7-5. Development of anti-idiotype antibodies as vaccines

SOURCE: Reprinted with permission from Ellis RW. New technologies for making vaccines. In: Plotkin SA, Mortimer EA Jr, eds. Vaccines. Philadelphia: W. B. Saunders Company; 1988:574.

anti-idiotypic antibodies were produced in rabbits that were administered monoclonal antibody (MoAb) to mouse HBsAg.[45] Thus, the anti-idiotypic antibodies represented an internal image of the HBsAg.

The protective effect of anti-idiotypes was first demonstrated by Sacks and associates, using a major surface glycoprotein (VAT 1.1) of a clone of *Trypanosoma rhodesiense* as the antigen.[46] MoAbs against VAT 1.1 were used as the antibody to prepare the anti-idiotypic antibodies. Pretreatment with anti-idiotypic antibodies 4 to 5 weeks before infection with the VAT 1.1 clone of trypanosomes prevented initial VAT 1.1 parasitemia.

Anti-idiotypes may also be useful in inducing an immune response when the corresponding antigens are not easily available. In addition, anti-idiotypes should enhance the induction of an immune response in young recipients of vaccines or when the antigens are poorly immunogenic. The use of anti-idiotypes may provide an opportunity to avoid the use of adjuvants; however, at present, most anti-idiotypes are produced in animals. Eventually, human anti-idiotypes produced through MoAb technology may be needed. The potential risk of anti-idiotypes, such as the potential for immunosuppression and the generation of antireceptor autoantibodies or immune complexes, should be evaluated.

Passive Immunization

This section reviews the history and use of passive immunization. In particular, the role of exogenous immunoglobulins in serotherapy is outlined. At the conclusion of this section, the many exciting new uses of immunoglobulin therapy, both intravenous and intramuscular, as a means of imparting passive immunity are described.

History of Passive Immunization

In active immunization, a relatively harmless antigenic form of an organism is given to a patient to impart memory to the immune system, thereby stimulating production of endogenous antibodies (see Chapter 2 for a review of the function of memory cells). In contrast, passive immunization protects individuals by facilitating the antigen-antibody reaction. Passive immunization is accomplished by administering exogenous immunoglobulin from an immune donor to an unprotected individual. The means by which an individual acquires specific passive immunity may be either natural or induced. An example of natural passive immunity is that provided by the immunoglobulins babies receive from their mothers; an example of induced passive immunity is that imparted to an individual by the administration of exogenous animal or human immunoglobulins.

Maternal-fetal immunity

It was first recognized in the late 1800s that certain diseases (e.g., diphtheria and tetanus) are caused by specific toxins secreted by organisms. Closely following this discovery was the realization that acquired immunity developed in animals exposed to these toxins and that antibodies in the serum were responsible for neutralizing the toxins. These antibodies are thus the source of immunity, and the serum containing these antibodies came to be known as antitoxins.

Antitoxins

Intramuscular Immunoglobulins (IMIgs)

Humoral immunity can be transferred from a sensitized person to a nonsensitized person through exogenous antibodies. Passive immunity occurs naturally in fetal life by placental transfer of maternal antibodies. The source of antibody for induced passive immunization may be immunoglobulin in serum from immunized animals (heterologous), or it may be antigen-specific or -nonspecific pooled human immunoglobulin (homologous). Table 7-7 lists the currently available animal antisera, and Table 7-8 lists the currently available human immunoglobulin products for passive immunization.

Passive immunization often involves injection of a specific immunoglobulin that is targeted for a specific antigen. This process is also referred to as seroprophylaxis or serotherapy. Serotherapy provides only temporary protection against an antigen, because it does not promote the formation of protective antibodies by the recipient. Normal body catabolism also contributes to the short duration of protection of exogenous immunoglobulin, as does the rapid depletion of antibody as it combines with antigen.[7,47]

Serotherapy

Table 7-7 Currently Available Animal Antisera for Passive Immunization

Disease	Product	Source
Black widow spider bite	Antivenin	Equine
Botulism	Botulism antitoxin	Equine
Diphtheria	Diphtheria antitoxin	Equine
Snakebite	Antivenin polyvalent; antivenin	Equine

Table 7-8 Currently Available Human Immunoglobulins for Passive Immunization

Disease	Product
Cytomegalovirus	Cytomegalovirus Ig
Hepatitis A; non-A, non-B hepatitis	IMIg
Hepatitis B	Hepatitis B Ig
Hypogammaglobulinemia	IMIg; IVIg
Measles	IMIg
Rabies	Rabies Ig
Rh isoimmunization	Rh O (D) Ig
Rubella	IMIg
Tetanus	Tetanus Ig
Varicella	Varicella-zoster Ig

Ig = immunoglobulin; IMIg = intramuscular immunoglobulin; IVIg = intravenous immunoglobulin.

Heterologous and homologous sera

Immunoglobulins for serotherapy are derived from either animal sources (heterologous) or human sources (homologous). Although antitoxins derived from active immunization of animals (i.e., horses and rabbits) neutralize the same toxins in humans, they are less desirable than those taken from human sources. Animal sera are seen as foreign proteins by the human immune system and frequently cause anaphylactic or serum sickness reactions because of the formation of precipitating antigen-antibody complexes.[47] Therefore, human immunoglobulin should be used whenever possible.

Patient history

When human sources are not available, animal sera may be given in life-threatening situations. However, patients or their relatives must be carefully questioned by the pharmacist or other health care provider to assess for preexisting hypersensitivity to animal sera and possible type I hypersensitivity reactions (see Chapter 4). A history of atopy or hypersensitivity greatly increases the likelihood that such a reaction will develop. Taking a history, along with the use of skin testing, to assess the risk of sera administration is critical to ensure patient safety.

Serotherapy with heterologous agents may provide immediate protection to a naive or specific antibody-free patient and has a variety of theoretical uses but only a limited number of current clinical uses. Its primary use is as prophylaxis in patients who have been exposed to diseases such as hepatitis and rabies.[47] Serotherapy is especially useful when the anticipated incubation period of the disease is shorter than the onset of protection with standard vaccination techniques, which usually take 7 to 10 days to become effective.[2,48] The effectiveness of passive immunization depends on prompt administration of immune sera. The sera must be given early in the incubation period to avoid onset of clinical illness in the exposed patient. For instance, diphtheria antitoxin must be given within 1 hour of symptom onset to prevent irreversible damage.[49]

Applications

The current uses of IMIgs outlined here include their use in treating established toxin-induced illnesses and in prophylaxis of viral infections.

IMIgs in Toxin-induced Diseases. This role of IMIgs is primarily limited to using antitoxins and antivenins in preventing onset of disease in exposed patients. Conditions that involve toxin production and may be treated with IMIgs include botulism, tetanus, diphtheria, black widow spider bites, and snakebite. Note in Table 7-7 that all IMIgs for this use are derived from horse sera.

IMIgs in Prophylaxis of Viral Infections. The WHO currently recommends using IMIgs only for patients exposed to hepatitis A; hepatitis B; non-A, non-B hepatitis; varicella-zoster; measles; rubella; and rabies. This use of IMIgs is much more common than for toxin-induced diseases.

IMIgs are useful for the prophylaxis of viral infections because of their capacity to decrease the severity or modify the effects of diseases for which no effective vaccine is available. As can be seen in Table 7-8, certain immunoglobulins are antigen specific: cytomegalovirus (CMV) Ig, hepatitis B Ig (HBIg), rabies Ig, tetanus Ig, and varicella-zoster Ig (VZIg). Antigen-specific immunoglobulins are derived from donors with very high circulating levels of a particular antibody. For example, VZIg is very specific for varicella because it is derived from the serum of convalescent patients with zoster.[2] However, in all other uses (i.e., hepatitis A; non-A, non-B hepatitis; measles; and rubella) nonspecific human IMIg is used for serotherapy. The two specific types of IMIg that are highlighted in this section are HBIg and VZIg.

HBIg is the preferred agent in postexposure prophylaxis against HBV. Active immunization with HBV vaccine is the ideal preventive tool in persons at risk for HBV exposure, such as health care workers. However, if an unvaccinated person is accidentally exposed, vaccination alone is inadequate because of the delayed onset of protection (it takes several weeks to develop hepatitis B antibody titers).[50]

HBIg advantage

The advantage of HBIg is that it can provide high levels of anti-hepatitis B antibody immediately. Because of its greater antigen specificity, it is more effective and preferred over nonspecific human IMIg, which provides only minimal anti-HBV antibodies.[50] HBIg should be administered intramuscularly immediately after exposure (preferably within 24 hours) as prophylaxis in patients at risk of developing HBV infection, including people exposed to materials contaminated with the virus, such as blood from a patient with HBV.[26,50-52] The prompt use of serotherapy provides immediate protection until vaccination can impart active immunity to the exposed individual.

Some studies have shown that HBIg alone administered to exposed individuals did not completely prevent the disease but merely attenuated the clinical illness by lengthening the incubation period.[50] Thus, the Immunization Practices Advisory Committee (ACIP) of the CDC has recommended that a combination approach consisting of administration of HBV vaccine and HBIg be used for postexposure prophylaxis in susceptible (unvaccinated) persons who have perinatal or needlestick exposure to persons known to have HBV or to their blood.[26]

In summary, the use of combined active (HBV vaccine) and passive (HBIg) immunization is thus recommended by the ACIP to prevent the onset of HBV.[26,50-52]

VZIg

Another example of the use of IMIgs in viral illness is the use of VZIg, the causative agent of chicken pox and herpes zoster. Because VZIg is prepared from the plasma of adults who have high titers of antivaricella antibodies, it has very high levels of antibody specifically directed at varicella-zoster. In contrast to HBIg, the use of VZIg is directed mainly at immunocompromised patients. Administration of VZIg (commercially produced by the Massachusetts Public Health Biologic Laboratories and available since 1978 through the American Red Cross) may be a lifesaving measure in certain high-risk patients, including those who are immunocompromised, those on drugs such as steroids or on radiation, and neonates who contract varicella.[53] Passive immunization with VZIg does not necessarily prevent the onset of chicken pox, but it modifies the clinical course of the disease by decreasing its severity.[53,54] Like all serotherapy, VZIg must be administered promptly (within 96 hours) after exposure to the varicella virus to be effective.[53,55,56] When used within this time frame in exposed immunodeficient children, VZIg significantly decreased the expected severity of chicken pox and decreased mortality, encephalitis, and pneumonia to less than 25% of the expected rate without treatment.[57]

The supply of VZIg is still somewhat limited. Because each adult dose costs several hundred dollars, it should not be used indiscriminately.[56] Table 7-9 lists the ACIP guidelines on which patients should receive VZIg.[53]

In summary, IMIgs have clinical utility in treating patients exposed to toxin-mediated diseases such as diphtheria and tetanus and viral diseases such as HBV and chicken pox.

Intravenous Immunoglobulins (IVIgs)

An important development in passive immunization in the past decade is the introduction of immunoglobulin suitable for intravenous use. Before the mid-1970s, no immunoglobulin products could be given intravenously, because they caused small IgG aggregate formation, anticomplement activity, and subsequent anaphylactic reactions. The formation of these aggregates was linked to the method of production. However, because of reformulation techniques, all IVIg products available in the United States can now be safely given intravenously.[58]

Production

IVIg is derived from IgG isolated from pooled human serum; although it contains primarily IgG, other antibody classes (IgE, IgM, and IgA) as well as other serum proteins may be present in trace amounts.[59] The larger the donor pool, the wider the spectrum of IgG antibodies contained in the serum. In fact, the WHO recommends that all IVIg products be derived from pools of at least 1,000 donors.[59]

Table 7-9 Guidelines of the Immunization Practices Advisory Committee, Centers for Disease Control, for Use of Varicella-zoster Immunoglobulin (VZIg)

1. Persons susceptible to varicella-zoster.
2. Persons with significant exposure within 96 hours of VZIg administration.
3. Persons younger than 15 years old (administration to immunocompromised adolescents and adults and to other older patients on an individualized basis).
4. Persons with one of the following underlying illnesses or conditions:
   a. Neoplastic disease (e.g., leukemia or lymphoma).
   b. Congenital or acquired immunodeficiency.
   c. Drug- or radiation-induced immunosuppression.
   d. Newborn of mother who had onset of chicken pox within 5 days before delivery or within 48 hours after delivery.
   e. Premature infant (gestation period > 28 weeks) whose mother lacks a prior history of chicken pox.
   f. Premature infant (gestation period < 28 weeks or birth weight ≤ 1,000 g) regardless of maternal history.

In the United States, all IVIg products must meet standards set by the FDA. All plasma donor units must be without HBsAg and antibody for HIV. All IVIg products contain no less than 90% of their immunoglobulin content as gamma globulin (as recommended by the WHO). Side effects occur after administration of IVIg in approximately 2% to 8% of patients, but they are generally mild (e.g., chills, nausea, abdominal pain) and can often be eliminated via premedication or by slowing the rate of intravenous infusion. The intravenous route for administering immunoglobulin has many advantages over the intramuscular route. The greatest advantage is that IVIgs can be given in much larger doses than was previously possible with IMIg products. Other advantages include immediate blood levels, greater bioavailability, ease of administration, relatively painless administration, fewer severe adverse reactions, and a half-life more closely

Side effects

IVIg advantages

resembling that of endogenous IgG (22 to 29 days).[51,60] Table 7-10 lists the six currently licensed IVIg products available in the United States.

The variables to consider when selecting a particular IVIg product are beyond the scope of this text. Therapeutic differences among the licensed products have never been studied in a controlled fashion, but because of their similarity these products are generally considered to be therapeutic equivalents. Factors the pharmacist should consider when making a product selection include plasma source, method of preparation, reconstitution time, storage requirements, available concentrations, available diluents, and cost. Unfortunately, all available IVIg products are quite expensive, especially because fairly substantial doses are commonly used. For example, a recommended dose of IVIg for idiopathic thrombocytopenia purpura (ITP) would average 400 mg/kg. This dose, 25 g to 35 g for an average-size adult, currently costs nearly $1,000 regardless of the manufacturer. Therefore, indiscriminate use of this product for non-FDA-approved uses should be closely monitored as a part of every institution's ongoing drug utilization evaluation program.

The IgG subclass profile varies slightly among the available products; this point is discussed more fully in the next section. Levels of antiviral antibody may also be considered, although the manufacturers often employ

Table 7-10 Intravenous Immunoglobulin Products Licensed in the United States

Product	Manufacturer	Sizes (g)	Formulation
Gamimune N®	Cutter Biologics	0.5, 2.5, 5.0, 12.5	Liquid in 10% maltose
Gammagard®	Hyland-Travenol	0.5, 2.5, 5.0, 10.0	Lyophilized powder
Gammar-IV®	Armour	0.5, 1.0, 2.5, 5.0	Lyophilized powder
Iveegam®	Immuno-U.S.	0.5, 1.0, 2.5, 5.0	Lyophilized powder
Sandoglobulin®	Sandoz	1.0, 3.0, 6.0	Lyophilized powder
Venoglobulin®	Alpha Therapeutics	0.5, 2.5, 5.0	Lyophilized powder

different immunologic assays to measure them, making strict comparison difficult.[61]

IgA deficiency

Patients with IgA deficiency should receive only IgA-free or IgA-poor preparations; this point should also be considered when an IVIg product is being selected.[61] IgA deficiency is the most common primary immunodeficiency, although it actually occurs in only 1 of every 400 patients.[62] Most IgA-deficient people are prone to frequent infections, especially respiratory tract infections.[62] These patients also often have low levels of IgG subclasses, especially the IgG2 subclass (combined IgA and IgG2 deficiency). From 10% to 60% of these patients have measurable titers of anti-IgA antibodies in their blood.[62,63] In these patients, administration of IVIg can be beneficial in correcting the IgG2 deficiency. However, their immune systems view the exogenous IgA found in many commercially available IVIg products as foreign, and their anti-IgA antibody titers can quickly increase in response. Because of these high levels of antibody, anaphylactic reactions can occur after infusion of any material containing IgA, such as blood, plasma, or IVIg products.[63] (See Chapter 4 for a review of the mechanism of anaphylactic reactions.) Therefore, to avoid unnecessary stimulation of the immune system and to decrease the incidence and severity of adverse reactions that still may occur in this very small population of patients who are IgA deficient, only immunoglobulin products low in IgA should be administered. In patients with IgA deficiencies who also have anti-IgA antibodies, IVIgs should not be used and alternate treatments should be considered. In addition, serum anti-IgA antibody titers should be closely monitored while patients are on immunoglobulin replacement therapy. An increase in antibody titers may indicate an enhanced risk of anaphylaxis.[64]

Applications

IVIg has many therapeutic uses. The three uses currently approved by the FDA are the treatment of hypogammaglobulinemia as a primary immunodeficiency, the treatment of ITP, and the treatment of hypogammaglobulinemia in patients with chronic lymphocytic leukemia (CLL). However, as can be seen from the partial list of potential uses shown in Table 7-11, IVIg is being studied in a wide variety of autoimmune and immunodeficient disease states.

IVIg is the preferred treatment in primary immunodeficiencies such as hypogammaglobulinemia, exerting therapeutic action through repletion of antibodies.[65] The diseases characterized as secondary or acquired immunodeficiencies vastly outnumber primary immunodeficiencies. IVIg has been studied in a variety of secondary immunodeficiencies, many of which are listed in Table 7-11.

Table 7-11 Potential and FDA-Approved Indications for Intravenous Immunoglobulins

Primary immunodeficiencies
Agammaglobulinemia
Hypogammaglobulinemia*
Secondary (acquired) immunodeficiencies
Malignancies associated with antibody deficiency
Chronic lymphocytic leukemia*
Multiple myeloma
Bacterial infections
Pseudomonas
Group B *Streptococcus*
Viral infections
Cytomegalovirus
Herpes simplex
Kidney, heart, and bone marrow transplant patients
High-risk premature infants and neonates
Acquired immunodeficiency syndrome patients
Burn patients
Thrombocytopenias
Autoimmune thrombocytopenia purpura
Idiopathic thrombocytopenia purpura*
Other autoimmune disorders
Collagen vascular diseases
Myasthenia gravis
Kawasaki's syndrome
Autoimmune neutropenia and hemolytic anemia

*FDA-approved.

IVIg has also been studied extensively in the treatment of ITP, a bleeding disorder characterized by destruction of platelets and easy bruising. ITP is now thought to be caused by an IgG-mediated autoimmune coating of platelets. The exact mechanism of action of IVIg in treating ITP is unclear. One suggested mechanism is that IVIg saturates Fc receptors on platelets, thus providing antibody-coated cells that are less susceptible to Fc-mediated phagocytosis and destruction by the reticuloendothelial system. Although several mechanisms may actually be involved, the important fact is that IVIg is clinically effective in raising platelet counts in both adults and children.[61] This increase in platelet counts is especially important before a surgical procedure or when there is active bleeding.[61] In responding

Efficacy

patients, the increase in platelet count is usually rapid (within 1 to 5 days) but the rise is generally only transient, lasting from several days to a month.[51]

The effectiveness of IVIg in other secondary (acquired) immunodeficiencies is thought to relate to both its immunomodulatory effect and its ability to replace specific antibodies. The infectious complications—bacterial, viral, and fungal—that often accompany these secondary immunodeficiencies can be devastating, especially in transplant patients and premature infants, among others. It is now known that hypogammaglobulinemia may be an important contributing factor in the development of these infectious complications. Based on this information and placebo-controlled clinical trials, the FDA approved use of IVIg in the prevention of recurrent bacterial infections in some patients with B-cell chronic lymphocytic leukemia.

Antigen-specific (hyperimmune) immunoglobulins have also shown promise in the management of specific infections. For example, the incidence and severity of CMV infections in transplant patients has been modulated by the administration of CMV-IVIg. CMV-IVIg has recently received FDA approval as an "orphan drug" for the attenuation of primary CMV disease associated with renal transplantation.[66] Use of CMV-IVIg is specifically targeted toward patients who are CMV seronegative but are receiving a kidney from a CMV-seropositive donor.[51] Prospective clinical studies have shown a 50% decrease in primary CMV disease in kidney transplant recipients who received CMV-IVIg versus untreated controls. CMV-IVIg is available from the Massachusetts Public Health Biologic Laboratories.[51,66]

In addition to clinical studies using CMV-IVIg in renal transplant recipients, CMV-IVIg has also been evaluated for its ability to decrease CMV pneumonitis and graft-versus-host disease in bone marrow, heart, and liver transplant recipients.[61,67-71] The use of hyperimmune CMV-IVIg to attenuate or prevent CMV infection in transplants other than kidney transplants remains controversial (see also Chapter 9). In addition, the high doses used in most of these trials would be prohibitively expensive outside a research setting.[72] The future use of antigen-specific hyperimmune IVIgs appears promising; however, further studies are warranted before therapeutic utility can be assessed.

In summary, IVIg has had great therapeutic impact not only in primary immunodeficiencies, but also in thrombocytopenias. Additional uses, such as in secondary immunodeficiencies and other autoimmune diseases, are under evaluation, and conclusive evidence regarding efficacy remains to be obtained.

IVIg Subclasses

Different subclasses of IgG are present in IVIg products as well as in normal human serum. These subclasses are important because they relate to disease etiology and are thus included as components of the various IVIg products available in the United States.

Four IgG subclasses have been identified which differ not only structurally but also functionally: IgG1, IgG2, IgG3, and IgG4. Structurally, the four subclasses have four different types of gamma heavy chains, which determine the subclass.[73] (See Chapter 2 for more on the structure of immunoglobulins.) Functionally, the specific roles of the IgG subclasses are still being actively investigated. The biologic properties of IgG1 are similar to those of IgG3; they include complement fixation and response to antigen.[73,74] IgG2 accounts for most immunoglobulin directed against the polysaccharide capsule of various bacteria, including *H. influenzae* and streptococci.[73] IgG4 has a role in the activation of mast cells of the respiratory tract, and its functions in the immune system are closely linked to those of IgG2.[74] Table 7-12 lists some of the presumed functions of each IgG subclass.

Deficiencies

The clinical impact of IgG subclasses relates to their unique roles in the normal human immune system (see Table 7-12). Deficiency in IgG subclasses in humans is now known to be associated with certain diseases. The first clinically defined subclass deficiency was noted in 1968.[75] Patients with an IgG subclass deficiency may be asymptomatic or very prone to severe infections. In addition, the deficiency may be in a single subclass or more than one. Most patients are lacking two subclasses; the predominant pattern is a lack of IgG1 and IgG3, followed in incidence by a deficiency of IgG2 and IgG4.[76] Among infection-prone adult patients with a single subclass deficiency, IgG3 accounts for the major deficiency; in children, IgG2 deficiency clearly dominates.[77,78]

Table 7-12 Functions of Gamma Globulin in Subclasses

Subclass	Presumed Functions
IgG1	Tissue protection, complement fixation, response to antigen
IgG2	Response to polysaccharide containing bacteria
IgG3	Complement fixation, virus neutralization
IgG4	Protection of the respiratory tract by harnessing mast cells and basophils

Disease association

The exact relationship of IgG subclass deficiency and increased susceptibility to infection is still unknown. However, it is postulated that the deficiency occurs secondary to a predominant T-cell defect or impaired T- and B-cell cooperation.[76] In one study, 75% of subclass-deficient adults studied also had impaired T- and B-cell function.[78] Patients with IgG2 or IgG4 deficiency have a higher incidence of severe infections than patients lacking IgG1 or IgG3.[76] IgG2-deficient patients are especially prone to respiratory tract infections by encapsulated bacteria, such as streptococcus,[73] whereas a deficiency of IgG4 has been associated with recurrent pyogenic respiratory infections.[74]

Recent studies have shown that subclass deficiencies can be clinically relevant and yet are underrecognized. Since IgG1 makes up more than 70% of the total IgG, a subclass deficiency of IgG2, IgG3, or IgG4 may not be identified if only the total IgG is measured. In fact, a documented subclass deficiency, especially IgG2, occurred in 24% of patients who had abnormal susceptibility to infections, normal total IgG levels, and no clear preexisting evidence of an immunodeficiency syndrome.[76] Therefore, workups of patients with frequent infections and a suspected immunodeficiency may need to include measurement of each subclass to document an IgG subclass deficiency.[73,79,80]

Measurements

Levels of IgG subclasses may be measured by a variety of techniques. The main variables among the tests are the types of reagents used and the assay method used. The reagents are usually either polyclonal antisera or MoAbs. Polyclonal antisera were the first reagents used to identify subclasses in early studies. The antisera are prepared by immunizing different animals with a single purified IgG subclass. Doing so involves an extremely complex production technique to prevent impurities of animal serum. Because the polyclonal antibodies are not subclass specific, their application is limited.

Because of the shortcomings of polyclonal antisera, MoAbs (see Chapter 11) have become the preferred reagents for detecting and quantifying IgG subclasses. Subclass-specific murine MoAbs have been available since the mid-1980s. They are preferred because they are more specific, more reproducible, and more available than polyclonal antisera.[81]

There are different assays to detect subclass levels. The radial immunodiffusion assay (see Chapter 5) was one of the first assays used to detect IgG subclasses. However, it lacks sensitivity for IgG3 and IgG4.[81] The enzyme-linked immunosorbent assay (ELISA) (see Chapter 5) is the preferred assay because of its improved sensitivity for subclasses with very minute levels in the serum. Therefore, most authors recommend the ELISA assay with MoAb reagents for evaluating subclass deficiencies of IgG.[76,78,81,82]

Measurements of subclass levels can vary depending on the laboratory for several reasons: (1) The different reagents assay procedures used by different laboratories may cause variable results. (2) Various MoAbs may be available for the same subclass (at least five specific antibodies are available for IgG1 alone).[81] (3) Results of assays may be reported only in relative percentages of subclasses, whereas the absolute values of the subclass levels may vary considerably.

Because standardized methods were not in place for the many studies that have been conducted on IgG subclass deficiencies, directly comparing patient populations among studies is difficult if not impossible.[81] Attention should be given to the reagents and assay methodology when evaluating the clinical literature on IgG subclasses.

Applications

The clinical utility of measuring the IgG subclass level relates to its application in diagnosing and treating immunodeficiency. Possible clinical applications include: (1) Early identification of IgG subclass deficiency can help to explain the cause of recurrent infections and assist with planning for the patient. (2) Subclass levels can be screened for preoperatively in patients with suspected immunodeficiency and history of severe infections, and the utility of postoperative IVIg replacement therapy can be assessed. (3) More exact treatments for specific deficiencies can be made.[81]

Commercially available IVIg products are clinically useful in treating symptomatic patients with subclass deficiency. To closely mimic normal serum, any IVIg product that is used should contain a proportion of each subclass similar to proportions found in normal serum. The WHO has recognized a "reference plasma" to act as a guideline for subclass distribution. The percentage of each subclass of six currently available IVIg products, in comparison to the WHO reference, is presented in Table 7-13.

Product evaluation

IVIg products should originate from large donor pools and should contain the IgG subclasses in their natural distribution. The products listed in Table 7-13 have been compared in several studies.[51,59,83-85] Specific quantification values and relative percentages differ among the studies, probably because of interlaboratory variability and differences in the donor pools. However, the relative differences and similarities among the available products is similarly described in most studies. Sandoglobulin® had lower levels of IgG1 and higher levels of IgG2.[83] Iveegam® had no detectable levels of IgG3, making this product probably unsuitable for replacement therapy according to the WHO standard. The greatest relative differences among the products was found in levels of IgG4. Gamimune® and Gammagard® had much lower levels of IgG4. This low level may be caused by one of the purification steps in the manufacturing process, which is designed to reduce the content of IGA.[83] Low levels of IgA are desirable in products given to patients with IgA deficiency and anti-IgA antibodies.

Table 7-13 Percentage of IgG Subclasses in Licensed Intravenous Immunoglobulin Products

Product	IgG1 (%)	IgG2 (%)	IgG3 (%)	IgG4 (%)
WHO reference plasma	60.0	29.4	6.5	4.1
Gamimune N®	66.7	27.0	5.4	0.9
Gammagard®	66.8	25.4	7.4	0.3
Gammar-IV®	69.0	23.0	6.0	2.0
Iveegam®	60–70	30–40	0	2.0
Sandoglobulin®	55.3	35.7	6.3	2.6
Venoglobulin®	60.9	29.4	5.3	4.4

SOURCE: Adapted with permission from the following:

[1] Skvaril F, Gardi A. Differences among available immunoglobulin preparations for intravenous use. *Pediatric Infectious Disease Journal.* 1988;7(suppl 5):543–8.
[2] Originally published in Knapp MJ, Colburn PA. Clinical uses of intravenous immune globulin. *Clinical Pharmacy.* 1990;9:509–29.

WHO = World Health Organization.

In fact, Gammagard® is the only IVIg product indicated in patients with IgA deficiency, because of its low content of IgA.[59] Historically, IgG products prepared by different methods had no IgG3 and very low levels of IgG4.[58] Lack of IgG4 in these older preparations was associated with increased incidence of pyogenic respiratory infections in patients.[74]

The clinical significance of the differing subclass distributions in these IVIg products is yet unknown. Four of the six products described in Table 7-13 (GamimuneN®, Gammagard®, Gammar-IV®, and Sandogobulin®) closely mimic the natural distribution of IgG, which accounts for the utility of these products in treating agammaglobulinemia[83] and the lack of infectious sequelae due to subclass imbalances. That Gammagard® has considerably lower levels of IgG4 than the other products may be of concern in treating patients with documented IgG4 subclass deficiency. The variations among products, as cited in the literature, may be due to differences in the manufacturing and purification processes, differences in assay procedures used by various investigators and laboratories, and differences in the pool of donors. Until these differences are standardized, it will be difficult to compare IVIg products reliably.

In conclusion, each IgG subclass plays an important role in the immune system. Clinical deficiency of a subclass may manifest itself as disease, most commonly as a chronic respiratory infection. Development and standardization of technology for quantification has added to our knowledge of IgG subclass deficiencies, especially with the advent of subclass-specific MoAbs. IVIg products with adequate subclass representation can normalize the plasma of patients with subclass deficiency.

Summary

Immunization may be achieved actively or passively. Active immunization exposes the immune system to a relatively harmless form of an antigen to stimulate the body's defenses against a specific disease. Passive immunization facilitates the antigen-antibody response by administering exogenous immunoglobulin from an immune donor to an unprotected individual.

Active immunization with live vaccines poses a risk that the patient will develop the disease rather than only an immune response. Allergic reactions are also possible, most frequently as a result of the culture medium. The risk of vaccination must be assessed within the context of the prevalence of disease and relative risk of adverse effects. Adverse effects to seven vaccines must be reported to VAERS.

Vaccines may contain live, attenuated organisms (generating lifelong immunity) or killed organisms. The latter require multiple administrations since they usually do not provide permanent protection with a single dose. Stability is crucial to live vaccines. Vaccines with killed organisms may, however, produce more adverse effects because of large quantities of extraneous material in the vaccine.

Hib disease is most prevalent in children younger than 2 years old. However, traditionally produced Hib vaccines are not very effective in this population. Vaccine conjugates can improve their performance with greater effectiveness in infants.

Biotechnologic methods of producing vaccine subunits include cloning (e.g., hepatitis B and malaria) and using synthetic peptides (e.g., influenza and malaria) to produce large amounts of a critical antigen. Recombinant technology is also used to produce attenuated vaccines that are genetically altered to a nonpathogenic state. Vaccinia viruses may be used as carrier organisms for introducing many different antigens through recombinant DNA technology. Adjuvants and anti-idiotypes are also being studied for immunologic effects.

Passive immunization vaccines, which provide only temporary protection, may be developed from animal or human sera. Passive immunization is more quickly effective, however, than active immunization. Animal sera may produce anaphylactic responses. Intramuscular immunoglobulin vaccines are presently used for treating toxin-induced illnesses and preventing viral infections. Intravenous immunoglobulin vaccines are used for many therapeutic purposes. They have several advantages over intramuscular vaccines but are much more costly.

References

1. Plotkin SL, Plotkin SA. A short history of vaccines. In: Plotkin SA, Mortimer EA Jr, eds. Vaccines. Philadelphia: W. B. Saunders Company; 1988.
2. Stites JP, Stobo JD, Fudenberg HH et al. Basic and clinical immunology. 5th ed. Los Altos, CA: Medical Publications; 1984.
3. Centers for Disease Control. Measles prevention: recommendations of the Immunization Practices Advisory Committee (ACIP). *MMWR.* 1989;38(suppl 9):1–18.
4. Centers for Disease Control. Discontinuation of duck embryo virus for rabies vaccines. *MMWR.* 1981;30:407–8.
5. Marks JS, Halpin TJ. Guillain-Barré syndrome in recipients of a New Jersey influenza vaccine. *JAMA.* 1980;243:2490–4.
6. Centers for Disease Control. Vaccine Adverse Event Reporting System (VAERS)—United States. *MMWR.* 1990;41:730–3.
7. Barret J. Textbook of immunology. 5th ed. St Louis: C. V. Mosby; 1988.
8. Hinman AR, Orenstein WA, Bart KJ et al. Immunization. In: Mandell GL, Douglas RG Jr, Bennett JE, eds. Principles and practice of infectious disease. 3rd ed. New York: Churchill Livingstone; 1990.
9. Ellis RW. New technologies for making vaccines. In: Plotkin SA, Mortimer EA Jr, eds. Vaccines. Philadelphia; W.B. Saunders Company; 1988.
10. Almond JW, Cann AJ. Attenuation. In: Roitt IM, ed. Immune intervention: new trends in vaccines. London: Academic Press; 1984:13–56.
11. Querfurth H, Swanson PD. Vaccine associated paralytic poliomyelitis: regional case series and review. *Arch Neurol.* 1990;47:541–4.
12. Nkowane BJ, Wassilak SGF, Orenstein WA et al. Vaccine-associated paralytic poliomyelitis. *JAMA.* 1987;257:1335–40.
13. Nathanson N, Langmuir AD. The Cutter incident: poliomyelitis following formaldehyde-inactivated poliovirus vaccination in the

United States during spring of 1955. I. Background. *Am J Hygiene.* 1963;78:16–28.
14. Ward J. Newer *Haemophilus influenzae* type b vaccines and passive prophylaxis. *Pediatric Infect Dis.* 1987;6:799–803.
15. Peltola H, Kayhty H, Virtanen M. Prevention of *H. influenzae* type b bacteremic infections with the capsular polysaccharide vaccine. *N Engl J Med.* 1984;310:1566–9.
16. Kayhty H, Karanko V, Peltola H et al. Serum antibodies after vaccination with *H. influenzae* type b capsular polysaccharide and responses to reimmunization: no evidence of immunologic tolerance or memory. *Pediatrics.* 1984;74:857–65.
17. Insel RA, Anderson P, Pichichero ME et al. Anticapsular antibody to *H. influenzae* type b. In: Sell SH, Wright PF, eds. *Haemophilus influenzae*: epidemiology, immunology, and prevention of disease. New York: Elsevier Biomedical; 1982:155–68.
18. Granoff DM, Shackelford PG, Suarex BK et al. *Haemophilus influenzae* type b disease in children vaccinated with type b polysaccharide vaccine. *N Engl J Med.* 1986;315:1583–90.
19. Shapiro ED. New vaccines against *Haemophilus influenzae* type B. *Pediatric Clinics N A.* 1990;37:567–82.
20. Eskola J, Peltola H, Takala AK et al. Efficacy of *Haemophilus influenzae* type b polysaccharide-diphtheria toxoid conjugate vaccine in infancy. *N Engl J Med.* 1987;317:717–22.
21. Ward J, Brenneman G, Letson GW et al. Limited efficacy of a *Haemophilus influenzae* type b conjugate vaccine in Alaska Native infants. *N Engl J Med.* 1990;323:1393–401.
22. Centers for Disease Control, Immunization Practices Advisory Committee. *Haemophilus* b conjugate vaccines for prevention of *Haemophilus influenzae* type b disease among infants and children two months of age and older. *MMWR.* 1991;40(RR-1):1–7.
23. Black SB, Shinefield HR, Fireman B et al. Efficacy in infancy of oligosaccharide conjugate *Haemophilus influenzae* type B (HbOC) vaccine in a United States population of 61080 children. *Pediatr Infect Dis.* 1991;10:97–104.
24. Anon. *H. influenzae* vaccine for infants. *The Medical Letter.* 33(836):5–7.
25. Centers for Disease Control, Advisory Committee of Immunization Practices. Update of hepatitis B prevention. *MMWR.* 1987;36:353–66.
26. Centers for Disease Control, Advisory Committee of Immunization Practices. Protection against viral hepatitis. *MMWR.* 1990;39:1–26.
27. Zahradink JM, Couch RB, Gerin JL. Safety and immunogenicity of a purified hepatitis B virus vaccine prepared by using recombinant DNA technology. *J Infect Dis.* 1987;155:903–8.
28. Goudeau A, Denis F, Mounier M et al. Comparative multicentre study of the immunogenicity of different hepatitis B vaccines in

health volunteers. *Postgraduate Medical Journal.* 1987;63(suppl 2):125–8.

29. Just M, Berger R, Just V. Reactogenicity and immunogenicity of a recombinant hepatitis B vaccine compared with a plasma-derived vaccine in young adults. *Postgraduate Medical Journal.* 1987;63(suppl 2):121–3.
30. Zajac BA, West DJ, McAleer WJ et al. Overview of clinical studies with hepatitis B vaccine made by recombinant DNA. *J Infection.* 1986;13(suppl A):39–45.
31. Stevens CE, Taylor PE, Tong MJ et al. Yeast-recombinant hepatitis B vaccine: efficacy with hepatitis B immune globulin in prevention of perinatal hepatitis B virus transmission. *JAMA.* 1987;257:2612–6.
32. Young JF, Hockmeyer WT, Gross M et al. Expression of *Plasmodium falciparum* circumsporozoite proteins in *Escherichia coli* for potential use in a human malaria vaccine. *Science.* 1985;228:958–62.
33. Ballou WR, Sherwood JA, Neva FA et al. Safety and efficacy of a recombinant DNA *Plasmodium falciparum* sporozoite vaccine. *Lancet.* 1987;1:1277–81.
34. Lerner RA. Synthetic vaccines. *Scientific American.* 1983;248:66–74.
35. Zavala F, Tam JP, Hollingdale MR et al. Rationale for development of a synthetic vaccine against *Plasmodium falciparum* malaria. *Science.* 1985;228:1436–40.
36. Herrington DA, Clyde DF, Losonsky M et al. Safety and immunogenicity in man of a synthetic peptide malaria vaccine against *Plasmodium falciparum* sporozoites. *Nature.* 1987;328:257–9.
37. Fields BN, Chanock RB. What biotechnology has to offer vaccine development. *Rev Infect Dis.* 1989;11(suppl 3):519–23.
38. Levine MM, Kaper JB, Herrington D et al. Safety, immunogenicity, and efficacy of recombinant live oral cholera vaccines, CVD 103 and CVD 103-HgR. *Lancet.* 1988;2:467–70.
39. Levine MM, Herrington D, Murphy JR et al. Safety, infectivity, immunogenicity, and in vivo stability of two attenuated auxotrophic mutant strains of Salmonella typhi, 541Ty and 543Ty, live oral vaccines in humans. *J Clin Invest.* 1987;79:888–902.
40. Paoletti E, Perkus ME, Piccini A et al. Vaccinia vectored vaccines. In: Quinnan GV Jr, ed. Vaccinia viruses as vectors for vaccine antigens. New York: Elsevier; 1985:137–51.
41. Karzon DT. Considerations of safety, efficacy and potential applications of vaccinia vectors for immunoprophylaxis: an alternative approach for control of human diseases for which vaccines are available. In: Quinnan GV Jr, ed. Vaccinia viruses as vectors for vaccine antigens. New York: Elsevier; 1985:231–6.

42. Perkus ME, Piccini BR, Lipinskas BR et al. Recombinant vaccinia virus: immunization against multiple pathogens. *Science.* 1985;229:981-4.
43. Arnon R. Synthetic vaccines. In: Roitt IM, ed. Immune intervention: new trends in vaccines. London: Academic Press; 1984:93-116.
44. Adam A, Lederer E. Muramyl dipeptides and analogues. In: Bell R, Torrigiani G, eds. Progress towards better vaccines. New York: Oxford University Press on behalf of the World Health Organization; 1986:185-203.
45. Lambert PH. Anti-idiotypic vaccines. In: Bell R, Torrigiani G, eds. Progress towards better vaccines. New York: Oxford University Press on behalf of the World Health Organization; 1986:89-96.
46. Sacks DL, Esser KM, Sher A. Immunization of mice against African trypanosomiasis using anti-idiotypic antibodies. *J Exper Med.* 1982;155:1108-19.
47. Roitt I. Essential immunology. 6th ed. Oxford: Blackwell Scientific Publications; 1987.
48. Sell S. Immunology, immunopathology and immunity. 3rd ed. New York: Harper & Row; 1980.
49. Rose RR, Milgrom F, van Oss CJ, eds. Principles of immunology. 2nd ed. New York: MacMillan; 1979.
50. Dienstag JL. Passive-active immunoprophylaxis after percutaneous exposure to hepatitis B virus. *Hepatology.* 1989;10:385-7.
51. American Hospital Formulary Service. Drug information 90. Bethesda, MD: American Society of Hospital Pharmacists; 1990:1880-1901, 1907-12, 2210.
52. Centers for Disease Control, Advisory Committee on Immunization Practices. Adult immunization: recommendations of the ACIP. *MMWR.* 1991;40:31-33, 70-71.
53. Centers for Disease Control, Advisory Committee on Immunization Practices Advisory Committee. Varicella-zoster immune globulin for the prevention of chicken pox: recommendations of the ACIP. *Ann Intern Med.* 1984;100:859-65.
54. Feldman S, Lott L. Varicella in children with cancer: impact of antiviral treatment and prophylaxis. *Pediatrics.* 1987;80:465-72.
55. Kastrup EK. Facts and comparisons. St Louis: J. B. Lippincott; 1990:445a-8a.
56. Bialecki C, Feder HM. Questions and controversies about varicella-zoster infections. *Hospital Practice.* 1989;24(suppl 3A):21-32.
57. Massachusetts Public Health Biologic Laboratories. Product Information: varicella zoster immune globulin (human). Boston; March 1989.
58. Skvaril F, Gardi A. Differences among available immunoglobulin preparations for intravenous use. *Pediatric Infectious Disease Journal.* 1988;7(suppl 5):S43-8.

59. Knapp MJ, Colburn PA. Clinical uses of intravenous immune globulin. *Clinical Pharmacy.* 1990;9:509–29.
60. Gordon DS. Intravenous immunoglobulin: a historical perspective. *Am J Med.* 1987;83(suppl 4A):1–2.
61. Stiehm ER. Intravenous immune globulins as therapeutic agents. *Ann Intern Med.* 1987;107:367–82.
62. Klemola T. Deficiency of immunoglobulin A. *Annals of Clinical Research.* 1987;19:248–57.
63. Burks AW, Sampson HA, Buckley RH. Anaphylactic reactions after gamma globulin administration in patients with hypogammaglobulinemia. *N Engl J Med.* 1986;314:560–4.
64. Bjorkander J, Hammarstrom L, Smith CI et al. Immunoglobulin prophylaxis in patients with antibody deficiency syndrome and anti-IGA antibodies. *Journal of Clinical Immunology.* 1987;7:8–15.
65. So A, Brenner MK, Hill ID et al. Intravenous gamma globulin treatment in patients with hypogammaglobulinemia. *Br Med J.* 1984;289:1171–8.
66. Anon. FDA approves marketing of CMVIG. *Clinical Pharmacy.* 1990;9:493.
67. Winston DJ, Pollard RB, Ho WG et al. Cytomegalovirus immune plasma in bone marrow transplant recipients. *Ann Intern Med.* 1982;97:11–18.
68. Sullivan KM, Kopecky KJ, Jocom J et al. Immunomodulatory and antimicrobial efficacy of IVIG in bone marrow transplantation. *N Engl J Med.* 1990;323:705–12.
69. Weimar W, Metselaar HJ, Balk A et al. Passive immunization to prevent CMV disease after kidney and heart transplantation. *Transplantation Proceedings.* 1990;22:229–32.
70. Snydman DR. CMVIG in the prevention and treatment of CMV disease. *Rev Infect Dis.* 1990;12(suppl 7):S839–48.
71. Meyers JD. Prevention of CMV infection after marrow transplantation. *Rev Infect Dis.* 1989;11(suppl 7):S1691–703.
72. Bailey TC. IVIG to prevent graft-versus-host disease after bone marrow transplantation. *N Engl J Med.* 1990;324:631–2. Letter.
73. Berger M. Immunoglobulin G subclass determination in diagnosis and management of antibody deficiency syndromes. *J Pediatr.* 1987;110:325–8.
74. Heiner DC. Significance of immunoglobulin (IgG) subclasses. *Am J Med.* 1984;76(suppl 3A):1–6.
75. Hansen LA, Soderstrom R, Avanzini A et al. Immunoglobulin subclass deficiency. *Pediatric Infectious Disease Journal.* 1988;7(suppl 5):S17–21.
76. Aucouturier P, Lacombe C, Bremard C et al. Serum IgG subclass levels in patients with primary immunodeficiency syndromes or abnormal susceptibility to infections. *Clinical Immunology and Immunopathology.* 1989;51:22–37.

77. Soderstrom T, Soderstrom R, Bengtsson U et al. Clinical and immunologic evaluation of patients low in single or multiple IgG subclasses. *Monographs in Allergy.* 1986;20:135-42.
78. Soderstrom T, Soderstrom R, Avanzini A et al. Immunoglobulin G subclass deficiencies. *International Archives of Allergy and Applied Immunology.* 1987;82:476-80.
79. Gordon DS. Intravenous immunoglobulin therapy: new directions and unanswered questions. *Am J Med.* 1987;83(suppl 4A):S2-6.
80. Heiner DC. Immunoglobulin subclass composition of intravenous immunoglobulin preparations: clinical relevance. *Rev Infect Dis.* 1986;8(suppl 4):S391-5.
81. Hamilton RG. Human IgG subclass measurements in the clinical laboratory. *Clinical Chemistry.* 1987;33:1707-25.
82. Ferrante A, Beard LJ. Immunoglobulin G subclass assays with polyclonal antisera and monoclonal antibodies. *Monographs in Allergy.* 1988;23:61-72.
83. Burckhardt JJ, Gardi A, Oxelius V et al. Immunoglobulin G subclass distribution in three human intravenous immunoglobulin preparations. *Vox Sanguinis.* 1989;57:10-4.
84. Lundblad JL, Londeree N, Mitra G. Characterization of various intravenous immunoglobulin preparations. *J Infection.* 1987;15(suppl 1):3-12.
85. Eibl MM, Leibl H, Mannhalter JW. IgG subclass distribution in intravenous immunoglobulin preparations. *J Infection.* 1988;17:271-76. Letter.

Self-Study Questions

1. Which of the following diseases is associated with a low enough incidence rate that the risk of adverse effects from a vaccination outweighs the possible benefits of disease prevention?

   A. Haemophilus influenzae.
   B. Hepatitis B.
   C. Smallpox.
   D. Polio.

   1. C

2. Specific adverse events following vaccination must be reported to the Vaccine Adverse Event Reporting System for which seven vaccinations?

   2. Diptheria, measles, mumps, pertussis, polio, rubella, and tetanus.

3. Which statement is true of live, attenuated vaccines? They stimulate...

   A. only the humoral immune response.
   B. only the cellular immune response.
   C. neither the cellular nor immune response.
   D. both the cellular and immune response.

   3. D

4. Conjugate vaccines such as PRP-D are effective in part because they produce a T-cell-independent immune response.

   A. True.
   B. False.

   4. B

5. What are two methods for producing subunit vaccines?

   5. Cloned proteins, synthetic peptides.

6. Hepatitis B virus vaccine has been cloned and expressed in three media. What are they?

   6. Yeast, *E. coli,* and mammalian cells.

7. Intramuscular immunoglobulin vaccines are more commonly used for preventing toxin-induced diseases than viral infections.

   A. True.
   B. False.

   7. B

8. Botulism, tetanus, diptheria, black widow spider bites, and snake bites.

8. Which five toxins may be treated with intramuscular immunoglobulin vaccines?

9. Serotherapy provides high levels of antibodies immediately. Standard vaccination therapy can take 7 to 10 days to become effective.

9. Why is serotherapy preferred over standard vaccination techniques for patients who have been exposed to diseases such as rabies or hepatitis?

10. A

10. A patient passively immunized with varicella zoster immunoglobulin may still develop chickenpox.

    A. True.
    B. False.

11. B

11. Which of the following statements is true about intravenous immunoglobulin use?

    A. IVIg raises patient platelet count slowly.
    B. Platelet count increase resulting from IVIg is transient.
    C. IVIg raises platelet count only in adult patients.
    D. Platelet count increase resulting from IVIg is long-lasting.

12. A

12. The composition of IVIg products should contain a proportion of each Ig subclass that closely resembles that in normal serum.

    A. True.
    B. False.

CHAPTER 8

Immunology of HIV Infection and AIDS

Bonnie D. Purdy, Pharm.D.
AIDS Clinical Specialist
Albany Medical Center
Albany, NY

Karen I. Plaisance, Pharm.D.
Associate Professor
Department of Clinical Pharmacy
University of Maryland School of Pharmacy
Baltimore, MD

Introduction

Since its recognition in 1981, acquired immunodeficiency syndrome (AIDS) has affected a substantial portion of the U.S. population. Approximately 200,000 cases of AIDS have been reported in the United States alone, largely reflecting infections that occurred during the 1970s and 1980s. Of the cases of AIDS reported to the Centers for Disease Control (CDC), more than 60% have resulted in death. While these numbers alone are staggering, it is estimated that approximately 1 million Americans are infected with human immunodeficiency virus (HIV), which causes AIDS. Of these 1 million Americans, an estimated 165,000 to 215,000 will die during the period 1991 to 1993.[1] The figures reported in the United States are frightening enough, yet the World Health Organization (WHO) indicates that cases of AIDS have been reported from approximately 130 countries.[2] However, the cases of AIDS reported to the CDC account for well over half the cases reported worldwide, reflecting both the substantial incidence of HIV infection in the United States and the usefulness of the established national surveillance program.[2]

As perhaps one of the most accessible members of the health care profession, the pharmacist can play an important role in educating communities and patients about HIV infection. In practice, pharmacists may be asked to advise individuals regarding high-risk behaviors, risk reduction strategies, and the appropriateness of HIV testing. For patients already suffering from AIDS, pharmacists may serve in a different capacity, advising them about adverse drug reactions, drug interactions, and the potential of investigational treatment strategies. With such a background, pharmacists should be able to provide sound counsel not only to patients with AIDS but also to the communities in which they live.

After reading this chapter, the learner will be able to—

Learning objectives

- Describe the pathogenesis of HIV infection.
- Discuss the epidemiology of HIV infection.
- Discuss testing methods used for detecting HIV infection.
- Describe symptomology of HIV-infected patients.
- Describe mechanisms of drug therapies used in treating HIV infection.
- Describe toxicities associated with HIV therapies.
- Discuss vaccination strategies being studied to prevent or cure HIV infection.

Chapter organization

This chapter highlights the immunologic aspects of HIV infection and discusses its etiology, pathogenesis, transmission, prevention, clinical manifestations, and treatment. First, the cause of AIDS, HIV infection, is discussed, followed by an explanation of the viral replicative cycle and the immunopathogenesis of HIV infection. The modes of transmission and potential means of preventing HIV are then summarized, followed by a description of the serologic tests currently available for detecting HIV antibodies. Included is a discussion of tests that may become useful in diagnosing HIV infection. The clinical manifestations of HIV disease and AIDS are briefly explained followed by a discussion of therapies used to prevent and treat diseases associated with HIV infection. The chapter concludes with a discussion of efforts to develop an HIV vaccine.

HIV Infection

Etiology

The causative agent of AIDS is HIV type 1 (HIV-1), first isolated in 1983 by groups in France and in the United States.[3,4] The virus is believed to have been present for several decades in localized areas of central Africa and has since spread extensively throughout both developed and undeveloped countries.

HIV is related to a group of nontransforming cytopathic retroviruses.[5] It is very closely related to a simian immunodeficiency virus (SIV), which causes a form of simian AIDS with encephalitis.[6] HIV type 2 (HIV-2), although relatively uncommon in the United States, produces an immunodeficiency syndrome similar to AIDS.[7] Isolates of HIV-2 appear to be more closely related, both antigenically and genetically, to SIV than to HIV-1.[6,8] Although there is cross-reactivity between the core proteins of HIV-1 and HIV-2, the envelope glycoproteins are not cross-reactive.[6,8]

HIV-1/HIV-2

During the late 1970s, infection with HIV began to spread in urban areas of central Africa. Globally, there now appear to be at least three epidemiologic patterns of HIV infection. Both the timing of the introduction of HIV into the population and the relative frequency of various routes of transmission in that population differentiate these patterns.[2]

Industrial nations

In the first pattern, prevalent in developed countries with large numbers of cases of AIDS (e.g., North America, Western Europe), HIV began to spread extensively through the population in the late 1970s. The majority of cases in this population occur in homosexual or bisexual males and users of illicit intravenous drugs, but heterosexual and perinatal transmission is increasing.

Africa and Caribbean

The second pattern occurs primarily in central, eastern, and southern Africa, and in the Caribbean basin. Like the first pattern, HIV began to spread through this population in the late 1970s; however, unlike the first pattern, the majority of AIDS cases in this population occur in heterosexuals, and perinatal transmission is frequent. Transmission through intravenous drug use or homosexual activity is virtually absent.

E. Europe and Asia

The third pattern of HIV infection is prominent in Eastern Europe and Asia. HIV was introduced into these populations in the early to mid-1980s, presumably through travel to, or contact with individuals from, countries with the first two patterns of infection. Only recently has transmission through indigenous homosexual and heterosexual practices and intravenous drug use been documented.

Mortality

The impact of the AIDS epidemic is partially reflected by the increase in adult mortality. During the 1980s, AIDS became a leading cause of death among young adults, especially between the ages of 25 and 44. More than 30,000 people with AIDS died in the year 1990 alone.[9] This number is almost one third of all CDC-reported deaths since the beginning of the AIDS epidemic. Among men between the ages of 25 and 44, HIV infection and AIDS was reported to be the second leading cause of death in 1989, surpassing heart disease, cancer, suicide, and homicide.[9] If the current trends continue, HIV infection and AIDS will be among the five leading causes of death for women aged 25 to 44 in 1991.[10]

U.S. populations

Most cases of AIDS in the United States have occurred in homosexual or bisexual men. In the heterosexual population, AIDS occurs most frequently in those with a history of intravenous drug use. In the United States in the past 2 years, the incidence of AIDS has increased in a linear fashion among homosexual and bisexual men, intravenous drug users, heterosexuals, and children. The incidence of AIDS is expected to continue to increase in these groups through 1993.[1] The proportion of cases of AIDS among blacks, Hispanics, and women also increased between 1987 and 1989. In 1989 the proportion of AIDS cases among those groups were 30% among blacks, 16% to 17% among Hispanics, and 11% among women.[1]

Viral Replicative Cycle

As demonstrated in Figure 8-1, infection with HIV begins with binding of the envelope glycoprotein of HIV, gp120, to the CD4+ receptor located on helper T cells and other populations of cells (e.g., monocytes and macrophages, glial cells, gut epithelium, bone marrow progenitors).[11] The virus is then internalized and uncoated. The precise mechanism by which the virus enters the cell has not been clearly established, but most recent evidence suggests that virus-mediated membrane fusion is the dominant pathway.[12,13]

With uncoating of the viral envelope, viral genomic RNA and the enzyme reverse transcriptase are released into the cytoplasm. The genomic RNA is then transcribed by the viral reverse transcriptase to proviral DNA. The proviral DNA may either remain in the cytoplasm in a linear or

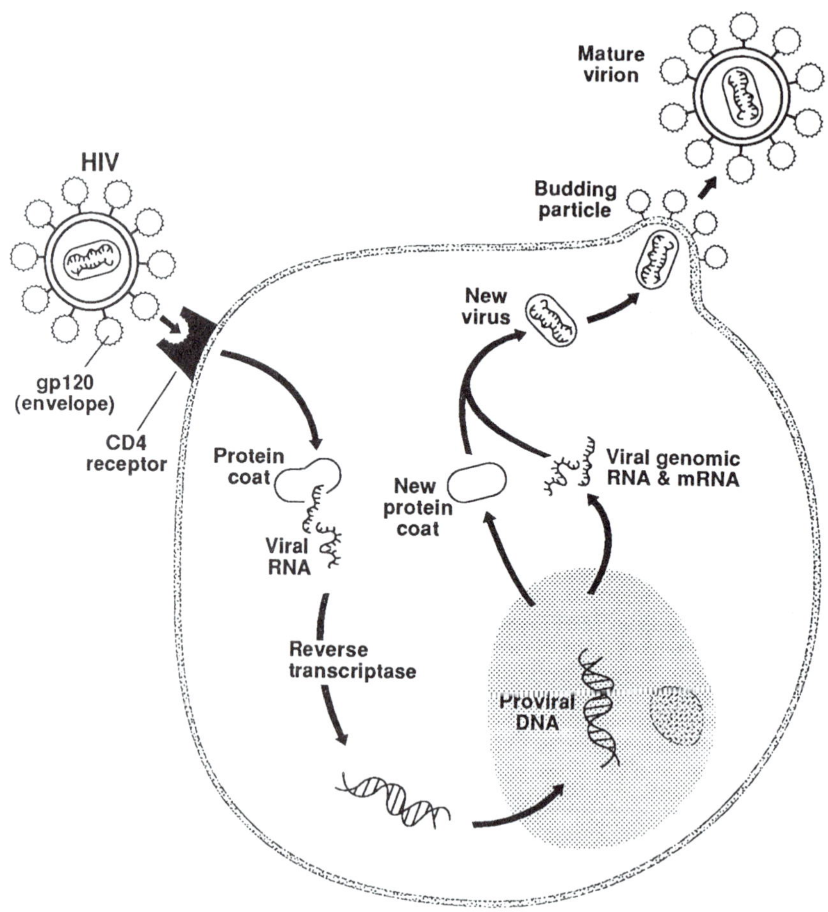

Figure 8-1. Replicative cycle of human immunodeficiency virus

circularized form or become integrated into the host's chromosomal DNA. Within the infected cell, large amounts of unintegrated viral DNA can accumulate. After the viral DNA is integrated into the host's chromosomal DNA, restricted gene expression allows the virus to remain latent until the cell is activated.[14] During this latent phase, the intracellular virus is protected from the host's immune system.[15]

Latent phase

With activation of the infected cell, the proviral DNA is transcribed into viral genomic RNA and messenger RNA (mRNA). Subsequently, translation of mRNA results in the formation of viral proteins. After protein modification and assembly of the viral proteins and genomic RNA, a mature virion is released by budding.[14]

CD4+ lymphocytes

With viral replication and release, the CD4+ lymphocyte is usually killed. This cytopathic effect may result from the accumulation of large amounts of unintegrated DNA or the weakening of the cellular membrane during budding of the mature virion.[16] In addition, cell-to-cell fusion and syncytia formation result in the cytolysis of both infected and uninfected cells. This mechanism may account for the disproportionate quantitative deficiency in CD4+ cells relative to the number of cells actually infected.[14]

Immunopathogenesis

The hallmark of the immunodeficiency found in patients infected with HIV is a quantitative deficiency of lymphocytes bearing the CD4 receptor, resulting in an imbalance of the CD4+-to-CD8+ (helper-to-suppressor) ratio.[17] In addition to this quantitative deficiency, functional abnormalities exist: inability to respond to soluble antigen (e.g., tetanus toxoid); impaired proliferative responses secondary either to abnormalities in antigen-presenting cells or to HIV infection itself; and suppressed lymphokine production.[18-20] The proliferative responses of lymphocytes not expressing the CD4 marker may also be suppressed.[20] Other functional defects in cellular immunity include impaired cytotoxic, natural killer (NK) cell, and cytomegalovirus (CMV)-specific cytotoxicity responses.[21] As the cellular response is progressively suppressed, the patient becomes at risk for the development of opportunistic infections and tumors.

The helper T cell plays a critical role in regulating the immune system; therefore, even a selective dysfunction of this cell would be expected to result in impairment of all arms of the immune system (see Chapters 1 and 2). Although the helper T cell is the major target of the virus, monocytes and macrophages can also be infected with HIV.[22,23] In addition to the ability of the monocyte to engulf the virus, certain subsets of these cells express the CD4 receptor and can subsequently bind to the gp120 glycoprotein of HIV.[24] Monocytes and macrophages infected with HIV demonstrate defective chemotaxis and altered monokine release.[14,25] With replication of the virus, monocytes and macrophages are not destroyed and may serve as a reservoir for latent infection.[23] Furthermore, the infected monocytes and macrophages probably play a dominant role in disseminating HIV infection.[23]

Monocyte/ macrophage role

Dysfunction in the humoral immune system results from helper T-cell dysregulation as well as abnormalities at the B-cell level. Although B cells are in an activated state, they are unable to mount a specific primary antibody response to new antigens. This humoral dysfunction is particularly evident in infants and children; some increased susceptibility to bacterial infections has also been observed in adults. Other anomalies of the humoral immune system include polyclonal activation, hypergammaglobulinemia, circulating immune complexes, and the formation of autoantibodies.[26] The polyclonal B-cell activation may be induced by either Epstein-Barr virus (EBV), CMV, or HIV. Table 8-1 summarizes the abnormalities in the various cells of the immune system resulting from infection with HIV.

Table 8-1 Abnormalities in the Immune System from Human Immunodeficiency Virus Infection

T cells
Quantitative decrease in the number of helper T cells
Inability to recognize and respond to soluble antigen
Diminished delayed-type hypersensitivity response
Decreased lymphokine production
Decreased natural killer cell activity
Decreased cytomegalovirus-specific cytotoxicity
Diminished ability to activate cells dependent on helper T cells
B cells
Elevated serum levels of nonspecific immunoglobulin (hypergammaglobulinemia)
Circulating immune complexes
Inability to produce antibody to new antigens
Monocytes and macrophages
Defective chemotaxis
Increased monokine release
Interleukin-1, tumor necrosis factor
Decreased in vitro killing of *Giardia lamblia* and *Toxoplasma gondii*

Transmission

HIV can be transmitted through sexual contact with an infected individual, through blood exposure through contaminated needles or infected blood products, and (perinatally) from an infected mother to her child. The virus has been isolated from essentially all body fluids including blood, semen, vaginal fluid, tears, breast milk, and saliva.[27-31] However, transmission of the virus to a susceptible host has been limited to blood, semen, and vaginal secretions.[32]

Sexual Exposure. AIDS was first identified in the homosexual population. In the United States, homosexual transmission of HIV is currently the predominant mode of transmission. A number of potential risk factors for the transmission of HIV in this setting have been evaluated. Rectal trauma was most strongly associated with HIV infection.[33] Seropositivity has been associated with both the number of sexual partners and the frequency with which the individual is the receptive partner in anal intercourse.[34-36]

HIV infection through female-to-female sexual contact has also been suggested.[37] Trauma resulting from sexual practices appears to have contributed to the transmission of HIV.

Infection with HIV should be considered fundamentally a sexually transmitted disease that is transmitted by both homosexual and heterosexual activity. Heterosexual transmission, first described in early 1983, may well be the predominant route of infection worldwide.[38,39] The number of cases of heterosexually transmitted AIDS is increasing faster in this country than the number of cases associated with other risk behaviors. The percentage of cases of AIDS attributed to heterosexual contact increased from 5% among the first 100,000 cases to 7% among the second 100,000 cases, representing a substantial increase in heterosexual transmission.[40]

Transmission efficacy

Transmission occurs from male to female and, although probably less efficiently, from female to male.[41] Sexual transmission appears to be facilitated by breaks in the vaginal or rectal mucosa.[42,43] Ulcerative sexually transmitted diseases, such as genital herpes simplex and syphilis, are significantly correlated with HIV infection, even after adjustment for numbers of sexual partners.[42]

Heterosexual transmission is more common in locations with a high prevalence of intravenous drug use.[39] The reported rate of infection is significantly higher in the female partners of infected male intravenous drug users (43 of 90 patients) than in the female partners of other index patients with AIDS (54 of 415 patients).[32] It may be that intravenous drug users are more efficient transmitters of HIV through sexual intercourse than persons with other risk behaviors.[42]

Parenteral Exposure. Transmission of HIV and the development of AIDS have been associated with intravenous drug use, blood and blood product transfusions, and occupational exposure.

Intravenous Drug Use. Transmission of HIV through intravenous drug use is linked to the heterosexual spread of HIV. Eighty-seven percent of heterosexually transmitted cases in New York City have occurred from a drug user to a non-drug-injecting partner.[44] Of women with AIDS, 30% to 50% acquired HIV infection through heterosexual activity.[45]

Infection with HIV in intravenous drug users appears related to the frequency of injection, the number of days of using unsterilized needles, and the median number of injections in shooting galleries.[39,44] Although the amount of blood contained in the needle is small, the syringe becomes contaminated with blood from multiple individuals.[39] With thousands of drug injections using potentially contaminated equipment, the combined risk associated with these variables is apparent.

Blood Transfusion and Organ Exposure. Receiving blood from an HIV seropositive donor is highly likely to result in infection. Seroconversion was reported in approximately 89% of recipients of HIV-positive transfusions.[46,47] Ward et al. found that once a donor transmitted HIV to a transfusion recipient, all subsequent recipients of that donor's blood seroconverted.[46,48] Seropositive recipients of HIV-infected blood develop immunologic parameters consistent with active HIV infection.[47] Lack of transmission may be related to the variability in the infectivity of the donor. In addition, packed red blood cells (RBCs) appear to have reduced infectivity when stored for more than 3 weeks. Therefore, the age of the product may also influence transmission.[49]

Blood/organ screening

Blood donations in the United States have been screened for antibody to HIV since early 1985; however, instances of HIV transmission from antibody-negative donations have been identified. Ward et al. investigated 13 persons seropositive for HIV who had received blood from seven donors screened as negative for antibody at the time of donation.[48] Twelve of the 13 recipients had no identifiable risk behaviors for HIV infection. Retrospectively, the seven donors were found to be infected with HIV. Most of these donors acknowledged a risk behavior associated with HIV infection or had reported a mononucleosis-like syndrome within 4 months before donating. The authors concluded that there is a small (1 in 40,000) but identifiable risk of acquiring HIV infection through antibody-negative blood. Important modifications regarding donor and unit exclusion occurred at the time of this study. Hence, this risk may well be overstated now. To further minimize this risk, the reasons for deferral of donation need to be communicated more effectively to blood donors who are at high risk, and new assays that detect HIV infection earlier should be evaluated.

Finally, transmission of HIV has been reported among recipients of various organ transplants, including kidney, bone, liver, heart, pancreas, and skin.[50] Currently, the Public Health Service recommends HIV antibody testing of all potential organ donors. Organs are also screened for the presence of HIV antibody as part of the procurement process.[50] With careful screening and deferral of donors with high-risk behaviors, the risk of acquiring HIV infection through transplantation is probably low.

Occupational Exposure. Health care workers constitute 5.4% of the work force in the United States and 5.5% of the patients with AIDS. Thus, they do not appear overrepresented among individuals with AIDS.[51]

In an ongoing, prospective study of health care workers at the National Institutes of Health, 1,344 participants have been enrolled in an effort to assess the risk of acquiring HIV infection secondary to occupational exposure (percutaneous, mucous membrane, or cutaneous) from patients with known or suspected HIV infection. Totals of 179 percutaneous, 346 mucous membrane, and 2,712 cutaneous exposures have been reported in these participants. Thus far, only one person has become seropositive, as a result of a deep cut with a sharp instrument contaminated with HIV-infected blood. No infections have occurred as a result of mucous membrane or cutaneous exposure. In combining the results from other prospective studies, the authors estimate that the risk of acquiring HIV infection secondary to a percutaneous exposure is 0.3% per exposure (95% confidence interval: 0.13% to 0.7%). The risk of HIV infection associated with mucous membrane or cutaneous exposure is much smaller.[52]

Exposure to Health Care Workers. Transmission of hepatitis B virus has been reported from infected health care workers to patients during invasive medical, surgical, and dental procedures. Until recently, no cases of HIV transmission from an HIV-infected health care worker to a patient had been reported. But in 1990, the CDC reported the first case consistent with possible transmission of HIV infection, from an HIV-infected dentist to a patient during an invasive dental procedure.[53] Since this report, two more persons under the care of this dentist have been reported to be HIV infected. Evidence including the similarity of the strains of HIV isolated from the dentist and these three patients strongly suggests that the patients were infected with HIV during their dental care. Although the risk of transmission in this setting has not been precisely defined, it is probably very low. However, this case does support the need for strict adherence to published guidelines for the prevention of transmission of HIV and other bloodborne pathogens in the health care setting.[53]

Perinatal Exposure. Transmission of HIV may occur in utero, at birth, and through breast-feeding. Although HIV has been isolated from breast milk and a small number of cases have been identified in which transmission through breast-feeding was likely, transmission is probably less efficient than in utero or during birth. It appears that infection with HIV occurs predominately in utero.[54]

Maternal antibodies

Studies of transmission and natural history of HIV infection are complicated in the newborn by lack of reliable diagnostic procedures. Infants born to HIV-infected mothers have maternally acquired antibodies to HIV. It is therefore necessary to follow these infants to detect the loss of maternal antibodies and development of serologic or virologic markers of infection. (See section on HIV testing.) The larger, prospective studies of seropositive mothers and their newborns have suggested a perinatal transmission rate in the range of 25% to 35%.[54]

Routes Not Associated with HIV Transmission. The lay press has devoted considerable attention to the potential for transmission of HIV by routes other than those that have been described. Large-scale epidemiologic investigations have repeatedly confirmed the association between transmission and sexual, blood, or perinatal exposure. Studies in family members of individuals with HIV infection have failed to document transmission of HIV through casual contact over periods of extensive and prolonged exposure.[55,56]

Prevention

Currently, there is no vaccine to prevent the spread of HIV infection. Therefore, education is our prime tool in containing the dissemination of HIV.

Changing lifestyles

Sexual Transmission. To reduce sexual transmission substantially, fundamental behavioral alterations are necessary. Health education should emphasize disease transmission, abstinence, monogamy, reduction in numbers of sexual partners, selection of sexual partners at low or no risk of infection, and correct and consistent use of latex condoms. Latex condoms have been shown to be effective in preventing in vitro passage of herpes simplex, CMV, and HIV.[57] Preliminary epidemiologic surveys also suggest that consistent use of condoms slows the spread of HIV via sexual transmission.[55,58] Spermicidal jellies and foams containing nonoxynol 9 may be a useful adjunct to condoms, because this agent has been shown to inactivate HIV and kill lymphocytes.[59] There is no risk of sexual exposure to individuals who practice sexual abstinence or are in a mutually monogamous relationship in which neither partner is infected or engages in high-risk behaviors.

Although a decline in the incidence of new HIV infections was observed in the 1980s, the projected incidence of AIDS among homosexuals is expected to continue to increase through 1993.[1] Furthermore, since 1985 there has been a rapid increase in the number of cases of syphilis among black men and women, especially in New York City, Philadelphia, Baltimore, Los Angeles, and certain parts of Texas and southern Florida. These increasing syphilis trends may not only be a marker for increasing sexual spread of HIV but may also be a co-factor facilitating HIV transmission.[42]

Parenteral Transmission. Intravenous drug use is becoming the behavior associated with the greatest risk of acquiring and transmitting HIV. Measures to reduce the transmission of HIV in this setting are urgently needed.

Interventions

Various groups have advocated innovative prevention strategies. The advisability of teaching methods of sterilizing equipment, providing injection materials, or legalizing recreational drug use have been questioned because of the potential role in magnifying our existing drug problem. Large-scale expansion of drug abuse treatment, one-on-one health promotion activities between current and former drug users, and efforts to promote safer sex practices and refusal to share needles are less controversial. Preliminary data from various programs suggest that facilitating safer injection practices and treating the underlying drug addiction are complementary rather than self-defeating.[60]

Blood-borne transmission of HIV through infected donated blood and blood products has virtually been eliminated through self-deferral of high-risk donors, testing of all blood and plasma for HIV antibodies, discarding of units that test positive, and use of heat-inactivated factor VIII. The process by which plasma-derived hepatitis B vaccine and immunoglobulin are manufactured either physically removes or chemically inactivates HIV, thus making these plasma-derived products safe.[61]

Perinatal Transmission. In the United States, reduction in perinatal transmission is linked to reducing heterosexual spread and transmission through intravenous drug use. Women seeking routine health care should be counseled regarding family planning and safer sexual practices, especially condom and spermicide use. In the United States, it is generally recommended that HIV-infected mothers avoid breast-feeding.

Testing

Serologic testing for antibody to HIV is the mainstay in the diagnosis of HIV infection in adults and children older than 18 months. However, seroconversion occurs on average 6 weeks after initial exposure to HIV. The range is 3 weeks to more than 9 months. An individual infected with HIV may have a negative test for antibody during this time.

Currently available antibody tests are generally inadequate for diagnosing infection in infants born to HIV-seropositive women. Almost all infants passively acquire maternal antibody in utero. Because maternal antibody may persist in infants as long as 15 to 18 months after birth, serologic tests for antibody during that time detect passively acquired antibody. True HIV infection of the infant cannot be detected serologically until maternal antibody has cleared. These tests therefore lack the specificity necessary for detecting infection in infants younger than 18 months.[62]

This section briefly summarizes the serologic tests currently available for detecting antibody to HIV and other diagnostic tests that may become useful in diagnosing HIV infection. See Chapter 5 for a more complete discussion of immunologic tests.

Antibody Testing.

Enzyme-linked Immunosorbent Assay (ELISA). ELISA was first licensed by the Food and Drug Administration (FDA) in 1985 primarily for the screening of blood and plasma products. Testing by ELISA is now the most useful screening tool for HIV infection. Ten commercially available ELISA kits are licensed by the FDA. Under optimal conditions, ELISA is 99.5% sensitive and 99.8% specific.[63]

Procedure

Serum samples positive by ELISA must be repeated in duplicate. Only samples tested by ELISA that are repeatedly reactive are considered to be positive. A positive ELISA is not sufficient to make the diagnosis of HIV infection, especially in low-prevalence populations; it must be followed by a confirmatory test. The Western blot is the most commonly used confirmatory test, although some laboratories have used a radioimmunoprecipitation assay.[64] A diagnosis of HIV infection is made when an individual has repeatedly positive ELISA results and a positive confirmatory test.

A window period of low sensitivity has been noted with ELISA.[65] This is the time between the initial infection and the production of antibody. Seroconversion generally occurs within six weeks. False-negative tests may occur during this window period in individuals recently infected with HIV who have not yet developed detectable antibody. An individual is still considered infectious during this time despite the absence of antibody to HIV. Children who are hypogammaglobulinemic and born of mothers who are HIV seropositive may have false-negative ELISA results because their immune systems are not capable of producing antibody to HIV.[66,67] Potential reasons for a false-positive ELISA are listed in Table 8-2.

Table 8-2 Possible Causes of False-positive Results on ELISA Testing

Autoimmune diseases
Collagen-vascular diseases
Liver disease
Chronic hepatitis
Alcoholic liver disease
Primary biliary cirrhosis
Primary sclerosing cholangitis
Hematologic malignancies
Multiple myeloma
Malaria
Acute DNA viral infections
Multiple blood transfusions
Certain HLA phenotypes

Western Blot. The Western blot assay is the most commonly used confirmatory test. Controversy exists among various groups as to the interpretation of a positive Western blot.[68] The CDC and the Association of State and Territorial Public Health Laboratory Directors suggest that a positive test should be defined by the presence of at least two of the following bands: p24, gp41, and/or gp120/160.[62] A negative test is the presence of zero bands. An indeterminant result is one in which fewer bands are present or bands are present other than the ones that define a positive result. An indeterminant result can be seen in individuals recently infected with HIV with incomplete serologic response and in patients with advanced disease.[68] An indeterminant result in persons whose physical examination and medical history are highly suggestive of HIV infection should be followed by a second Western blot in 6 months; it will likely yield a positive result. Conversely, repeat testing of an indeterminant result in individuals at low risk for infection generally yields the same banding pattern as their previous indeterminant result did. These individuals are rarely, if ever, truly infected with HIV.[69]

Interpretation

Investigational Methods.

Assay for p24 Antigen. The detection of p24 antigen, which is one of the HIV core proteins, in the serum of an HIV-infected person is an indicator of active viral replication. Serum p24 antigen can be detected during two different phases of HIV infection: immediately after HIV infection has been acquired and before the antibody to HIV has developed, and in the late stages of illness.[70-72] The p24 antigen assay is now used primarily as a

Application

research tool. One of the major disadvantages of this assay is its inability to detect serum p24 antigen in the presence of high titers of HIV-specific antibodies secondary to the formation of antibody-antigen complexes.[62] This assay may be valuable in detecting serum p24 antigen during the window period before people have developed antibody to HIV and in children who are hypogammaglobulinemic.[62,73] Assays of p24 antigen have also been used to monitor the progression of disease and the effect of antiviral therapy in patients with advanced disease.[74,75]

HIV Culture. The use of viral culture is restricted to the research setting. These cultures are costly and labor-intensive, often taking 28 days or more to complete.[76] Special precautions are required to prevent exposing laboratory personnel. The amount of blood required for viral cultures limits its utility in infants younger than 18 months.[62] The sensitivity of the viral culture varies among different laboratories and during the course of the illness. In individuals with AIDS, culture yield may be as high as 100% versus 10% in asymptomatic individuals with HIV infection.[77]

Polymerase Chain Reaction. Polymerase chain reaction (PCR) is a new diagnostic technique that shows promising results. PCR is a method of amplifying the viral DNA up to 1 million times or more to increase the probability of detection.[62] This method offers several advantages over other diagnostic tests, including its potential use in detecting virus in infants younger than 18 months. In addition, PCR is not affected by the presence of maternal antibody.[78] Preliminary results in this setting are encouraging. The assay is less labor-intensive than culturing and can be completed in 1 day.

Antigen detection

Since PCR detects antigen, not antibody, infection with HIV may be detected earlier. However, the sensitivity of PCR can vary with the course of HIV illness, and it may be less sensitive during asymptomatic period and highly sensitive in patients with AIDS.[79] Continued testing of PCR is under way.

Spectrum of Disease

The spectrum of HIV illness ranges from asymptomatic infection to the severe symptoms associated with AIDS. The interval between initial infection with HIV and the development of AIDS appears to be long and variable. Early studies from 1984 of patients who developed AIDS associated with blood transfusions suggested incubation periods of 21 months for children and 31 months for adults.[32] More recent data suggest that the incubation period may exceed 8 years for infection acquired by both transfusion-related and homosexual exposures.[32] Prognostic indicators, such as the decline of antibody to p24, the appearance or persistent presence of HIV antigenemia, and oral candidiasis, suggest progression of HIV infection to AIDS.[80,81] In one study, the mean cumulative survival of individuals with AIDS was approximately 50% at 1 year and 15% at 15 years, although sex, race, age, and AIDS-defining illness appeared to contribute to the overall survival of specific subgroups of this population.[82]

The most severe consequence of advanced HIV infection is AIDS, often resulting in death within 2 years. The various manifestations of HIV infection are briefly discussed here.

Acute Infection

Acute infection with HIV occurs before seroconversion and may or may not be associated with symptoms.[83] Seroconversion usually occurs in approximately 6 weeks, with a range of 3 weeks to 15 months, after initial exposure to HIV.

Symptoms

In those who experience symptoms, a mononucleosis-like illness is most frequently reported after exposure to HIV. During the acute illness, the individual may have fever, sweats, lethargy, malaise, myalgias, arthralgias, headaches, photophobia, diarrhea, sore throat, lymphadenopathy, and a truncal maculopapular rash. Thrombocytopenia and lymphopenia have also been reported in the first several days; inversion of the ratio of CD4+ to CD8+ cells occurs shortly thereafter.[84] Central nervous system abnormalities such as aseptic meningitis, encephalopathy, and peripheral neuropathy have also been reported during acute infection.[85]

It is unclear what percentage of primarily infected persons experience this mononucleosislike illness and whether the illness is a reliable and consistent indicator of infection with HIV. However, Tindall et al.[84] investigated the clinical and immunologic findings during seroconversion in a group of homosexual men. Approximately 92% of the patients who had seroconverted experienced signs of acute illness versus 40% in the control group. Fifty percent of seroconverted subjects had an inverted ratio of CD4+ to CD8+ cells versus none of the control subjects. The mean duration of this acute illness was approximately 3 weeks.

Asymptomatic Infection

The guidelines established by the CDC define asymptomatic infection as the absence of clinical signs and symptoms of HIV infection in persons with laboratory evidence of antibody to HIV.[86] Individuals may or may not have the hematologic abnormalities often associated with HIV infection, such as lymphopenia, thrombocytopenia, and decrease in CD4+ lymphocytes.

Persistent Generalized Lymphadenopathy

Persistent generalized lymphadenopathy (PGL) is the presence of a palpable lymph node greater than or equal to 1 cm at two or more extrainguinal sites persisting for more than 3 months with no other illness. PGL indicates progression of HIV infection and may herald the development of an AIDS-defining illness.

Clinical Definition of AIDS

Opportunistic infections

The CDC surveillance definition of AIDS is based on the occurrence of opportunistic infections or neoplasms indicative of cellular immune deficiency. The current definition, revised in 1987, also includes HIV encephalopathy and wasting syndrome and recognizes the increasing frequency of presumptive methods for diagnosing the opportunistic infections associated with AIDS.[87] Diseases included in the CDC definition of AIDS are listed in Table 8-3. This section discusses certain opportunistic infections and neoplasms.

Table 8-3 Diseases Indicative of Acquired Immunodeficiency Syndrome

Opportunistic Infections	Other Diseases	Neoplasms
Cryptosporidiosis	Lymphoid pneumonia	Kaposi's sarcoma
Cytomegalovirus	Progressive multifocal leukoencephalopathy	Lymphoma
Isosporiasis	HIV encephalopathy	
Pneumocystis carinii	HIV wasting syndrome	
Toxoplasmosis		
Candidiasis		
Coccidioidomycosis		
Herpes simplex		
Histoplasmosis		
Tuberculosis		
Other mycobacterial infections		
Salmonellosis		

SOURCE: Adapted from Centers for Disease Control. Revision of the CDC surveillance case definition for acquired immunodeficiency syndrome. *MMWR.* 1987;36(suppl 1s):3–15.

Many of the opportunistic infections and neoplasms seen in patients infected with HIV are a direct result of a severely impaired cellular immune function. The cell-mediated arm of the immune system is responsible for protecting the individual from developing these infections and neoplasms. The presence of these infections and neoplasms can be correlated with the total number of CD4 cells. In a healthy adult, the normal number of CD4 cells is about 1,000/mm^3.[88] This number declines in an HIV-infected individual, on average, by approximately 40 to 80/mm^3 or more per year.[88] The first infections generally begin to appear when the CD4 cells are between 200 and 500/mm^3. Once the CD4 count falls below 200/mm^3, the more severe, life-threatening infections and neoplasms develop.[88-90] This progression is illustrated in Figure 8-2.

CD4 cells

Opportunistic Infections. Because of the profound, irreversible immunodeficiency in AIDS patients, opportunistic infections are generally less responsive to conventional therapy and frequently relapse when therapy is discontinued. Lifelong suppressive therapy is often required for many of these infections. Opportunistic infections are the leading cause of death in patients with AIDS.

Pneumocystis carinii Pneumonia (PCP). PCP occurs in up to 80% of patients with AIDS and is the initial opportunistic infection in approximately 60%. The rate of occurrence in individuals with less than 200 CD4 cells is approximately 8% after 6 months and 18% after 1 year.[91] Like other infections, PCP may represent reactivation of latent infection.[92]

PCP

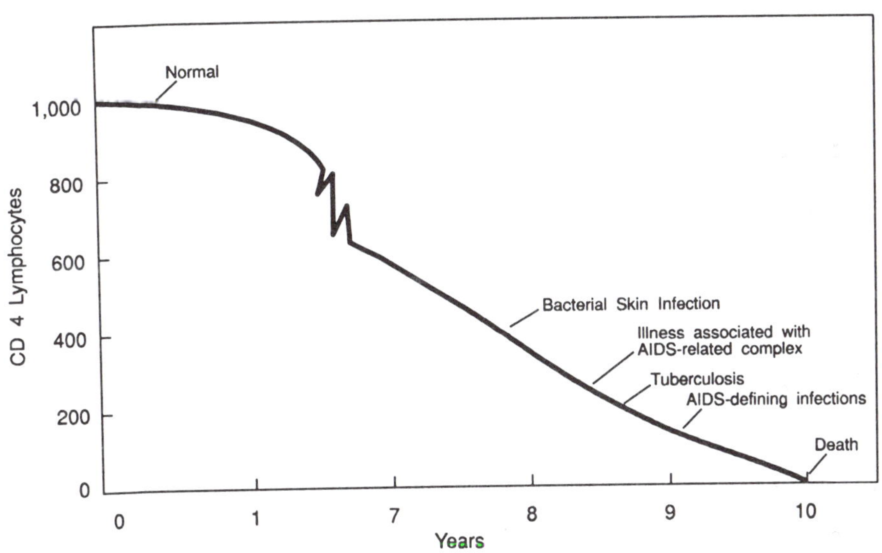

Figure 8-2. Relationship between CD4 count and progression of HIV illness

In contrast to other immunocompromised patients, PCP is characterized by a more subtle, indolent process. In one study the median duration of symptoms at the time of diagnosis was 28 days in AIDS patients versus 5 days in other immunocompromised patients.[93] Clinical manifestations of PCP include fever, shortness of breath, and nonproductive cough, with only subtle changes on chest roentgenography. Definitive diagnosis is made by identifying the organism in the sputum, or by bronchoscopy with either broncho-alveolar lavage or biopsy.[94,95] Although 80% of patients survive their initial hospitalization, 60% of patients relapse within 1 year.[91,96] Survival decreases to 40% to 60% with recurrent episodes.[96]

Cryptococcal Meningitis. This infection occurs in approximately 5% to 10% of patients infected with HIV. Cryptococcal infection can occur not only in the central nervous system but also in the lungs, skin, genitourinary tract, bone marrow, and blood.[97-99] Manifestations of cryptococcal meningitis may be subtle; fever and headache are the most common findings. Meningismus, photophobia, changes in mental status, and seizures occur less frequently.[97-100] The interval between onset of symptoms and diagnosis ranges from 1 day to 4 months with a mean of 31 days.[100] The diagnosis is established by detecting (1) yeast cells by India ink stain and culture or (2) cryptococcal antigen in the cerebrospinal fluid, or both.[97-100] Also, the presence of cryptococcal antigen can usually be detected in the serum. Even with therapy, cryptococcal antigen titers may remain elevated. Antigen titers of 1:8 or more in the cerebrospinal fluid after therapy are associated with higher rates of relapse.[97] Once acute therapy is completed, suppressive therapy is usually indicated.

Focal encephalitis

Toxoplasmosis. Toxoplasmosis is the most common cause of focal encephalitis in patients with AIDS.[101] Symptoms include fever, confusion, hemispheric signs such as hemiparesis and aphasia, meningeal signs, coma, and seizures. The most useful tool in diagnosing toxoplasmosis has been the computed tomography scan, which reveals multiple low-density lesions or rings or nodular-enhancing lesions.[101,102] Serology has proved to be of limited value. Definitive diagnosis requires the demonstration of tachyzoites in brain tissue obtained at biopsy.

Empiric therapy may be considered in patients with positive serology and a clinical picture suggestive of toxoplasmosis. An initial response is usually observed after 2 weeks of therapy.[101,102] Again, as with many of the opportunistic infections, relapse is common when treatment is stopped.

MAC

Mycobacterium avium-intracellulare (MAC) and M. tuberculosis. Both of these infections occur frequently in AIDS patients and often occur as part of disseminated disease.[103] Before the AIDS epidemic, MAC infection was rare and was seen occasionally in patients with chronic pulmonary disease. MAC is usually diagnosed in the late stages of HIV illness and has been documented in as many as 53% of patients with AIDS at autopsy.[103-105] The manifestations of MAC range from no symptoms to a constellation of nonspecific findings including diarrhea, abdominal pain, malabsorption, persistent fevers, anemia, and weight loss.[103-105] Cultures of bone marrow, lymph node, and liver biopsies may be employed to guide in the diagnosis of disseminated infection. In addition, positive cultures are seen in respiratory secretions, urine, and stool and have been reported to precede disseminated infection.[103]

TB

Tuberculosis is prevalent among individuals infected with HIV, particularly those in areas where tuberculosis is known to be endemic.[103,106] Tuberculosis typically precedes the development of other opportunistic infections that contribute to the diagnosis of AIDS. As in the general population, tuberculosis usually represents reactivation of latent infection acquired earlier in life. Disseminated, extrapulmonary disease is encountered frequently, representing 67% of tuberculosis seen in patients with AIDS.[103,106] Clinical manifestations vary depending on the site involved. Like MAC, the diagnosis is made by finding M. tuberculosis in the affected tissues or secretions. The CDC has recommended administering tuberculin skin tests to people infected with HIV. However, because of depressed cellular responses, a negative reaction does not rule out infection.[107]

Candidiasis. Candidiasis often presents as oral thrush or esophagitis and is the most common fungal infection in patients infected with HIV.[108] In addition, unexplained oral candidiasis in individuals at risk for HIV infection may indicate impending progression of HIV infection. Approximately 60% of these patients develop an opportunistic infection or Kaposi's sarcoma (KS) within a median of 3 months after the diagnosis of oral candidiasis.[109]

Retinitis

Herpesvirus. Infections with herpes group viruses, such as herpes simplex and CMV, are frequent in individuals infected with HIV. Mucocutaneous herpes simplex can be painful, and patients may experience frequent relapses.[110] CMV is particularly common in the homosexual population and is a frequent cause of morbidity and mortality.[111-114] Like other herpesviruses, CMV can cause persistent infection with viral shedding from a number of body sites.[112,113] Viremia occurs in approximately 50% of patients; more than 90% have evidence of CMV at autopsy.[110] Retinitis is the most common manifestation of CMV infection and is a leading cause of blindness in patients with AIDS. In addition to CMV retinitis, other clinical syndromes seen with CMV include colitis, esophagitis, encephalitis, adrenalitis, pneumonitis, sclerosing cholangitis, and hepatitis. Relapse rates are high, especially with CMV retinitis; therefore, long-term suppressive therapy is often necessary.[111-114]

Neoplasms. Severe cellular suppression and polyclonal B-cell activation may contribute to the development of cancers in patients with AIDS. Although both KS and non-Hodgkin's lymphoma are relatively uncommon outside the HIV setting, these tumors occur more frequently and often present atypically in patients with AIDS.

Kaposi's Sarcoma. KS, one of the first-described clinical manifestations of AIDS,[115,116] occurs in 21% of homosexual men, up to 8% of heterosexual men, and 1% to 3% of patients with parenterally acquired HIV infection.[117] KS rarely occurs in women infected with HIV. Although the number of cases of KS continues to increase, the number of new cases per year appears to be decreasing in homosexual men.[117,118] The natural history of KS is not completely known, and considerable research is under way to identify viral, environmental, or other factors that may increase the risk for KS. That partners of women with KS are usually bisexual men, not users of intravenous drugs, suggests that a sexually transmitted cofactor may play a role.[117] A possible relationship may also exist between HIV and KS. The tat gene of HIV is a regulatory protein that promotes viral gene expression and replication. It has been proposed that HIV, through expression of the tat gene, may up-regulate the progression of KS through a similar process.[119]

G.I. lesions

Before the AIDS epidemic, KS was a rare tumor that occurred predominantly among middle-aged men of Eastern European or Mediterranean extraction. The clinical presentation of KS in AIDS patients is very diverse and differs from the classic, localized presentation. In patients with AIDS, KS tends to involve the skin, especially the head, neck, and trunk; lymph nodes; mucous membranes; and the entire gastrointestinal tract.[120] More than 50% of patients have visceral lesions, particularly in the gastrointestinal tract, at initial presentation.[121] The rate of progression varies among patients. Most individuals with KS have rapid, progressive disease with multiple organ involvement, particularly the gastrointestinal tract and pulmonary parenchyma. However, a small percentage experience a slow and indolent process similar to that seen in the classic form. The mortality rate associated with KS is approximately 20%. Patients with cutaneous KS and no history of opportunistic infections or symptomatic HIV infection have the most favorable prognosis. Patients with gastrointestinal KS have a slightly reduced survival rate, and those with pulmonary KS have the worst prognosis.[121]

Non-Hodgkin's Lymphoma. Non-Hodgkin's lymphoma occurs in approximately 5% to 10% of patients with AIDS.[122] Non-Hodgkin's lymphoma has been reported in homosexual men, male and female users of intravenous drugs, and hemophiliacs.[122-124] While the reason for the increased incidence of aggressive lymphomas in AIDS patients is unclear, the presence of EBV, resulting in polyclonal B-cell proliferation, may have a permissive effect.[120] AIDS-related lymphoma differs from lymphomas in other populations because these lymphomas occur in a younger population, are often disseminated, are predominantly high- or intermediate-grade B-cell type, and generally follow a rapidly progressive clinical course.[125,126] More than 70% of these patients have involvement of extranodal sites, especially the brain, bone marrow, and bowel.[127–129] Primary lymphoma of the brain in patients with AIDS carries a poor prognosis, especially if it is of high grade with immunoblastic histology.[120,130] Treatment of patients with AIDS-related non-Hodgkin's lymphoma is associated with a complete response rate of 33% to 50% and high relapse and mortality rates.[130] Decisions regarding aggressive chemotherapy are made on an individual basis.

Treatment Approaches for HIV Infection

An intensive program has been undertaken to develop strategies aimed at preventing HIV infection and altering the progression of HIV illness. This section reviews both antiviral and immunomodulatory approaches under investigation and summarizes current efforts to develop vaccine candidates.

Antiviral Therapy

The potential targets in the viral replicative cycle against which antiviral intervention may be directed are summarized in Table 8-4. These targets include inhibition of binding to the CD4 receptor, prevention of viral entry or uncoating, inhibition of the enzyme reverse transcriptase, inhibition of viral protein synthesis and processing, inhibition of viral assembly, and inhibition of viral release.[131,132]

Inhibitors of Viral Binding. A number of approaches to inhibiting viral binding are being investigated. Perhaps the greatest interest has been generated by the production of soluble, truncated forms of the CD4 molecule. The rationale for this approach is to present HIV with excess soluble recombinant CD4 (rCD4) and thereby bind the virus extracellularly before it can bind to the native CD4 molecule on susceptible target cells. This approach should be useful in inhibiting portions of the replicative cycle that require the CD4 receptor and block the cytolysis of uninfected cells induced by syncytia.[131,132] The phase I trials suggested that, at least at the doses used, rCD4 was nontoxic and had no measurable adverse effect on immune function.[133,134] In addition, suggestion of antiviral effect with a decrease in p24 antigenemia was observed at the highest doses.[133] The potential for the host to recognize rCD4 as foreign and develop antibodies that may iatrogenically destroy the host's own CD4-bearing cells has raised

rCD4

Table 8-4 Potential Target Mechanisms of Antiretroviral Therapy

Mechanism	Agent
Inhibition of viral binding	Sulfated polysaccharides (dextran, pentosan, carrageenans) Soluble CD4 (sCD4) sCD4 hybrids Peptide T Monoclonal antienvelope antibodies
Inhibition of membrane fusion	
Inhibition of reverse transcriptase	Dideoxynucleosides (zidovudine, ddI, ddC, d4T) Foscarnet Nonnucleoside inhibitors
Inhibition of integration of provirus	Integrase inhibitors
Inhibition of transcription of provirus	Tat inhibitors
Inhibition of translation of viral mRNA	Antisense oligonucleotides
Inhibition of posttranslational processing	Glycosylation inhibitors (castanospermine) Protease inhibitors (pepstatin A)
Inhibition of budding and release	Interferon, ampligen

concern. Posttherapeutic induction of anti-CD4 antibody was observed in three volunteers in the two trials.[133,134] The appearance of this antibody did not have any apparent adverse clinical consequences.

Because of the relatively short half-life (45 minutes) and the suboptimal antiviral effects observed in the phase I trials of rCD4, second-generation versions of rCD4 hybrids are now under study. By linking domains of the rCD4 molecule with the Fc portion of immunoglobulin, the dual goals of extending the half-life and incorporating specific functions of immunoglobulin may be achieved.[135] Recombinant CD4 has also been linked to cellular toxins such as Pseudomonas exotoxin A and ricin. These compounds should selectively bind to cells expressing HIV and, through the toxin, kill the infected cells. This may be a particularly attractive approach to targeting cells, such as macrophages, that are relatively resistant to the cytopathic effect of HIV.[131,132]

Reverse Transcriptase Inhibitors. Because reverse transcriptase, which uses RNA to make DNA, is an essential and relatively unique feature of HIV, inhibition of this enzyme was recognized early as an important target

Dideoxynucleosides

for antiretroviral therapy. In 1985 it was observed that the dideoxynucleosides had potent in vitro activity against HIV. These compounds must be activated to the 5'-triphosphate by the biochemical machinery of the cell. This anabolic phosphorylation involves a series of kinases. Substantial differences in the rates at which human cells phosphorylate these compounds are reflected in their antiretroviral activity.[131,132,136]

Two mechanisms may contribute to the activity of the dideoxynucleosides. First, as triphosphates, they compete with cellular deoxynucleoside 5'-triphosphates, which are the essential substrates for formation of proviral DNA. Inhibition constants, generally within the range of 0.005 to 0.2 μmol, are achievable intracellularly. In addition, because of the 3' modification, no additional nucleotides can be added once reverse transcriptase adds these nucleotides to a growing chain of DNA, and HIV replication is halted.[136]

Zidovudine

In July 1985, a phase I trial was begun to determine toxicity and pharmacokinetics of zidovudine in patients with AIDS or AIDS-related complex (ARC). On the basis of these preliminary results, a multicenter phase II trial was begun in February 1986. A total of 282 patients with AIDS or advanced ARC were randomized to receive either zidovudine (250 mg orally every 4 hours) or placebo. By September, 1 patient receiving zidovudine had died versus 19 placebo recipients. Patients receiving zidovudine had fewer opportunistic infections, gained weight, and had improved intellectual functioning and overall better prognosis. Zidovudine recipients had at least transient increases in CD4 counts and decreases in p24 antigen. After 36 weeks, mortality was 39.3% in those receiving placebo versus 6.2% in those receiving zidovudine.[137] On the basis of this trial, zidovudine was approved in the United States in March 1987 for the treatment of patients who had PCP or whose CD4 counts were less than 200 cells/mm^3. In patients diagnosed with AIDS between April 1987 and June 1989, median survival was four times greater among zidovudine recipients (770 days) than among those who had never received zidovudine (190 days).[138] The dosages that were initially approved by the FDA, however, resulted in substantial bone marrow toxicity.

These dose-limiting toxicities prompted evaluation of the efficacy of lower dosages of zidovudine in the maintenance of those with advanced HIV illness. After a median follow-up of approximately 2 years, a significantly better survival rate was noted in the group receiving 600 mg of zidovudine per day (72%) versus the patients receiving the standard higher dose therapy of 1,200 to 1,500 mg per day (65%). No significant differences in occurrences of opportunistic infections, times to next infection, declines in CD4+ counts, or p24 antigen levels were noted. However, serious anemia and neutropenia occurred earlier and more frequently in those receiving the higher doses.[139]

The utility of zidovudine to delay the onset of AIDS or ARC was examined in a group of asymptomatic individuals infected with HIV. Persons with CD4+ counts below 500 cells/mm^3 had a significantly lower rate of disease progression if they received zidovudine versus placebo. The efficacy was equivalent for the low-dose (500 mg) and high-dose (1,500 mg) groups. Lower baseline platelet counts, higher levels of p24 antigen, and lower baseline CD4 counts were significantly correlated with risk of progression to AIDS. Again, hematologic toxicity was a problem for the group receiving the high doses of zidovudine.[140]

The efficacy of zidovudine in early symptomatic HIV illness was assessed in 711 patients with mildly symptomatic disease. Significant differences in the time to first critical event were apparent in the 513 subjects with baseline CD4 counts of 200 to 500, but not for the 198 subjects with initial CD4 counts of 500 to 799.[141] The current FDA labeling reflects the results of these studies as well as studies performed in the pediatric population.

ddC and ddI

Both dideoxycytidine (ddC) and didanosine (dideoxyinosine [ddI]) have reached the latter stages of clinical evaluation. Two phase I studies suggested that ddC would reduce viral load as well as produce immunologic improvements. However, painful peripheral neuropathy developed in patients receiving higher doses for longer periods. Virologic improvement has now been suggested at lower doses (0.03 mg/kg), which have been better tolerated. Significant suppression of serum p24 antigen was observed in most patients receiving 0.01 mg/kg and less frequently at 0.005 mg/kg.[136,142] Phase II studies at lower doses and alternating regimens with zidovudine are nearing completion.

Didanosine has progressed rapidly into clinical trials because of its relatively large therapeutic index. The active moiety of didanosine—dideoxyadenosine (ddA) triphosphate—has a rather long intracellular half-life, which supports the potential utility of dosing intervals of 12 to 24 hours.[136] The maximum tolerated oral doses observed in the phase I trials were 12 mg/kg per day when given twice daily and 20.4 mg/kg per day when given once daily.[143,144] Significant declines in p24 antigenemia, increases in CD4 counts, and symptomatic improvement were observed. Didanosine therapy appeared to be limited by peripheral neuropathy and pancreatitis. Neuropathy or pancreatitis developed in 10 of 22 patients receiving more than 12 mg/kg versus 2 of 15 patients who received 12 mg/kg or less.[144] Overall, toxicity was much less pronounced in the study when daily dosing was used, perhaps reflecting reduced bioavailability of larger dose sizes. Overall, in the phase II and III studies and the expanded access program, the incidence of pancreatitis is less than 2%; the mortality rate is less than 2% of those developing pancreatitis. Factors that appear to increase the risk of developing pancreatitis include a history of pancreatitis, advanced HIV infection (especially with disseminated CMV or MAC infection), and elevated serum transaminases. Other drugs that have been associated with the development of pancreatitis, such as pentamidine and sulfonamides, should be used cautiously, if at all, in patients who are receiving didanosine. Finally, because of the risk of pancreatitis, alcohol use should be discouraged.[132]

Protease (Proteinase) and Integrase Inhibition. HIV encodes for enzymes, in addition to reverse transcriptase, which are important in viral replication. The enzyme proteinase appears to be essential for the processing of core proteins and viral infectivity. Proteinase processes the precursors of gag and pol to the mature virion components by cleaving the polyprotein precursors. Inhibiting this enzyme therefore prevents the formation of mature core proteins as well as reverse transcriptase. Thus, inhibition of this target may have impact at multiple steps in the viral replicative cycle.[131,132] Specific inhibitors of this enzyme are under development.

Retroviral integrases are the enzymes necessary for integration of the proviral DNA into the cellular DNA. Mutants that lack integrase do not appear able to replicate in cell culture.[131,132] Thus, inhibition of retroviral integrase may be an important target for antiviral strategies.

Later Stages of Viral Replication. Once the proviral DNA has become integrated within the host's DNA, a number of factors regulate expression of mature virion. A variety of stimuli may activate the infected cell. After activation the proviral DNA is transcribed into RNA, which is then translated into viral proteins, modified, and assembled, and mature virion is finally released from the cell. Viral proteins, including tat, rev, and nef, are believed to be regulators of these processes. Strategies that target these regulatory proteins are being explored.[131,132] Another interesting approach to inhibiting protein synthesis is the use of antisense segments of modified DNA (phosphorothioate oligodeoxynucleosides). These complementary strands of DNA are modified to prevent degradation and bind to viral RNA, blocking the movement of ribosomes along the RNA and thus preventing protein synthesis.[131,132]

Protein regulators

After synthesis, the viral proteins must be modified to allow for assembly. Sugar residues are added to form glycoproteins and during this process, terminal sugars are cleaved by trimming glucosidases. Castanospermine, an inhibitor of glucosidases, has been found to inhibit HIV replication in vitro. Glucosidase inhibition results in the production of

Castanospermine

viral glycoproteins that are of greater molecular weight. These glycoproteins are reduced in viral infectivity and are less able to form syncytia. More specific analogs, such as N-butyl deoxynojirimycin, are now under evaluation.[131,132]

Finally, viral components must assemble at the cell surface and be released from the cell as a mature viral particle. Interferons (IFNs)—alfa, beta, and gamma—are known to inhibit HIV replication in both acute and chronic infection. The precise mechanisms of the antiviral effects of IFNs are unclear in chronic infection, but IFN alfa probably acts, at least in part, by inhibiting the release of mature virions. IFN therapy is discussed in greater depth in the following paragraphs (also see Chapter 10).

Immunologic Treatment

The presence of immunologic defects associated with HIV has stimulated the development of novel approaches to its treatment. Combining the ability to replace or enhance the immune system with potent antiviral agents holds real promise for management of HIV infection. Immunomodulators may act by either restoring or enhancing the immune system. Some immunomodulators may actually modulate the toxicities associated with other medications. Examples of these approaches are listed in Table 8-5.

Table 8-5 Immunomodulation Strategies for Human Immunodeficiency Virus Infection

Immune replacement therapy
Bone marrow transplantation
Intravenous immunoglobulin
Passive immunization
Thymic hormones
Transfer factor
Immune enhancement
Interferon
Ditiocarb
Inosine pranobex
IMREG-1
Colony-stimulating factors
Erythropoietin (EPO)
Granulocyte-macrophage colony-stimulating factor (GM-CSF)
Granulocyte colony-stimulating factor (G-CSF)

Immune Replacement.

Bone Marrow Transplantation (BMT). Interest in BMT (see Chapter 9) has continued from the early days of the AIDS epidemic. In 1984 the National Institute of Allergy and Infectious Diseases attempted to reconstitute the immune system of a patient with AIDS by adoptive transfer of lymphocytes and BMT from an identical twin. Although the patient died, immunologic improvement was documented and suggested the potential utility of this approach.[145] Recently, BMT was combined with antiviral therapy in a patient with AIDS-related non-Hodgkin's lymphoma. This case report used ablative chemoradiotherapy, BMT, and aggressive antiviral therapy both before and after the transplant. Engraftment occurred by day 17, and peripheral blood mononuclear cells and bone marrow were culture negative for HIV. Again, the patient died of recurrent tumor. However, at autopsy there was no evidence of HIV by culture or by PCR gene amplification techniques.[146] These preliminary results suggest that the antiviral therapy prevented HIV infection in donor-derived hematopoietic cells.

HIV control

Intravenous Immunoglobulin (IVIg) and Passive Immunotherapy. The intravenous administration of immunoglobulin has been used to treat immune-mediated cytopenias, particularly thrombocytopenia, and to prevent bacterial infections in pediatric patients. No comparative trials have been reported to date, but one interesting report suggested clinical benefit from administration of high-dose IVIg. Eight children received 200 mg/kg every 3 weeks. In the year before the study, these children experienced 34 serious infections necessitating 220 total hospital days. During the first 12 months of the study, only 6 infections occurred, requiring only 56 hospital days. Four of the eight children were antigenemic before the study; all became antigen negative while receiving IVIg. One of the four subsequently reverted to antigen positive.[147] Whether this reversion resulted from neutralizing antibody in the immunoglobulin is unclear.

Infection control

Some intriguing observations have been noted in patients receiving passive immunotherapy with human plasma containing high titers of anti-HIV neutralizing antibody. These two reports described antigenemic patients with AIDS who were rendered p24 antigen negative after the plasma infusions. Whether this result implies antiviral effect or a transient artifact is uncertain.[148,149]

Other Replacement Strategies. Thymic hormones have also been used in an attempt to replace defective cellular immunity. The results of one small study are somewhat discouraging. Neither immunologic nor clinical benefit was observed.[150] Perhaps administering these compounds would be most effective earlier in the course of HIV illness.

Immune Enhancement. Multiple strategies to enhance the immune deficiency present in HIV infection are also under evaluation: IFNs, ditiocarb, inosine pranobex, interleukin-2 (IL-2), IMREG-1, ampligen, and AS-101. Hematopoietic growth factors are also under evaluation and may be able to minimize leukopenia that occurs as a consequence of either HIV infection or treatment.

Antiviral/ immunomodulation

Interferons. IFNs gained early attention because of their triad of antiviral, immunomodulatory, and antiproliferative activities. The antiviral and immunomodulatory potential of IFN alfa in patients with asymptomatic HIV infection was recently evaluated. The study enrolled 34 individuals with CD4+ counts of more than 400 cells/mm^3 and either positive cultures for HIV or positive p24 antigen. Patients received either placebo or 35 million units (MU) per day of IFN alfa subcutaneously for 12 weeks. Of the patients assigned to IFN, 35% withdrew because of toxicity. The average maximum tolerated daily dose of IFN was 17.5 MU/day. While receiving IFN, 41% of patients became HIV culture negative versus 13% in the placebo group. No opportunistic infections developed in the IFN recipients, whereas five placebo recipients developed opportunistic infections during the study. During the treatment period, CD4+ cells were at or above baseline levels while the CD4+ counts declined in the placebo recipients. However, all IFN recipients developed a flulike syndrome early during treatment. Other toxicities included granulocytopenia (55%) and elevated liver enzymes (45%).[151] Thus, IFN may have a role in the early management of HIV illness. Future strategies to optimize therapeutic effect while modulating toxicities are under evaluation.

One such strategy takes advantage of the synergistic antiretroviral activity of IFN alfa combined with zidovudine. Because optimal response of KS depends partly on immunologic integrity, preliminary data suggested that greater tumor response might be observed with this combination. An evaluation of one such regimen was recently reported. The maximum tolerated dose of the two agents was 18 MU per day of IFN alfa combined with 600 mg per day of zidovudine. Tumor regression was observed in 17 of 37 patients. Immunologic and virologic improvement was also observed.[152] This enhanced tumor activity has been reported in other studies as well. The overall response rate to relatively high doses of IFN (20 MU) is 30%.[153] The combination approach with lower doses of IFN alfa and zidovudine is capable of eliciting somewhat higher response rates of 40% to 50%.[153]

Combination therapy

Dose-related toxicities may be a limitation of these combination approaches. Strategies such as the use of still lower doses, combining with colony-stimulating factors (CSFs), and the use of other retroviral agents or other immunomodulators may be necessary. The combination of IFN alfa, zidovudine, and granulocyte-macrophage colony-stimulating factor (GM-CSF) is currently under investigation. Results obtained in two small studies suggest some promise for this approach.[154,155]

Both IFN beta and IFN gamma are also under evaluation in HIV illness. IFN beta is associated with less hematologic toxicity and, therefore, larger doses may be tolerated. The results of a phase II trial with IFN beta in poor-prognosis KS suggested some antiviral effect. However, the major response rate in this disease was disappointing: only 16% of patients had a clinical response. Toxicities were minimal; the major one was skin related. Eight patients developed local skin necrosis at the injection sites. This necrosis would often occur 1 week or more after injection and resulted in ulceration of the skin penetrating to the subcutaneous tissues.[156]

Ditiocarb efficacy

Ditiocarb and Inosine Pranobex. Ditiocarb and inosine pranobex are compounds that act as nonspecific enhancers of immune function. Ditiocarb appears to exhibit both antiviral and immunomodulatory activity primarily through induction of T-cell differentiation. Eighty-three patients with HIV infection were randomized to receive ditiocarb or placebo for 16 weeks in a crossover fashion. Patients receiving ditiocarb had significant improvement in constitutional symptoms and improvement in lymphadenopathy and immune function. Fewer patients progressed to AIDS while receiving ditiocarb. These effects were transient, apparent only during ditiocarb therapy.[157] The German Ditiocarb Study Group reported an evaluation of 60 patients who were randomized to receive either oral or intravenous ditiocarb and placebo for 24 weeks. Significantly delayed disease progression was observed in the intravenous group versus matched placebo. The benefit in the oral group was not statistically significant. However, over the 18-month follow-up, ditiocarb administration was associated with a greater proportion of patients remaining free of AIDS.[158] A multicenter study conducted in the United States randomized 389 symptomatic patients to receive either ditiocarb (400 mg/m^2 orally once weekly) or placebo. Significantly fewer new opportunistic infections occurred among the 191 patients receiving ditiocarb (5.2%) versus placebo recipients (11%). No immunologic improvement was attributable to ditiocarb in this study.[159]

Inosine pranobex may confer immunomodulatory activity also. Early reports suggested that daily doses of 3 g to 4 g may improve NK cell activity and lymphocyte transformation, perhaps through improved production of IL-1 or IL-2. Results from a large multicenter trial recently suggested that inosine pranobex delayed progression to AIDS, but it had no effect on the number of CD4+ cells or the development of other HIV related conditions.[160] Other controlled trials with inosine pranobex have yielded less positive results. A multicenter study conducted in the United

States and United Kingdom showed no benefit from 4 g of inosine pranobex given daily for 6 months.[161] With the conflicting results of these trials, the role of inosine pranobex remains unclear.

Colony-stimulating Factors. CSFs are glycoproteins that regulate hematopoietic cellular development (see Chapter 2). Preliminary results suggest that these proteins may be useful in stimulating the production of both erythrocytes and neutrophils. A decrease in RBC transfusion requirements has been observed in patients with AIDS and low endogenous erythropoietin levels concomitantly receiving recombinant erythropoietin and zidovudine.[162] A phase I and II trial of GM-CSF was undertaken in 16 patients with AIDS and leukopenia. This study revealed dose-dependent increases in circulating granulocytes. Mature neutrophils, band forms, and eosinophils accounted for most of the increase. Circulating monocytes increased by two to four times over baseline. Dose-related changes in lymphocyte counts were not observed.[163] The use of GM-CSF may reduce the morbidity associated with either disease-related or therapy-related neutropenia in patients with AIDS. However, the ability of GM-CSF to stimulate HIV replication in monocytes is a cause for concern. Whether CSFs can sustain hematopoiesis in a setting of continued suppression is also uncertain. A small study of GM-CSF used as a single agent followed by an alternating regimen with zidovudine lends support for these concerns. In this study, GM-CSF increased both circulating monocyte numbers and function and increased HIV replication (as measured by increased p24 antigen) in six of nine patients. Furthermore, bone marrow evaluations performed at 14 weeks revealed increased cellularity and increased myeloid precursors in only three of seven patients.[164] Because of the potential for enhancement of viral replication, it is likely that the ultimate role of GM-CSF will be in combination with antiviral therapy. However, in vitro studies suggest that GM-CSF may lower the intracellular concentrations of zidovudine triphosphate.[165] The potential clinical significance of this point is unknown. Further evaluations of both GM-CSF and granulocyte-CSF in combination with zidovudine are under way.

Combination therapy

Other Immunomodulators. Other immunomodulators under evaluation in HIV-infected patients are listed in Table 8-5. Impaired production of IL-2 has been described in patients with AIDS. Immunoenhancing effects of IL-2 have been observed in vitro, but results in patients have been disappointing, perhaps because of suboptimal dosing.[166] In some patients to whom IL-2 was administered, temporary increases in circulating lymphocytes were observed. Studies with combinations of IL-2 and zidovudine are under way.

IL-2

IMREG-1

IMREG-1 is derived from the white blood cells of healthy individuals and appears to confer immunoenhancing effects when administered to patients with symptomatic HIV infection. In a randomized multicenter trial, individuals receiving IMREG-1 had a lower incidence of AIDS-defining illnesses (5 of 95 patients) versus placebo recipients (12 of 48 patients). Immunologic improvement was also observed; a greater percentage of IMREG-1 recipients showed a trend toward an increase in CD4+ cells.[167]

Ampligen

Ampligen is a double-stranded RNA molecule that stimulates IFN production. In vitro, ampligen has exhibited both antiviral and immunomodulatory properties. A small study of 10 patients suggested that twice-weekly doses of 200 to 250 mg appeared to increase immunologic function.[168] Larger scale trials are currently under way.

AS-101

AS-101 is an organotellurium compound that appears to stimulate the production of IL-2, CSFs, IFN gamma, and tumor necrosis factor. Preliminary studies again suggest some immunologic improvement. Phase I and II studies and studies with zidovudine are under way.

Because stimulation of the immune system may also activate HIV replication, combination approaches using antiviral agents with immunomodulatory agents are likely to be more effective than either modality alone.

Vaccine Development

Vaccine development is probably crucial to the ultimate containment of HIV, but to develop an effective and safe vaccine is a formidable challenge. Optimism has been stimulated by recent advances in the molecular understanding of viral variability and immunologic response to specific epitopes. In addition, meaningful progress in development of a suitable animal model has been achieved with experimental trials of SIV infection. These models make it possible to evaluate the cross-protection afforded to isolates that are dissimilar to those contained in the vaccine. Mucosal models of infection are also under development.[169] Although these advances are important in the evolution of a vaccine for HIV, several developmental considerations remain.

Animal testing

Developmental Considerations. Although progress has been made in the development of animal models, HIV is uniquely pathogenic for humans and, therefore, no exact animal model exists in which to study the spectrum of the disease. The only animal known to be susceptible to HIV infection is the chimpanzee.[170] Once infected, chimpanzees produce an antibody profile similar to that of humans, shed virus, and demonstrate cytopathic changes in CD4+ cells. Chimpanzees occasionally develop lymphadenopathy and temporary CD4+ depression, but they do not develop an AIDS-like illness. Hence, although the chimpanzee appears to be an adequate model in which to assess the efficacy of a vaccine against primary HIV infection, this model may not accurately reflect the ability of the vaccine to prevent AIDS in humans. Adding to the problem is the severely limited availability of chimpanzees for research in vaccine development. Given these limitations, a great deal of excitement has been generated regarding the progress made with the SIV model. However, genetic and biologic differences between HIV and SIV may limit the value of this model, particularly with respect to extent of virus variability.[169,171]

Antigenic variation

HIV is notable for the high degree of antigenic variation found among HIV isolates. The region of greatest variability is the external envelope glycoprotein.[172] The extent of protection conferred by vaccine candidates against divergent isolates must be evaluated. Infection with HIV-2 has been well described. Although HIV-1 and HIV-2 share common core proteins, their envelope proteins differ. Finally, both phenotypic and genotypic mixing are known to exist in some retroviral systems, allowing for the possibility that mutations are constantly occurring in nature. It will be necessary to determine whether an immunogen selected from a single virus is group specific, or whether it will stimulate the formation of antibodies capable of neutralizing less related variants.[173]

The role of antibody protection from HIV infection is not completely understood. Some patients with HIV infection have neutralizing antibody against HIV. However, in vitro viral neutralization may not reflect in vivo activity. The presence of neutralizing antibody in the sera of both asymptomatic seropositive people and patients with AIDS suggests that these antibodies do not extend adequate protection.[174]

Vaccines

Other retroviral systems suggest that the major antigens important for vaccine development are the external envelope glycoproteins. Since the antigens are found on the exterior portion of the virion, they are the first to be exposed to the immune system.[175] However, infected cells may express on their cell surface other gene products internalized within the whole virion.[173,175] Therefore, antigens defined by genes critical for viral growth and cytopathogenicity, even if not located on the outside of the virus, should be considered potential immunogens. These genes are summarized in Table 8-6.

Strategies for optimizing the presentation of immunogen need to be evaluated. The only adjuvant systems approved for human use are aluminum hydroxide and aluminum phosphate. Although alum is effective in some vaccines, a more efficient stimulator of humoral and cellular response may be needed for a vaccine effective against HIV. Alternative systems such as muramyl dipeptides, liposomes, and immune-stimulating complexes are under development. The immunogenicity of the preparation may be enhanced by several orders of magnitude if a potent adjuvant system is used.[173]

Table 8-6 Viral Gene Products for Vaccine Consideration

Gene	Size	Function
env	gp160 gp120 gp41	External structural proteins Envelope glycoprotein Transmembrane anchor
pol	p66, p51, p31	Viral enzymes (reverse transcriptase, integrase, protease)
gag	p55, p24, p17	Structural capsid proteins
tat	p14	Viral transactivator
rev	p20	RNA transport and stability factor

It is necessary to be able to distinguish between antibody production in response to natural infection and antibody production in response to vaccination. The traditional role of vaccines is to *prevent* disease. The role of a vaccine to treat people already infected with HIV is under evaluation. Because HIV is pathogenic for the cells that are necessary for the development of an immune response to the vaccine, the vaccine may not be able to elicit an adequate immune response. Furthermore, if administered to individuals already infected with HIV, the vaccine, by stimulating infected cells, could potentially have deleterious effects by enhancing infectivity and the progression of disease.

To test the efficacy of vaccine candidates, phase II studies enrolling seronegative individuals who engage in high-risk behaviors are necessary. Investigators in these studies must balance their ability to obtain HIV vaccine efficacy data with their ethical obligations to inform and educate their subjects regarding the avoidance of risky behaviors. The implication of maintaining this equilibrium is that the reported efficacy of the vaccine may be clouded by the impact of the investigators' counseling.

Vaccine Approaches. The approaches that appear to hold greatest promise for HIV are subunit vaccines consisting of cloned, purified, or synthetic HIV proteins, and recombinant vaccines (see Chapter 7). These subunits may be presented with a suitable adjuvant, or the gene encoding for the desired subunit can be inserted into an attenuated vector. Both these approaches have focused on the envelope glycoprotein as the cloned antigen. Finally, anti-idiotype vaccines are in the early stages of human evaluation. These vaccines (see Chapter 7) directed at CD4 should stimulate the production of antibodies that resemble CD4, potentially interfering with viral binding to CD4 receptors on host cells. The approaches currently under investigation are listed in Table 8-7.

Table 8-7 General Approaches to Vaccine Development for Human Immunodeficiency Virus

Purified natural products
Synthetic peptide or subunit + adjuvant
Subunit in viral vector
Anti-idiotype

Human Trials.

Whole Virus Vaccines. Although a whole virus approach to vaccination is more controversial than a genetically engineered vaccine, whole-virus vaccines are under evaluation. A small number of HIV-infected subjects with PGL were immunized with 20 μg of a gamma-irradiated HIV immunogen emulsified in Freund's adjuvant.[171] A booster injection was administered 3 months after the first inoculation. These subjects have been observed for at least 8 months. Thus far, no adverse immunologic consequences have been observed. The total CD4+ counts and the ratio of CD4+ to CD8+ remained stable in eight of nine patients immunized, and these patients remained clinically well during follow-up. One patient with profound antigenemia at entry continued the progressive decline in CD4+ count and developed an AIDS-defining illness 5 months after vaccination. These preliminary results suggest that HIV-specific cytotoxic lymphocytes may be induced by vaccination and may destroy HIV-infected cells. Preexisting neutralizing antibody would then prevent cell-free virus from infecting susceptible cells. Further studies in asymptomatic HIV-infected persons and seronegative individuals are being planned.[171]

CD4+ to CD8+ ratio

HIV Subunit Recombinant Vaccines. Zagury et al.[176] reported the results of primary immunization of one seronegative human volunteer with a recombinant HIV-vaccinia virus.[176] No local or systemic reactions after immunization were noted. No immune defects, assessed by the ratio of CD4+ to CD8+ cells and in vitro IL-2 production, were detected in a 9-week period. Neutralizing antibody was detected on days 30 and 63 to human T lymphotropic virus type IIIB (HTLV-IIIB) (1:40), but not against a divergent subtype, HTLV-IIIRF. In vitro cellular immune response was studied 63 days after immunization. Stimulation with HTLV-IIIB produced a high level of response as measured by the proliferative index and the number of IL-2 receptor-positive cells. HTLV-IIIRF stimulation also activated the cells, but to a lesser extent. This research clearly demonstrates that immunization with a recombinant vaccinia virus expressing HTLV-IIIB envelope glycoproteins was capable of inducing a primary immune response against the immunizing strain and also, to a lesser extent, against a divergent strain.

Efficacy on divergent strains

The phase I trials of an HIV-1 recombinant envelope glycoprotein (gp160) expressed in baculovirus and formulated with alum was recently reported.[177] In this multicenter trial, 72 subjects were randomized to receive the gp160 vaccine (either 40 μg or 80 μg) recombinant hepatitis B vaccine, or alum adjuvant as a placebo. Immunization did not have any adverse consequences on lymphocyte counts, mitogenic responses, or delayed-type hypersensitivity reactions. Weakly reactive antibody responses were detected in 91% of the subjects receiving the candidate vaccine, usually after the second dose. Antibody levels increased dramatically after the subsequent dose or doses and then declined over the ensuing 12 to 18 months. Serum-neutralizing antibody and complement-mediated antibody enhancement was present in 20% to 25% of individuals after the fourth dose. These findings suggest the need for multiple-dose immunization regimens and, perhaps, higher doses of this recombinant gp160 candidate. Dose-ranging trials of gp160 vaccines are under way.[178] Finally, phase I trials of an envelope recombinant (gp120) combined with an alternative adjuvant, muramyl tripeptide, suggested the safety and immunogenicity of nontraditional adjuvants.[179]

Summary

HIV is transmitted through sexual exposure and through infected blood products, organ transplants, shared intravenous drug needles, and perinatally from mother to fetus. Once infection is established, HIV may lie dormant for years before being activated. When activated, the virus selectively destroys CD4+ cells, creating an imbalance of the CD4+ to CD8+ ratio and suppressing production of lymphokines and NK cells. The ELISA and Western blot tests are most commonly used to detect antibodies to HIV, although other testing methods are being investigated. Antibodies to HIV are usually detectable within weeks to months after exposure. Infants will usually acquire maternal antibodies in utero but may not be HIV infected themselves.

Symptoms of acute disease may include a mononucleosis-like syndrome or central nervous system abnormalities. AIDS-defining illnesses include opportunistic infections such as PCP, wasting syndrome, and some neoplasms such as KS. Suppressive therapy is required for many opportunistic infections, including PCP and cryptococcal meningitis. A number of antiviral and immunologic strategies have been investigated in an attempt to halt or reverse the destruction of the immune system. Early antiviral development focused on inhibiting reverse transcriptase. Other sites in the viral replicative cycle are now being explored.

Vaccine development is frustrated by lack of an exact animal model and the extreme antigenic variation of HIV. Both whole virus and recombinant vaccines are being tested.

References

1. Centers for Disease Control. HIV prevalence estimates and AIDS case projections for the United States: report based upon a workshop. *MMWR.* 1990;39:1-31.
2. Piot P, Plummer FA, Mhalu FS et al. AIDS: an international perspective. *Science.* 1988;239:573-9.
3. Gallo RC, Salahuddin SZ, Popovic M et al. Frequent detection and isolation of cytopathic retroviruses (HTLV III) from patients with AIDS and at risk for AIDS. *Science.* 1984;224:500-3.
4. Barre-Sinoussi F, Chermann JC, Rey F et al. Isolation of a T-lymphotropic retrovirus from a patient at risk for the acquired immune deficiency syndrome (AIDS). *Science.* 1983;220:868-71.
5. Clavel F, Guetard D, Brun-Vezinet F et al. Isolation of a new human retrovirus from West African patients with AIDS. *Science.* 1986;233:343-6.
6. Franchini G, Gurgo C, Guo H-G et al. Sequence of simian immunodeficiency virus and its relationship to the human immunodeficiency viruses. *Nature.* 1987;238:539-43.
7. Clavel F, Mansinho K, Chamaret S et al. Human immunodeficiency virus type 2 infection associated with AIDS in West Africa. *N Engl J Med.* 1987;316:1180-5.
8. Kanki PJ, Barin F, M'Boup S et al. New human T-lymphotropic retrovirus related to simian T-lymphotropic virus type III (STLV-III_{AGM}). *Science.* 1986;232:238-43.
9. Centers for Disease Control. Mortality attributable to HIV infection/AIDS—United States, 1981-90. *MMWR.* 1991;40:41-4.
10. Chu SY, Buehler JW, Berkelman RL. Impact of the human immunodeficiency virus epidemic on mortality in women of reproductive age, United States. *JAMA.* 1990;264:225-9.
11. Castro BA, Cheng-Mayer C, Evans LA et al. HIV heterogeneity and viral pathogenesis. *AIDS.* 1988;2(suppl 1):s17-s27.
12. Stein BS, Gowda SD, Lifson JD et al. pH-independent HIV entry into CD4-positive T-cells via virus envelope fusion to the plasma membrane. *Cell.* 1987;49:659-68.
13. Bedinger P, Moriarty A, von Borstel RC II et al. Internalization of the human immunodeficiency virus does not require the cytoplasmic domain of CD4. *Nature.* 1988;334:162-5.
14. Ho DD, Pomerantz RJ, Kaplan JC. Pathogenesis of infection with human immunodeficiency virus. *N Engl J Med.* 1987;317:278-86.

15. Southern P, Oldstone MBA. Medical consequences of persistent viral infection. *N Engl J Med.* 1986;314:356–67.

16. Fauci AS. The human immunodeficiency virus: infectivity and mechanisms of pathogenesis. *Science.* 1988;239:617–22.

17. Klatzmann D, Barre-Sinoussi F, Nugeyre MT et al. Selective tropism of lymphadenopathy associated virus (LAV) for helper-inducer T-lymphocytes. *Science.* 1984;225:59–64.

18. Lane HC, Depper JM, Greene WC et al. Qualitative analysis of immune function in patients with the acquired immunodeficiency syndrome: evidence for a selective defect in soluble antigen recognition. *N Engl J Med.* 1985;313:79–84.

19. Murray HW, Rubin BY, Masur H et al. Impaired production of lymphokines and immune (gamma) interferon in the acquired immunodeficiency syndrome. *N Engl J Med.* 1984;310:883–9.

20. Margolick JB, Volkman DJ, Folks TM et al. Amplification of HTLV-III/LAV infection by antigen-induced activation of T-cells and direct suppression by virus of lymphocyte blastogenic responses. *J Immunol.* 1987;138:1719–23.

21. Rook RH, Masur H, Lane HC et al. Interleukin-2 enhances the depressed natural killer and cytomegalovirus-specific cytotoxic activities of lymphocytes from patients with the acquired immunodeficiency syndrome. *J Clin Invest.* 1983;72:398–403.

22. Ho DD, Rota TR, Hirsch MS. Infection of monocyte/macrophage by human T-lymphotropic virus type III. *J Clin Invest.* 1986;77:1712–5.

23. Gartner S, Markovits P, Markovits DM et al. The role of mononuclear phagocytes in HTLV-III/LAV infection. *Science.* 1985;233:215–9.

24. Talle MA, Rao PE, Westberg E et al. Patterns of antigenic expression on human monocytes as defined by monoclonal antibodies. *Cell Immunology.* 1983;78:83–99.

25. Smith PD, Ohura K, Masur H et al. Monocyte function in the acquired immunodeficiency syndrome: defective chemotaxis. *J Clin Invest.* 1984;74:2121–8.

26. Lane HC, Masur H, Edgar LC et al. Abnormalities of B-cell activation and immunoregulation in patients with the acquired immunodeficiency syndrome. *N Engl J Med.* 1983;309:453–8.

27. Gallo RC, Salahuddin SZ, Popovic M et al. Frequent detection and isolation of cytopathic retroviruses (HTLV-III) from patients with AIDS and at risk for AIDS. *Science.* 1984;224:500–3.

28. Ho DD, Schooley TI, Rota TR et al. HTLV-III in semen and blood of a healthy homosexual man. *Science.* 1984;226:451–3.

29. Wofsy CB, Cohen JB, Hauer LB et al. Isolation of AIDS-associated retrovirus from genital secretions of women with antibodies to the virus. *Lancet.* 1986;1:527–9.

30. Fujikawa LS, Palestine AG, Nussenblatt RB et al. Isolation of human T-lymphotropic virus type III from the tears of a patient with the acquired immunodeficiency syndrome. *Lancet.* 1985;2:529-30.
31. Ho DD, Byington RE, Schooley RT et al. Infrequency of isolation of HTLV-III virus from saliva in AIDS. *N Engl J Med.* 1985;313:1606. Letter.
32. Curran JW, Jaffe HW, Hardy AM et al. Epidemiology of HIV infection and AIDS in the United States. *Science.* 1988;239:610-6.
33. Chmiel JS, Detels R, Kaslow RA et al. Factors associated with prevalent human immunodeficiency virus (HIV) infection in the multicenter AIDS cohort study. *Am J Epidemiol.* 1987;126:568-77.
34. Darrow WW, Echenberg DF, Jaffe HW et al. Risk factors for human immunodeficiency virus (HIV) infections in homosexual men. *Am J Public Health.* 1987;77:479-83.
35. Winkelstein W, Lyman DM, Padian N et al. Sexual practices and risk of infection by the human immunodeficiency virus: the San Francisco Men's Health Study. *JAMA.* 1987;257:321-5.
36. Moss AR, Osmond D, Bacchetti P et al. Risk factors for AIDS and HIV seropositivity in homosexual men. *Am J Epidemiol.* 1987;125:1035-47.
37. Marmar M, Weiss LR, Lyden M et al. Possible female-to-female transmission of human immunodeficiency virus. *Ann Intern Med.* 1986;105:969.
38. Harris C, Butkus C, Klein RS et al. Immunodeficiency in female sexual partners of men with the acquired immunodeficiency syndrome. *N Engl J Med.* 1983;308:1181-4.
39. Friedland GH, Klein RS. Transmission of the human immunodeficiency virus. *N Engl J Med.* 1987;317:1125-35.
40. Centers for Disease Control. The second 100,000 cases of acquired immunodeficiency syndrome—United States, June 1981-December 1991. *MMWR.* 1992; 41:28-31.
41. Al-Nozha M, Ramia S, Al-Frayh A et al. Female to male: an inefficient mode of transmission of human immunodeficiency virus. *J Acquired Immunodeficiency Syndrome.* 1990;3:193-4.
42. Holmberg SD, Horsburgh CR Jr, Ward JW et al. Biologic factors in the sexual transmission of human immunodeficiency virus. *J Infect Dis.* 1989;160:116-25.
43. Padian NS, Shiboski SC, Jewell NP. The effect of number of exposures on the risk of heterosexual HIV transmission. *J Infect Dis.* 1990;161:883-7.
44. Des Jarlais DC, Friedman SR, Stoneburner RL. HIV infection and intravenous drug use: critical issues in transmission dynamics, infection outcomes, and prevention. *Rev Infect Dis.* 1988;10:151-8.
45. Guinan ME, Hardy A. Epidemiology of AIDS in women in the United States: 1981-1986. *JAMA.* 1987;257:2039-42.

46. Ward JW, Deppe DA, Samson S et al. Risk of human immunodeficiency virus infection from blood donors who later developed the acquired immunodeficiency syndrome. *Ann Intern Med.* 1987;106:61–2.
47. Donegan E, Stuart M, Niland JC et al. Infection with human immunodeficiency virus type 1 (HIV-1) among recipients of antibody-positive blood donations. *Ann Intern Med.* 1990;113:733–9.
48. Ward JW, Holmberg SD, Allen JR et al. Transmission of human immunodeficiency virus (HIV) by blood transfusions screened as negative for HIV antibody. *N Engl J Med.* 1988;318:473–8.
49. Donegan E, Lenes BA, Tomasulo PA et al. Transmission of HIV-1 by component type and duration of shelf storage before transfusion. *Transfusion.* 1990;30:839–40.
50. Rivers EP, Buse SM, Bivins BA et al. Organ and tissue procurement in the acute care setting: principles and practice—part 2. *Ann Emerg Med.* 1990;19:193–200.
51. Lifson AR, Castro KG, McCray E et al. National surveillance of AIDS in health care workers. *JAMA.* 1986;256:3231–4.
52. Henderson DK, Fahey BS, Willy M et al. Risk for occupational transmission of human immunodeficiency virus type 1 (HIV-1) associated with exposures. *Ann Intern Med.* 1990;113:740–6.
53. Centers for Disease Control. Update: transmission of HIV infection during an invasive dental procedure—Florida. *MMWR.* 1991;40:21–7.
54. Oxtoby MJ. Perinatally acquired HIV infection. In: Pizzo PA, Wilfert CM, eds. Pediatric AIDS: the challenge of HIV infection in infants, children, and adolescents. Baltimore: Williams and Wilkins; 1991:3–21.
55. Fischl MA, Dickinson GM, Scott GM et al. Evaluation of heterosexual partners, children, and household contacts of adults with AIDS. *JAMA.* 1987;257:640–4.
56. Friedland GH, Saltzman BR, Rogers MF et al. Lack of transmission of HTLV-III/LAV infection to household contacts of patients with AIDS or AIDS-related complex with oral candidiasis. *N Engl J Med.* 1986;314:344–9.
57. Rietmeijer CM, Krebs WJ, Feorino PM et al. Condoms as physical and chemical barriers against human immunodeficiency virus. *JAMA.* 1988;259:1851–3.
58. Mann J, Quinn TC, Piot P et al. Condom use and HIV infection among prostitutes in Zaire. *N Engl J Med.* 1987;316:345.
59. Hicks DR, Martin LS, Voeller B et al. Inactivation of LAV/HTLV-III infected cultures of normal human lymphocytes by nonoxynol-9 in vitro. *Lancet.* 1985;2:1422–3.
60. Brickner PW, Torres RA, Barnes M et al. Recommendations for control and prevention of human immunodeficiency virus (HIV) infection in intravenous drug users. *Ann Intern Med.* 1989;110:833–7.

61. Centers for Disease Control. Hepatitis B virus vaccine safety: report of an interagency group. *MMWR.* 1982;31:465–7.
62. Rogers MF, Ou CY, Kilbourne B et al. Advances and problems in the diagnosis of HIV infection in infants. In: Pizzo PA, Wilfert CM, eds. Pediatric AIDS: the challenge of HIV infection in infants, children, and adolescents. Baltimore: Williams and Wilkins; 1991:159–74.
63. Centers for Disease Control. Serologic testing for antibody to human immunodeficiency virus. *MMWR.* 1987;36:833–45.
64. Centers for Disease Control. Public Health Service guidelines for counseling and antibody testing to prevent HIV infection and AIDS. *MMWR.* 1987;36:509–15.
65. Marlink RG, Allan JS, McLane MP et al. Low sensitivity of ELISA testing in early HIV infection. *N Engl J Med.* 1986;315:1549. Letter.
66. Parks WP, Scott GB. An overview of pediatric AIDS: approaches to diagnosis and outcome assessment. In: Broder S, ed. AIDS—modern concepts and therapeutic challenges. New York: Marcel Dekker; 1987:245–62.
67. Purdy BD, Plaisance KI. Infection with the human immunodeficiency virus: epidemiology, pathogenesis, transmission, diagnosis, and manifestations. *Am J Hosp Pharm.* 1989;46:1185–209.
68. Steckelberg JM, Cockerill FR. Subspeciality clinics: infectious diseases: serologic testing for human immunodeficiency virus antibodies. *Mayo Clin Proc.* 1988;63:373–80.
69. Centers for Disease Control. Interpretation and use of the Western blot assay for serodiagnosis of human immunodeficiency virus type 1 infections. *MMWR.* 1989:38(suppl 7):s1–7.
70. Kessler HA, Baauw B, Spear J et al. Diagnosis of human immunodeficiency virus infection in seronegative homosexuals presenting with an acute viral syndrome. *JAMA.* 1987;258:1196–9.
71. Wittek AE, Phelan MA, Wells MA et al. Detection of human immunodeficiency virus core protein in plasma by enzyme immunoassay: association of antigenemia with symptomatic disease and T-helper cell depletion. *Ann Intern Med.* 1987;107:286–92.
72. Allain JP, Laurian Y, Paul DA et al. Long-term evaluation of HIV antigen and antibodies to p24 and gp41 in patients with hemophilia: potential clinical importance. *N Engl J Med.* 1987;317:1114–21.
73. Borkowksy W, Krasinski K, Paul D et al. Human-immunodeficiency-virus infections in infants negative for anti-HIV by enzyme-linked immunoassay. *Lancet.* 1987;1:1168–71.
74. Chaisson RE, Allain J, Volberding PA. Significant changes in HIV antigen level in the serum of patients treated with azidothymidine. *N Engl J Med.* 1986;315:1610–11.
75. Fahey JL, Taylor JMG, Detels R et al. The prognostic value for cellular and serologic markers in infection with human immunodeficiency virus type 1. *N Engl J Med.* 1990;322:166–72.

76. Michalski FT. The diagnosis of human immunodeficiency virus infection: progress in less than five years. *Yale J Biol Med.* 1989;62:93–102.
77. Schochetman G, Epstein JS, Zuck TF. Serodiagnosis of infection with the AIDS virus and other human retroviruses. *Ann Rev Microbiol.* 1989;43:629–59.
78. Rogers MF, Ou CY, Rayfield M et al. Use of the polymerase chain reaction for early detection of proviral sequences of human immunodeficiency virus in infants born to seropositive mothers. *N Engl J Med.* 1989;320:1649–54.
79. Simmonds P, Balfe P, Peutherer JF et al. Human immunodeficiency virus-infected individuals contain provirus in small numbers of peripheral mononuclear cells and at low copy numbers. *J Virol.* 1990;64:864–72.
80. Rothenberg R, Woelfel M, Stoneburner R et al. Survival with the acquired immunodeficiency syndrome: experience with 5833 cases in New York City. *N Engl J Med.* 1987;317:1297–302.
81. Pederson C, Nielsen CM, Vestergaard BF et al. Temporal relation of antigenemia and loss of antibodies to core antigens to development of clinical disease in HIV infection. *Br Med J* (Clinical Research Ed.). 1987;295:567–9.
82. Klein RS, Harris CA, Small CB et al. Oral candidiasis in high-risk patients as the initial manifestation of acquired immunodeficiency syndrome. *N Engl J Med.* 1984;311:354–8.
83. Nicholson JKA, McDougal S, Jaffe HW et al. Exposure to human T-lymphotropic virus type III/lymphadenopathy-associated virus and immunologic abnormalities in asymptomatic homosexual men. *Ann Intern Med.* 1985;103:37–42.
84. Tindall B, Barker S, Donovan B et al. Characterization of the acute clinical illness associated with human immunodeficiency virus infection. *Arch Intern Med.* 1988;148:945–9.
85. Ho DD, Sarngadharan MG, Resnick L et al. Primary human T-lymphotropic virus type III infection. *Ann Intern Med.* 1985;103:880–3.
86. Centers for Disease Control. Classification system for human T-lymphotropic virus type III/lymphadenopathy-associated virus infections. *Ann Intern Med.* 1986;105:234–7.
87. Centers for Disease Control. Revision of the CDC surveillance case definition for acquired immunodeficiency syndrome. *MMWR.* 1987;36(suppl 1s):3–15.
88. Crowe S, Stewart K, Carlin J et al. Relationship between opportunistic infections (OI) and malignancy (OM) in HIV patients and CD4 lymphocyte number. Paper presented at the Sixth International Conference on AIDS. San Francisco: June 1990.
89. Mills J, Masur H. AIDS-related infections. *Scientific American.* 1990;263:50–7.

90. Masur H, Ognibene FP, Yarchoan R et al. CD4 counts as predictor of opportunistic pneumonias in human immunodeficiency virus (HIV) infection. *Ann Intern Med.* 1989;111:223-31.
91. Phair T, Munoz A, Detels R et al. The risk of *Pneumocystis carinii* pneumonia among men infected with human immunodeficiency virus type 1. *N Engl J Med.* 1990;322:161-5.
92. Hughes WT. *Pneumocystis carinii* pneumonitis. *N Engl J Med.* 1987;317:1021-3.
93. Kovacs JA, Hiemenz JW, Macher AM et al. *Pneumocystis carinii* pneumonia: a comparison between patients with the acquired immunodeficiency syndrome and patients with other immunodeficiencies. *Ann Intern Med.* 1984;100:663-71.
94. Ognibene FP, Shelhamer J, Gill V et al. The diagnosis of *Pneumocystis carinii* syndrome using subsegmental bronchoalveolar lavage. *Am Rev Resp Dis.* 1986;133:226-9.
95. Bigby TD, Margolskee D, Curtis JL et al. The usefulness of induced sputum in the diagnosis of *Pneumocystis carinii* pneumonia in patients with the acquired immunodeficiency syndrome. *Am Rev Resp Dis.* 1986;133:515-8.
96. Allegra CJ, Chabner BA, Tuazon CU et al. Trimetrexate for the treatment of *Pneumocystis carinii* pneumonia in patients with the acquired immunodeficiency syndrome. *N Engl J Med.* 1987;317:978-85.
97. Dismukes WE. Cryptococcal meningitis in patients with AIDS. *J Infect Dis.* 1988;157:624-8.
98. Kovacs JA, Kovacs AA, Polis M et al. Cryptococcosis in the acquired immunodeficiency syndrome. *Ann Intern Med.* 1985;103:533-8.
99. Zuger A, Louie E, Holzmann RS et al. Cryptococcal disease in patients with the acquired immunodeficiency syndrome: diagnostic features and outcome of treatment. *Ann Intern Med.* 1986;104:234-40.
100. Chuck SL, Sande MA. Infections with *Cryptococcus neoformans* in the acquired immunodeficiency syndrome. *N Engl J Med.* 1989;321:794-9.
101. Wong B, Gold JWM, Brown AE et al. Central-nervous system toxoplasmosis in homosexual men and parenteral drug abusers. *Ann Intern Med.* 1984;100:36-42.
102. Leport C, Raffi F, Matheron S et al. Treatment of central nervous system toxoplasmosis with pyrimethamine/sulfadiazine combination in 35 patients with the acquired immunodeficiency syndrome: efficacy of long-term continuous therapy. *Am J Med.* 1988;84:94-100.
103. Hawkins CC. Managing mycobacterial infections in AIDS patients. *Infections in Medicine.* 1988;5:157-9,207-8.

104. Hawkins CC, Gold JWM, Whimbey E et al. Mycobacterium avium complex infections in patients with the acquired immunodeficiency syndrome. *Ann Intern Med.* 1986;105:184–8.
105. Young LS. Mycobacterium avium complex infection. *J Infect Dis.* 1988;157:863–67.
106. Chaisson RE, Slutkin G. Tuberculosis and human immunodeficiency virus infection. *J Infect Dis.* 1989;159:96–100.
107. Centers for Disease Control. Diagnosis and management of mycobacterium infections and disease in persons with human immunodeficiency virus infection. *Ann Intern Med.* 1987;106:254–6.
108. Glatt AE, Chirgwin K, Landesman SH. Current concepts: treatment of infections with human immunodeficiency virus. *N Engl J Med.* 1988;318:1439–48.
109. Klein RS, Harris CA, Small CB et al. Oral candidiasis in high-risk patients as the initial manifestation of acquired immunodeficiency syndrome. *N Engl J Med.* 1984;311:354–8.
110. Quinnan GV Jr, Masur H, Rook AH et al. Herpes virus infections in the acquired immunodeficiency syndrome. *JAMA.* 1984;252:72–7.
111. Macher AM, Reichert CM, Straus SE et al. Death in the AIDS patient: role of cytomegalovirus. *N Engl J Med.* 1983;309:1454. Letter.
112. Jacobson MA, Mill J. Serious cytomegalovirus disease in the acquired immunodeficiency syndrome (AIDS): clinical findings, diagnosis, and treatment. *Ann Intern Med.* 1988;108:585–94.
113. Drew WL. Cytomegalovirus infection in patients with AIDS. *J Infect Dis.* 1988;158:449–55.
114. Pau AK, Pitrak DL. Management of cytomegalovirus infection in patients with acquired immunodeficiency syndrome. *Clin Pharm.* 1990;9:613–31.
115. Center for Disease Control. Kaposi's sarcoma and pneumocystis pneumonia among homosexual men—New York City and California. *MMWR.* 1981;30:305–8.
116. Hymes KB, Cheung T, Greene JB et al. Kaposi's sarcoma in homosexual men: a report of eight cases. *Lancet.* 1981;2:598–600.
117. Beral V, Peterman TA, Berkelman RL et al. Kaposi's sarcoma among persons with AIDS: a sexually transmitted infection? *Lancet.* 1990;335:123–8.
118. Des Jarlais DC, Stoneburner R, Thomas P et al. Declines in proportions of Kaposi's sarcoma among cases of AIDS in multiple-risk groups in New York City. *Lancet.* 1987;1:1024–5.
119. Vogel J, Hinrichs SH, Reynolds RK et al. The HIV tat gene induces dermal lesions resembling Kaposi's sarcoma in transgenic mice. *Nature.* 1988;335:606–11.
120. Safai B, Lowenthal DA, Koziner B. Malignant neoplasms associated with the HTLV-III/LAV infection. *Antibiotics and Chemotherapy.* 1987;38:80–98.

121. Groopman JE, Broder S. Cancer in AIDS and other immunodeficiency states. In: Devita VT, Hellman S, Rosenberg SA, eds. Cancer: principles and practice of oncology. Vol. 2. Philadelphia: J. B. Lippincott Company;1989:1953–70.
122. Ziegler JR, Beckstead JA, Volberding PA et al. Non-Hodgkin's lymphoma in 90 homosexual men. *N Engl J Med.* 1984;311:565–70.
123. Levine AM, Meyer PR, Begandy MK et al. Development of B-cell lymphoma in homosexual men. *Ann Intern Med.* 1984;100:7–13.
124. Gill PS, Meyer PR, Pavlova Z et al. B-cell ALL in adults: clinical, morphologic, and immunologic findings. *J Clin Oncol.* 1986;4:737–43.
125. Kalter SP, Riggs SA, Cabanillas F et al. Aggressive non-Hodgkin's lymphoma in immunocompromised homosexual males. *Blood.* 1985;66:655–9.
126. Levine AM. Non-Hodgkin's lymphomas and other malignancies in the acquired immunodeficiency syndrome. *Semin Oncol.* 1987;14(suppl 3):34–8.
127. Bermudez MA, Grant KM, Rodvien R et al. Non-Hodgkin's lymphoma in a population with or at risk for acquired immunodeficiency syndrome. *Am J Med.* 1989;86:71–6.
128. Lamb R, Gonzales R, Myers A et al. Aggressive non-Hodgkin's lymphoma in AIDS: the University of Colorado experience. *Am J Med Sci.* 1990;300:345–9.
129. Kaplan LD, Abrams DI, Feigal E et al. AIDS-associated non-Hodgkin's lymphoma in San Francisco. *JAMA.* 1989;261:719–24.
130. Goldstein J, Dickson D, Valentine E et al. Radiation therapy (RT) of the central nervous system (CNS) in AIDS-related non-Hodgkin's lymphoma (NHL). Paper presented at the Sixth International Conference on AIDS, San Francisco. June 1990. Abstract No. 2102.
131. Hirsch MS. Chemotherapy of human immunodeficiency virus infections: current practice and future prospects. *J Infect Dis.* 1990;161:845–57.
132. Broder S, Mitsuya H, Yarchoan R et al. Antiretroviral therapy in AIDS. *Ann Intern Med.* 1990;113:604–18.
133. Schooley RT, Merigan TC, Gaut P et al. Recombinant soluble CD4 therapy in patients with the acquired immunodeficiency syndrome (AIDS) and AIDS-related complex. *Ann Intern Med.* 1990;112:247–53.
134. Kahn JO, Allan JD, Hodges TL et al. The safety and pharmacokinetics of recombinant soluble CD4 (rCD4) in subjects with the acquired immunodeficiency syndrome (AIDS) and AIDS-related complex. *Ann Intern Med.* 1990;112:254–61.
135. Capon DJ, Chamow SM, Mordenti J et al. Designing CD4 immunoadhesins for AIDS therapy. *Nature.* 1989;337:525–31.

136. Yarchoan R, Mitsuya H, Myers C et al. Clinical pharmacology of 3'-azido-2',3'-dideoxythymidine (zidovudine) and related dideoxynucleosides. *New Engl J Med.* 1989;321:726–38.

137. Fischl MA, Richman DD, Grieco MH et al. The efficacy of 3'-azido-3'deoxythymidine (azidothymidine) in the treatment of patients with AIDS and AIDS-related complex: a double-blind placebo-controlled trial. *N Engl J Med.* 1987;317:185–91.

138. Moore RD, Hidalgo J, Sugland BW et al. Zidovudine and the natural history of the acquired immunodeficiency syndrome. *N Engl J Med.* 1991;324:1412–6.

139. Fischl MA, Parker CB, Pettinelli C et al. A randomized controlled trial of a reduced daily dose of zidovudine in patients with the acquired immunodeficiency syndrome. *N Engl J Med.* 1990;323:1009–14.

140. Volberding PA, Lagakos SW, Koch MA et al. Zidovudine in asymptomatic human immunodeficiency virus infection. *N Engl J Med.* 1990;322:941–9.

141. Fischl MA, Richman DD, Hansen M et al. The safety and efficacy of zidovudine (AZT) in the treatment of subjects with mildly symptomatic human immunodeficiency virus type 1 (HIV) infection. *Ann Intern Med.* 1990;112:727–37.

142. Broder S, Yarchoan R. Dideoxycytidine: current clinical experience and future prospects. *Am J Med.* 1990;88(suppl 5B):31s–33s.

143. Cooley TP, Kunches LM, Saunders CA et al. Once daily administration of 2',3'-dideoxyinosine (ddI) in patients with the acquired immunodeficiency syndrome or AIDS-related complex. *N Engl J Med.* 1990;322:1340–5.

144. Lambert JS, Seidlin M, Reichman RC et al. 2',3'-Dideoxyinosine (ddI) in patients with the acquired immunodeficiency syndrome or AIDS-related complex. *N Engl J Med.* 1990;322:1333–40.

145. Lane HC, Masur H, Longo DL et al. Partial immune reconstitution in a patient with the acquired immunodeficiency syndrome. *N Engl J Med.* 1984;311:1099–1103.

146. Holland HK, Saral R, Rossi JJ et al. Allogeneic bone marrow transplantation, zidovudine, and human immunodeficiency virus type 1 (HIV-1) infection: studies in a patient with non-Hodgkins lymphoma. *Ann Intern Med.* 1989;111:973–81.

147. Hague RA, Yap PL, Mok JYQ et al. Intravenous immunoglobulin in HIV infection: evidence for the efficacy of treatment. *Arch Dis Child.* 1989;64:1146–50.

148. Jackson GG, Perkins JT, Rubenis M et al. Passive immunoneutralization of human immunodeficiency virus in patients with advanced AIDS. *Lancet.* 1988;2:647–52.

149. Karpas A, Hill F, Youle M et al. Effects of passive immunization in patients with the acquired immunodeficiency syndrome-related complex and acquired immunodeficiency syndrome. *Proc Natl Acad Sci USA.* 1988;85:9234-37.

150. Chachoua A, Green MD, Valentine F et al. Phase I/II trial of thymostimulin in opportunistic infections of the acquired immune deficiency syndrome. *Cancer Invest.* 1989;7:225-9.

151. Lane HC, Davey V, Kovacs JA et al. Interferon-alfa in patients with asymptomatic human immunodeficiency virus infection. *Ann Intern Med.* 1990;112:805-11.

152. Krown SE, Gold JWM, Niedzwiecki D et al. Interferon-alfa with zidovudine: safety, tolerance and clinical and virologic effects in patients with Kaposi sarcoma associated with the acquired immunodeficiency syndrome. *Ann Intern Med.* 1990;112:812-21.

153. Krown SE. Approaches to interferon combination therapy in the treatment of AIDS. *Seminars in Oncology.* 1990;17(suppl 1):11-5.

154. Scadden DT, Bering HA, Levine JD et al. Granulocyte-macrophage colony-stimulating factor mitigates the neutropenia of combined interferon alfa and zidovudine treatment of acquired immune deficiency syndrome-associated Kaposi's sarcoma. *J Clin Oncol.* 1991;9:802-8.

155. Davey, RT Jr, Davey VJ, Metcalf JA et al. A phase I/II trial of zidovudine, interferon alfa, and granulocyte-macrophage colony-stimulating factor in the treatment of human immunodeficiency virus type 1 infection. *J Infect Dis.* 1991;164:43-52.

156. Miles SA, Wang HJ, Cortes E et al. Beta-interferon therapy in patients with poor-prognosis Kaposi's sarcoma related to the acquired immunodeficiency syndrome (AIDS): a phase II trial with preliminary evidence of antiviral activity and low incidence of opportunistic infections. *Ann Intern Med.* 1990;112:582-9.

157. Lang JM, Touraine JL, Trepo C et al. Randomized, double-blind, placebo controlled trial of ditiocarb sodium ("Imuthiol") in human immunodeficiency virus infection. *Lancet.* 1988;2:702-6.

158. Reisinger EC, Kern P, Ernst M et al. Inhibition of HIV progression by dithiocarb. *Lancet.* 1990;1:679-82.

159. Hersh EM, Brewton G, Abrams D et al. Ditiocarb sodium (diethyldithiocarbamate) therapy in patients with symptomatic HIV infection and AIDS. *JAMA.* 1991;265:1538-44.

160. Pedersen C, Sandstrom E, Petersen CS et al. The efficacy of inosine pranobex in preventing the acquired immunodeficiency syndrome in patients with human immunodeficiency virus infection. *N Engl J Med.* 1990;322:1757-63.

161. Kweder SL, Schnur RA, Cooper EC. Inosine pranobex—is a single positive trial enough? *N Engl J Med.* 1990;322:1807-9.

162. Fischl M, Galpin JE, Levine JD et al. Recombinant erythropoietin for patients with AIDS treated with zidovudine. *N Engl J Med.* 1990;322:1488–93.

163. Groopman JE, Mitsuyasu RT, DeLeo MJ et al. Effect of recombinant human granulocyte-macrophage colony-stimulating factor in the acquired immunodeficiency syndrome. *N Engl J Med.* 1987;317:593–8.

164. Pluda JM, Yarchoan R, Smith PD et al. Subcutaneous recombinant granulocyte-macrophage colony-stimulating factor used as a single agent and in an alternating regimen with azidothymidine in leukopenic patients with severe human immunodeficiency virus infection. *Blood.* 1990;76:463–72.

165. Bhalla K, Birkhofer M, Grant S et al. The effect of recombinant human granulocyte-macrophage colony-stimulating factor (GM-CSF) on 3'-azido-3'-deoxythymidine (AZT) mediated biochemical and cytotoxic effects on normal human myeloid progenitor cells. *Exp Hematol.* 1989;17:17–20.

166. Lotze MT, Franan LW, Sharrow DO et al. In vivo administration of purified human interleukin 2. I. Half-life and immunologic effects of the Jurkat cell line-derived interleukin 2. *J Immunol.* 1985;134:157–66.

167. Gottlieb MS, Zackin RA, Fiala M et al. Response to treatment with the leukocyte-derived immunomodulator IMREG-1 in immunocompromised patients with AIDS-related complex: a multicenter, double-blind, placebo-controlled trial. *Ann Intern Med.* 1991;115:84–91.

168. Carter WA, Strayer DR, Brodsky I et al. Clinical, immunological and virological effects of ampligen, a mismatched double-stranded RNA in patients with AIDS or AIDS-related complex. *Lancet.* 1987;1:1286–92.

169. Bolognesi DP. AIDS vaccines: progress and unmet challenges. *Ann Intern Med.* 1991;114:161–2.

170. Goudsmit J, Smit L, Krone WJA et al. IgG response to human immunodeficiency virus in experimentally infected chimpanzees mimics the IgG response in humans. *J Infect Dis.* 1987;155:327–31.

171. Fauci AS, Gallo RC, Koenig S et al. Development and evaluation of a vaccine for human immunodeficiency virus (HIV) infection. *Ann Intern Med.* 1989;110:373–85.

172. Starcich BR, Hahn BH, Shaw GM et al. Identification and characterization of conserved and variable regions in the envelope gene of HTLV-III/LAV, the retrovirus of AIDS. *Cell.* 1986;45:637–48.

173. Koff WC, Hoth DF. Development and testing of AIDS vaccines. *Science.* 1988;241:426–32.

174. Robert-Guroff M, Brown M, Gallo RC. HTLV-III-neutralizing antibodies in patients with AIDS and AIDS-related complex. *Nature.* 1985;361:72–4.
175. Fischinger PJ, Gallo RC, Bolognesi DP. Toward a vaccine against AIDS: rationale and current progress. *Mt Sinai J Med.* 1986;53:639–47.
176. Zagury D, Leonard R, Fouchard M et al. Immunization against AIDS in humans. *Nature.* 1987;326:249–50.
177. Dolin R, Graham BS, Greenberg SB et al. The safety and immunogenicity of a human immunodeficiency virus type 1 (HIV-1) recombinant gp160 candidate vaccine in humans. *Ann Intern Med.* 1991;114:119–27.
178. Kovacs H, Easter ME, Davey R et al. Safety and immunogenicity of recombinant gp160, a candidate AIDS vaccine. Paper presented to 30th Interscience Conference on Antimicrobial Agents and Chemotherapy, Atlanta. 1990.
179. Wintsch J, Chaignant CL, Braun DG et al. Safety and immunogenicity of a genetically engineered human immunodeficiency virus vaccine. *J Infect Dis.* 1991;163:219–25.

Self-Study Questions

1. List the three types of cells that can be infected with HIV.

    1. Helper T cells; suppressor T cells, monocytes/ macrophages.

2. Which of the following is the initial event in the HIV replicative cycle?

    A. p24 attaches to reverse transcriptase.
    B. gp120 binds to CD4 receptor.
    C. The virus is internalized.
    D. The CD4+/CD8+ ratio is inverted.

    2. B

3. Health care workers, as a demographic group for epidemiologic study, are disproportionately represented among the HIV-infected population in the United States.

    A. True.
    B. False.

    3. B

4. Which of the following demographic groups represents the fastest-growing subpopulation of HIV-infected patients in the United States?

    A. Intravenous drug users.
    B. Homosexuals.
    C. Heterosexuals.
    D. Infants.

    4. C

5. A high-risk patient with an indeterminant result from a Western blot should be tested again for HIV in ____________months.

    5. Six.

6. During what two phases of HIV infection is serum p24 antigen detectable using the p24 antigen assay?

    6. Immediately after HIV infection; in the late stages of illness.

7. What is the most common fungal infection found in patients with HIV?

    7. Candidiasis.

Answer	Question
8. A	8. Opportunistic infections are the leading cause of death for patients with HIV. A. True. B. False.
9. B	9. How does soluble recombinant CD4 exert antiviral activity? A. Protease inhibition. B. Viral binding inhibition. C. Integrase inhibition. D. Reverse transcriptase inhibition.
10. Erythrocytes; neutrophils.	10. The results of preliminary studies suggest that colony-stimulating factors may be useful in stimulating the production of ____________ and ____________ in treating HIV infection.
11. D	11. What is the most common toxicity associated with interferon therapy for HIV infection? A. Hepatitis. B. Peripheral neuropathy. C. Local skin necrosis. D. Flulike syndrome.
12. A	12. Painful peripheral neuropathy is a toxicity associated with some, but not all, reverse transcriptase inhibitors. A. True. B. False.
13. B	13. The chimpanzee is the only exact animal model that exists for the study of HIV vaccination effects. A. True. B. False.
14. Natural infection with HIV occurred.	14. Assuming the results are accurate, an HIV antibody test could be positive in a volunteer immunized with an HIV vaccine if (a) the volunteer developed antibodies to the vaccine, or (b)________________________.

CHAPTER 9

Solid-Organ and Bone Marrow Transplantation

Kathleen D. Lake, Pharm.D.
Program Director, Cardiothoracic Transplantation and Research
Minneapolis Heart Institute
Abbott Northwestern Hospital
Minneapolis, MN

Timothy R. McGuire, Pharm.D.
Assistant Professor, Pharmacy Practice
College of Pharmacy
University of Nebraska Medical Center
Omaha, NE

Introduction

For many years, scientists were unsuccessful in their attempts to replace diseased and injured organs with donated healthy organs. As discussed in the chapter on the major histocompatibility complex (MHC), only an organ donated from an identical twin was acceptable to the host's immune system. Organs donated from family members or cadavers were not likely to be sufficiently compatible to avoid rejection.

New drugs, genetic engineering techniques, surgical procedures, MHC typing, and an advanced understanding of the mechanisms of the immune system have promoted organ transplant procedures from the realm of experiment to that of an accepted treatment for many patients. Problems still remain, however, with immunosuppressive agents adding their own complications to patient therapy. Suppressing the host's immune system reduces the incidence of graft rejection but also leaves the host vulnerable to opportunistic infections. Immunosuppressive agents can also have detrimental side effects that increase the host's risk for complications. Donor marrow can be treated to reduce the risk of the transplant rejecting the host, but the treatment may reduce the effectiveness of the grafting process.

The pharmacist's job in treating the transplant patient is a crucial one, being concerned with immunosuppressive therapy, postoperative antibiotic therapy, nutritional therapy, palliative therapy to adverse reactions, monitoring drug levels, interactions, and adverse reactions, and providing advice about appropriate experimental agents.

Learning objectives

After reading this chapter, the learner will be able to—

- Describe the immunosuppressive effects of various agents.
- Discuss immunosuppressive therapies for solid organ transplant procedures.
- Discuss patient selection criteria for various solid organ transplants.
- Discuss rescue therapies for acute solid organ transplant rejection.
- Discuss postoperative complications and side effects of solid organ transplants.
- Discuss immunosuppressive therapy for bone marrow transplant patients.
- Discuss post-bone marrow transplant complications and their therapies.

Chapter organization

This chapter begins with an overview of the development of solid organ and bone marrow transplantation. Immunosuppressive agents (cyclosporine, azathioprine, corticosteroids, OKT3, antilymphocyte and antithymocyte globulins, methotrexate, cyclophosphamide, FK506, rapamycin, RS61443, deoxyspergualin, cyclosporine G, thalidomide, and investigational monoclonal antibodies), their mechanisms, side effects, and applications are discussed next. Nonpharmacologic therapies are briefly covered.

Solid organ transplant procedures are discussed in the following order: heart, lung and heart-lung, liver, kidney, pancreas and islet cell, islet-thymic, and small intestine. The history, indications, patient selection criteria, immunosuppressive therapy, complications, and postoperative care are discussed for each type of transplant. The discussion of solid organ transplants concludes with an expanded section about complications.

The discussion of bone marrow transplants provides background information about the history and patient populations, which includes strategies for increasing the donor pool. Pathophysiology and therapy for graft-versus-host disease are covered as well as other possible complications of bone marrow transplant such as infections, venocclusive disease, and interstitial pneumonitis.

Early Efforts in Transplantation

Solid Organs

Although the idea of solid-organ transplantation dates back to ancient times, the first major milestone was the development of the vascular anastomosis technique by Alexis Carrel and Charley Claude Guthrie in 1902.[1] Using this technique, a variety of tissue and organ grafts were performed in various animal species.

Kidney

The first attempt at kidney transplantation occurred in 1933, although it was not until 1954, in Boston, that the first long-term surviving kidney transplant was performed between identical twins. The first successful attempts at intentionally suppressing the immune system in humans occurred between 1958 and 1962 when Murray[2,3] in Boston and Hamburger in Paris used varying dosages of total body irradiation to circumvent rejection of transplanted kidneys in nonidentical twins. This was the beginning of immunosuppression, and the developments in transplantation have paralleled those in immunosuppressive therapy.

Subsequent major milestones in organ transplantation occurred in the 1960s with the development of tissue-typing techniques and new immunosuppressive agents. Early work with the antimetabolite 6-mercaptopurine (6-MP) by Schwartz and Dameshek[4] led to the development of an imidazole derivative of this drug, azathioprine, by Hitchings and Elion[5] of the Burroughs Wellcome Research Laboratories. The combination of this agent with corticosteroids demonstrated increased efficacy in preventing rejection.[6] During the next decade, a variety of techniques and agents including thoracic duct drainage, splenectomy, thymectomy, lymphoid or graft irradiation, cyclophosphamide (CTX), and the polyclonal antilymphocyte and antithymocyte globulins were used in attempts to suppress the immune response.

CsA

The next major milestone occurred in the mid-1970s with the discovery of cyclosporine (CsA). The success seen with heart, liver, pancreas, pancreas-kidney, heart-lung, and lung transplantation during the past decade has been credited to the introduction of CsA (Table 9-1). By the mid-1980s, combinations of two, three, and four drugs were being used to augment immunosuppression while minimizing the toxicity of the individual agents.

MoAbs

The discovery by Kohler and Milstein[7] of the technique to produce monoclonal antibodies (MoAbs) heralded a new era of immunosuppressive therapy for clinical organ transplantation in the 1980s. Their contribution was recognized with the Nobel Prize in 1984. The development of new agents using MoAb technology is being stimulated by the selectivity and specificity of MoAbs against specific immunologic targets.

Perhaps the most recent milestone was the recognition of clinical transplantation specialists E.D. Thomas and J.E. Murray, who were awarded the Nobel Prize in 1990 for their achievements in bone marrow transplantation (BMT) and renal transplantation, respectively.

Despite a dramatic increase in the number of transplants performed each year and the number of centers performing them, the major limitation is the availability of donor organs relative to the number of patients in need of a

Table 9-1 Success of Organ Transplantation, United States, 1990

Organ	Number of Programs	Number of Transplants Performed	One-Year Actuarial Survival Rate (%)	
			Graft	Patient
Heart	151	2,085 (6 DT*)		81
Heart-lung	81	50		58
Lung	71			59
Double		62		67
Single		200		
Kidney	235	9,560 (1,773 LRD)	CAD, 81	92
			LRD, 91	96
Liver	87	2,656 (9 LRD)	69	76
Pancreas	86	549 (0 LRD)	53	84

(From United Network for Organ Sharing.)

CAD = cadaveric donor; DT = domino transplant (heart-lung); LRD = living related donor.

*In the domino transplant, only six of which were performed in 1990, the lung transplant patient's heart is removed along with the lungs and the patient receives both a transplanted heart and transplanted lungs; the healthy heart is then donated to another recipient.

transplant. Future efforts need to be directed at maximizing the use of donor organs and developing other options such as the use of xenografts or implantable artificial organs to meet the needs of these patients.

Bone Marrow Transplantation

GVHD

The initial work leading to the development of BMT was performed in the 1950s, when it was found that heavily irradiated mice would transiently accept bone marrow and that this marrow protected against the lethal effects of radiation. However, animals died from a disease that severely affected the gut, skin, and liver and caused cachexia. Because of the severe growth retardation, this disease became known as runt disease and was later recognized as acute graft-versus-host disease (GVHD).

BMT is a potentially curative treatment in acute and chronic leukemias, lymphomas, aplastic anemia, and various genetic disorders. There are two major types of BMT, allogeneic and autologous. An uncommon form of BMT between identical twins is called syngeneic. In autologous BMT the donor and the recipient are the same person; thus, there are no immunologic barriers to the transplant. Conversely, in allogeneic BMT the transplant is between immunologically distinct individuals. This immunologic disparity manifests itself in two ways: the patient can reject the donor's marrow and fail to engraft, or the patient can develop acute GVHD.[8]

Allogeneic and autologous

Most of the early work with allogeneic BMT in humans was performed in Seattle. While approximately 90% of the first cohort of patients who received transplants for advanced leukemia died, about 10% survived who otherwise would not have. These cures in patients with advanced disease supported the use of BMT earlier in the disease process, when patients still have a good performance status.[8]

Immunosuppressive Agents

Efforts to succeed with solid organ and bone marrow transplants have been frustrated by the human immune response to allogeneic transplants. Therefore, a primary concern is to minimize the rejection process and the toxicities often associated with immunosuppressive agents.

The following discussion on immunosuppressive agents provides information about the pharmacology of the transplantation process; specific organ transplants are discussed later in this chapter.

Cyclosporine

Effects and Uses. Cyclosporine (CsA) is an 11-amino-acid cyclic peptide with reversible immunosuppressive activity. It blocks the production of interleukin 2 (IL-2) from CD4+ cells while sparing function of CD8+ cells, B cells, macrophages, and granulocytes. It inhibits CD4+ cell production of IL-2 without causing death of the cell. It also inhibits clonal expansion of allosensitized T cells by decreasing the numbers of IL-2 surface receptors.

IL-2 inhibition

Because CsA inhibits the synthesis of IL-2, it works early in the cascade of events leading to organ rejection or acute GVHD. It inhibits the clonal expansion of alloantigen-sensitized CD4+ and CD8+ T cells. It is not active against preformed cytotoxic T lymphocytes (CD8+) or in non-T-cell-related rejection.

The mechanism by which CsA inhibits the synthesis of IL-2 is unclear. However, the mechanism may involve CsA's binding to a cytosolic binding protein (cyclophilin), which may be important in signal transmission for de novo IL-2 production. There is indirect support for this mechanism in that very similar immunosuppression is seen with the investigational macrolide FK506, which binds to a distinct but similar protein.

Pharmacokinetic variability

Dosing and Monitoring. CsA pharmacokinetics are complex and vary among transplant populations.[9] In the BMT setting, CsA pharmacokinetics may be altered by low hematocrit. Red blood cells (RBCs) bind CsA, and in a drug with a low to intermediate extraction ratio like CsA, clearance increases with decreased binding. Age seems also to be an important factor in the disposition of CsA; pediatric patients have higher clearance values than older patients. A group of researchers has suggested that this age-related difference in clearance may result from lower serum lipoprotein concentrations and CsA binding in younger patients.[10] In addition, many drugs are capable of altering the clearance of CsA (see Table 9-2).[11-13]

The use of therapeutic drug monitoring to reduce the risk of nephrotoxicity associated with CsA remains controversial. A number of studies have demonstrated an association between elevated CsA concentrations and renal dysfunction, but a therapeutic range has not been identified. The therapeutic drug monitoring of CsA is complicated by important assay and biologic fluid considerations. One of the difficulties in assessing CsA concentrations comes from the fact that many of the early studies used a polyclonal RIA that is now unavailable. The current polyclonal assay using a fluorescence polarization immunoassay (FPIA) has different metabolite-binding affinities and demonstrates about 1.6 times higher concentrations in plasma than the polyclonal radioimmunoassay

Table 9-2 Representative Drug Interactions with Cyclosporine[11–13]

Drugs That Increase Levels of Cyclosporine	Drugs That Decrease Levels of Cyclosporine	Drugs That Cause Additive Nephrotoxicity
Ketoconazole, fluconazole	Phenytoin	Amphotericin B
Erythromycin	Carbamazepine	Aminoglycosides
Oral contraceptive hormones	Phenobarbital	Melphalan
Diltiazem	Primidone	Nonsteroidal anti-inflammatory drugs
Verapamil	Rifampin	
Nicardipine	Nafcillin	
Metoclopramide	Octreotide	
FK506		

(RIA). In whole blood the FPIA and RIA give about the same value. Whether a specific (i.e., HPLC) or nonspecific (i.e., FPIA) assay should be used is still controversial. The more complete studies have been performed using nonspecific assays and have shown the most convincing positive correlation between concentration and effect.[14]

In most investigations of the relationship between CsA concentrations and efficacy or toxicity, serum or plasma concentrations have been measured. The question regarding the use of whole blood versus serum or plasma remains controversial. CsA is highly bound to RBCs. This binding is temperature dependent. As the temperature of blood is lowered from body temperature to room temperature, the CsA increasingly partitions into the RBCs. Thus, serum or plasma levels are affected by temperature variations. Because of this temperature-dependent effect, it may be advantageous to use whole-blood assays if the samples cannot be handled with consistent temperature restrictions. However, with appropriate sample handling—which means that one consistent temperature is used to separate serum or plasma, such as a 2-hour equilibration at room temperature—consistent results can be obtained. Until more is known about the activity of the metabolites, it is difficult to recommend one assay method or biologic matrix over another; it may be reasonable to use the assay and matrix that is most convenient for the given institution.

Side Effects and Toxicity. CsA has a number of important toxicities, the most common and clinically relevant of which is renal dysfunction. CsA nephrotoxicity can manifest as an acute renal failure or chronic nephrotoxicity. The acute renal dysfunction associated with CsA is characterized by decreased glomerular filtration within days of starting the drug. A number of drugs have also been reported to produce additive nephrotoxicity with CsA (see Table 9-2).[11-13]

Renal dysfunction

A number of renal protectants have been investigated to decrease the acute renal failure syndrome: prostaglandin E2, clonidine, and pentoxifylline. A recent article reported that patients on amphotericin and CsA and receiving pentoxifylline were able to receive significantly higher CsA doses with lower serum creatinine values than patients not receiving pentoxifylline. Most important, there was significantly less acute GVHD in the pentoxifylline group, perhaps as a result of higher CsA doses in that group.[15] Calcium antagonists are also being evaluated for their renal protective effects.[16,17]

In addition to nephrotoxicity, CsA can cause liver dysfunction, neurotoxicity, hirsutism, and infusion-related reactions characterized by burning of the soles and palms.

Azathioprine

Effects and Uses. Azathioprine is a purine analog that has been used as a component of immunosuppressive regimens since 1961.[3] Its popularity has fluctuated through the decades as newer immunosuppressive agents have surfaced, but it is of great importance in the evolution of clinical transplantation. The Burroughs Wellcome Research Foundation synthesized azathioprine in an attempt to develop a more stable compound capable of resisting enzymatic deactivation in tissues. It was determined later, however, that azathioprine had a better therapeutic index than 6-mercaptopurine (6-MP), an antineoplastic agent used in treating leukemia.[5]

Rejection prevention

Azathioprine is an imidazolyl derivative of 6-MP. It has been considered a slow-release prodrug of 6-MP because it is readily metabolized to 6-MP and other metabolites.[18] It acts through its incorporation into cellular DNA, inhibiting purine nucleotide synthesis and metabolism and altering the synthesis and function of RNA. It inhibits humoral and cellular immunity during the initial stages of lymphoid differentiation. Thus, it is useful in preventing the onset of acute rejection, but it is of no value in treating acute rejection. Azathioprine may also reduce neutrophil production and macrophage function and thereby reduce the nonspecific inflammatory aspect of the immune reaction.[19]

Dosing and Monitoring. Even though azathioprine has been used for more than 25 years, its pharmacokinetics have not been fully characterized. The development of sensitive and specific assays has allowed better definition of the pharmacokinetics of azathioprine and its metabolites.[20-25]

IV vs. oral

The absorption of orally administered azathioprine is rapid but incomplete. It is rapidly converted by glutathione to 6-MP in the liver and the RBCs; peak plasma concentrations of 6-MP after oral and intravenous administration occur within 1 to 2 hours and 5 to 15 minutes, respectively.[20-22,25,26] Bioavailability of 6-MP after administration of azathioprine has been estimated to be 41% to 44%.[27] On the basis of these findings, the dose of azathioprine should be doubled in converting from the intravenous to the oral route of administration.[18]

Half-life

Because of the extensive biotransformation, both azathioprine and 6-MP disappear rapidly from the blood after intravenous or oral administration.[22,23,28,29] Concentrations of both azathioprine and 6-MP are unquantifiable beyond 8 hours after a dose of azathioprine.[21] Both azathioprine and 6-MP have a short half-life—12.5 ± 3.0 minutes and 50.4 ± 36.6 minutes, respectively. Clearance is not affected by renal impairment.[22] This fact does not exclude the possibility that some of azathioprine's metabolites may accumulate with renal impairment and thus may contribute to its myelosuppressive effect.

6-MP is further broken down to 6-thiouric acid, an inactive end product primarily eliminated by the kidneys, or further transformed intracellularly to thioinosinic acid and 6-thioguanine nucleotides (TGNs). Thioinosinic acid and TGNs (active moieties) are largely responsible for the immunosuppressive and myelotoxic effects of azathioprine.[25] The half-life of RBC TGN appears to be quite long (e.g., 13 days), allowing for once-daily dosing of azathioprine.[25]

An initial dose of 3 to 5 mg/kg per day of azathioprine is administered preoperatively. Immediately after transplantation, the dose is usually tapered to a maintenance dose of 1 to 3 mg/kg per day or titrated to patient tolerance as determined by a desired white blood cell (WBC) count in the range of 3,500 to 6,000 cells/mm^3. Azathioprine has been used extensively in double-, triple-, and quadruple-drug regimens for organ transplantation and for treating autoimmune diseases. Clinical studies using azathioprine are reviewed elsewhere.[18]

Drug interactions

A reduction of 75% to 80% of the azathioprine dose is necessary in patients receiving the xanthine-oxidase inhibitor allopurinol, which blocks the metabolism of azathioprine and other purines.[30-32] Other drug interactants include muscle relaxants. Azathioprine has been associated with increased requirements of the nondepolarizing muscle relaxant pancuronium, but it potentiates the activity of succinylcholine, a depolarizing muscle relaxant.[33,34] Increased warfarin requirements have been reported for patients receiving 6-MP and may be expected with azathioprine.[35] An interaction may be anticipated between azathioprine and other drugs known to cause leukopenia.

Side Effects and Toxicity. The primary toxicity of azathioprine is its dose-related bone marrow suppression, characterized by leukopenia,[36,37] thrombocytopenia, macrocytic anemia,[38] pure red cell aplasia, and reticulocytopenia.[39] Myelosuppression is usually delayed, with hematologic disorders appearing 7 to 14 days after initiation of therapy.[40] Other adverse effects include increased predisposition to infections (viral, bacterial, and fungal),[41] hepatic dysfunction and jaundice,[42-45] alopecia, stomatitis,[46] acute pancreatitis,[47] and increased risk of malignancy.[48] The adverse effects of azathioprine are reviewed in greater detail elsewhere.[18]

Corticosteroids

Mechanisms

Effects and Uses. The usefulness of corticosteroids in solid-organ transplantation and BMT results from three of their pharmacologic effects: (1) a direct effect on circulating lymphocytes, (2) modulation of specific cellular immune functions, and (3) a nonspecific anti-inflammatory effect.

Corticosteroids cause a rapid and profound drop in circulating T lymphocytes, not as a result of direct destruction of lymphocytes but, rather, from sequestration of lymphocytes in the bone marrow. Besides decreasing the number of circulating monocytes and lymphocytes (particularly CD4+ T lymphocytes) and increasing the number of circulating neutrophils, corticosteroids have major effects on lymphocyte, monocyte, and neutrophil function. Corticosteroids bind to an intracytosolic steroid receptor and are transported to the nucleus, where they alter DNA and RNA synthesis (Figure 9-1). They are also potent phosphodiesterase inhibitors leading to accumulation of intracellular cyclic adenosine monophosphate and inhibition of lymphocyte activation. Inhibition of IL-1 secretion from macrophages and IL-2 secretion from T lymphocytes inhibits the generation of cytotoxic T lymphocytes. The nonspecific, potent anti-inflammatory effect is a result of the inhibition of arachidonic acid release and suppression of macrophage phagocytosis.

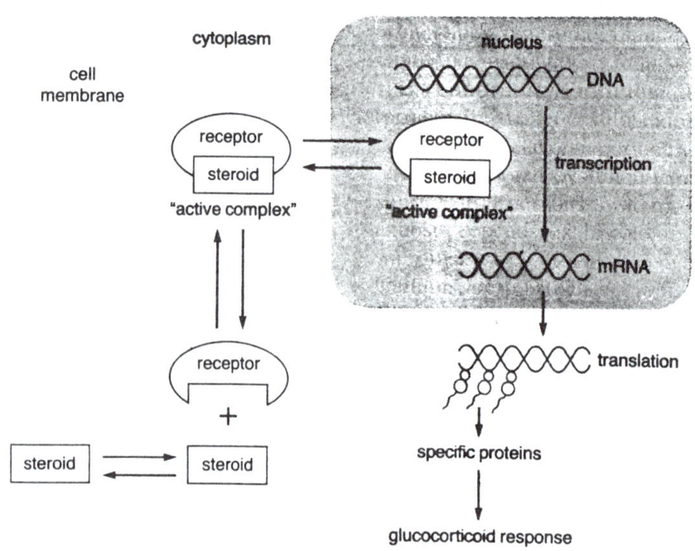

Figure 9-1. Mechanism of action of steroid hormones on the molecular level

Dosing and Monitoring. Corticosteroids have a broad spectrum of use in clinical transplantation. They are used in both preventing and treating graft rejection and acute GVHD. In general, prophylactic doses in solid-organ transplantation are in the range of 1 to 2 mg/kg per day and tapered over months to 0.1 to 0.3 mg/kg per day. In BMT, corticosteroids are used for both the treatment and prophylaxis of acute GVHD. Unlike solid-organ transplantation patients, BMT patients who do not develop acute or chronic GVHD may discontinue immunosuppressive prophylaxis by 6 months after transplant. A recent paper reported that the use of corticosteroids in BMT patients may actually increase the incidence of acute GVHD in those receiving methotrexate (MTX) and CsA.[49] The thought is that steroids inhibit the antiproliferative effect of MTX by interfering with its cell-cycle-dependent suppression of T-cell proliferation. The investigators then looked at the effect of delaying the initiation of steroids until day 14 after transplant (the last dose of MTX was given on day 11). The rate of acute GVHD in the delay group was equivalent to that of patients not receiving steroids. This study suggests that in BMT patients receiving MTX and CsA, the addition of corticosteroids for GVHD prophylaxis is not helpful and may actually be detrimental.

MTX and CsA

Side Effects and Toxicity. Because of the significant toxicities associated with long-term corticosteroid use, there has been a more aggressive use of steroid-sparing drugs such as CsA, so that lower doses of steroids can be given. Table 9-3 lists some of the side effects associated with corticosteroid therapy.

OKT3

Effects and Uses. Muromonab OKT3 (OKT3) is a murine MoAb of the IgG2a isotype[50] that binds to the CD3 receptor found only on mature circulating T cells and medullary thymocytes.[50-52] The CD3 receptor complex is situated next to the T-cell antigen recognition site. By binding to the CD3 receptor, OKT3 blocks the ability of cells to become stimulated by foreign antigens, thus inhibiting both the generation and function of cytotoxic T cells responsible for graft rejection. After the initial dose of OKT3, T cells virtually disappear from the circulation within minutes to hours. During treatment with OKT3, T cells bearing the usual array of surface markers (CD2, CD4, CD8) reappear but are devoid of the OKT3 target, the CD3 receptor.[53-55] Within 48 hours of discontinuing therapy, the normal array of surface markers, including CD3, reappears on T cells. Proposed mechanisms for OKT3's action include opsonization of circulating T cells and subsequent removal by the reticuloendothelial system;[56] modulation (internalization) of the T-lymphocyte

Mechanism

Table 9-3 Selective Side Effects of Corticosteroid Therapy

Central nervous system
Euphoria
Depression
Adrenal axis suppression
Hypertension
Sodium and water retention
Myopathy
Avascular necrosis
Infection
Impaired wound healing
Increased appetite
Osteoporosis
Cataracts
Hyperglycemia

antigen-receptor-CD3 complex, rendering the T cell nonfunctional;[57] and coating of the T-cell receptor, inhibiting T-lymphocyte antigen recognition for the duration of the therapy.[58,59]

OKT3 is effective in reversing and preventing rejection in solid-organ transplantation. Immunologic monitoring should be performed during and after OKT3 therapy to monitor the efficacy of treatment and to assess whether retreatment with OKT3 is possible. It is particularly important that immune monitoring be performed during retreatment with OKT3 so that appropriate dose adjustments can be made.[60] OKT3 is an important prototype of MoAbs and can be considered the gold standard against which newer agents should be compared.

Dosing and Monitoring. Limited information is available on the pharmacokinetics of OKT3. The 18-hour half-life of OKT3 is significantly less than the half-life of inert immunoglobulin in humans (20 days).[61,62] This discrepancy may be due to the continuous adsorption of OKT3 onto newly developing CD3 receptors of T lymphocytes or to the development of human antimouse antibodies, which may complex with the compound and cause its consumption.[63] The volume of distribution for OKT3 appears to be similar to that of albumin, but the binding and distribution characteristics of OKT3 have not been fully characterized.

The therapeutic effectiveness of OKT3 in reversing acute allograft rejection is related to its ability to block the action of cytotoxic T lymphocytes against the allograft. Potential causes for failure of OKT3 or subsequent need for higher OKT3 doses include immune clearance of the agent as a result of human antimurine antibody production, increased consumption from high antigen production rates, an abnormally high clearance rate of mouse immunoglobulin, and an escape of T-cell functional dependence on the CD3 antigen.[55]

The efficacy of OKT3 therapy can be monitored by measuring peripheral T-cell subsets (CD2+, CD3+, CD4+, CD8+),[53-55] serum OKT3 levels,[51,64,65] and the production of human antimurine antibodies.

Goal

With regard to monitoring T-cell subsets, the goal of therapy is to maintain the percentage of CD3+ at less than 5% (absolute CD3+ cells less than 20 to 30/mm^3). The reappearance of CD3+ T lymphocytes is usually the first indication of an ineffective OKT3 response. The dosage of OKT3 may need to be increased if the first three or four doses do not effectively remove all CD3+ cells. The OKT3 dose can be increased by 2.5-mg increments to help overcome circulating anti-OKT3 antibodies. Some patients have safely received 15 mg per day—three times the usual dose.[66]

ELISA monitoring

Using enzyme-linked immunosorbent assay (ELISA) to measure OKT3 serum concentrations may prove useful as a more precise method of monitoring therapy.[67] Peak serum concentrations in excess of 1,000 ng/mL are achieved after the initial dose. After rapid elimination of the first dose, usual trough concentrations of 100 ng/mL are seen by 24 hours. The desired trough serum concentration of more than 800 ng/mL is usually achieved by the third or fourth day of therapy, but it may not be achieved until the seventh day in some patients. Usual doses of OKT3 produce steady-state trough concentrations of 800 to 1,000 ng/mL.[60]

Pediatric dose

The usual dosage regimen for OKT3 is 5 mg intravenously daily for 10 to 14 days. Before administration, OKT3 must be filtered through a 0.20- to 0.22-micron low-protein-binding filter to remove particulate matter. After filtering, OKT3 should be administered as an intravenous bolus via a peripheral vein. Lower doses have proved equally effective in some patients.[67] The manufacturer originally recommended that a dose of 2.5 mg be administered daily in children who weigh less than 30 kg, but it has been observed recently that children may actually require larger doses (5 to 7.5 mg daily) to achieve therapeutic concentrations and maintain efficacy.[68-70] Clinical studies of OKT3 are reviewed elsewhere.[63,71]

The development of anti-OKT3 antibodies by the recipient may seriously limit the use of OKT3. Initial reports indicated that 67% to 100% of patients treated with OKT3 alone or with concomitant low-dose prednisone and azathioprine developed antimurine antibodies.[72-75] More recent data indicate that antimurine antibodies develop in 18% to 29% of patients treated with OKT3 in combination with triple-drug immunosuppression.[72] The incidence of antibody formation has been reported to vary between heart and kidney recipients,[76] but, more important, the incidence may be related to the overall level of immunosuppression imposed by the concomitant administration of other immunosuppressive drugs and the patient's underlying immune status.[60,74-77] Azathioprine (2 to 2.5 mg/kg per day) or cyclophosphamide (CTX) (400 mg intravenously for three doses) prevented antibody production in 60% of patients.[72,78] The appearance of antimurine antibodies is highly variable and may occur as early as 8 to 10 days after the initiation of therapy, but they may not appear until the third or fourth week after therapy is discontinued.[72,79-81] In addition, the use of antibody titers to predict future efficacy of OKT3 is limited by the variability of different analytical techniques used at various centers. Ortho Biotech is currently conducting a multicenter trial to standardize the technique for measuring antibodies and to determine the optimal interval at which titers should be measured. Until the results of the study are known, the current recommendation is to monitor antibody titers 21 to 28 days after initiation of therapy. Titers of 1 to 1,000 or more suggest significant antibody formation and preclude subsequent administration of OKT3.

Monitoring

Side Effects and Toxicity. Most patients experience a mild to severe flu-like syndrome with the first two or three doses of OKT3. Symptoms include fever, chills, headache, nausea, vomiting, diarrhea, and myalgias. This reaction may be secondary to the clearance and lysis of opsonized T cells by mononuclear phagocytes or due to the activation of T cells and monocytes by OKT3,[82] resulting in the release of cytokines such as IL-2, IL-3, IL-6, interferon (IFN) gamma, and tumor necrosis factor (TNF).[83,84] With subsequent doses, the severity of the reaction is lessened or the syndrome disappears because of the substantial reduction in the number of CD3+ T cells, the amount of cytokines released, and the depletion of cytokine receptors. Less frequent side effects include pulmonary edema in fluid-overloaded patients (more than 3% over dry weight),[82,85] marked hypotension,[86] aseptic meningitis,[87-89] and seizures.[90] An acute decline in glomerular filtration rate, causing a reversible rise in serum creatinine during the first 1 to 3 days of OKT3 therapy, may be the result of cytokine-induced renal toxicity.[78] Conflicting data exist regarding the efficacy of prophylactic agents (antihistamines, antipyretics, steroids) in blocking the cytokine release syndrome.[66,91] Recent experience with investigational MoAbs, anti-TNF, and anti-INF gamma appear promising in their ability to minimize OKT3's first-dose side effects.[92] A protocol using 50 mg of indomethacin before OKT3 and then 25 mg every 8 hours for 48 hours is under investigation and appears to be effective in blocking the first-dose side effects.[93] Pentoxifylline may also prove useful in reducing the OKT3-induced cytokine release syndrome.[94]

Prophylaxis

As with other immunosuppressive agents, a higher incidence of infection and malignancy has been observed after OKT3 therapy. However, this finding is most likely related to the degree and duration of the overall level of immunosuppression rather than to the specific type of agent.[95-98]

Antilymphocyte Globulin and Antithymocyte Globulin

Effects and Uses. The immunosuppressive qualities of heterologous antilymphocyte serum were first described by Woodruff in 1963.[99] Antilymphocyte antibodies were the first form of selective immunosuppression to be used as anti-T-cell therapy. Polyclonal antilymphocyte antibodies have since been used, both alone and in combination with other immunosuppressive agents, to prevent and treat rejection episodes in organ transplantation.[100-108]

Production technique

Antilymphocyte globulin (ALG) and antithymocyte globulin (ATG) are produced by first injecting a series of ALG human spleen cells or ATG thymocytes into various animals (e.g., horse, goat, or rabbit). Antibodies are then isolated from the animal sera.[109,110] Their potency lies primarily in the IgG antibody fraction. Their action is directed not only against T cells but also against B cells and nonlymphoid cells, and they cause marked lymphocytopenia. ALG acts by binding to surface antigens on host T or B lymphocytes, causing (1) opsonization and removal by the reticuloendothelial system or (2) direct, complement-assisted lysing of lymphocytes.

Dosing and Monitoring. The pharmacokinetics of ALGs and ATGs have not been fully elucidated. The plasma half-life of equine IgG averages 6 days (range 1.5 to 12 days). ALG is poorly distributed in lymphoid tissue but binds avidly to bone marrow cells, to circulating lymphocytes, granulocytes, platelets, and visceral tissues (e.g., thymus, tonsil, kidney, breast, liver, lung, intestine, and testes). The plasma concentrations and half-life of IgG vary depending on the patient's ability to catabolize foreign IgG. Approximately 1% of a dose of ATG is excreted in urine as unchanged equine IgG.

ALGs and ATGs are produced for investigational use by various institutions around the world. The only commercially available product, ATGAM, has had very limited availability until just recently. Minnesota ALG (MALG) is administered in doses of 15 to 20 mg/kg per day for 8 to 14 days after transplantation. The dose is diluted in 250 mL of saline and infused through a central line at a rate of 60 mL per hour for 4 hours. The recommended dose for ATGAM is 10 to 15 mg/kg per day for up to 14 days but varies according to institutional protocol and type of transplant. The required dose should be diluted in 250 to 1,000 mL of saline and administered through a central line for 4 to 8 hours. The dose of rabbit ATG varies from 1.5 to 3.0 mg/kg per day and is administered intramuscularly using the Z-track method in two to four divided doses. One milliliter of 0.25% Marcaine (no epinephrine) is added to each syringe. Ultrasonic massage and a heating pad should be applied 30 minutes before and after injection. For all of these agents, efficacy is monitored by measuring the T-cell count. Depression of the circulating T-cell count should be maintained below 5% of the total fraction of circulating lymphocytes or below 50 to 100 cells/mm^3.

Quadruple therapy

Although CsA has become the mainstay of posttransplant immunosuppression, quadruple immunosuppressive therapy has evolved to minimize toxicity of the individual agents. Quadruple therapy using sequential MALG and CsA in combination with azathioprine and prednisone is now widely used in cadaver-donor kidney[111,112] and liver transplantation.[111] Compared with conventional therapy, quadruple immunosuppression significantly reduces early rejection episodes, resulting in enhanced hepatic allograft survival and fewer retransplants. However, initial hospitalization expense is increased, as is the potential for infection and malignancy related to the overimmunosuppression.

In cadaver-donor renal transplant patients, MALG is routinely administered initially after transplant in place of CsA and continued until appropriate renal function is documented.[113] This approach avoids the early use of CsA during the period of recovery from preservation injury, because CsA may enhance the ischemic injury that occurs during graft retrieval and preservation.[113]

Several investigators have compared ALG with OKT3 as a rejection therapy.[114,115] OKT3 has proved to be more effective than ALG for initial rescue therapy, since it is more homogeneous and specific.[114] Because of its heterogeneity, MALG may require an additional course of therapy or longer initial course (14 to 21 days) to achieve results equivalent to OKT3.[114] OKT3 has the advantage of ease of administration, whereas MALG requires infusion by central venous access for at least 4 hours. In contrast, rabbit ATG is administered intramuscularly and causes substantial pain and discomfort necessitating the use of heat and massage.

Side Effects and Toxicity. Antilymphocyte sera are composed of antibodies directed against multiple-surface antigens. This nonspecificity predisposes the patient to significant side effects related to the seras' cross-reactivity with nonlymphocytic blood cells and other human tissues.[116-118] Side effects seen with ALG include fever, chills, erythema, pruritus, leukopenia, thrombocytopenia, arthralgias, myalgias, and (rarely) allergic reactions such as anaphylaxis and serum sickness.

Premedication

Premedication with acetaminophen, antihistamines, and steroids decreases the incidence of adverse reactions. Switching to a different source (e.g., goat or rabbit) may be necessary if the reactions are severe. Like other immunosuppressants, ALG and ATG have been associated with increased incidence of infections and neoplasms, including lymphomas at the site of injection.

Limitations

The major limitations associated with ATG and ALG use relate to their (1) batch-to-batch variability in potency and purity, (2) variable immunosuppressive efficacy among different preparations, (3) lack of commercial availability, (4) contamination with other globulins, resulting in substantial side effects, and (5) derivation from animal sources, incurring the risk of potentially serious allergic reactions.

Methotrexate

Effects and Uses. Methotrexate (MTX) is an antimetabolic folic acid analog that inhibits DNA synthesis in cell division and suppresses both cellular and humoral immunity. MTX prevents dihydrofolic acid from converting to tetrahydrofolic acid by inhibiting the enzyme dihydrofolate reductase. This inhibition ultimately interferes with DNA and protein synthesis. This agent has been employed in autoimmune disease and in preventing GVHD in BMT patients,[119] but it has had limited use in solid-organ transplantation.[120,121]

MTX has been used for BMT in combination with cyclosporine or methylprednisolone and ATG to prevent GVHD. Dosage regimens usually consist of 15 mg/m^2 per day on day 1 after transplant, 10 mg/m^2 per day on days 3, 6, and 11. It is either discontinued at day 11 when used in combination with other agents or administered weekly thereafter for 100 days when used alone. The combination of ATG and methylprednisolone appears more effective than MTX alone in preventing GVHD (21% versus 48%). A comparative study between MTX alone and CsA alone showed no difference in preventing GVHD;[122] however, the combination of CsA and MTX is superior to either agent alone.[119]

Side Effects and Toxicity. MTX is minimally metabolized, and only small amounts are excreted via the bile.[123] Elimination occurs primarily by renal excretion via glomerular filtration, absorption in the proximal tubule (blocked by probenecid), and active tubular secretion in the distal tubule (blocked by salicylates). In patients with compromised renal function, serum concentrations should be monitored to avoid excessive toxicity. The toxicity may depend more on the duration of exposure than on the peak concentration. Because of MTX's action on rapidly proliferating cells—such as in the bone marrow, intestine, and mouth—it produces side effects such as myelosuppression, diarrhea, and mucositis. Methotrexate may increase the incidence of venooclusive disease of the liver, and doses are held in patients with severe mucositis. The administration of methotrexate in patients with third spore fluid (i.e. pulmonary effusion) may be hazardous due to sequestration of the drug in the fluid and slow release into the systemic circulation.

Cyclophosphamide

Effects and Uses. Since its development in 1958,[124] cyclophosphamide (CTX) has proved to be a unique drug, owing to its multifunctional properties. In addition to its anticancer cytotoxicity, CTX may function as both an immunosuppressive and immunostimulating drug.

Classified as an alkylating agent, CTX is metabolically activated in the liver by phosphoamidases to active alkylating metabolites. The main active metabolite is phosphoramide mustard, which inhibits the cross-linking of DNA, leading to cell death.

Low doses

CTX suppresses both humoral and cell-mediated immunity.[125,126] In low doses it is toxic to precursors of suppressor T cells, and it enhances natural killer cell activity and macrophage activation.[127,128]

It has been employed as a conditioning agent as a treatment for rejection in both solid-organ transplantation and BMT patients, and as therapy in chronic GVHD.[129,130] Infrequently, it may be used as a substitute agent in organ transplantation when azathioprine has to be withdrawn because of hepatotoxicity or leukopenia.[131] CTX has been used in transplant recipients with severe, prolonged, and uncontrollable rejection that has failed to respond to standard therapy.[132]

Allopurinol

Dosing and Monitoring. After oral administration, CTX is well absorbed (90% bioavailability), and maximal plasma concentrations are achieved after 1 hour.[122] The volume of distribution is 0.64 L/kg. Most of the drug is metabolized by the liver, and only 20% or less is excreted as unchanged drug.[128] Both the parent drug and its metabolites are eliminated primarily via the kidneys. The half-life of CTX after intravenous administration ranges from 4 to 7 hours; however, CTX or its metabolites or both may be detected in the plasma for up to 72 hours. Allopurinol has been found to prolong the half-life substantially by affecting CTX's metabolism.[128] Renal impairment also prolongs plasma-alkylating activity. Microsomal enzyme-inducing drugs seem to vary only the half-life without modifying the overall toxicity.[128]

WBC count

Doses of CTX up to 3 to 4 mg/kg per day for 4 days followed by a reduction to 1 mg/kg per day have been used to treat graft rejection. The nadir in WBC count usually occurs within 1 to 2 weeks, and the dosage needs to be titrated to maintain the WBC count between 4,000 and 6,000/mm^3.

Side Effects and Toxicity. The toxicity of CTX differs from that of other antineoplastic agents in that significant thrombocytopenia is much less common than leukopenia, but alopecia occurs very frequently. It is believed that the toxic metabolites phosphoramide mustard and acrolein account for the cytotoxic properties of the parent drug. Nausea and vomiting is common and severe when CTX is administered intravenously at high doses. CTX causes no local irritation upon extravasation. CTX commonly causes hemorrhagic cystitis, which can usually be prevented by vigorous intravenous hydration or the use of MESNA. With oral CTX, adequate water intake must be maintained to avoid this complication. Other side effects include syndrome of inappropriate antidiuretic hormone, chronic pulmonary fibrosis, and bone marrow suppression.[122] Acute myocardial necrosis has been observed in patients who received high-dose (more than 100) CTX mg/kg before BMT; most instances of cardiac toxicity occur at total doses of more than 1.55 g/m^2.[133]

Nausea and vomiting

Investigational Agents

Various agents are currently under investigation for their immunosuppressive potential. FK506 and rapamycin (RPM) are two macrolides that appear promising.

FK506. FK506 (Fujisawa), a product of a screening program designed to detect fermentation products, has immunosuppressive ability similar to that of CsA. FK506 has been in phase I and II clinical trials for solid-organ transplantation and autoimmune disorders since February 1989 at the University of Pittsburgh. Multicenter, randomized, prospective clinical trials using FK506 in liver transplantation began in the fall of 1990. Preliminary results appear promising.[134-138]

CsA similarities

FK506 binds to the peptidyl-prolyl cis-trans isomerase receptor and has a mechanism of action similar to that of CsA. Both agents block the secretion of IL-2 and other lymphokines.[139-141] Their pharmacokinetic profiles are also similar. Reported clinical pharmacokinetic parameters include a half-life of 8.7 hours (range 5.5 to 16.6 hours), mean volume of distribution of 1,342 L, and mean clearance of 143 L per hour (range 88 to 269 L per hour). After oral administration FK506 is poorly, erratically, and incompletely absorbed. Unlike CsA, it does not require bile to ensure adequate absorption.[142] After an oral dose of 0.15 mg/kg, peak plasma concentrations of 0.4 to 3.7 ng/mL were achieved. The time to peak varied from 1 to 4 hours. The mean bioavailability is 27%. FK506 is metabolized by the cytochrome P450 enzyme system, as is CsA,[142] which accounts for the similar drug interactions (e.g., ketoconazole, erythromycin, phenytoin) that have been reported.[142-144]

Dose

Therapy is initiated with a parenteral dose of 0.075 to 0.15 mg/kg administered intravenously for 4 hours. When the patient is able to ingest the oral form, a total dosage of 0.3 mg/kg per day is administered in two equally divided doses. Therapy is adjusted based on serum trough levels as measured by ELISA.[145]

FK506 appears to be particularly beneficial in liver transplantation and autoimmune liver disease, in which its hepatotrophic effects allow for the repair and regeneration of damaged liver tissue.[146,147] Other advantages are its steroid-sparing effects as evidenced by the ability of 50% to 60% of patients to be tapered off prednisone and the lesser incidence of side effects (e.g., hypertension, hypercholesterolemia, hirsutism, and gingival hyperplasia).[148] The propensity of FK506 to cause neurotoxicity,[149,150] nephrotoxicity, and diabetes and predispose patients to opportunistic infections is similar to that of CsA.[138,148,151]

Rapamycin. RPM (Wyeth-Ayerst) was discovered in the mid-1970s during a screening program intended to identify novel antifungal agents. However, further development was not pursued at that time. Once the structure of FK506 was elucidated, RPM was found to be structurally similar, and investigations into its use as an antirejection agent were revived. Although its effects are not fully elucidated, RPM may act at multiple stages in the activation process of lymphocytes. It is known to be a more potent agent than FK506 or CsA.[152] Animal trials are ongoing to clarify its dose-response relationship, toxicology profile, and potential for drug interactions.[153,154]

Purine antagonist

RS61443. RS61443 (Syntex) is a purine antagonist that has recently completed phase I and II clinical trials in kidney and heart transplantation. Preliminary data suggest its efficacy to be dose related. A pilot study using RS61443 for intractable rejection in heart, kidney, and liver transplantation is currently under way. Unlike most of these investigational agents, which have had limited use in humans, RS61443 is a synthetic derivative of mycophenolic acid, which has been used to treat psoriasis for more than 10 years.[155] Preliminary studies indicate that RS61443 causes less bone marrow toxicity than azathioprine, another purine antagonist.[156,157]

Deoxyspergualin. Deoxyspergualin (15-DSG) (Bristol-Myers) entered phase I and II clinical trials for kidney transplantation in 1991. This guanidine derivative has been found to exert a powerful immunosuppressive effect in animal models. Since 15-DSG must be given parenterally, its clinical potential lies in the management of rejection. Its mechanism of action has not been completely elucidated, but it may suppress the functions of macrophages and monocytes and may also inhibit clonal amplification of T and B cells. Multicenter trials in Japan have reported a variety of tolerable side effects, including headache, fatigue, facial and perioral numbness, mild leukopenia, thrombocytopenia, and gastrointestinal discomfort.[158-163]

Cyclosporine G. Cyclosporine G (Sandoz) also entered multicenter phase II clinical trials for kidney transplantation in 1991. This compound is structurally identical to CsA except for the position 2 amino acid, where 1-nor-valine is substituted for alpha amino butyric acid. This agent causes less nephrotoxicity in animal models than CsA; however, this finding has not been confirmed in human trials.[164,165]

Thalidomide. Thalidomide was first produced in 1953 and was initially used as a sedative. Its neurologic and teratogenic toxicity was not reported until 1961. Thalidomide has been known for more than 20 years to have immunosuppressive activity. It has remained in clinical use because of its value in Hansen's disease (leprosy). Its value in acute and chronic GVHD was suggested in the mid-1980s, and it has been particularly useful in patients with chronic GVHD.

Thalidomide inhibits neutrophil phagocytosis, chemotaxis, and production of oxygen radicals. It also increases suppressor T-cell activity (CD8+) and inhibits helper T-cell (CD4+) function.

Most patients with chronic GVHD respond to thalidomide, but the results in patients with acute GVHD have been disappointing. Heney et al.[166] reviewed the course of 16 patients with GVHD who were given thalidomide. Five of six patients with chronic GVHD showed a good response. The sole nonresponder dropped out because of severe constipation. Only one of nine patients with acute GVHD had a good response. However, this finding might have been a function of the patients' poor performance status. All had severe GVHD and were severely immunocompromised.

Nonmyelo-suppressive

The nonmyelosuppressive character of thalidomide makes it an interesting investigational agent. Its acute toxicities, which are not severe, include sedation, headache, and constipation. The most important side effect other than its teratogenicity is a polyneuropathy characterized by paresthesias of the hands and feet, usually with pallor and associated coldness. It usually develops over months and may be related to cumulative doses rather than to duration of therapy. There are reports that the neuropathy begins after a total dose of 40 to 50 grams. Some of the symptoms are reversible, but there is evidence that the abnormalities can be long lasting.[166]

Investigational Monoclonals. The introduction of OKT3 has spurred production of new MoAbs, including $T_{10}B_{9}$.1A-3A,[167] 33B3.1,[168] OKT4A,[169] and Anti Tac,[170] among others.[171,172] The major advantage of these agents is that they do not cause the troublesome adverse effects associated with the first few doses of OKT3. Research is being conducted to limit the immunogenicity of murine MoAb therapy. In the future, MoAbs may be chimeric (i.e., human-mouse hybrids) so that the molecule would be a human protein except for the antigen-binding site, which would be collected from either mice or humans.[173] These modifications should decrease the incidence of side effects experienced with murine MoAbs (see Chapter 11).

Xomazyme

MoAbs directed against CD5+ T cells are being used to treat steroid-resistant acute GVHD. Xomazyme, a MoAb directed against CD5+ T cells, is conjugated to a toxin (ricin A chain). Unlike monoclonals against CD3+ cells, Xomazyme destroys its T-cell target. There has been a response rate of about 60% compared with 30% for historical controls who were treated with ATG.[174] Other MoAbs, particularly those effective against various cytokines and perhaps antiendotoxin antibodies, have potential for decreasing the incidence and severity of acute GVHD and organ rejection. Anti-TNF antibody has been used successfully in animal models for acute GVHD. The use of MoAbs directed against CD3+ cells has resulted in about an 80% complete and partial response in patients with steroid-resistant severe acute GVHD. However, most cases of GVHD have recurred when MoAb therapy was stopped.

Investigations are also under way using a variety of fusion proteins that contain exotoxins such as diphtheria and ricin A.[173,175] Although these fusion proteins are not MoAbs, their ability to specifically target cells is similar. Recombinant DNA technology has enabled us to link together two genes that do not occur naturally. Linking together IL-2 and diphtheria toxin genes yields a product that will selectively bind to cells expressing high-affinity IL-2 receptors with subsequent killing of the cell by the endocytosed diphtheria toxin.

Miscellaneous. Other investigational agents undergoing animal trials in the United States or clinical trials in Europe or both include mizoribine[176-178] and succinylacetone.[169,179]

Nonpharmacologic Means of Immunosuppression

A number of nonpharmacologic methods used to prevent and treat graft rejection have been investigated over the years, including local graft irradiation, total lymphoid irradiation, plasmapheresis, and a variety of methods that decrease the severity of rejection by causing lymphoid depletion, such as splenectomy, leukapheresis, and thoracic duct drainage.

Transfusion

Blood transfusions have become the most widely used form of pretransplant immunosuppression. Ample evidence exists that pretransplant blood transfusions improve survival rates of cadaver-donor kidney allografts.[180] In addition, donor-specific transfusions may be obtained from the living related donor. Azathioprine and CsA may be started at the time of pretransplant transfusions to reduce the incidence of sensitization associated with donor-specific transfusions. Possible mechanisms for the transfusion immunosuppressant effect are the generation of suppressor T lymphocytes, anti-idiotype antibodies, and clonal depletion.[180] About half of the total immunosuppressive effect seems to be conferred by one transfusion,[181] and the peak effect occurs with about 14 transfusions.[180] The optimal number of pretransplant transfusions remains debatable.[180]

Splenectomy

Pretransplant splenectomy was found to have a beneficial effect for at least the first 2 years after kidney transplantation with no decrease in patient survival.[182] However, long-term follow-up showed no significant difference in graft survival between splenectomized and nonsplenectomized recipients, and the incidence of death from sepsis was higher among splenectomized recipients.[182] Therefore, routine pretransplant splenectomy is currently not recommended.

Irradiation

In the late 1950s, whole-body irradiation was abandoned and replaced with total lymphoid irradiation, a technique directed at the small fraction of the entire lymphocyte pool that is responsible for the rejection reaction toward a transplanted graft.[183] Targeting irradiation in this manner limits toxicity and allows for reduction in posttransplant immunosuppression.

As a mode of immunosuppression, total lymphoid irradiation has been a major therapeutic advance in the treatment of Hodgkin's disease, in which it was found to produce a selective and prolonged reduction in the number and function of circulating helper T cells and certain subsets of B cells.[184]

The dose used in organ transplantation is considerably lower than that used in Hodgkin's disease. Patients awaiting transplants are treated with a course of total lymphoid irradiation and monitored for suppression of their T cells. Thereafter, patients can receive transplants with markedly reduced immunosuppressive requirements.[185] Recent reports have shown the technique to be a useful adjunct for the intermediate-term control of early or recurrent acute cardiac rejection.[186] It has also been used as "salvage" therapy for cardiac allograft rejection that is unresponsive to conventional therapy.[187]

Heart Transplantation

History

The era of human cardiac transplantation was initiated in 1964 by Dr. James Hardy[188] at the University of Mississippi, using a chimpanzee as the organ donor. In 1967, Dr. Christian Barnard[189] of South Africa performed the first human-to-human cardiac transplant. The initial success of this procedure produced a brief flurry of activity, but the clinical results were disappointing because of the high incidence of complications and low survival rates. By 1978 fewer than 15 cardiac transplantation programs were operating worldwide.

The introduction of CsA in 1978 and the widespread clinical adoption of CsA-based immunosuppressive regimens by 1983 resulted in dramatic improvement in survival and reduction in complications after cardiac transplantation.[190] Other factors, including improvements in organ preservation allowing for distant procurement,[191] introduction of the endomyocardial biopsy for diagnosis of rejection,[192] and advances in the prevention and treatment of opportunistic infections, also contributed to the improved survival rates.[193]

Indications and Candidates

Potential cardiac transplant recipients are patients with end-stage cardiac failure who have New York Heart Association class III or IV symptoms refractory to conventional medical management and no coexisting conditions that might preclude a successful clinical outcome. Life expectancy in heart transplant candidates is generally less than 1 year. Patient selection criteria are listed in Table 9-4.[194]

Etiology

The most common causes of heart failure in potential recipients are idiopathic dilated cardiomyopathy in 50% of patients and ischemic heart disease in 41%. Other causes include congenital, valvular, postpartum, viral, and drug-induced (e.g., ethanol) cardiomyopathies.

Preexisting factors that may increase the risk of complications after transplantation include insulin-dependent diabetes, hyperlipidemia, renal insufficiency, symptomatic cerebrovascular disease, neuropsychiatric disease, and recent myocarditis. Multiorgan and permanent system failure are contraindications for transplantation. Reversible degrees of renal and hepatic dysfunction are not absolute contraindications, however, because they may be seen as sequelae of chronic heart failure.

Table 9-4 Selection and Exclusion Criteria for Heart Transplantation Recipients

Indications
Age, newborn to 60 years
Irremediable cardiac disease, class IV New York Heart Association
Normal function or irreversible dysfunction of liver, kidneys, lungs, or central nervous system
Pulmonary vascular resistance less than 6 to 8 Woods units or pharmacologically irreversible
Contraindications
Active malignancy or infection
Recent pulmonary infarction
Active peptic ulcer disease
Severe peripheral or cerebrovascular disease
Insulin-dependent diabetes mellitus, unless under excellent medical control and without renal and neurological dysfunction

SOURCE: Adapted from Burdine J, Fischel RJ, Bolman RM III. Cardiac transplantation. *Crit Care Clin.* 1990;6[4]:932.

Absolute contraindications to orthotopic cardiac transplantation are (1) the presence of severe, irreversible pulmonary hypertension that may result in right-sided donor failure after transplantation, (2) preformed antibodies against the donor organ, and (3) the presence of other diseases (infection, malignancy) that may limit survival. Patients with elevated pulmonary vascular resistances may be considered candidates for heart-lung or single-lung transplantation.

Transplantation Technique

Surgical procedure

The diseased heart is removed and replaced with a donor heart while the patient is on cardiopulmonary bypass. Once the cross-clamp is removed and rewarming is under way, the heart often enters sinus rhythm spontaneously. The heart is subjected to numerous insults during the transplant process, including cold cardioplegia, surgical trauma, and anoxia. The total ischemic time should be limited to 4 hours to minimize these insults. Lidocaine is used to treat any arrhythmias that may arise after the procedure. Because cardiac output is depressed immediately after transplantation, isoproterenol is titrated to maintain a heart rate of approximately 110 beats per minute for up to 7 days after surgery. A limited number of patients, including those who received amiodarone preoperatively, may require temporary or permanent atrial pacing during the postoperative period.[195-197]

The transplanted human heart is denervated, and patients therefore do not usually experience the anginal pain typically associated with ischemia. Denervation removes the cholinergic influence provided by the autonomic nervous system, resulting in a higher-than-normal resting heart rate. Thus, atropine, carotid sinus pressure, and the Valsalva maneuver have no effect on the donor heart rate.[198] Adrenergic receptors remain intact and respond normally to catecholamines, beta blockers, and glucagon.[199]

Mechanical bridging

In addition to intravenous inotropic support, critically ill heart failure patients may require mechanical "bridging" to transplantation to buy time to find a suitable donor. Various devices have been used to bridge patients, including the intra-aortic balloon pump, the Symbion-7 Total Artificial Heart, the Penn State Heart, and a number of ventricular assist devices.[200,201]

Immunosuppressive Treatment

Pre-op regimens

Current preoperative immunosuppressive regimens consist primarily of azathioprine (2 to 4 mg/kg orally or intravenously) and varying dosages of CsA (0 to 10 mg/kg) administered orally within 4 to 6 hours of surgery. All patients receive 500 mg of methylprednisolone immediately after the cardiopulmonary bypass is discontinued and for the first 36 hours after surgery (125 mg intravenously every 12 hours).

Post-op protocols

Postoperative care of the uncomplicated transplant recipient is similar to that provided for other cardiac surgical patients in that time to extubation, duration of stay in the intensive care unit, and length of total hospitalization are comparable. CsA is either initiated on day 1 or delayed until day 3 or 4 to decrease potential nephrotoxicity in the immediate postoperative period. For that reason, the postoperative dosage of CsA varies from center to center (4 to 12 mg/kg per day); however, it is usually titrated to achieve CsA whole-blood levels as assayed by high-pressure liquid chromatography (HPLC) in the range of 175 to 250 ng/mL or plasma levels by RIA of 180 to 250 ng/mL. Intravenous CsA (0.5 to 4 mg/kg per day) may be used in patients with absorption problems.[202-204] However, controversy exists about what steady-state concentrations are desirable (e.g., 300 to 450 ng/mL). Azathioprine is initiated at 2 mg/kg per day and is adjusted to maintain a peripheral WBC count of 3,500 to 7,000 cells/mm^3. Prednisone is tapered from an initial dose of 1.5 mg/kg per day to 0.2 mg/kg per day by the end of 3 months and then tapered to approximately 0.1 mg/kg per day by 6 to 12 months.[205-208]

Some centers use cytolytic agents—for example, OKT3 5 mg per day, ALG 20 mg/kg per day, ATG 10 to 15 mg/kg per day, or rabbit ATG 1 to 3 mg/kg per day—as induction therapy during the first 7 to 14 postoperative days to minimize the adverse side effects (e.g., CsA nephrotoxicity) observed with the other agents.[209-220] To date, pooled data series show no clear-cut survival improvements with induction therapy, although it appears that a higher percentage of patients may be weaned from prednisone, thereby reducing the incidence of long-term steroid-associated complications.[214,217,221-223] These protocols usually result in the discontinuation of prednisone by 3 to 6 months after transplantation. Controversy exists about whether prophylactic therapy with these cytolytic agents confers any added benefits.[224] In addition, cytolytic therapy is expensive, difficult to administer, may alter the incidence and character of infectious complications, and may result in a higher incidence of malignancy.[95,225]

Postoperative Complications

Acute rejection

Rejection and infection remain the major causes of morbidity and mortality in the postoperative period. Endomyocardial biopsies are performed frequently after transplantation to monitor for acute rejection. Histologic features consistent with rejection include diffuse mononuclear infiltrate with cellular necrosis.[226] Depending on the severity of the rejection, the patient may be asymptomatic or manifest a variety of clinical signs and symptoms (e.g., fever, lethargy, weakness, dyspnea, hypotension, S3 gallop, or arrhythmias). Initial treatment of rejection usually consists of a steroid pulse (1.0 g daily for 3 days) or prednisone taper or both.[227,228] OKT3, ALG, or ATG is used to treat refractory rejection episodes.[229-231]

Steroid pulse

Eighty percent of all infections in heart transplantation recipients occur within the first 3 months after transplantation and after episodes of augmented immunosuppression during rejection episodes.[232] The increased risk lasts for 3 months after treatment and is highest when combinations of high-dose steroids and other agents (e.g., ATG) are used.[233] Since the introduction of CsA and triple drug regimens, the overall incidence and severity of bacterial infection have decreased,[232] while the incidence of viral infections has increased.

Chronic rejection

The major cause of late morbidity and mortality in the cardiac transplant recipient is the development of transplant coronary artery disease (chronic rejection), which is characterized by a diffuse and often rapidly progressive form of occlusive coronary artery disease. Because the transplanted heart is denervated, patients are usually asymptomatic until sufficient myocardial damage has occurred to cause congestive heart failure. This process may be caused by chronic rejection, but cytomegalovirus (CMV) infection has also been identified as a risk factor.[234,235] Because percutaneous transluminal coronary angiography and coronary bypass surgery are not usually options for treating diffuse coronary artery disease, retransplantation remains the only viable option. The prognosis after retransplantation is suboptimal; the 1-year actuarial survival rate is 49%.[236]

Other complications that are troublesome after cardiac transplantation are hypertension, hyperlipidemia, nephrotoxicity, and malignancy.[237]

Lung and Heart-lung Transplantation

History

The first human lung transplant was attempted by Hardy in 1963. For 20 years, experimental lung transplantation was plagued by a variety of complications including respiratory insufficiency caused by denervation of the lung, dehiscence of the bronchial or tracheal anastomosis associated with high-dose steroid therapy, and the difficulty of diagnosing rejection. The first successful heart-lung transplant was performed in 1981 at Stanford,[238] and the first single-lung transplant was performed at Toronto in 1983.[239]

Indications and Candidates

Lung transplantation has been successfully extended to a variety of advanced lung diseases including pulmonary fibrosis, chronic obstructive lung disease, cystic fibrosis, primary pulmonary hypertension, and selected forms of Eisenmenger's syndrome. Current selection criteria for lung transplantation in general and heart-lung, double-lung, and single-lung transplantation in particular are listed in Tables 9-5 through 9-8.[240]

Immunosuppressive Treatment

The lung is one of the largest transplantable organs and has an extensive intrinsic immune apparatus. The lung may be more susceptible to rejection because of its large population of T lymphocytes and macrophages, its constant contact with external antigens, and its extensive vascular bed. Immunosuppressive therapy for lung transplantation has been patterned after earlier experience with other solid organs.

CsA

Preoperative immunosuppression in the lung transplant recipient usually consists of varying dosages of CsA (4 to 8 mg/kg) and azathioprine (2 to 4 mg/kg orally or intravenously). Early postoperative induction regimens are based on the use of ALG (15 mg/kg per day), ATG (10 to 15 mg/kg per day), or OKT3 (5 mg per day) to provide a steroid-sparing effect. These agents are used for a minimum of 7 to 14 days, at which point CsA levels are predictably in the therapeutic range.

Corticosteroids are avoided during the first 1 to 2 weeks in an effort to improve tracheal or bronchial anastamotic healing. Prednisone (1.5 mg/kg

Table 9-5 Medical and Psychosocial Selection Criteria for Lung Transplantation

- Medical criteria
  - Life expectancy <18 months
  - Age <60 years (single-lung), <50 years (double-lung), <50 years (heart-lung)
  - Absence of systemic disease with end-organ damage other than lung
  - No previous major abdominal surgery
  - Right ventricular ejection fraction >25%
  - Non-steroid dependent
  - Adequate nutrition and nonobese
  - Ambulatory
  - No surgical violation of the pleural space (double-lung and heart-lung only)
- Psychosocial criteria
  - No major psychiatric disturbance
  - No drug abuse problem
  - Good motivation
  - Adequate social support
  - Adequate financial resources

SOURCE: Adapted from Morrison DL, Maurer JR, Grossman RF. Preoperative assessment for lung transplantation. *Clin Chest Med.* 1990;2[2]:210.

Table 9-6 Selection Criteria for Heart-lung Transplantation

- Pulmonary vascular disease
  - Primary pulmonary hypertension
  - Eisenmenger's syndrome with congenital heart defect
  - Chronic pulmonary emboli (if thromboendarterectomy is not feasible)
- Pulmonary parenchymal disease (with nonrecoverable cardiac function)
  - Chronic obstructive pulmonary disease
  - Bronchiectasis
  - Cystic fibrosis
  - Others
    - Sarcoidosis
    - Fibrosing alveolitis
    - Eosinophilic granuloma
    - Lymphangioleiomyomatosis
- Pulmonary parenchymal disease with separate cardiac dysfunction

SOURCE: Reprinted from Morrison DL, Maurer JR, Grossman RF. Preoperative assessment for lung transplantation. *Clin Chest Med.* 1990;2[2]:210.

Table 9-7 Selection Criteria for Double-lung Transplantation

End-stage chronic obstructive pulmonary disease
Emphysema
Alpha-1 antitrypsin deficiency
Familial emphysema
Bronchiolitis obliterans
Pulmonary sepsis
Cystic fibrosis
Bronchiectasis
Pulmonary hypertension (with recoverable right ventricular function)
Miscellaneous
Eosinophilic granuloma
Lymphangioleiomyomatosis
Other (individually assessed)

SOURCE: Reprinted from Morrison DL, Maurer JR, Grossman RF. Preoperative assessment for lung transplantation. *Clin Chest Med.* 1990;2[2]:209.

Table 9-8 Selection Criteria for Single-lung Transplantation

End-stage fibrotic lung disease
Idiopathic pulmonary fibrosis
Familial pulmonary fibrosis
Extrinsic allergic alveolitis
Occupational lung disease
Drug- or toxin-induced lung disease
Sarcoidosis
Limited scleroderma
Other
Pulmonary hypertension (with reversible right ventricular function)
Primary pulmonary hypertension
Eisenmenger physiology (selected cases)
Limited scleroderma
Chronic obstructive pulmonary disease

SOURCE: Reprinted from Morrison DL, Maurer JR, Grossman RF. Preoperative assessment for lung transplantation. *Clin Chest Med.* 1990;2[2]:208.

per day) is usually initiated at the end of the second to third week and tapered to a maintenance dose of 0.1 to 0.2 mg/kg per day. Alternatively, prednisone (0.15 to 0.2 mg/kg per day) may be initiated as early as 5 to 7

Post-op protocols

days after surgery unless a major airway complication is apparent. The dose is then increased to 0.5 mg/kg per day by 3 weeks after transplantation and maintained until 3 to 6 months, when the dose is tapered to 0.2 mg/kg per day and slowly modified to an alternate-day schedule (0.2 mg/kg per day every other day).

CsA is initiated after surgery, either orally (6 to 8 mg/kg per day) or intravenously (2 to 4 mg per hour) and adjusted to achieve therapeutic concentrations. CsA concentrations are maintained in the high-therapeutic-to-supratherapeutic range unless renal function declines. The azathioprine dose is adjusted to maintain the WBC count in the range of 3,500 to 6,000/mm^3. Despite aggressive immunosuppressive therapy, rejection episodes requiring bolus administration of 1 g of methylprednisolone daily for 3 days occur frequently.

Postoperative Complications

Lung transplant recipients are predisposed to the same long-term complications as other immunosuppressed patients (e.g., hypertension, hyperlipidemia, obesity, rejection, infection, and malignancy). Differentiating rejection from infection remains a challenging dilemma. There is still no reliable marker for rejection, except for the response to a bolus of steroids, which may be deleterious to anastamotic healing. Transbronchial lung biopsy and simultaneous bronchoalveolar lavage may become useful adjuncts. Because CMV pneumonia can be life threatening in a lung transplant patient, most centers use various prophylactic regimens consisting of immune globulin (e.g., 500 mg/kg on days 0, 1, 2, and 7, and then weekly for 3 months) or CMV hyperimmune globulin (100 to 150 mg/kg weekly to monthly for 8 doses), and ganciclovir (5 mg/kg every 12 hours for 2 weeks or 5 mg/kg every 24 hours while hospitalized, then Monday through Friday for 3 months) in negative recipients of CMV-positive organs.[241-243] The efficacy of one protocol over another has not been confirmed, but randomized trials are under way.

Fluid overload

The lung transplant recipient undergoes considerable intraoperative trauma and is at high risk for early postoperative complications including hemorrhage, pulmonary edema, volume overload, hemodynamic instability, infection, and rejection.[244] Double-lung recipients may develop a hyperdynamic profile with a high cardiac output and a low peripheral vascular resistance. Alpha-adrenergic agents (norepinephrine, phenylephrine) should be used cautiously so that blood flow does not become compromised and interfere with subsequent healing of the tracheal or bronchial anastomosis.[245]

Most lung transplant recipients are cachectic before transplantation because of hypermetabolism and long-standing pulmonary disease. Postoperative nutritional replacement may be complicated by fluid restrictions, hypermetabolism, malabsorption, or a prolonged postoperative ileus (i.e., in patients in whom a laparotomy was performed to mobilize the omentum). Gastric atony or outlet obstruction may also occur if the vagus nerve is severed or damaged during surgical manipulation.[241] Postoperative nutritional support provided by intravenous alimentation or a feeding jejunostomy and oral supplementation is imperative to facilitate weaning from the respirator, promote tissue healing, and prevent infection.

OB

The most devastating complication and threat to long-term survival after lung transplantation is the development of obstructive airway disease as a result of obliterative bronchiolitis (OB). OB is characterized clinically by a relatively rapid and progressive form of obstructive airway disease that is frequently fatal. Early detection through the use of serial measurements of pulmonary function, serial transbronchial lung biopsies, and a trial of augmented immunosuppression may slow the progression of the disease.[246] Therapy for OB has included high-dose steroids, ATG, ALG, and OKT3, none of which has emerged as superior to the others. Trials are under way to evaluate the efficacy of MTX, which has been used for treating recalcitrant cardiac rejection.[120]

Liver Transplantation

History

The initial work that led to the current success with liver transplantation occurred more than 30 years ago. Unlike renal transplantation techniques, the surgical techniques for liver transplantation are relatively complex; early work centered on the technical aspects of the surgery itself. Surgical complications were the cause of death in the few patients who were transplanted in the early 1960s. The technical problems associated with liver transplant surgery were overcome relatively rapidly, at which point it became apparent that other problems such as organ availability, preservation of organs, and graft rejection would be more difficult to solve. One-year patient survival rates throughout the 1960s and nearly all of the 1970s hovered around 20% to 30%. With the availability of CsA at the end of 1979, 1-year actuarial graft survival increased to 70%. With the development of University of Wisconsin solution for organ preservation and CsA for immunosuppression the modern era of liver transplantation had arrived.[247]

Indications and Candidates

Table 9-9 lists the diseases for which liver transplantation is a major treatment modality and reflects the Pittsburgh experience in more than 1,200 adult and pediatric patients who received transplants between 1981 and 1988.[248] Currently there is no upper age limit for patients undergoing liver transplantation. Patients older than 70 years and newborns have undergone transplants successfully.

Table 9-9 Native Liver Disease in 400 Pediatric and 858 Adult Recipients of Liver Transplants at the University of Pittsburgh, 1981–1988

Disease	No. of Cases
Parenchymal	522
Postnecrotic cirrhosis	348
Alcoholic cirrhosis	76
Acute liver failure	54
Budd-Chiari syndrome	18
Congenital hepatic fibrosis	9
Cystic fibrosis	6
Neonatal hepatitis	8
Hepatic trauma	3
Cholestatic	544
Biliary atresia	217
Primary biliary cirrhosis	186
Sclerosing cholangitis	100
Secondary biliary cirrhosis	25
Familial cholestasis	16
Inborn errors of metabolism	114
Tumors	78
Benign	10
Primary malignant	60
Metastatic	8
Total	1258

SOURCE: Reprinted with permission from Starzl TE, Demetris AJ, Van Thiel DV. Liver transplantation. *N Engl J Med.* 1989;321:1014–22, 1092.

Patient selection

Controversy persists regarding which patients should undergo liver transplantation. This controversy results partly from having too few organs for the number of transplant candidates. Transplants for patients with liver carcinoma are very controversial because of the high incidence of nonhepatic tumor involvement and tumor relapse. Less controversial are transplants for patients with the hepatitis B virus or alcoholic liver disease. Recent data indicate that the use of passive immunoprophylaxis with anti-hepatitis B immunoglobulin can decrease 2-year actuarial reinfection rates from the historical 80% to 90% to about 30%.[249]

Hepatitis

The use of liver transplantation for fulminant hepatitis (sudden onset of liver failure) is well established. Common causes include type A, B, and C hepatitis and various forms of toxic hepatitis induced by drug and nondrug chemicals. It is important to recognize when to perform transplants in these patients. Conditions that predict rapid progression to death include grade III and IV hepatic encephalopathy, metabolic acidosis, severe irreversible coagulopathy, sepsis, and cardiovascular compromise. It is also important to confirm that liver dysfunction is irreversible before considering transplantation. Therefore, most patients who are at the point of receiving transplants have some or all of these complications. Despite the severely compromised condition of these patients, an impressive 50% to 80% of patients will survive in the long term after liver transplantation. In comparison, only about 20% are long-term survivors with medical management alone.[250]

Chronic disease

Liver transplantation is also indicated for treating end-stage chronic liver disease. The decision to transplant is often more subtle than in the case of acute liver failure and involves issues of worsening dementia, frequent hospital admissions, and—in children—mental and physical growth retardation. Not all patients have the jaundiced appearance that is so typical. When hepatocellular disease is involved, patients often appear minimally jaundiced, but profound hypoalbuminemia and coagulopathy are always present. In comparison, cholestatic disease (biliary atresia and primary biliary cirrhosis) always presents with jaundice.[250]

One of the major predictors for a successful outcome is the pretransplant performance status of the patient. For example, patients without severe complications before transplant have an 80% 2-year survival rate versus 55% in patients with major complications. The difference between these groups is the high perioperative mortality.[250]

Immunology of the Transplanted Liver

Hyperacute rejection is a result of lymphocytotoxic antibodies directed against lymphocytes in the donor organ. It is not well understood why the liver is relatively resistant to this form of rejection even though it affects heart and kidney transplants. Certain anatomic characteristics of the liver may protect it against immune injury. For example, the dual blood supply of the hepatic artery and portal vein provides protection against ischemia. In addition, much of the vasculature of the liver has endothelium that is different from other vascular beds and that may make the liver relatively resistant to immune complex-mediated injury. A very interesting observation is that lymphocytotoxic antibodies disappear from the circulation shortly after liver transplantation. Consequently, a transplanted liver can actually protect other transplanted solid organs from undergoing hyperacute rejection.

Evidence that the immunology of rejection associated with liver transplantation is different from other solid organs is suggested by the lack of correlation between HLA matching and the incidence of rejection. A number of studies have actually demonstrated an inverse relationship between the degree of HLA matching and graft survival.

Chronic rejection is distinctly different from acute rejection. Chronic rejection develops slowly and is not effectively treated by intensifying immunosuppressive therapy. Chronic rejection frequently presents as obstructive jaundice without other major liver abnormalities.

The role of endotoxemia and TNF in primary nonfunction of the liver is being actively investigated. Endotoxin stimulates the production of various inflammatory cytokines, including TNF and IL-1. These cytokines can cause direct endothelial damage, and their activation of coagulation pathways can lead to vascular congestion and ischemia of the graft. The normal liver serves as a protective organ against endotoxemia, but this ability may be impaired after transplant, exposing the graft to damage from released cytokines.[248]

Immunosuppressive Treatment

CsA

CsA has been the single most important factor accounting for the routine performance of liver transplants. About 10 years ago, only 20% to 30% of patients were alive 1 year after liver transplant, whereas current 1-year survival rates are in the range of 80%. Immunosuppressive agents before the CsA era included total body irradiation, corticosteroids, azathioprine, and ATG. The combination of azathioprine and corticosteroid produced about a 20% 5-year survival versus current CsA and steroid combinations, with which more than 60% of patients are alive at 5 years. Improvements in surgical techniques have also had a modest impact on current survival rates. Quadruple therapy using sequential MALG and CsA in combination with azathioprine and prednisone is now widely used in cadaver-donor kidney[111,112] and liver transplantation.[112]

Azathioprine

Drug combinations currently used to prevent graft rejection in liver transplantation usually include CsA and corticosteroids with or without azathioprine. The addition of azathioprine may allow a reduction in CsA dose to minimize nephrotoxicity. OKT3 can also be used for rejection prophylaxis, although its major role continues to be in treating allograft rejection along with agents such as ATG and corticosteroids.

One method of induction used in adults involves administering 1 g of methylprednisolone at the time of transplant, then later switching to 200 mg per day in four equal doses every 6 hours and tapered by 40 mg per day. The dose is then stabilized at 20 mg per day by the end of the first week. In addition, CsA is used, starting at a dose of 4 to 6 mg/kg per day intravenously; subsequent doses are based on concentrations. Once the patient's digestive tract begins functioning normally, the patient is converted to oral CsA at about 8.75 mg/kg twice daily. When CsA is being instituted, part of the daily dose continues to be given intravenously and slowly tapered until the entire dose is administered orally.[247]

Assays

Because of the high variability of CsA absorption in liver transplant patients, the development of assays that measure concentrations in the blood was very important in the appropriate use of this drug. CsA whole-blood concentrations are usually maintained at higher levels than in BMT patients. The dose is adjusted to maintain trough levels in the range of 800 to 1,200 ng/mL as measured by a polyclonal antibody assay.

Rejection episodes are often treated with high-dose "pulse" steroid therapy (1 g methylprednisolone); the steroids are then cycled in a manner similar to induction after surgery. In patients with whom high-dose steroids are ineffective, a 10- to 14-day course of OKT3 (5 mg per day) or ATG (10 to 20 mg/kg) may be used.

Postoperative Complications

Ischemia

Posttransplant complications that increase the risk of early graft loss (or primary nonfunction) include ischemic injury to the liver and acute rejection. Ischemia is the main cause for graft loss during the early posttransplant period. Ischemia can occur to the organ after the death of the donor or after transplantation in the recipient. The University of Wisconsin solution, which allows the liver to be refrigerated for at least 24 hours, has significantly decreased the incidence of primary nonfunction of the liver.

Although hyperacute rejection of the transplanted kidney and heart is well recognized clinically, it is not so in liver transplantation. However, some of the primary nonfunction seen in liver transplantation is likely a result of hyperacute rejection of the liver.

Kidney Transplantation

History

The first successful kidney transplants were performed between identical twins in 1954[251] and then between nonidentical twins in 1961 using total body irradiation as immunosuppression.[2,3] Dramatic strides have been made in renal transplantation in the past 35 years. One-year graft and patient survival rates in recipients of a kidney from a living related donor (HLA-identical sibling) are 91% and 96%, respectively,[252] whereas in recipients of cadaver-donor kidneys survival rates are 81% and 92%, respectively. In addition to improved survival, the economic ramifications of kidney transplantation have also been recognized. Transplantation is more cost-effective than chronic hemodialysis.[253,254] More important, survival,[255] degree of rehabilitation, and quality of life are far better than with hemodialysis.[256]

Indications and Candidates

On the basis of these findings, most patients presenting with end-stage renal disease should be considered potential transplant recipients. Specific and relative contraindications to renal transplantation are listed in Tables 9-10 and 9-11.[252]

Histocompatibility matching

Contraindications to kidney donation are summarized in Table 9-12. Living related donors are preferred for transplantation because of improved survival rates attributable to histocompatibility matching. An additional benefit of using living donors includes the opportunity to schedule surgery electively, which allows for optimization of the recipient's medical condition and minimization of the allograft preservation time. A kidney donated by a living unrelated donor (e.g., spouse) can also be used in patients for whom no genetically related individual is a suitable donor.[257] Management of living related donors and their postoperative course are described in detail elsewhere.[252,258] Recipients of living related donor kidneys are admitted 2 days before transplantation for final evaluation and dialysis if necessary.

Even though living organ donors are preferred, most transplanted kidneys continue to come from cadaver donors. Cadaver kidneys are tissue typed by six HLA loci (A, B, C, DQ, DP, and DR) and are transported nationwide to be matched with a recipient of identical HLA type. This process evolved from studies indicating that recipients of kidneys from donors with a six-antigen match and recipients of kidneys from HLA-identical siblings are comparable in allograft survival.[259] Lesser

Table 9-10 Specific Contraindications to Renal Transplantation

Potentially reversible renal failure
Immunologic incompatibility
Active infection
Acute myocardial infarction within 3 to 6 months, unstable angina, or cardiac rhythm
Recent cardiovascular accident or frequent transient ischemic attacks
Metastatic or symptomatic cancer or both
Active connective tissue or immunologic disease
Systemic lupus erythematosus
Scleroderma
Wegener's granulomatosis
Amyloidosis
Anti-glomerular basement membrane disease (Goodpasture's)
Hemolytic-uremic syndrome or thrombotic idiopathic purpura
Vasculitis
Inability to anastamose to pelvic vessels
Inability to create ileal or sigmoid loop in absence of functioning bladder
Positive for human immunodeficiency virus
Primary hyperoxalosis
Fabry's disease
Mental incompetence to consent
Active gastrointestinal bleeding

SOURCE: Courtesy of Michael Lazarus, M.D., associate professor of medicine, Harvard Medical School, Brigham and Women's Hospital, Boston.

antigen-matched kidneys are allocated by the United Network for Organ Sharing on the basis of points scored for sensitization against various HLA specificities, length of time waiting, medical urgency, and other factors.[258]

Transplantation Technique

Recipients of cadaver donors are admitted to the hospital approximately 12 to 24 hours before transplantation. Current preservation techniques allow kidney storage for up to 72 hours, but all possible attempts are made to minimize cold storage time to reduce the incidence of delayed graft function.

Preoperative

Preoperative management of the kidney transplant recipient includes insertion of a central venous pressure monitoring line, instillation of antibiotic solution into the bladder via a Foley catheter, and administration

Table 9-11 Relative Contraindications to Renal Transplantation

- Age >65 years
- History of myocardial infarction and coronary artery disease, now stable
- Previous cardiovascular accident, now stable
- Cancer (apparent cure with follow-up of >1 year)
- Psychiatric or emotional disorder sufficient to interfere with treatment
- Hepatic disease (chronic active hepatitis or cirrhosis)
- Pulmonary disease (chronic obstructive pulmonary disease or bronchiectasis)
- Severe bone disease (osteitis fibrosa cystica)
- Aluminum osteomalacia
- Subacute infections (osteomyelitis, diverticulitis, cholecystitis)
- Severe peptic ulcer disease

SOURCE: Courtesy of Michael Lazarus, M.D., associate professor of medicine, Harvard Medical School, Brigham and Women's Hospital, Boston.

Table 9-12 Potential Contraindications to Kidney Donation

- Psychologic
  - Coercion
  - Strong opposition from family or spouse
  - Significant psychiatric disturbance
- Physical
  - Obesity
  - Hypertension
  - Systemic disease
  - Renal disease
  - Diabetes mellitus
  - Cardiac, pulmonary, or hepatic disease
  - Significant atherosclerosis
  - Active infection
  - Smoker
- Radiologic
  - Multiple renal vessels (>2)
  - Unilateral renal disease
  - Multiple cysts

SOURCE: Courtesy of Michael Lazarus, M.D., associate professor of medicine, Harvard Medical School, Brigham and Women's Hospital, Boston.

of immunosuppressive medications and prophylactic antibiotics. Since its inception in the 1950s, the retroperitoneal iliac approach has become the standard technique for kidney transplantation in adults.[2] The transplanted kidney is usually placed in the contralateral iliac fossa of the recipient to keep the ureter and collecting system medial. Vascularization is performed as quickly as possible to minimize ischemic time to the kidney. Before the kidneys are unclamped and revascularized, the patient is fluid resuscitated to maintain a systolic blood pressure of 140 mm Hg and central venous pressure of 10 to 15 mm Hg. Either furosemide (1 mg/kg) or bumetanide (2.5 to 5 mg) is administered with mannitol (0.24 to 1.0 g/kg).[258] When the procedure has been completed, most patients are extubated and transported to an intensive care unit for the first 24 hours. The patient's vital signs and hemodynamic status are monitored closely, and electrolytes and minerals are replaced as needed.

Immunosuppressive Treatment

Prophylactic immunosuppressive regimens for renal transplantation are usually based on the use of triple-drug therapy (i.e., CsA, azathioprine, and prednisone) for cadaver and mismatched living related grafts,[260-262] whereas alternative regimens may be used for living related HLA-identical siblings.[263] Some centers use induction therapy with OKT3 (5 mg per day), ALG (15 to 20 mg/kg), or ATG (15 mg/kg) for 7 days to delay the administration of CsA until renal function is well established.[264-267] Initial doses of CsA—8 to 10 mg/kg per day orally or 1 to 2 mg/kg per day intravenously—are adjusted according to CsA drug concentrations. In living related recipients, CsA may actually be administered 48 hours before transplantation. Azathioprine (4 to 5 mg/kg) is given preoperatively and adjusted postoperatively to keep the WBC count higher than 4,000/mm^3. Prednisone (0.5 to 2 mg/kg per day) is used initially and then tapered to 0.1 to 0.2 mg/kg per day by 12 months.

The treatment of acute rejection episodes is usually initiated with steroid "pulse" therapy (e.g., 500 to 1,000 mg intravenously every day for 3 days) and a prednisone taper, which is effective in treating 60% to 70% of first rejections. If the patient does not respond, ALG (20 mg/kg per day), ATG (15 mg/kg per day), or OKT3 (5 mg per day) for 7 to 10 days can be used. Alternatively, mild rejection in patients who are ambulatory and in whom CsA toxicity is unlikely can be treated with a minipulse of prednisone (100 mg orally each day for 3 days).

Postoperative Complications

Allograft rejection

Although the success rates following renal transplantation have improved in the past 2 decades, allograft rejection continues to be a major problem and is the leading cause of graft loss in renal transplant recipients. Despite the use of multidrug immunosuppressive regimens, most patients experience one or two clinically evident rejection episodes during the first year after transplantation. Renal allograft rejection episodes are of five types (Table 9-13) based on time of onset, clinical criteria, histologic findings, and response to antirejection.

Early postoperative complications in the renal transplant recipient include delayed graft function secondary to mechanical causes (ureteral, arterial, or venous occlusions or thrombosis, renal artery stenosis, or fluid collections) and nonmechanical causes (e.g., hypovolemia and acute tubular necrosis, CsA nephrotoxicity, or rejection).[252] Various laboratory tests have been used to evaluate renal compromise in transplanted kidneys, but most of them are nonspecific, expensive, and impractical for routine bedside monitoring.[268] In a patient with acute oliguric renal failure, an iodine 131 hippuran renogram can identify other causes of graft dysfunction such as renal artery thrombosis, ureteral necrosis with urine leak, and an obstruction along the urinary tract. A renal perfusion scan can be used to determine the adequacy of blood flow to the graft. Ultrasound shows dilation of the pelvicalyceal system if the patient has an obstructive uropathy and reveals perirenal fluid collections that might compress the kidney or the ureter. On the basis of these test findings, an antegrade pyelography may be used to

Table 9-13 Types of Renal Allograft Rejection

Type	Time of Damage	Effector Mechanism	Cause
Hyperacute	Minutes to hours	Ab	Preformed cytotoxic antibodies directed against donor antigens
Accelerated	2 to 5 days	CMI(± Ab)	Previous sensitization to donor
Acute	7 to 21 days	CMI(± Ab)	Development of allogeneic reaction to donor antigens
Chronic	>3 months	CMI(± Ab)	Disturbance of host's or graft's tolerance
Immuno-pathologic	>3 months		New organ damaged by immunopathologic events related to those that necessitated the transplant

Ab = antibody (humoral)-mediated immunity; CMI = cellular-mediated immunity.

delineate the level and nature of obstruction, or a renal arteriogram may be used to confirm a thromboembolic event.[268]

Hyperacute rejection

Hyperacute rejection occurs within minutes to a few hours of renal transplantation. This type of rejection is prevented by ensuring that the patient and donor are ABO and HLA compatible. The clinical findings include acute anuria, hypertension, hyperkalemia, metabolic acidosis, pulmonary edema, and possible disseminated intravascular coagulation. Hyperacute rejection must be distinguished from other causes of anuria such as obstruction of the urinary tract, renal pelvic necrosis, ureteral necrosis with urine leak, ischemic acute tubular necrosis, and severe intravascular volume depletion.[268] Once the diagnosis of hyperacute rejection is confirmed, the graft must be removed immediately.

Accelerated rejection

Accelerated rejection usually occurs before day 6 after transplantation. At first the patient has good renal function but then develops acute oliguric renal failure. This type of rejection occurs in a patient who has previously been sensitized to antigens similar to those in the donor kidney (through blood transfusions, multiple pregnancies, or a previous transplant). Most patients who experience accelerated acute rejection do not respond to antirejection therapy and require nephrectomy, but OKT3 or high-dose steroids are occasionally effective.

Acute cellular rejection

Acute cellular rejection usually presents within 7 to 10 days of transplantation but may be delayed up to the fifth week in patients receiving prophylactic ALG.[269] Clinical manifestations may vary from an asymptomatic mild reduction in renal function to acute oliguric renal failure, hypertension, and pulmonary edema.[268] Other clinical events associated with acute cellular rejection include fever, malaise, anorexia, myalgia, oliguria, weight gain, edema, and congestive heart failure.[268] Clinically, it is difficult to differentiate acute rejection from CsA-induced nephrotoxicity. The differentiation can be made by noting that patients with CsA nephrotoxicity are usually afebrile, demonstrate only mild oliguria, have increased ratios of blood urea nitrogen to creatinine, and possibly elevated CsA levels. A renal biopsy is helpful for differentiating between rejection and CsA nephrotoxicity. Biopsies are usually performed when the initial presentation of oligoanuria occurs 7 to 14 days after transplantation, when renal function deteriorates acutely or gradually without obvious cause, or when the serum creatinine does not return to baseline after treatment of a rejection episode. Histologically, the renal biopsy specimen shows a perivascular mononuclear cell infiltration with acute graft rejection.

Chronic rejection

Chronic rejection can occur months to years after transplantation. It is the predominant cause of graft loss in the late posttransplant period (after 1 year). Chronic rejection is characterized by the classic triad of hypertension, proteinuria, and progressive decline in renal function. Histologically, two types of lesions are observed. The first primarily involves the medium-sized and larger vessels, showing progressive thickening of the vessel walls and occlusion of the lumen. The other histologic pattern mainly affects the glomeruli, which have a lobular appearance on light microscopy.[268] Because there is no effective treatment for chronic rejection other than retransplantation, therapy is based on delaying the progression of chronic renal failure (i.e., controlling hypertension, adopting a low-protein diet, correcting acidosis, and initiating dialysis when the creatinine clearance approaches 15 mL per minute). Lower 1-year graft survival rates of 70% or less have been reported after multiple transplants.[270]

Immunopathologic destruction of the kidney graft can occur any time after 3 months and is related to the immunologic process that damaged the original organ. Immunologic diseases that recur after transplantation include membranoproliferative glomerulonephritis, focal glomerulosclerosis, and lupus nephropathy (see Table 9-10).

Pancreas and Islet Cell Transplantation

History

The first pancreas transplant was performed at the University of Minnesota in 1966.[271] Very poor results were seen between 1966 and 1977, during which time graft and recipient survival rates were only 3% and 39%, respectively. Changes in surgical technique, the introduction of CsA, and improvements in the diagnosis of rejection have led to a progressive improvement in pancreas transplant graft and patient survival rates. ABO-identical blood group and HLA-DR matching have also improved allograft survival after cadaveric pancreas transplantation.[272,273] During the past 5 years, graft function and patient survival rates of 63% and 89%, respectively, have been reported by the International Pancreas Transplant Registry.[273] Functional survival for pancreas grafts (defined as insulin independence and normoglycemia) is more than 74% at 1 year for recipients of simultaneous cadaver-donor kidney transplants.[274]

Indications and Candidates

Pancreas transplantation is indicated for patients who already have or are likely to develop complications of diabetes that are more serious than the adverse effects associated with immunosuppressive therapy.[274] It is also indicated in nonuremic diabetic patients with other complications (e.g., retinopathy, albuminuria, or diabetic nephropathy) and in those who have extreme difficulty with diabetic control (Table 9-14).[275] The intent of pancreas transplantation is to establish an insulin-independent

Diabetes

normoglycemic state in type I (insulin-dependent) diabetic patients and to prevent the onset or halt the progression of secondary complications of diabetes.[276] After successful pancreas transplantation, exogenous insulin can be discontinued and the patient's quality of life improved. Contraindications to pancreas transplantation include coronary artery disease, active infections, and malignancy (see Table 9-14).[275]

Transplantation Technique

Transplantation of the pancreas mandates diverting the pancreatic exocrine secretions into the recipient's intestine or bladder. The latter is preferable

Table 9-14 Indications and Contraindications for Pancreas Transplantation

Indications
Combined kidney-pancreas
Type I diabetes with end-stage renal disease
Pancreas alone
Type I diabetes with a functioning renal transplant or with one or more of the following.*
Preuremic nephropathy (albuminuria with creatine clearance >50 mL per minute)
Progressive retinopathy
Brittle diabetes
Marked Insulin resistance
Severe neuropathic pain
Pancreatectomy for benign disease
Contraindications
Drug abuse
Psychosis
Concurrent malignancy or infection
Ongoing peripheral gangrene
Incapacitating neuropathy (bedridden)
Incapacitating gastropathy (unable to take oral medication)
Severe coronary artery disease or cardiomyopathy

SOURCE: Adapted from Grundfest-Broniatowski S. Pancreas transplantation: state of the art. *Cleve Clin J Med.* 1990;57[6]:566.

*These criteria are not routinely used in all institutions doing pancreas transplantation.

because it allows for monitoring rejection by measuring the decrease in urine amylase activity that precedes deterioration of endocrine function.[277] Postoperative management includes fluid and electrolyte monitoring. An infusion of regular human insulin is used to maintain plasma glucose concentrations at less than 150 mg/dL, because chronic hyperglycemia is detrimental to beta cells. The Foley catheter is removed after 7 days. Plasma glucose is monitored every 4 hours; complete blood cell count, electrolytes, and serum and 24-hour urinary amylase and pH are monitored daily. Patients receive prophylactic antibiotics for the first postoperative week and are maintained on nystatin for 6 months. Uncomplicated pancreas transplant recipients are usually discharged from the hospital during the third postoperative week.[276]

Immunosuppressive Treatment

Increased immuno-suppression

The immunosuppressive management of the pancreas transplant recipient is the same as for recipients of other solid organ allografts, but pancreas recipients require a higher level of immunosuppression. Regimens usually include ALG (20 mg/kg per day) or OKT3 (5 mg per day) for 14 days, CsA targeted to maintain HPLC whole-blood levels at 200 ng/mL, azathioprine (2.5 mg/kg per day) to maintain WBC count at 4,000 cells/mm^3 or better, and prednisone (1 to 2 mg/kg per day tapered to 0.5 mg/kg per day by 1 to 2 months and then tapered to a long-term maintenance dose of 0.2 mg/kg per day or less by 1 year).

Rejection is routinely treated with ALG (20 mg/kg per day) or OKT3 (5 mg per day) for 7 days along with a rapid prednisone taper of 2 mg/kg per day for 2 days, 1.5 mg/kg per day for 2 days, 1.0 mg/kg per day for 2 days, 0.75 mg/kg per day for 2 days, and 0.5 mg/kg per day for 2 days and then back to baseline.[276] Attempts are made to limit the amount of ALG or OKT3 during the first 4 months to 21 doses; if there is a second rejection episode in this interval, high-dose steroids (1.0 g per day for 3 days) are used.

Postoperative Complications

New surgical techniques have lowered the incidence of many postoperative complications. Technical failures (e.g., loss of graft due to thrombosis) occurred in 16% of 1,855 transplants performed between 1986 and 1990. Thrombosis also appears to be somewhat less frequent with whole-organ versus segmental pancreas transplantation. Diversion of exocrine secretions of the pancreas into the bladder instead of the intestine has decreased the incidence of infection and increased survival. The use of newer preservation solutions (e.g., University of Wisconsin or plasma-based solutions) has also decreased the incidence of postoperative pancreatitis and allowed for storage from 24 to 30 hours.

Rejection

Other postoperative complications include rejection and opportunistic infections. Rejection remains the most common cause of graft loss and is more difficult to diagnose than liver, kidney, or heart transplant rejection. Rejection may mimic infection or graft pancreatitis. It may manifest as a greater than 25% decrease in urine amylase activity (to less than 10,000 international units (IU)/L), a drop in serum amylase, hyperglycemia, or deterioration in renal function in combined kidney-pancreas recipients. Percutaneous pancreas biopsy may assist in the diagnosis of rejection[278] but is not performed routinely. Other tests being evaluated as markers of rejection include measurement of C peptide, serum IL-2 receptors, pancreas-specific protein, urinary pH, insulin, trypsin, and pancreatic juice volume. Analysis of pancreatic juice for inflammatory and blast cells also is used, as well as imaging studies such as radionuclide flow scans, angiography, and magnetic resonance.[279-284]

Islet Cell Transplantation

Investigations of islet cell transplantation are under way. Successful long-term transplantation of sufficient numbers of human islets to allow withdrawal of insulin has not yet been achieved, however.[285] This procedure may be an alternative to whole or partial pancreas transplantation as endocrine replacement therapy in type I diabetic patients.[286] It has been proposed that islet cells can be transplanted into the liver, spleen, brain, testes, peritoneal cavity, kidney, muscle beds, and subcutaneous spaces.[287] Limitations to successful islet cell transplantation at this time include the ineffectiveness of current immunosuppressive regimens, the inability to diagnose early graft rejection, and not knowing how much beta cell mass is necessary to restore normal glucose utilization.[287]

Islet-thymic Transplantation

Immunoalteration

A unique, strategic method of transplantation has been experimented with to improve our understanding of the mechanisms involved in the development of immune tolerance. Pancreatic islet cells have been successfully transplanted into the thymus gland of type I diabetic patients. In the thymus, thymocytes mature and are educated to respond to certain foreign antigens. When the islet cells (antigens) are transplanted into this area, the maturing lymphocytes accept foreign tissue as being part of the self.[288]

Theoretically, a piece of heart, kidney, or liver tissue transplanted into the thymus should produce the same immunologic tolerance so that the entire organ can later be transplanted, evading an attack by the immune system.

Immunoisolation

In addition to this "immunoalteration" technique, another promising method called immunoisolation is being investigated. This method involves encapsulating islet cells in a membrane so as to keep them out of reach of the body's immune cells but still allow insulin to diffuse outward.[286,289] It is hoped that this procedure may allow animal islet cells to be transplanted into humans and solve the donor shortage problem.[286]

Small-intestine Transplantation

History

Bowel transplantation was first attempted in 1901 by Carrel and developed successfully in the dog model in 1959 by Lillehei. Despite recent major improvements in surgical techniques and the introduction of new immunosuppressive regimens, the clinical results of small-intestine transplantation (SIT) remain dismal. Less than 25% long-term functional graft survival has been achieved with CsA-based regimens.[290] Greater success could possibly be achieved by simultaneously transplanting other visceral organs such as the liver,[291] or with the use of new immunosuppressive agents (e.g., FK506).[292]

Indications and Candidates

For several decades, transplantation of the small intestine has been proposed as a means of increasing intestinal absorption in patients who have undergone extensive small-bowel resection and become dependent on total parenteral nutrition. The recent renewed interest in SIT has been generated primarily by the success of CsA as an immunosuppressant in solid-organ transplantation.

Indications for SIT include failure of home parenteral nutrition to sustain a patient with short-bowel syndrome (e.g., Crohn's disease, radiation enteritis) and congenital causes of small-bowel failure (e.g., microvillus atrophy).[293]

Immunosuppressive Treatment

IV CsA

Achieving an effective but not excessive level of immunosuppression remains a major challenge after SIT. Because of abnormal absorption in the immediate postoperative period, CsA must be administered intravenously. The use of CsA after SIT in humans has been disappointing.[294-297] Treatment with CsA alone or in combination with OKT3, ALG, azathioprine, prednisone, and graft irradiation has not reliably prevented rejection and GVHD.[291,298]

Combined small-bowel and liver transplantation appears to reduce the risk of intestinal rejection. In addition, donor RBC transfusions and intravenous pretreatment of the donor with methylprednisolone (1 mg/kg), OKT3 (10 mg), and ALG (30 mg/kg) over 6 to 12 hours may be useful to reduce the number of lymphoreticular cells in the graft.[291] Postoperative immunosuppressive regimens have included continuous intravenous CsA (3 mg/kg per 24 hours) and OKT3 (5 mg per day for 10 to 14 days). Maintenance immunosuppression has included intravenous CsA followed by oral CsA starting 4 weeks after transplant, methylprednisolone (0.5 mg/kg per day), gradually tapered to 0.1 mg/kg per day, and azathioprine (0.7 mg/kg per day). Monoclonal RIA for CsA levels have been targeted at 300 to 500 ng/mL for the first 3 months and 200 ng/mL thereafter. Graft monitoring after clinical small-bowel transplantation includes daily biopsies during the early postoperative course and at less frequent intervals thereafter.

FK506

Preliminary reports with FK506 suggest that it may be a more effective agent for SIT than CsA-based regimens.[292,299] Initial intravenous doses of 0.1 mg/kg per day followed by oral doses of 0.3 mg/kg per day in divided doses were successful in preventing rejection. Maintenance doses of FK506 were lower. Prednisolone was given initially and later tapered or discontinued.

Postoperative Complications

GVHD

Two major problems were identified early and continue to plague intestinal transplantation. First is the complex immunologic response that occurs after small-bowel transplantation, which includes both classic cell-mediated graft rejection by the recipient and GVHD, in which graft lymphocytes within lymphoid tissues in the gut wall attack the recipient.[293] GVHD can be reduced or even abolished if the lymphoid tissue in the graft is reduced by irradiation before transplantation or by resection of mesenteric lymph nodes.[293,300] Secondly, the physiologic functions of the graft are severely disturbed by the process of transplantation, and further immunologic damage not only hampers recovery but also destroys the barrier functions vital to recipient survival.[293] If the patient survives the perioperative period, the next major obstacle is surviving infection. Rejection of the small intestine may increase intestinal permeability and result in bacterial translocation and sepsis.[291,301]

Denervation

An inevitable consequence of small-bowel transplantation is graft denervation. This is important because salt and water absorption is under neurologic control by the autonomic nervous system. Motor function is also disturbed by denervation.[293]

Additional challenges for successful small-bowel transplantation include (1) the technical aspects of small-vessel anastomoses, (2) the risks of infection related to complications due to routine colonization of the small intestine with microorganisms, (3) the lack of uniform approach to small intestine preservation, and (4) the lack of a consistent method of identifying rejection.[293,302]

Complications After Solid-organ Transplantation

During the past decade, dramatic increases in graft and patient survival were witnessed following solid-organ transplantation. These increases are due to a variety of factors: identification of better patient selection parameters, improvements in tissue-typing techniques, development of more specific immunosuppressive regimens, improvements in organ preservation, refinement of surgical technique, improvements in the recognition, distinction, and treatment of allograft rejection, and introduction of effective agents for both the prophylaxis and treatment of all types of opportunistic infections. Despite the improved survival rates, the development of complications continues to plague long-term survival after solid-organ transplantation.[237,241,261,262,303-307] The major complications arise from an imbalance in the recipient's overall level of immunosuppression. Preventing rejection increases the risk of infection and malignancy. The ultimate goal of immunosuppressive therapy is to develop tolerance to the graft while leaving intact the host's defenses against microbial pathogens and tumors.

Goal

Acute Rejection

Despite dramatic strides in the advancement of organ transplantation, acute rejection is one of the leading causes of morbidity and mortality. The immune response to an allograft almost invariably results in rejection if not prevented by appropriate treatment. Not only are grafts lost in the early weeks or months after transplantation, but in surviving grafts the lesions may lead to permanent damage and to a gradual deterioration of function months to years later. The accurate diagnosis and effective treatment of allograft rejection remains one of the most critical determinants of both short- and long-term survival. Development of noninvasive means for detecting early rejection is desired.

Chronic Rejection

Although survival rates after transplantation continue to improve (see Table 9-1), long-term survival in all types of organ transplantation is limited by the development of chronic rejection. Regardless of organ type, chronic rejection is the common denominator that eventually causes graft failure with resultant ischemia and fibrosis secondary to progressive effects on the arterial and arteriolar circulation. This progressive process is the main cause of long-term kidney graft failure, graft atherosclerosis of transplanted hearts, bile duct obliteration in liver transplants, and bronchiolitis obliterans in lung grafts. Until this process is better understood and can be controlled, indefinite graft survival will remain unattainable in most cases.[252]

Infections

Risk factors

Various factors increase the risk of acquiring an infection after solid-organ transplantation: diabetes mellitus, hepatitis, splenectomy, persistent uremia, cadaveric allograft transplantation, and repeated treatment of persistent or recurrent rejection.[308,309] In addition, immunosuppressive agents can cause a variety of effects, such as leukopenia, lymphopenia, and the breakdown of the mucosal barriers, thus increasing the risk of infection.

The risk of acquiring an infection is greatest during the first 3 months after transplantation and again after a rejection episode is treated. This risk correlates with the overall level of immunosuppression associated with high-dose steroid therapy and the use of OKT3, ALG, and ATG in addition to triple-drug immunosuppression.[260,310-312]

The potential sources of infection and the range of microorganisms capable of causing invasive infection in immunocompromised patients are immense, encompassing the patient's endogenous microbial flora and organisms present in the environment, ingested with food or water, and conveyed with an organ transplant or blood product.[313] The types of infection most commonly seen in the immunocompromised host range from bacterial to opportunistic fungal, viral, and protozoal infections. Since the introduction of CsA and triple-drug regimens, the incidence and severity of bacterial infections has decreased, while the incidence of viral infections has increased. The clinical presentation of many of these infections is relatively benign in comparison with the severity of the disease process and extent of involvement.

Prevention

Successful treatment of infections in the transplant recipient depends on how quickly the specific diagnosis is made and on the availability of effective therapy. In most situations, preventing an infection is better than attempting to treat it later. Infection prophylaxis consists of perioperative antibiotics and both systemic and local irrigation therapy.[314] Choice of antibiotic varies according to the type of organ transplanted and center preference.

Long-term trimethoprim-sulfamethoxazole (1 double-strength tablet daily for 6 months, 2 double-strength tablets twice daily 3 days per week for 3 months)[315] is used to protect against *Pneumocystis carinii, Toxoplasma, Nocardia, Listeria,* and *Legionella* infection. Trials are also under way to evaluate the use of dapsone (50 mg twice monthly) and inhaled pentamidine therapy for prevention of *Pneumocystis* infection. High-dose acyclovir (up to 1,600 mg per day) adjusted according to renal function has been advocated for prophylaxis against CMV and other herpes infections in renal transplant recipients.[316] Randomized trials are ongoing to evaluate the efficacy of both immune globulin and CMV hyperimmune globulin with and without ganciclovir in the prevention of CMV in other types of solid-organ transplantation.[317] Either nystatin (administered as swish-and-swallow suspension or lozenge) or clotrimazole troches (three times daily for 6 months) are used to prevent fungal colonization and infection.

Specific types of infections and their treatment in the transplant recipient are reviewed elsewhere.[308,309,318-323]

Hypertension

The incidence of hypertension following solid-organ transplantation and BMT has increased dramatically since the routine incorporation of CsA into immunosuppressive regimens.[324-326] Corticosteroids may exacerbate hypertension after transplantation, but the incidence of hypertension with regimens based on the combination of azathioprine and prednisone is one third that of the CsA era. Cyclosporine-associated hypertension (CAH) CAH
occurs in 50% to 100% of transplant recipients; the incidence may be highest in heart transplant recipients.[327,328] Its development is independent of race, sex, age, and prior history of hypertension.[324,329] The onset of CAH is evident within 4 to 6 weeks after transplantation. Heart transplant recipients typically require antihypertensive therapy indefinitely,[208,328] whereas the percentage of renal transplant patients requiring treatment has been reported to decrease over time.[330]

Various mechanisms for CAH have been proposed, including enhanced sympathetic activity,[325] altered renin activity,[331,332] enhanced vasoconstrictor prostaglandins,[333] and hypomagnesemia.[334] Treatment of CAH frequently requires the use of multiple agents. Calcium antagonists may be the most effective.[335] Variable efficacy has been observed with diuretics, vasodilators, and beta blockers. Laboratory data have shown that angiotensin-converting enzyme inhibitors are unable to block the effect;

many centers have reported reasonable efficacy, however. Further research is needed to clarify CsA's role in the development of this form of hypertension and to identify effective treatment strategies.

Hyperlipidemia

Hyperlipidemia and obesity are ongoing problems that occur after transplantation. The major concern is the increased risk associated with these variables for the development of coronary artery disease and the subsequent need for coronary bypass surgery in a transplant recipient. It is not clear whether these factors contribute to the chronic graft atherosclerosis seen in cardiac transplant recipients. Elevation of plasma lipids has been associated with the use of both corticosteroids and CsA. Several studies have demonstrated that prednisone is the primary culprit[336-338] and that prednisone withdrawal lowers cholesterol levels,[339,340] but conflicting reports also exist.[341-344] CsA has also been implicated as the causative factor in the development of hyperlipidemia after transplantation. A possible mechanism may be a direct toxic effect imposed by CsA on the hepatocyte, resulting in impaired cellular clearance of low-density lipoprotein by the liver.[343] Withdrawing CsA after converting to azathioprine-based regimens has resulted in significant decreases in total cholesterol and triglycerides.[345] The finding that withdrawing either CsA or prednisone produces a decline in lipid levels may actually reflect an additive or synergistic hyperlipidemic response produced by this combination of drugs.

Causative agents

Transplant patients are treated for hyperlipidemia like other patients. Before drug therapy is implemented, a low-fat diet in combination with a weight reduction and exercise program should be instituted. If necessary, drug therapy can be added to these basic interventions. The treatment of hyperlipidemia has varied, and there are no controlled, randomized trials evaluating the efficacy of the available agents. Lovastatin appears to be safe and effective provided the daily dose does not exceed 20 mg.[346] Higher doses may be useful, but because CsA inhibits the metabolism of lovastatin, it is desirable to measure the serum concentrations of lovastatin and its metabolites. Higher doses of lovastatin in combination with CsA have resulted in elevated creatinine phosphokinase levels and rhabdomyolysis.[347-349] If necessary, the use of alternate-day steroids or discontinuation of prednisone[339,340] or CsA[345] may be considered, but the efficacy of these methods has not been fully evaluated in all types of organ transplants.

Finally, it is unclear whether improved control of plasma lipids and obesity will prevent chronic graft rejection in the heart transplant recipient and coronary artery disease in other organ recipients to the same magnitude that has been observed in nontransplant patients.

Malignancy

Successful maintenance of allograft function requires continuous therapy with potent immunosuppressive agents that interfere with normal immune surveillance and function. The biologic activity of these agents may engender diminished immune surveillance, direct carcinogenic or mutagenic action, chronic antigenic stimulation, or activation of oncogenic viruses resulting in increased potential for tumor development.[48,350-353] Malignant neoplasms are an unfortunate consequence of chronic immunosuppression and may be an unavoidable complication of modifying the normal immune process. Cancers that occur most frequently in the general population (e.g., carcinomas of the lung, prostate, breast, and colon and invasive carcinomas of the uterine cervix) are not increased among transplant recipients. However, various cancers that are uncommon in the general population are often more prevalent in transplant recipients: lymphomas, squamous cell carcinomas of the lip and skin, Kaposi's sarcoma, other sarcomas, carcinomas of the vulva and perineum, carcinomas of the kidney, and hepatobiliary tumors.[354,355]

Consequential effects

The incidence of lymphoma appears to correlate with the intensity of immunosuppression. The use of more intensive immunosuppression in extrarenal transplant recipients is particularly common and is reflected in the higher incidence of lymphomas seen in cardiac recipients versus renal recipients.[356] The incidence, time to occurrence, and features of the tumors appear to vary with use of various immunosuppressive agents. Azathioprine-based immunosuppressive regimens have been associated with a high incidence of cutaneous malignancies. One possible mechanism to explain this unusually high incidence of skin cancer involves azathioprine's metabolite, nitroimidazole, which causes significant photosensitivity resulting in subsequent skin cancer.[357,358] With the introduction of CsA, one study found the incidence of non-Hodgkin's lymphoma or lymphoproliferative disorder (LPD) increased to 29% versus 11% with regimens based on azathioprine or CTX.[355] Among patients treated with OKT3 and other MoAbs, lymphomas account for 64% of all tumors. These lymphomas frequently develop soon after transplantation (7 months on the average), and 68% occur within the first 4 months.[354,355] In a recent report, LPD developed in 1.3% of patients receiving triple-drug immunosuppression versus 11.4% of patients receiving the MoAb OKT3.[95] This report conflicts with experiences of other centers.[96-98] Similarly, the use of ATG was found to increase the risk of LPD.[359]

Lymphoma correlation

The pathogenesis of this process may be related to T-cell-specific agents (e.g., CsA, OKT3, or ATG) that directly impair T-cell function, causing a reduction in host response to viral infections, particularly Epstein-Barr virus

(EBV) and CMV.[360] EBV has been shown to have infectious as well as oncogenic properties.[361-363] Reduction in immunosuppression intensity and concomitant therapy with acyclovir have resolved some forms of LPD.[356,364]

The clinical presentation of LPD may vary from a flu-like syndrome to multisystem organ failure.[365] Extranodal involvement occurs in 69% of cases in transplant recipients versus 24% to 48% in the general population. Central nervous system involvement occurs more frequently in patients with conventional immunosuppression (39%) versus CsA-based regimens (14%).[352]

The diagnosis of LPD is made by a tissue biopsy. The histologic types of LPD have been described elsewhere.[364] Treatment depends on symptoms, presentation, and extent of involvement. In general, reduction of immunosuppression and concomitant therapy with acyclovir have been associated with resolution and remission of LPD.[356,365] Radiotherapy, chemotherapy, and surgical excision may be necessary in certain situations as palliative therapy, but these steps are rarely curative. Optimal preventive therapy is to avoid overimmunosuppression in transplant recipients. A 5-year mortality rate of 37% has been reported in patients with LPD.[356]

Bone Marrow Transplantation

Candidates

More than 4,000 allogeneic BMTs were performed in 1990.[366] Allogeneic BMT is the preferred treatment for chronic myelogenous leukemia, acute myelogenous leukemia out of first remission, and aplastic anemia. It has a very important but more controversial role in acute myelogenous leukemia in first remission and acute lymphocytic leukemia out of first remission. Allogeneic BMT has been used successfully in multiple myeloma, Hodgkin's and non-Hodgkin's lymphoma, breast cancer, and various inherited disorders. More experimentally, it has been used in sickle cell anemia and acquired immune deficiency syndrome. BMT is likely to be used to treat an increasing number of diseases in the next few years, increasing the demand on acceptable donor sources.

Gene therapy

In a very exciting area of active research, gene therapy is being coupled with allogeneic BMT. The gene that encodes for a missing protein is integrated into donor stem cells by means of a retroviral carrier. The transvected gene is then given to the subject who has been prepared for transplant with conventional preparative regimens. This process has been performed successfully in mice but has been unsuccessful to date in larger animals. However, once this relatively new technology is optimized, gene therapy may be able to cure human disease.[367,368]

Health care rationing

Despite the increasing number of transplants performed each year, many people have focused on the high cost of the procedure in a time when health care rationing has become a reality. A recent study examined the cost-effectiveness of performing BMT in patients with acute nonlymphocytic leukemia. The average expense (over 5 years) was nearly $200,000 for the BMT group versus $140,000 for the conventional treatment group, but the longer survival of the BMT patients resulted in an equivalent cost per year.[369] It may be possible to reduce the costs of BMT with the appropriate use of the colony-stimulating factors (CSFs) by shortening the period of neutropenia and thrombocytopenia. In the future, BMT may become a short-stay procedure.

Even with a reduction in posttransplant complications in allogeneic BMT and a reduction in its expense, general application of this procedure will be limited by the fact that only about 30% to 35% of patients who require an HLA-identical allogeneic BMT have a matched sibling. To increase the pool of acceptable donors, many centers have gone to performing HLA-matched unrelated transplants. Other methods of increasing the pool of donors include using mismatched siblings with and without T-cell depletion, using autologous bone marrow, and doing peripheral stem cell transplants.

Increasing the Donor Pool

Partial match

Many candidates for allogeneic BMT do not have an HLA-identical sibling donor and are denied this potentially curative procedure. The use of partially matched related donors has been extensively investigated by the Seattle group,[370] who have found that two- and three-antigen mismatches have an unacceptably high incidence of graft failure and severe acute GVHD, but one-antigen mismatches do not. The one exception is aplastic anemia, in which one-antigen mismatches have a very high rate of graft rejection. At best, related donors with one-antigen mismatches can increase the donor pool by 10%.[371]

Another method of increasing the number of acceptable donors is to use unrelated HLA-matched transplants. Large registries have cataloged the HLA phenotype of thousands of potential donors, significantly increasing the availability of this type of marrow donor. In unrelated matched transplants, donor and recipient are phenotypically matched at the major histocompatibility complex loci but not necessarily at the minor histocompatibility loci. Because of potential mismatch at the minor loci, patients are more likely to reject the donor marrow and to develop severe GVHD. Methods of decreasing rejection of donor marrow and acute GVHD have centered on optimizing preparative regimens and posttransplant immunosuppressive regimens.[372]

Complete matches between unrelated individuals at HLA-A, -B, and -DR along with a nonreactive mixed lymphocyte reaction are very uncommon. It is estimated that for a registry with 100,000 entries a patient has only a 45% chance of a match. As in the situation with related donors, if one-antigen mismatches could be used, the number of acceptable donors could be increased. The use of one-antigen mismatched unrelated donors is an active area of current research.

CSFs

Autologous BMT has been used in treating various solid tumors and acute leukemia. With solid tumors it is frequently possible to harvest bone marrow that does not contain contaminating cancer cells. In patients with solid tumors that have spread to the bone marrow, stem cells can be collected from the peripheral blood. Peripheral stem cells are harvested by multiple leukopheresis. The difficulty with peripheral stem cell transplants is the relatively low number of stem cells in the peripheral blood versus the bone marrow. It has been observed that treatment with chemotherapy (high-dose CTX) before leukopheresis increases the number of peripheral stem cells obtained per collection. Pretreatment with CTX results in adequate stem cell numbers with fewer phereses and less volume infused into the patient. More recently, the CSFs granulocyte macrophage-colony stimulating factor (GM-CSF), granulocyte colony-stimulating factor (G-CSF), and IL-3 (multi-CSF) have been used to increase the number of stem cells that can be harvested per pheresis.

Preparative Regimens

CTX

Patients receive various combinations of cytotoxic chemotherapy with or without radiation as preparation for BMT. Table 9-15 lists a few of the preparative regimens used in allogeneic BMT. Agents used to prepare patients for allogeneic BMT have differing antitumor and immunosuppressive activities. For example, etoposide and cytarabine are effective antitumor agents; however, CTX is superior to either agent in suppressing immunity and allowing acceptance of donor marrow.[129] The addition of radiation is particularly valuable in treating areas of disease where drugs may penetrate poorly. It also can reduce graft rejection because of its potent immunosuppressive activity. Busulfan is a drug that, added to CTX, results in engraftment rates equivalent to CTX and total body irradiation.[373]

Acute Graft-versus-host Disease

Patients who undergo allogeneic BMT are at risk for acute GVHD. Acute GVHD results from immunocompetent cells in the donor bone marrow recognizing the major or minor histocompatibility antigens of the recipient's tissue as foreign. This recognition sets in motion a cascade of

Table 9-15 Representative Preparative Regimens for Leukemia

Preparative Regimen	Dose and Frequency
Cyclophosphamide	60 mg/kg/day for 2 days
TBI	1,200–1,575 rad over 6–7 days
Cytarabine	3 gm/m^2 for 12 doses
TBI	850–1,200 rad single dose or over 6 days
Cyclophosphamide	60 mg/kg for 2 doses
Busulfan	4 mg/kg/day for 4 days
Etoposide	60 mg/kg for 1 dose
Cyclophosphamide	60 mg/kg for 2 doses
Busulfan	4 mg/kg/day for 4 days

TBI = total body irradiation.

Susceptible tissues

immunologic events leading to the destruction of tissues in the skin, gastrointestinal tract, and liver. Why these three organs are most affected is unclear; however, they do have a higher concentration of surface DR antigens.

Biopsies of the tissues affected by acute GVHD show a high concentration of CD8+ (cytotoxic/suppressor) T cells. The other major subset of T cells, the CD4+ (helper/inducer) cells, are also involved in the acute GVHD reaction. While many of the steps in the development of acute GVHD are not well understood, it is known that CD4+ T cells interact with class II antigens, including DR antigens, thus leading to the release of IL-2 and the clonal expansion of cytotoxic T cells (CD8+). CD8+ cells can recognize differences in class I antigens (HLA-A and HLA-B). Either the CD4+ T-cell subset or the CD8+ subset can initiate the acute GVHD reaction. The interaction between foreign class I and II antigens and T cells occurs at the surface of an antigen-presenting cell, usually a monocyte or macrophage. IL-1 released from the monocytes activates T cells, resulting in release of IL-2 from CD4+ cells and clonal expansion and differentiation. IL-2 can stimulate the expression of its own receptor, leading to an amplification of the IL-2 system.[366] Other cytokines are released during this process, including TNF alpha and interferon (IFN) gamma, which can worsen the graft-versus-host reaction by increasing the expression of HLA-A, HLA-B, and HLA-DR on tissues of the recipient (Figure 9-2).[366]

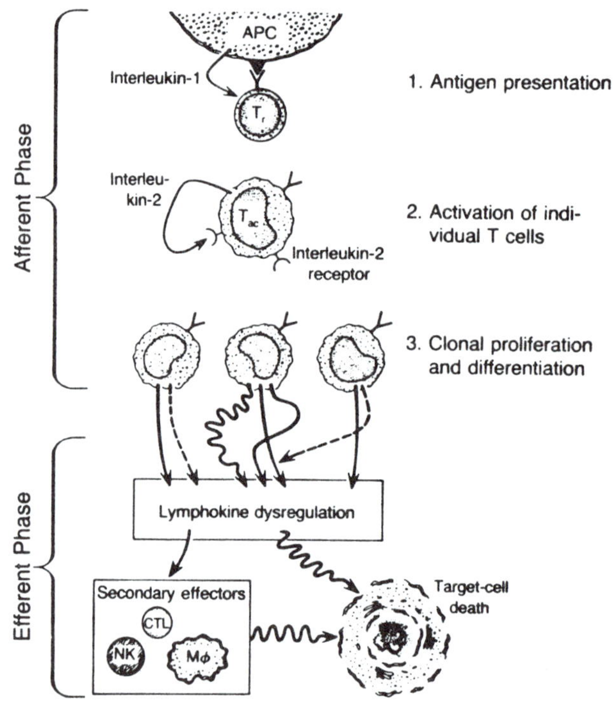

Figure 9-2. The two-phase immunopathophysiologic process of graft-versus-host disease

SOURCE: Reprinted with permission from Ferrara JL, Deeg HJ. Graft-versus-host disease. *N Engl J Med.* 1991;324:670.

GVHD staging

Table 9-16 is a summary of the Seattle scheme for staging the tissues affected by acute GVHD.[374] An overall grade from I (mild) to IV (severe) is assigned based on a composite staging score. As the grade of disease increases, patient survival decreases. Even patients with grade I acute GVHD are at higher risk for chronic GVHD and infection than patients without acute GVHD.

Without immunosuppression nearly all patients would develop severe acute GVHD within the first 10 days after transplant.[375] With appropriate prophylactic immunosuppression the incidence of grade II to grade IV acute GVHD is reduced to about 10% to 50% in HLA-matched sibling transplants. Drugs that have been used in the prophylaxis of acute GVHD include CsA, MTX, ATG, CTX, and corticosteroids. Nearly all BMT centers use combinations of these drugs to prevent acute GVHD. Table 9-17 lists the common combinations of prophylactic immunosuppressive regimens used to prevent acute GVHD.[174]

Table 9-16 Summary of the Seattle Scheme for Staging Acute Graft-versus-host Disease

Stage	Skin	Liver	Gastrointestinal Tract
+	Maculopapular rash <25% body surface	Serum bilirubin 2 to 3 mg/dL	>500 mL diarrhea/day
+ +	Maculopapular rash 25% to 50% body surface	Serum bilirubin 3 to 6 mg/dL	<1,000 mL diarrhea/day
+ ++	Generalized erythroderma	Serum bilirubin 6 to 15 mg/dL	>1,500 mL diarrhea/day
++ ++	Generalized erythroderma with bullous formation and desquamation	Serum bilirubin >15 mg/dL	Severe abdominal pain with or without ileus

SOURCE: Reprinted from Garovoy MR, Melzer JS, Ascher N et al. Clinical transplantation. In: Sittes DR, Teit AI, eds. Basic and clinical immunology. East Norwalk, CT: Appleton and Lange; 1991:761.

Prophylaxis

Aggressive prophylactic immunosuppression is used because, once established, acute GVHD is difficult to treat. The mortality from grades III and IV acute GVHD is very high, ranging from 60% to 100%. Unrelated matched transplants or mismatched related transplants can result in an unacceptably high incidence of severe acute GVHD. Methods to improve the results of non-HLA-matched sibling transplants include T-cell depletion of donor marrow and the use of more aggressive prophylactic immunosuppression.

Graft-versus-leukemia

Since the graft-versus-host reaction is initiated by immunocompetent cells in the infused donor marrow, it is possible to nearly eliminate acute GVHD by depleting the marrow of T cells. Unfortunately, besides initiating acute GVHD, T cells are involved in facilitating marrow engraftment, and T-cell depletion increases the rate of graft rejection. Developing some acute GVHD has an advantage in patients with acute and chronic myelogenous leukemia, in which a graft-versus-leukemia effect has been recognized. Because relapse remains the major source of mortality in leukemia patients, the loss of a graft-versus-leukemia effect increases mortality after BMT. Some centers are investigating the feasibility of selectively depleting T-cell

Table 9-17 Representative Immunosuppressive Regimens for Bone Marrow Transplantation

Prophylactic Regimen		Treatment Regimen
In vitro	In vivo	
None	MTX	Glucocorticoids
	CTX	ATG ± CsA
		MoAb or immunotoxin
None	CsA	Glucocorticoids
	CsA + MTX	Increased CsA dose
	CsA + CTX	ATG
		MoAb or immunotoxin
None	Glucocorticoids	Glucocorticoids, increased dose
	MoAb or immunotoxin	ATG ± CsA
MoAb, rosetting, elutriation	None or with any of the drugs above	Glucocorticoids ATG ± CsA MoAb or immunotoxin

SOURCE: Adapted from Deeg HJ, Henslee-Downey PJ. Management of acute graft-versus-host disease. *Bone Marrow Transplant.* 1990;6:2.

ATG = antithymocyte globulin; CsA = cyclosporine; CTX = cyclophosphamide; MoAb = monoclonal antibody; MTX = methotrexate.

subsets by using anti-CD8 antibody and complement in an attempt to get the advantage of graft-versus-leukemia effect while limiting the severity of acute GVHD.[376]

Steroids

When acute GVHD develops, treatment often requires increasing the doses of drugs being used for prophylaxis and adding other agents. Steroids are always included and are among the most active agents for treating acute GVHD. Comparative studies have shown ATG or CsA to be less effective than steroids for treating acute GVHD.

Chronic Graft-versus-host Disease

Acute GVHD is the major risk factor for developing chronic GVHD, but the pathophysiology of the two diseases is significantly different. The traditional definition of chronic GVHD is disease that continues or begins after day 100. Unlike acute GVHD, chronic GVHD can affect any organ and is similar to various connective tissue diseases. There is a suggestion that chronic GVHD results from autosensitized T cells that are not eliminated from the patient because of abnormal thymus function. Thymic dysfunction occurs in many patients from the conditioning regimen or acute GVHD.[366]

Incidences

Chronic GVHD occurs in about 25% to 50% of patients receiving HLA-identical grafts. Chronic GVHD can be graded as either limited (localized skin involvement or liver abnormalities or both) or extensive (many organs affected). In the majority of patients with chronic GVHD the disease is extensive and, without treatment, would result in death. The major source of mortality in patients with chronic GVHD is infection resulting from severe immunosuppression. Chronic GVHD produces severe lymphoid and splenic atrophy. The splenic atrophy is one of the reasons why there is a relatively high incidence of pneumococcal infections in patients with chronic GVHD. Chronic GVHD treatment usually includes corticosteroids with or without CsA, but may also include azathioprine. Thalidomide is being used investigationally for cutaneous chronic GVHD.[377]

Syngeneic and Autologous Graft-versus-host Disease

Animals that receive marrow from an identical twin or self after a course of radiation and CsA may develop acute GVHD. This type of GVHD is thought to result from interaction of one's own T cells with class II antigens. It can be induced in patients who have been prepared with high-dose chemoradiation and given a short course of CsA. It is probably due to autoreactive T cell release from a damaged thymus. These autoreactive cells, in response to a deficiency of immunoregulatory cells caused by chemoradiation, can produce syngeneic GVHD. The disease can be grade II to III in severity, but it is usually easily treated with corticosteroids. The initial induction of syngeneic GVHD is currently being performed in a few centers in an attempt to obtain a potential benefit on relapse rates as a result of the graft-versus-leukemia effect.[366,378]

Infectious Complications

Post-BMT infectious complications result from granulocytopenia and lymphopenia. Recovery from granulocytopenia usually occurs within the first month of transplant, whereas abnormalities in lymphocyte number and function last for months after transplant.

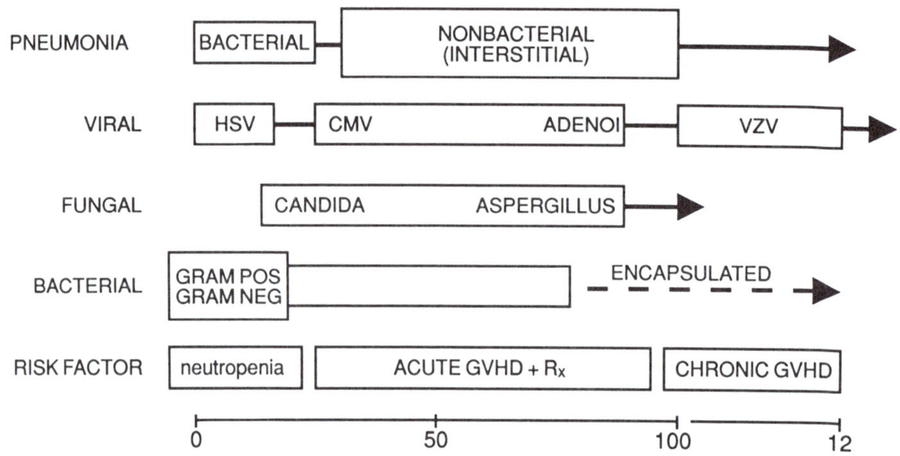

Figure 9-3. Predisposing risk factors and common infections by time after marrow transplant

SOURCE: Reprinted with permission from Meyers JD. Infections in marrow recipients. In: Mandell GL, et al., eds. Principles and practice of infectious diseases. New York: Wiley; 1984:28.

Risk periods

There are three identifiable risk periods for infectious complications.[379] The first month is characterized by profound leukopenia, and patients are predisposed to bacterial and fungal infections. This risk is lowered as granulocytes begin to increase; empiric antibacterials and antifungals can usually be stopped when granulocytes reach 500/mm^3. The second period of risk is the time from granulocyte engraftment to about day 100. The risk of infection during this stage results from the immaturity of the lymphocyte arm of the immune response. The major infection during this period is cytomegalovirus (CMV). The third phase, occurring after day 100, is a result of continued T-cell dysfunction—in particular an abnormal CD4-to-CD8 ratio. Patients are at high risk of infection from varicella-zoster virus. Because of low immunoglobulin concentrations, infections from encapsulated organisms, particularly *Pneumococcus,* become a problem. Figure 9-3 depicts the relationship between time since transplant and risk of infection.

Antibacterial agents

Phase I. Shortly after transplant, patients' granulocytes drop below 500/mm^3, and as soon as fever develops, empiric antibacterial agents are begun. There is substantial variation in the agents used, but they often include drugs (e.g., vancomycin) effective against Gram-positive bacteria and Gram-negative bacteria. Many centers use single-agent empiric antibiotics, which usually consist of an antipseudomonal beta-lactam drug (e.g., ceftazidime), but a point of concern is the reported mortality from Gram-positive infections in BMT patients. There have been sporadic reports of fatal infections from *Streptococcus viridians* with death occurring within hours of the first positive blood culture. While coagulase-negative (i.e., *S. epidermidis*) and -positive (*S. aureus*) staphylococci are the most common bacterial infections after marrow transplantation and cause significant morbidity, they seldom result in death.

Antifungal drugs

Neutropenic patients who continue to be febrile while on appropriate antibacterials are begun on empiric antifungal drugs. In the early 1960s, Bodey et al.[380] demonstrated that fungal infections were often found only at autopsy and that patients who were febrile in the face of appropriate antibacterial therapy were likely to have fungal infections. They found that when the period of severe neutropenia extended beyond 3 weeks, the risk of developing a bacterial or fungal infection increased to nearly 100% (Figure 9-4).[380] This relationship between the length of neutropenia and serious infection is one of the reasons why the general availability of the CSFs was eagerly awaited.

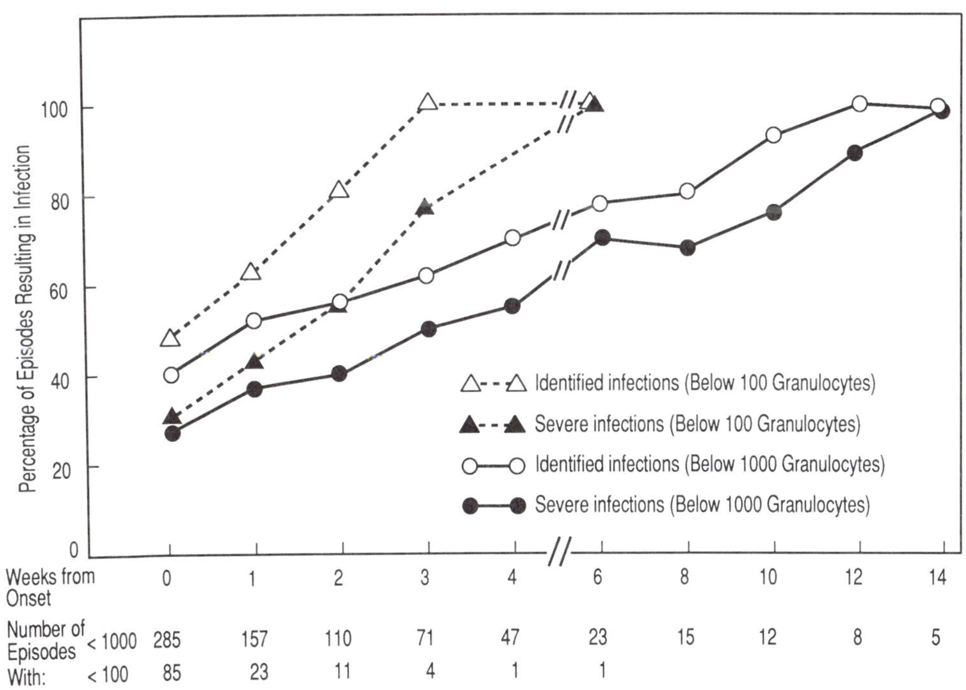

Figure 9-4. Relationship between length of neutropenia and serious infection

SOURCE: Reprinted with permission from Body GP, Buckley M, Sathe YS et al. Quantitative relationship between circulating leukocytes and infection in patients with acute leukemia. *Ann Intern Med.* 1966;64:334.

Although granulocytopenia is the major risk factor for infection during the early posttransplant period, severe mucositis from preparative regimen toxicity also disrupts a major barrier to infection. The disruption of the barrier function of the oral mucosa (mucositis) can lead to systemic fungal and bacterial infections and is a major risk factor for the reactivation of herpes simplex virus (HSV) infections. The development of oral HSV infection can cause substantial morbidity and prolong hospitalization. Uncommonly, HSV infections can evolve into esophagitis and, more rarely, pneumonia. Because the majority of patients undergoing transplantation are HSV positive, most receive prophylactic acyclovir.

Acyclovir

The use of appropriate empiric antibacterials and antifungals along with the use of prophylactic acyclovir substantially reduces the risk of early infection. The source of the infections is usually endogenous flora. HSV infections nearly always result from virus reactivation. The source of bacterial infections is usually the patient's own skin or gastrointestinal tract. Similar to the relationship between mucositis and the risk of HSV infections, the disruption of the lower gastrointestinal tract by preparative regimen toxicity predisposes patients to Gram-negative bacteremia and fungemia. Many of the drugs used in the preparative regimens (e.g., thiotepa, busulfan, and ARA-C) can disrupt skin integrity, increasing the likelihood of Gram-positive infections. The major risk factor for Gram-positive infections is the use of central venous catheters. It is very common for Gram-positive organisms on the skin to produce tunnel infections and line infections.

Catheter risk

In an attempt to reduce exposure to exogenous and endogenous flora, some centers use laminar airflow isolation coupled with gut and skin decontamination. This method has been shown to decrease the incidence of bacterial infections but has not substantially reduced fungal infections. There is a single report that this method reduces the incidence and severity of acute GVHD in patients with aplastic anemia.[381] While this observation has not been confirmed by other studies, it may be consistent with a growing body of evidence that TNF alpha is an important mediator of acute GVHD. Reducing lipopolysaccharide (LPS) in the gastrointestinal tract (from cell walls of Gram-negative bacteria) by using nonabsorbable antibiotics and laminar airflow isolation may decrease release of TNF from LPS-stimulated tissue macrophages and thus decrease the incidence of acute GVHD.[382] The role of cytokines in the development of posttransplant complications is a very active area of research.

CSFs

The CSFs have their major effect during the early posttransplant period. Three CSFs are currently available commercially: erythropoietin, G-CSF, and GM-CSF (see Chapter 10). In brief, G-CSF obtained a wide labeling indication and is being used in BMT. It has been used at varying doses (2 to 64 μg/kg per day) for 2 to 3 weeks, starting the day of bone marrow infusion. Studies report a reduction in septic episodes, days of fever, and number of days to achieve 500 granulocytes. GM-CSF has a more restricted Food and Drug Administration-approved indication in accelerating engraftment after autologous BMT. Results with GM-CSF and G-CSF in the BMT setting are very similar. However, a few studies have reported more rapid platelet recovery in the GM-CSF-treated patients, which has not been reported with G-CSF. Both CSFs have been used in allogeneic BMT and have been reported to shorten the time to engraftment by approximately 5 to 7 days.[383] The CSFs have demonstrated a beneficial effect in decreasing the severity of mucositis. The concern in using the CSFs in allogeneic BMT is the potential for increasing acute GVHD or stimulating a malignant clone. To date, there has been no increased incidence of either complication. These concerns will have to be evaluated in subsequent studies, and the CSFs should be used under protocol in the setting of allogeneic BMT.[384]

Pentoxifylline

The methylxanthine derivative pentoxifylline is being used in BMT patients to prevent the development of amphotericin- and CsA-induced nephrotoxicity.[15] In addition, pentoxifylline (by virtue of its ability to modulate TNF) may decrease the incidence of acute GVHD. Like the CSFs, pentoxifylline may also enhance engraftment. Its potential role in enhancing engraftment is inferred from animal studies in which anti-TNF antibody has been found to speed hematopoietic recovery after intensive treatment.[382]

TNF alpha

It has been demonstrated that macrophages in various tissues, including the lung and liver, continue to secrete cytokines after BMT. Two of these cytokines, IFN gamma and TNF alpha, can increase the expression of HLA class I and class II proteins on the surface of endothelial cells. This increased expression of major histocompatibility complex proteins on cell surfaces may increase the incidence and severity of acute GVHD. Anti-TNF antibodies have been reported to prevent and reverse acute GVHD, suggesting an important role for the cytokines in the pathophysiology of acute GVHD.[382] The modulation of the TNF alpha may account for the decreased acute GVHD reported in a recent article investigating the effect of pentoxifylline on amphotericin and CsA nephrotoxicity.[15] However, because patients treated with pentoxifylline were able to receive higher doses of CsA, this effect was difficult to assess.

The role of pentoxifylline in decreasing the period of neutropenia after engraftment remains very experimental. In vitro data show that TNF alpha inhibits colony-forming unit granulocyte-monocyte formation. Neutralizing TNF alpha may block this effect. A large randomized study is currently under way that may be able to answer some of the questions regarding the ability of pentoxifylline to prevent cyclosporine and amphotericin nephrotoxicity, prevent acute GVHD, and shorten the period of neutropenia.

CMV disease

Phase II. From the time of engraftment to about day 100, patients are at risk for CMV disease. CMV pneumonia is the third leading cause of overall mortality in allogeneic BMT behind disease relapse and acute GVHD, and it is the leading cause of infectious mortality. CMV pneumonia, although relatively common in allogeneic BMT, is exceedingly uncommon in autologous and syngeneic BMT. Part of the reason may be the increased incidence of CMV infection in patients who develop acute GVHD. In the BMT population, CMV can usually be acquired from one of three sources: reactivation of latent virus, infusion of CMV-positive bone marrow, or infusion of CMV-positive blood products.[385]

Acyclovir

Various methods have been used to prevent and treat CMV infection. High-dose acyclovir has been used in patients who present at transplant with latent CMV, as determined by a positive antibody titre against the virus (seropositive). Similarly, in patients who receive CMV-positive marrow, high-dose acyclovir can be used to reduce risk of CMV pneumonia. High-dose acyclovir has been reported to decrease the incidence of CMV pneumonia by about 40%.[386] Recently, ganciclovir plus biweekly immunoglobulin has been shown to be highly successful in decreasing the incidence of CMV infection.[387] In this study, prophylactic ganciclovir was begun in patients who had a positive CMV rapid antigen test on bronchoalveolar lavage fluid on day 35 after transplant. The results showed a reduction in CMV pneumonia from around 70% to 25%. Since the median day of onset for CMV infection is about day 60, this study design may be more reasonable than starting prophylaxis before transplant and continuing until engraftment. Using ganciclovir prophylaxis before engraftment is not ideal because marrow suppression is associated with the drug. The only drawback to the routine use of this combination in BMT patients is the lack of an oral form of ganciclovir, which requires that daily intravenous infusions be administered on an outpatient basis.

Ganciclovir

Ig

The results of using either prophylactic immunoglobulin or CMV hyperimmunoglobulin alone against CMV have been mixed. Most of the studies show a significant effect on the incidence of CMV infection, but fewer have demonstrated a significant reduction in CMV interstitial pneumonia. Bowden et al.[388] demonstrated that, while CMV hyperimmune globulin was not successful in reducing the incidence of CMV pneumonitis in seronegative patients, screening blood products and giving patients who received a seronegative graft only CMV-negative blood eliminated the risk of CMV pneumonitis.

CMV disease develops in about 20% of BMT patients and can cause hepatitis, pneumonitis, gastroenteritis, and retinitis. The course of the disease depends on whether the patient also has acute GVHD and on the immunosuppressive agents the patient is receiving. The most devastating form of CMV disease is interstitial pneumonitis, which historically has had a 90% fatality rate. However, recent use of the combination of ganciclovir and immunoglobulin has considerably improved the outcome of patients with CMV pneumonia.

The pathophysiology of CMV is poorly understood, but there is significant indirect evidence to suggest that, although the virus is responsible for the initial disease pathology, a secondary autoimmune response causes much of the progressive damage associated with CMV disease. Steroids have not been helpful in CMV disease, but dual pathology is suggested by the fact that immunoglobulin preparations that are relatively low in CMV titres when coupled with ganciclovir produce responses significantly greater than are seen with either agent alone. The association of CMV with acute GVHD and vascular rejection in solid-organ transplants also suggests that CMV affects immune responses.

Steroids

Phase III. This phase can last for 1 to 2 years and is characterized by abnormal T- and B-cell function. During this period, lymphocytes are poorly responsive to antigenic stimulation, and immunoglobulin concentrations are lower than normal. The poor immunoglobulin response leads to infections from encapsulated bacteria, particularly *Pneumococcus.* The T-cell dysfunction predisposes patients to viral infections, particularly varicella-zoster virus (VZV).[389] Patients are often given oral prophylactic antibiotics, such as twice-weekly trimethoprim and sulfamethoxazole or daily penicillin VK, to prevent infections from encapsulated bacteria. Preventive therapy for VZV infections is not routinely given, but some centers are investigating the use of outpatient oral acyclovir to prevent HSV and VZV infections. However, some clinicians believe that, once the period of profound immunosuppression is over, it is important for patients to reconstitute their immunity against these latent viruses and that routine prophylaxis should not be given. Treatment of VZV is often initiated at the first sign of vesicals in a dermatome distribution. High doses of acyclovir every 8 hours (500 mg/m^2) are effective in decreasing time to resolution and stopping systemic spread of the disease.

Venoocclusive Disease of the Liver

The pathology of venoocclusive disease (VOD) is characterized by a concentric, nonthrombotic occlusion of the small intrahepatic veins. It is uncommon to use liver biopsy to diagnose VOD because of high false negatives and potential complications in the neutropenic and thrombocytopenic patient. Therefore, the diagnosis of VOD is primarily a clinical one and is characterized by right upper quadrant pain, unexplained weight gain, and elevated liver function tests usually occurring within the first 2 weeks after transplant. The cause of VOD is the use of high-dose chemotherapy with or without total body irradiation.

Support therapy

Treatment of VOD has been largely supportive. Diuretics are used to mobilize edema; commonly used agents include spironolactone and careful use of furosemide. The use of albumin in patients with normal albumin is not helpful. The use of nephrotoxic drugs including CsA, amphotericin, and aminoglycosides should be minimized to avoid hepatorenal syndrome. The majority of patients survive VOD and their liver function usually normalizes over weeks to months, but mortality has ranged between 7% and 50%.[390]

Idiopathic Interstitial Pneumonia

The pathophysiology and treatment of CMV pneumonia have already been discussed. Other forms of interstitial pneumonitis can occur, usually as a result of the high-dose chemotherapy and radiation used to prepare patients for transplant. This so-called idiopathic pneumonitis occurs in about 10% of both allogeneic and syngeneic transplant patients. It has also been described in autologous transplant patients. Mortality is about 50% to 60% in idiopathic interstitial pneumonitis.

Risk factors

Patients receiving total body irradiation and CTX as their preparative regimen are at higher risk for idiopathic pneumonitis than patients receiving only CTX. Older patients also are at higher risk for idiopathic pneumonitis. A specific type of idiopathic pneumonia called diffuse alveolar hemorrhage has been described.[391] The pneumonitis is preceded by various systemic effects including elevations in serum creatinine and platelet consumption. It is characterized by blood return on bronchoaveolar lavage and occurs at about the time neutrophils begin to be seen in the peripheral blood.

Summary

Many new drugs, the foremost of which is cyclosporine (CsA), have improved the success rate of solid organ transplants. Other immunosuppressive agents include azathioprine, corticosteroids, OKT3, ALG, ATG, methotrexate, and cyclophosphamide. Investigational agents include FK506, rapamycin, RS61443, deoxyspergualin, cyclosporine G, thalidomide, and several MoAbs.

The number of successful heart, lung, liver, kidney, pancreas, and islet cell transplants has increased during the past 10 years as improvements have been made in the effectiveness of immunomodulating agents, surgical techniques, organ donor programs, and preservation fluids for organ transportation. CsA and azathioprine are often used preoperatively to prophylactically suppress the immune system. CsA is usually used postoperatively as well in combination with OKT3, ALG, or ATG.

Postoperative complications of solid organ transplants can include acute or chronic rejection, infections, hypertension, hyperlipidemia, or malignancies. Acute rejection is frequently treated with steroids with or without prednisone. Chronic rejection may require retransplantation.

There are three types of bone marrow transplants—allogeneic, autologous, and syngeneic. The most common type of allogeneic transplant is between HLA-identical siblings. Like kidney transplants between unrelated persons, unrelated allogeneic transplants are coordinated through donor registries. Cyclophosphamide and radiation may be used to prepare a patient for allogeneic BMT to decrease the incidence of graft rejection. Immunosuppressive regimens are aggressive to prevent severe acute GVHD since it is difficult to treat and often fatal.

References

1. Carrel A, Guthrie CC. The transplantation of veins and organs. *Am J Med.* 1905;10:1101-2.
2. Murray JE, Merrill JP, Dammin GJ et al. Studies on transplantation immunity after total body irradiation: clinical and experimental investigations. *Surgery.* 1960;48:272-84.
3. Murray JE, Harrison JH. Surgical management of fifty patients with kidney transplants including eighteen pairs of twins. *Am J Surgery.* 1963;105:205-18.
4. Schwartz R, Dameschek W. Drug-induced immunological tolerance. *Nature.* 1959;183:1682.
5. Hitchings GH, Elion BG, Falco EA et al. Antagonists of nucleic acid derivatives. I. The *Lactobacillus casei* model. *J Bio Chem.* 1950;183:1.
6. Starzl TE, Marchioro TL, Waddell WR. The reversal of rejection in human renal homografts with subsequent development of homograft tolerance. *Surg Gynecol Obstet.* 1963;117:385-95.
7. Kohler G, Milstein C. Continuous cultures of fused cells secreting antibody of predefined specificity. *Nature.* 1975;256:495-7.
8. Thomas ED, Storb R, Clift RA et al. Bone marrow transplantation. *N Engl J Med.* 1975;292:832-43,895-902.
9. Venkataramanan R, Habucky K, Burckart GJ et al. Clinical pharmacokinetics in organ transplant patients. *Clin Pharmacokin.* 1989;116(3):134-61.
10. Yee GC, McGuire TR, Gmur DJ et al. Blood cyclosporine pharmacokinetics in patients undergoing marrow transplantation. *Transplantation.* 1988;46:399-402.
11. Lake KD. Cyclosporine drug interactions: a review. *Cardiac Surgery: State of the Art Reviews.* 1988;2(4):617-30.

12. Lake KD. Update and management of CsA drug interactions. *Pharmacotherapy.* 1991;11(5):110S–118S.
13. Yee GC, McGuire TR. Pharmacokinetic interactions with cyclosporine. Parts I and II. *Clin Pharmacokin.* 1990;19:319–32, 400–15.
14. Yee GC, Self SG, McGuire TR et al. Serum cyclosporine concentrations and risk of acute GVHD after allogeneic marrow transplantation. *N Engl J Med.* 1988;319:65–70.
15. Bianco JA, Almgren J, Kern DC et al. Evidence that oral pentoxifylline reverses acute renal dysfunction in bone marrow transplant recipients receiving amphotericin B and cyclosporine. *Transplantation.* 1991;51:925–27.
16. Dawidson I, Rooth P, Fry WR et al. Prevention of acute cyclosporine-induced renal blood flow inhibition and improved immunosuppression with verapamil. *Transplantation.* 1989;48(4):575–80.
17. Morales JM, Andres A, Alvarez C et al. Calcium channel blockers and early cyclosporine nephrotoxicity after renal transplantation: a prospective randomized study. *Transplant Proc.* 1990;22(4):1733–5.
18. Chan GL, Canafax DM, Johnson CA. The therapeutic use of azathioprine in renal transplantation. *Pharmacotherapy.* 1987;7(5):165–77.
19. Van Scoik KG, Johnson CA, Porter WR. The pharmacology and metabolism of the thiopurine drugs 6-mercaptopurine and azathioprine. *Drug Metab Rev.* 1985;16(1 & 2):157–74.
20. Odlind B, Grefberg N, Hartvig P et al. Pharmacokinetics of azathioprine and 6-mercaptopurine: methodological aspects and preliminary results in uremic patients. *Scand J Urol and Nephrol.* 1981;64(suppl):213–9.
21. Odlind B, Hartvig P, Lindstrom B et al. Serum azathioprine and 6-mercaptopurine levels and immunosuppression activity after azathioprine in uremic patients. *Int J Immunopharmacol.* 1986;8:1–11.
22. Lin SN, Jessup K, Floyd M et al. Quantitation of plasma azathioprine and 6-mercaptopurine levels in renal transplant patients. *Transplantation.* 1980;29:290–4.
23. Maddocks JL. Clinical pharmacological observations on azathioprine in kidney transplant patients. *Clinical Science and Molecular Medicine.* 1978;55:20P. Abstract.
24. Chan GL, Erdmann GR, Gruber SA et al. Pharmacokinetics of 6-thiouric acid and 6-mercaptopurine in renal allograft recipients after oral administration of azathioprine. *Eur J Clin Pharmacol.* 1989:36(3):265–71.
25. Chan GL, Gruber SA, Skjei KL et al. Principles of immunosuppression. *Crit Care Clin.* 1990;6(4):841–92.

26. Ding TL, Benet LZ. Determination of 6-mercaptopurine and azathioprine in plasma by high-performance liquid chromatography. *J Chromatogr.* 1979;163:281–8.
27. Ding TL, Gamberatoglio JG, Amend WJC et al. Azathioprine (AZA) bioavailability and pharmacokinetics in kidney transplant patients. *Clin Pharmacol Ther.* 1980;27(2):250. Abstract.
28. Maddock JL. Assay of azathioprine, 6-mercaptopurine and a novel thiopurine metabolite in human plasma. *Br J Clin Pharmacol.* 1979;8:273–8.
29. Houston JB. Drug metabolite kinetics. *Pharmacotherapy.* 1982;15:521–52.
30. Watts GF, Corston R. Hypersensitivity to azathioprine in myasthenia gravis. *Postgrad Med J.* 1984;60:362–3.
31. Brooks RJ, Dorr RT, Durie BGM. Interaction of allopurinol with 6-mercaptopurine and azathioprine. *Biomedicine.* 1982;36:217–22.
32. Coffey JJ, White CA, Lesk AB et al. Effect of allopurinol on the pharmacokinetics of 6-mercaptopurine (MSC 775) in cancer patients. *Cancer Res.* 1972;32:1283–9.
33. Vetten KB: Immunosuppressive therapy and anesthesia. *South African Medical Journal.* 1973;47:767–70.
34. Dretchen KL, Morgenroth VH III, Standaert FG et al. Azathioprine: effects on neuromuscular transmission. *Anesthesiology.* 1976;45:604–9.
35. Spiers ASD, Mibashan PS. Increased warfarin requirement during mercaptopurine therapy: a new drug interaction. *Lancet.* 1974;2:221–2.
36. Maddocks JL, Lennard L, Amess J et al. Azathioprine and severe bone marrow depression. *Lancet.* 1986;1:156. Letter.
37. Simmons RL, Moberg AW, Gerwurz H et al. Immunosuppression by antihuman lymphocyte globulin: correlation of human and animals assay systems with clinical results. *Transplant Proc.* 1971;3:745–8.
38. Lennard L, Murphy MF, Maddocks JL et al. Severe megaloblastic anaemia associated with abnormal azathioprine metabolism. *Br J Clin Pharmacol.* 1984;17:171–2.
39. Old CW, Flannery EP, Grogan TM et al. Azathioprine-induced pure red blood cell aplasia. *JAMA.* 1978;240:552–4.
40. Winklestein A. The effects of azathioprine and 6MP on immunity. *J Immunopharmacol.* 1979;1:429–54.
41. Rosman M, Bertino JR. Azathioprine. *Ann Intern Med.* 1973;79:694–700.
42. Stuart FP, Torrs E, Hester WJ et al. Orthotopic autotransplantation and allotransplantation of the liver: functional and structural patterns in the dog. *Ann Surg.* 1967;165:325–9.
43. Starzl TE, Torrs E, Hester WJ et al. Factors determining short- and long-term survival after orthotopic liver homotransplantation in the dog. *Surgery.* 1965;58:131–53.

44. Berne TV, Chatterjee SN, Craig JR et al. Hepatic dysfunction in recipients of renal allografts. *Surg Gynecol Obstet.* 1975;141:171-5.
45. Zarday Z, Veith FJ, Gliedman ML et al. Irreversible liver damage after azathioprine. *JAMA.* 1972;222:690-1.
46. McCormack JJ, Johns DG. Purine antimetabolites. In: Chabner B, ed. Pharmacologic principles of cancer treatment. Philadelphia: W. B. Saunders Company; 1982:213-8.
47. Nakashima Y, Howard JM. Drug-induced acute pancreatitis. *Surg Gynecol Obstet.* 1977;145:105-9.
48. Penn I. Cancer is a complication of severe immunosuppression. *Surg Gynecol Obstet.* 1986;162:603-10.
49. Storb R, Pepe M, Anasetti C et al. What role for prednisone in prevention of acute graft-versus-host disease in patients undergoing marrow transplants. *Blood.* 1990;76:1037-45.
50. Kung PC, Goldstein G, Reinherz EL et al. Monoclonal antibodies defining distinctive human T-cell surface antigens. *Science.* 1979;206:347-9.
51. Chang TW, Kung PC, Gingras SP et al. Does OKT3 monoclonal antibody react with an antigen-recognition structure on human T cells? *Proc Natl Acad Sci USA.* 1981;78(3):1805-8.
52. Reinherz EL, Meuer S, Fitzgerald KA et al. Antigen recognition by human T lymphocytes is linked to surface expression of the T-3 molecular complex. *Cell.* 1982;30:735-43.
53. Chatenoud L, Bandrihaye MF, Krefs H et al. Human in vivo antigenic modulation induced by the anti-T-cell OKT3 monoclonal antibody. *Eur J Immunol.* 1982;12:979-82.
54. Delmonico FL, Cosimi AB. Monoclonal antibody treatment of human allograft recipients. *Surg Gynecol Obstet.* 1988;166(1):89-98.
55. Shield CF, Norman DJ. Immunologic monitoring during and after OKT3 therapy. *Am J Kidney Dis.* 1988;11:112-9.
56. Miller RA, Maloney DG, McKillop J et al. In vivo effects of murine hybridoma monoclonal antibody in a patient with T-cell leukemia. *Blood.* 1981;58:78-86.
57. Rinnooy Kan EA, Wright SD, Welte K et al. Fc receptors on monocytes cause OKT3-treated lymphocytes to internalize T3 and to secrete IL-2. *Cell Immunol.* 1986;98:181.
58. Carreno M, Miller J, Fuller NL. Are OKT3 binding sites on T-cells modulated or merely converted (blind-folded) by OKT3 during therapy? *Transplant Proc.* 1989;21(1):987-8.
59. Gedel H, Lebeck LL, Jensik FC. Discordant expression of CD3 and T-cell receptor antigen on lymphocytes from patients treated with OKT3. *Transplant Proc.* 1989;21(1):1745-6.
60. Schroeder TJ, First MR, Hurtubise PE et al. Immunologic monitoring with orthoclone OKT3 therapy. *J Heart Transplant.* 1989;8:371-80.

61. Goldstein G, Norman DJ, Hennell KR et al. Pharmacokinetic study of Orthoclone OKT3 serum levels during treatment of acute renal allograft rejection. *Transplantation.* 1988;46(4):587–9.
62. Waldman TA, Strober W, Blaese RM. Immunoglobulins. Washington, DC: National Academy of Sciences; 1970.
63. Hooks MA, Wade CS, Millikan WJ Jr. Muromonab CD-3: a review of its pharmacology, pharmacokinetics, and clinical use in transplantation. *Pharmacotherapy.* 1991;11(1):26–37.
64. Biddison WE, Rao PE, Talle MA et al. Possible involvement of the T4 molecule in T cell recognition of class II HLA antigens: evidence from studies of CTL-target cell binding. *J Exp Med.* 1984;159:783–97.
65. Biddison WE, Rao PE, Talle MA et al. Distinct epitopes on the T-8 molecule are differentially involved in cytotoxic T-cell function. *Hum Immunol.* 1984;9:117–30.
66. Norman W. The clinical role of OKT3. *Cardiol Clin.* 1990;8(1):97–105.
67. Norman W, Barry JM, Bennett WM et al. OKT3 for induction immunosuppression in renal transplantation: a comparative study of high versus low doses. *Transplant Proc.* 1991;23(1):1052–4.
68. Leone MR, Barry JM, Alexander SR et al. Monoclonal antibody OKT3 therapy in pediatric kidney transplant patients. *J Pediatr.* 1990;116(suppl 5):S86–S91.
69. Schroeder TJ, Ryckman FC, Hurtubise PE et al. Immunological monitoring during and following OKT3 therapy in children. *Clinical Transplantation.* 1991;5:191–6.
70. Ryckman FC, Schroeder TJ, Pedersen SH et al. Use of monoclonal antibody immunosuppressive therapy in pediatric renal and liner transplantation. *Clinical Transplantation.* 1991;5:186–90.
71. Todd PA, Brogden RN. Muromonab CD3: a review of its pharmacology and therapeutic potential. *Drugs.* 1989;37:871–99.
72. Goldstein G, Fucello AJ, Norman DJ et al. OKT3 monoclonal antibody plasma levels during therapy and the subsequent development of host antibodies to OKT3. *Transplantation.* 1986;42(5):507–11.
73. Ortho Multicenter Transplant Study Group. A randomized clinical trial of OKT3 monoclonal antibody for acute rejection of cadaveric renal transplants. *N Engl J Med.* 1985;313:337–42.
74. Shield CF, Fucello AJ, Marlett P et al. Human antibody response to antilymphocytic preparations in renal transplant patients. *Transplant Proc.* 1987;19:2217–21.
75. Shield CF, Norman W, Marlett R et al. Comparison of antimurine and antihorse antibody production during the treatment of allograft rejection and OKT3 or antithymocyte globulin. *Nephron.* 1987;46(suppl 1):48–51.

76. Hesse CJ, Heyse P, Stolk BJM et al. Differences in antibody formation to OKT3 between kidney and heart transplant recipients. *Transplant Proc.* 1989;12(1):979–80.
77. Nelson PW, Jaffers GJ, Fuller TC et al. Reduction of immune response to OKT3 monoclonal antibody. *Transplant Proc.* 1985;18:644–9.
78. Norman W, Shield CF, Barry J et al. A U.S. clinical study of orthoclone OKT3 in renal transplantation. *Transplant Proc.* 1987;19(suppl 1):21–7.
79. Chatenoud L, Bandrihaye MF, Kreis H et al. The restricted human response to the murine monoclonal OKT3 antibody. *Transplant Proc.* 1985;17:558–9.
80. Bach JF, Chatenoud L. Immunologic monitoring of orthoclone OKT3-treated patients: the problem of antimonoclonal immune response. *Transplant Proc.* 1987;19(suppl 1):17–20.
81. Bandrihaye MF, Chantenoud L, Kreis H et al. Unusually restricted anti-isotype human immune response to OKT3 antibody. *Eur J Immunol.* 1984;14:686–91.
82. Cosimi AB. Clinical development of orthoclone OKT3. *Transplant Proc.* 1987;19(suppl 1):7–16.
83. Chatenoud L, Ferran C, Legendre C et al. In vivo cell activation following OKT3 administration. Systemic cytokine release and modulation by corticosteroids. *Transplantation.* 1990;49(4):697–702.
84. Abramowicz D, Schandene L, Goldman M et al. Release of tumor necrosis factor, interleukin-2, and gamma-interferon in serum after injection of OKT3 monoclonal antibody in kidney transplant recipients. *Transplantation.* 1989;47:606–8.
85. Rowe PA, Rocker GM, Morgan AG et al. OKT3 and pulmonary capillary permeability. *Br Med J.* 1987;255:1099.
86. Hosenpud JD, Norman DJ, Pantley GA et al. OKT3-induced hypotension in cardiac allograft recipients treated for resistant rejection. *J Heart Transplant.* 1989;8:159–66.
87. Emmons C, Smith J, Flanigan M. Cerebrospinal fluid inflammation during OKT3 therapy. *Lancet.* 1986;2:510. Letter.
88. Martin MA, Massanaari RM, Nghiem DD et al. Nosocomial aseptic meningitis associated with administration of OKT3. *JAMA.* 1988;259:2002–5.
89. Thomas DM, Nicholls AJ, Feest TG et al. OKT3 and cerebral oedema. *Br Med J.* 1987;295:1486.
90. Thistlethwaite JR, Gaber AO, Haag BW et al. OKT3 treatment of steroid resistant renal allograft rejection. *Transplantation.* 1987;43(2):176–84.
91. Chatenoud L, Legendre C, Ferran C et al. Corticosteroid inhibition of the OKT3-induced cytokine-related syndrome—dosage and kinetics prerequisites. *Transplantation.* 1991;51(2):334–8.

92. Ferran C, Sheehan R, Schreiber JF et al. Anti-TNF abrogates the cytokine-related anti-CD3 induced syndrome. *Transplant Proc.* 1991;23(1):849–50.
93. First MR, Schroeder TJ, Hariharan S et al. The use of indomethacin to decrease the early adverse effects of OKT_3. Paper presented to the American Society of Transplant Physicians 10th Annual Meeting. Chicago, IL: May 29, 1991;123A.
94. Richard E, Lorber MI, Marks WH et al. Are calcium channel blockers protective against first dose reactions to OKT_3? Paper presented to the American Society of Transplant Physicians 10th Annual Meeting. Chicago, IL: May 29, 1991;124A.
95. Swinnen LJ, Costanzo-Nordin MR, Fisher SG et al. Increased incidence of lymphoproliferative disorder after immunosuppression with the monoclonal antibody of OKT3 in cardiac transplant recipients. *N Engl J Med.* 1990;323:1723–8.
96. Emery RW, Lake KD. Post-transplantation lymphoproliferative disorder and OKT3. *N Engl J Med.* 1991;324(20):1437. Letter.
97. Cosimi AB, Rubin RH. Post-transplantation lymphoproliferative disorder and OKT3. *N Engl J Med.* 1991;324(20):1438. Letter.
98. Abramowicz D, Goldman M, De Pauw L et al. Posttransplantation lymphoproliferative disorder and OKT3. *N Engl J Med.* 1991;324(20):1439. Letter.
99. Woodruff MFA, Anderson NF. Effect of lymphocyte depletion by thoracic duct fistula and administration of anti-lymphocyte serum on the survival of skin homografts in rats. *Nature.* 1963;200:702–4.
100. Delmonico FL, Auchincloss H, Rubin RH et al. The selective use of antilymphocyte serum for cyclosporine treated patients with renal allograft dysfunction. *Ann Surg.* 1987;206:649–54.
101. Fassbinder W, Scheuermann EH, Stutte HJ et al. Improved graft prognosis by treatment of steroid-resistant rejections with ATG and plasmapheresis. *Proceedings of the European Dialysis and Transplant Association.* 1983;20:362–7.
102. Hardy MA, Nowygrod R, Elberg A et al. Use of ATG in treatment of steroid-resistant rejection. *Transplantation.* 1980;29:162–4.
103. Kreis H, Mansoum R, Descamps JM et al. Antithymocyte globulin in cadaver kidney transplantation: a randomized trial based on T cell monitoring. *Kidney Int.* 1981;19:438–44.
104. Nelson PW, Cosimi AB, Delmonico FL et al. Antithymocyte globulin as the primary treatment for renal allograft rejection. *Transplantation.* 1983; 36:587–9.
105. Sheil GR, Mears D, Kelly GE et al. A controlled trial of antilymphocyte globulin therapy (ALG) in man. *Transplant Proc.* 1972;4:501–5.
106. Shield CF, Cosimi AB, Tolkoff-Rubin N et al. Use of antithymocyte globulin for reversal of acute allograft rejection. *Transplantation.* 1979;28:461–9.

107. Starzl TE, Marchioro TL, Porter KKA et al. The use of heterologous antilymphoid agents in canine renal and liver homotransplantation and human renal homotransplantation. *Surg Gynecol Obstet.* 1967;124(2):301-8.

108. Fries D, Hiesse C, Lantz O et al. Optimization of antilymphocytes globulin in renal transplantation. *Transplant Proc.* 1990;22(4):1793-4.

109. Cosimi AB. Antilymphocyte globulin: a final (?) look. In: Morris PJ, Tilney NL, eds. Progress in transplantation. Edinburgh: Churchill Livingstone; 1985:167-88.

110. Cosimi AB, Delmonico FL. Anti-lymphocyte antibody immunosuppressive therapy. In: Williams GM, Burdick JF, Solez K, eds. Kidney transplant rejection. New York: Marcel Dekker; 1986:335-40.

111. Kalayoglu M, Strathe RJ, Hoffman RM et al. Quadruple immunosuppressive therapy for liver transplantation. *Transplant Proc.* 1988;20(suppl 1):524-9.

112. Deirhoi MH, Sollinger HW, Kalayoglu M et al. Quadruple immunosuppression in 305 consecutive cadaver renal allografts. *Clinical Transplantation.* 1987;1:71-4.

113. Stratta RJ, D'Alessandro AM, Armbrust MIJ et al. Sequential antilymphoctye globulin/cyclosporine immunosuppression in cadaveric renal transplantation. *Transplantation.* 1989;47(1):96-102.

114. Deeb GM, Bolling SF, Steimle CN et al. A randomized prospective comparison of MALG with OKT3 for rescue therapy of acute myocardial rejection. *Transplantation.* 1991;51:180-3.

115. Hesse UJ, Weinand P, Baldamus C et al. Preliminary results of a prospectively randomized trial of ALG vs OKT3 for steroid resistant rejection after renal transplantation in the early postoperative period. *Transplant Proc.* 1990;22(5):2273-4.

116. Cerilli G, Brastle L, Clarke J et al. Correlation of cell reaction patterns and in vitro immunosuppression capabilities of six ATG products used clinically. *Transplant Proc.* 1985;17:2760.

117. Lawley TJ, Bielory L, Gascon P et al. A prospective clinical and immunologic analysis of patients with serum sickness. *N Engl J Med.* 1984;311:1407-13.

118. Vermnier I, Giraud P, Eche JP et al. Hematologic side effects of antilymphocyte globulins: prevalence and impact on therapeutic protocol. *Transplant Proc.* 1985;17:2765-6.

119. Storb R, Deeg HJ, Whitehead J et al. Marrow transplantation in aplastic anemia: two controlled trials of a combination of methotrexate and cyclosporine versus cyclosporine alone or methotrexate alone for prophylaxis of acute graft vs. host disease. *Transplant Proc.* 1987;19:2608-2613.

120. Costanzo-Nordin MR, Grusk BB, Silver MA et al. Reversal of recalcitrant cardiac allograft rejection with methotrexate. *Circulation.* 1988; 78(suppl 3):47–57.
121. Olsen SL, O'Connell JB, Bristow MR et al. Methotrexate as an adjunct in the treatment of persistent mild cardiac allograft rejection. *Transplantation.* 1990;50(5):773–5.
122. Yau JC, LeMaistre CF, Zagars GK et al. Methylprednisolone, cyclosporine and methotrexate for prophylaxis of acute graft-versus-host disease. *Bone Marrow Transplant.* 1990;5:269–72.
123. Chabner BA, Myers CE. Clinical pharmacology of cancer chemotherapy. In: DeVita VT Jr, Hellman S, Rosenberg SA, eds. Cancer principles and practice of oncology. Philadelphia: J. B. Lippincott Company; 1989:349–95.
124. Arnold H, Bourseaux R, Brock N. Chemotherapeutic action of a cyclic nitrogen mustard phosphamide ester (B158-ASTA) in experimental tumors of the rat. *Nature.* 1958;181:931.
125. Kaufmann SHE, Han H, Diamanstein T. Relative susceptibilities of T cell subsets involved in delayed type hypersensitivity to sheep red cells to the in vitro action of 4-hydroperoxycyclophosphamide. *J Immunol.* 1980;125:1304–8.
126. Ozer H, Cowens JW, Colvin M et al. In vitro effects of 4-hydroperoxycyclophosphamide on human immunoregulatory T subset function. *J Exp Med.* 1982;155:276–90.
127. Connors TA. Alkylating drugs, nitrosourea and dialkyl triazenes. In: Pinedo HM, ed. Cancer chemotherapy. Amsterdam: Elsevier-North Holland; 1979:25–55.
128. Hengst JCD, Kempf RA. Immunomodulation by cyclophosphamide. *Clinics in Immunology and Allergy.* 1984;4(2):199–216.
129. Gassmann W, Uharek L, Wottge HU et al. Comparison of cyclophosphamide, cytarabine, and etoposide as immunosuppressive agents before allogeneic bone marrow transplantation. *Blood.* 1988;72:1574–9.
130. Yadav RVS, Indudhara R, Kumar P et al. Cyclophosphamide in renal transplantation. *Transplantation.* 1988;45(2):421–4.
131. Starzl TE, Halgrimson CG, Penn I. Cyclosphophamide and human organ transplantation. *Lancet.* 1971;2:70–4.
132. Evrard HM, Miller C, Schwartz M et al. Resistant hepatic allograft rejection successfully treated with cyclophosphamide and plasmapheresis. *Transplantation.* 1990;50(4):702–20.
133. Steinherz IJ, Steinherz PG. Cyclophosphamide cardiotoxicity. *Cancer Bulletin.* 1985;37:231–4.
134. Fung JJ, Todo S, Jain A et al. Conversion from cyclosporine to FK506 in liver allograft recipients with cyclosporine-related complications. *Transplant Proc.* 1990;22(1):6–12.
135. Fung JJ, Todo S, Tzakis A et al. Current status of FK506 in liver transplantation. *Transplant Proc.* 1991;23(3):1902–5.

136. Armitage JM, Kormos RL, Fung J et al. Preliminary experience with FK-506 in thoracic transplantation. *Transplant Proc.* 1991;52(1):164-7.
137. Shapiro R, Jordan M, Fung J et al. Kidney transplantation under FK-506 immunosuppression. *Transplant Proc.* 1991;23(1):920-3.
138. Todo S, Fung JJ, Tzakis A et al. One hundred ten consecutive primary orthotopic liver transplants under FK506 in adults. *Transplant Proc.* 1991;23(1):1397-1402.
139. Kino T, Hatanaka H, Miyata S et al. FK-506, a novel immunosuppressant isolated from a Streptomyces. II. Immunosuppressive effect of FK-506 in vitro. *J Antibiot.* 1987;40:1256-65.
140. Sawada S, Suzuki G, Kawase Y et al. Novel immunosuppressive agent, FK506 in vitro effects on the cloned T cell activation. *J Immunol.* 1987;139:1797-1803.
141. Zeevi A, Duquesnoy R, Eiras G et al. Immunosuppressive effect on FK-506 on in vitro lymphocyte alloactivation: synergism with cyclosporine A. *Transplant Proc.* 1987;19(suppl 6):40-4.
142. Venkataramanan R, Jain A, Cadoff E et al. Pharmacokinetics of FK506 preclinical and clinical studies. *Transplant Proc.* 1990;22(1):52-6.
143. Starzl TE, Todo S, Fung JJ et al. FK-506 for liver, kidney and pancreas transplantation. *Lancet.* 1989;2:1000-4.
144. Burke MD, Omar G, Thomson AW et al. Inhibition of the metabolism of cyclosporine by human liver microsomes by FK506. *Transplantation.* 1990;50(5):901-2.
145. Tamura K, Kobayashi M, Hashimoto K et al. A highly sensitive method to assay FK-506 levels in plasma. *Transplant Proc.* 1987;5(suppl 6):23-9.
146. Francavilla A, Barone M, Starzl TE et al. FK506 as a growth control factor. *Transplant Proc.* 1990;23(1):90-2.
147. Mazzaferro V, Scotti C, Porter KA et al. Studies of the hepatotrophic qualities of FK506 and CyA. *Transplant Proc.* 1990;22(1):93-5.
148. Starzl TE, Abu-Elmagd K, Tzakis A et al. Selected topics on FK506, with special references to rescue of extrahepatic whole organs grafts, transplantation of "forbidden organs," side effects, mechanisms and practical pharmacokinetics. *Transplant Proc.* 1991;23(1):914-9.
149. Reyes J, Gayoiski T, Fung JJ et al. Expressive dysphasia possibly related to FK506 in two liver transplant recipients. *Transplantation.* 1990;50(6):1043-4.
150. Abu-Elmagd K, Fung JJ, Alessiani M et al. The effect of graft function on FK-506 plasma levels, doses and renal function with particular reference to the liver. *Transplantation.* 1991;52:71-7.
151. Alessiani M, Kusne S, Martin M et al. Infection in adult liver transplantation under FK-506 immunosuppression. *Transplant Proc.* 1991;23(1):1501-3.

152. Morris RE, Wu J, Shorthouse R. A study of the contrasting effects of cyclosporine, FK506, and rapamycin on the suppression of allograft rejection. *Transplant Proc.* 1990;22(4):1638–41.
153. Morris RE, Meiser BM, Wu J et al. Use of rapamycin for the suppression of alloimmune reactions in vivo: schedule dependence, tolerance induction, synergy with cyclosporine and FK506, and effect on host-versus-graft and graft-versus-host reactions. *Transplant Proc.* 1991;23(1):521–4.
154. Stepkowski SM, Chen H, Daloze P et al. Rapamycin, a potent immunosuppressive drug for vascularized heart, kidney, and small bowel transplantation in the rat. *Transplantation.* 1991;51(1):22–6.
155. Epinette WW, Parker CM, Jones EL et al. Mycophenolic acid for psoriasis. *J Am Acad Dermatol.* 1987;17:962–71.
156. Morris RE, Hoyt EG, Murphy MP et al. Mycophenolic acid morpholinoethylester (RS-61442) is a new immunosuppressant that prevents and halts heart allograft rejection by selective inhibition of T- and B-cell purine synthesis. *Transplant Proc.* 1990;22(4):1659–62.
157. Platz, KP, Sollinger HW, Hullett DA et al. RS-61443—a new, potent immunosuppressive agent. *Transplantation.* 1991;51(1):27–31.
158. Amemiya H, Suzuki S, Ota K et al. A novel rescue drug, 15 deoxyspergualin. First clinical trials for recurrent graft rejection in renal recipients. *Transplantation.* 1990;49(2):337–43.
159. Amemiya H, Dohi K, Otsubo O et al. Markedly enhanced therapeutic effect of deoxyspergualin on acute rejection when combined with methylprednisolone in kidney recipients. *Transplant Proc.* 1991;23:1087–9.
160. Takahashi K, Ota K, Tanabe K et al. Effect of a novel immunosuppressive agent, deoxyspergualin on rejection in kidney transplant recipients. *Transplant Proc.* 1990;22(4):1606–12.
161. Groth CG, Ohlman S, Ericson BG et al. Deoxyspergualin for liver graft rejection. *Lancet.* 1990;336(8715):626. Letter.
162. Okazaki H, Sato T, Jimbo M et al. Prophylactic use of deoxyspergualin in living related renal transplantation. *Transplant Proc.* 1991;23:1094–5.
163. Koyama I, Amemiya H, Taguchi Y et al. Prophylactic use of deoxyspergualin in a quadruple immunosuppressive protocol in renal transplantation. *Transplant Proc.* 1991;23:1096–8.
164. Huser B, Landmann J, Mihatsch MJ et al. Clinical pilot study with cyclosporine G (CyG) in kidney transplant recipients. *Kidney Int.* 1987;32:431.
165. Todo S, Porter KA, Kam I et al. Canine liver transplantation under Nva^2 cyclosporine versus cyclosporine. *Transplantation.* 1986;41:296–300.
166. Heney D, Bailey CC, Lewis IJ. Thalidomide in the treatment of graft-versus-host disease. *Biomed Pharmacother.* 1990;44:199–204.

167. Waid TH, Lucas BA, Thompson JS et al. Treatment of acute rejection with anti-T-cell antigen receptor complex T1OB9.1A31 or anti-CD3 (OKT3) monoclonal antibody: results of a prospective randomized double-blind trial. *Transplant Proc.* 1991;23(1):1062–5.
168. Soulillou JP, Cantarovich D, LeMauff B et al. Randomized controlled trial of a monoclonal antibody against the interleukin-2 receptor (33B3.1) as compared with rabbit antithymocyte globulin for prophylaxis against rejection of renal allografts. *N Engl J Med.* 1990;322:1175–82.
169. Goldsmith MF. Researchers follow varied molecular paths toward better control of organ rejection. *JAMA.* 1990;263(9):1184–7.
170. Kirkman RL, Shapiro ME, Carpenter CB. A randomized prospective trial of Anti-Tac monoclonal antibody in human renal transplantation. *Transplantation.* 1991:51(1):107–13.
171. Carpenter CB, Suthanthiran M, eds. The prophylactic use of monoclonal antibodies in renal transplantation. *Am J Kidney Dis.* 1989;14(suppl 2):1–77.
172. Junghans RP, Waldmann TA, Landolfi NF et al. Anti-Tac-H, a humanized antibody to the interleukin 2 receptor with new features for immunotherapy in malignant and immune disorders. *Cancer Res.* 1990;50:1495–1502.
173. Kirkman RL, Bacha P, Barret LV et al. Prolongation of cardiac allograft survival in murine recipients treated with a diphtheria toxin-related interleukin-2 fusion protein. *Transplantation.* 1989;47(2):327–30.
174. Deeg HJ, Henslee-Downey PJ. Management of acute graft-versus-host disease. *Bone Marrow Transplant.* 1990;6:1–9.
175. Bastos MG, Pankewycz O, Rubin-Kelley VE et al. Concomitant administration of hapten and Il-2-toxin (DAB_{486}-IL-2) results in specific deletion of antigen-activated T-cell clones. *J Immunol.* 1990;145(11):3535–9.
176. Takahara S, Fununishi T, Kokado Y et al. Combined immunosuppression with low-dose cyclosporine, mizoribine, and prednisone. *Transplant Proc.* 1988;20(3):147–51.
177. Kokado Y, Isjibashi M, Jiang H et al. A new triple-drug induction therapy with low-dose cyclosporine, mizoribine and prednisone in renal transplantation. *Transplant Proc.* 1989;21(1):1575–8.
178. Marumo F, Okuba M, Yokota K. A clinical study of renal transplant patient receiving triple-drug therapy—cyclosporine A, mizoribine, and prednisone. *Transplant Proc.* 1988;20(suppl 1):406–9.
179. Hess RA, Tschudy DP, Blaese RM. Immunosuppression by Succinylacetone. II. Prevention of graft-vs-host disease. *J Immunol.* 1987;139:2845–9.
180. Fine RN, Terasaki PI, Ettenger RB et al. Renal transplantation update. *Ann Intern Med.* 1984;100:246–57.

181. Opelz G, Graver B, Terasaki PI. Induction of high kidney graft survival rate by multiple transfusion. *Lancet.* 1981;1:223-5.
182. Sutherland DER, Fryd DS, So SKS et al. Long-term effect of splenectomy versus no splenectomy in renal transplant patients. *Transplantation.* 1984;38(6):619-24.
183. Flye MW. Immunosuppressive therapy. In: Flye MW, ed. Principles of organ transplantation. Philadelphia: W. B. Saunders Company; 1989:155-75.
184. Struber S. Total lymphoid irradiation in alloimmunity and autoimmunity. II. *J Pediatr.* 1987;3(6):1051-5.
185. Monaco AP. Development of clinical immunosuppressants for organ transplantation. *Jpn J Surg.* 1988;18(2):119-30.
186. Salter M, Bourge R, Kirklin JK et al. Total lymphoid irradiation as therapy for recurrent allograft rejection. *J Heart Transplant.* 1991;10:176. Abstract.
187. Hunt SA, Strober S, Hoppe RT et al. Total lymphoid irradiation for treatment of intractable cardiac allograft rejection. *Heart Transplant.* 1991;10:211-6.
188. Hardy JD, Chavez CM, Kurrus FD et al. Heart transplantation in man: developmental studies and report of a case. *JAMA.* 1964;188:1132-40.
189. Barnard CN. The operation. *South African Medical Journal.* 1967;41:1271-4.
190. Gorensek MJ, Stewart RW, Keys TF et al. Decreased infections in cardiac transplant recipients on cyclosporine with reduced corticosteroid use. *Cleve Clin J Med.* 1989;56(7):690-5.
191. Thomas FT, Szentpetery SS, Mammana RE et al. Long distance transportation of human hearts for transplantation. *Ann Thorac Surg.* 1978;26:344-50.
192. Caves PK, Billingham ME, Stinson EB et al. Diagnosis of human cardiac allograft rejection by serial cardiac biopsy. *J Thorac Cardiovasc Surg.* 1973;66:461-6.
193. Dunn DL, Mayoral JL, Gillingham KJ et al. Treatment of invasive cytomegalovirus disease in solid organ transplant patients with ganciclovir. *Transplantation.* 1991;51(1):98-106.
194. Burdine J, Fischel RJ, Bolman RM III. Cardiac transplantation. *Crit Care Clin.* 1990;6(4):927-45.
195. Cameron DE, Augustine SM, Gardner TJ et al. Preoperative amiodarone therapy causes graft bradycardia following orthotopic heart transplantation. *J Heart Transplant.* 1988;7(1):67. Abstract.
196. MacDonald P, Hackworthy R, Keogh A et al. Effect of chronic amiodarone therapy prior to transplantation on early cardiac allograft function. *J Heart Transplant.* 1990;9(1):68. Abstract.
197. Rosvold D, Narins B, McClurken J et al. Permanent pacemakers after cardiac transplantation: reasons to delay insertion. *J Heart Transplant.* 1990;9:77. Abstract.

198. Stinson EB, Schroeder JS, Griepp RB et al. Observations on the behavior of recipient atria after cardiac transplantation in man. *Am J Cardiol.* 1972;30:615–22.

199. Stinson EB, Griepp RB, Schroeder JS et al. Hemodynamic observations one and two years after cardiac transplantation in man. *Circulation.* 1972;45:1183–94.

200. Pennington DG, McBride LR, Kanter KR et al. Bridging to heart transplantation with circulatory support devices. *J Heart Transplant.* 1989;8:116–23.

201. Reedy JE, Swartz MT, Termuhlen DF et al. Bridge to heart transplantation: importance of patient selection. *J Heart Transplant.* 1990;9:473–81.

202. Bolman RM, Cance CG. Intravenous cyclosporine for heart transplantation. *Transplant Proc.* 1989;21(1):2488.

203. Macris MP, Frazier OH, VanBuren CT et al. Improved immunosuppression for heart transplant patients using intravenous doses of cyclosporine. *Transplantation.* 1989;47:311–4.

204. Schroeder TJ, Myre SA, Melvin DB et al. Efficacy and safety of constant-rate intravenous cyclosporine infusion immediately after heart transplantation. *J Heart Transplant.* 1989;8:5–10.

205. Walker AM, ed. Transplant protocols. Chestnut Hill, MA: Epidemiology Resources, Inc.; 1990.

206. Bolman RM, Elick B, Olivari MT et al. Improved immunosuppression for heart transplantation. *J Heart Transplant.* 1985;4:315–8.

207. Bolman RM, Olivari MT, Saffitz J et al. Current results with triple therapy for heart transplantation. *Transplant Proc.* 1987;19:249–51.

208. Olivari MT, Kubo SH, Braunlin EA et al. Five-year experience with triple-drug immunosuppression therapy in cardiac transplantation. *Circulation.* 1990;82(suppl 4):264–8.

209. Bolling SF, Deeb GM, Miska PT. Comparison of polyclonal antibody, sera for early prophylaxis following cardiac transplantation. *J Surg Res.* 1989;47:292–6.

210. Carey JA, Frist WH. Use of polyclonal antilymphocytic preparations for prophylaxis in heart transplantation. *J Heart Transplant.* 1990;9:297–300.

211. Copeland JG, Icenogle TB, Williams RJ et al. Rabbit antithymocyte globulin: a 10-year experience in cardiac transplantation. *J Thorac Cardiovasc Surg.* 1990;99:852–60.

212. Costanzo-Nordin MR, O'Sullivan EJ, Hubbell EA et al. Longterm follow-up of heart transplant recipients treated with murine antihuman mature T cell monoclonal antibody (OKT3): the Loyola experience. *J Heart Transplant.* 1989;8:288–95.

213. Costanzo-Nordin MR, O'Sullivan JE, Johnson MR et al. Prospective randomized trial of OKT3-versus horse antithymocyte globulin-based immunosuppressive prophylaxis in heart transplantation. *J Heart Transplant.* 1990;9:306–15.

214. Emery RW, Joyce LD, Pritzker MR. Induction immunosuppression for patients bridged to transplantation. *J Heart Transplant.* 1990;9:316–20.

215. Gay, WA, O'Connell JG, Burton NA et al. OKT3 monoclonal antibody in cardiac transplantation: experience with 102 patients. *Ann Surg.* 1988;208:287–90.

216. Macris MP, Frazier OH, Lammermeier D et al. Clinical experience with muromonab-CD3 monoclonal antibody (OKT3) in heart transplantation. *J Heart Transplant.* 1989;8:281–7.

217. Prieto M, Lake KD, Pritzker MR et al. OKT3 induction and steroid free maintenance immunosuppression for treatment of high risk heart transplant recipients. *Journal of Heart and Lung Transplantation* 1991;10:901–911.

218. Barr ML, Sanchez JA, Seche LA et al. Anti-CD3 monoclonal antibody induction therapy immunological equivalency with triple-drug therapy in heart transplantation. *Circulation.* 1990;82(suppl 4):291–4.

219. Kirklin JK, Bourge RC, White-Williams C et al. Prophylactic therapy for rejection after cardiac transplantation: a comparison of rabbit antithymocyte globulin and OKT3. *J Thorac Cardiovasc Surg.* 1990;99(4):716–24.

220. Kormos RL, Herlan DB, Armitage JM et al. Monoclonal versus polyclonal therapy for prophylaxis against rejection after heart transplantation. *J Heart Transplant.* 1990;9:1–10.

221. Moore CK, Renlund DG, Rasmussen LG et al. Long-term morbidity of cyclosporine with corticosteroid-free maintenance immunosuppression in cardiac transplantation. *Transplant Proc.* 1990;22:25–9.

222. O'Connell JB, Bristow MR, Rasmussen LG et al. Cardiac allograft function with corticosteroid-free maintenance immunosuppression. *Circulation.* 1990;82(suppl 4):318–21.

223. Renlund DG, O'Connell JB, Gilbert EM et al. A prospective comparison of murine monoclonal CD3 (OKT3) antibody-based and equine antithymocyte globulin-based rejection prophylaxis in cardiac transplantation. *Transplantation.* 1989;47:599–605.

224. Renlund DG, O'Connell JB, Bristow MR. Early rejection prophylaxis in heart transplantation: is cytolytic therapy necessary? *J Heart Transplant.* 1989;8(3):191–2.

225. Oh CS, Stratta RJ, Fox BC et al. Increased infections associated with the use of OKT3 for treatment of steroid-resistant rejection in renal transplantation. *Transplantation.* 1988;45:68–73.

226. Billingham ME, Cary NRB, Hammond ME et al. A working formulation for the standardization of nomenclature in the diagnosis of heart and lung rejection. *J Heart Transplant.* 1990;9(6):587–93.

227. Hosenpud JD, Norman DJ, Pantley GA. Low-dose oral prednisone in the treatment of acute cardiac allograft rejection not associated with hemodynamic compromise. *J Heart Transplant.* 1990;9:292–6.

228. Miller LW. Treatment of cardiac allograft rejection with intravenous steroids. II. *J Heart Transplant.* 1990;9(3):283–7.

229. Costanzo-Nordin MR, Silver MA, O'Connell JB et al. Successful reversal of acute cardiac allograft rejection with OKT3 monoclonal antibody. *Circulation.* 1987;76(suppl 5):71–80.

230. Gilbert EM, Eiswirth CC, Renlund DG et al. Use of Orthoclone OKT3 monoclonal antibody in cardiac transplantation: early experience with rejection prophylaxis and treatment of refractory rejection. *Transplant Proc.* 1987;21(suppl 1):45–53.

231. Sweeney MS, Sinnott JT, Cullison JP et al. The use of OKT3 for stubborn heart allograft rejection: an advance in clinical immunotherapy? *J Heart Transplant.* 1987;6:324–8.

232. Andreone PA, Olivari MT, Elick B et al. Reduction of infectious complications following heart transplantation with triple-drug immunotherapy. *J Heart Transplant.* 1986;5:13–9.

233. Mason JW, Stinson EB, Hunt SA et al. Infections after cardiac transplantation: relation to rejection therapy. *Ann Intern Med.* 1976;85:69–72.

234. Grattan MT, Moreno-Cabral CE, Starnes VA et al. Cytomegalovirus infection is associated with cardiac allograft rejection and atherosclerosis. *JAMA.* 1989;261:3561–6.

235. McDonald K, Rector TJ, Braunlin EA et al. Association of coronary artery disease in cardiac transplant recipients with cytomegalovirus infection. *Am J Cardiol.* 1989;64:359–62.

236. Kriett JM, Kaye MP. The registry of the international society for heart transplantation: seventh official report—1990. *J Heart Transplant.* 1990;9:323–30.

237. Miller LW. Long-term complications of cardiac transplantation. *Prog in Cardiovasc Dis.* 1991;33(4):229–82.

238. Reitz BA, Wallwork JL, Hunt SA et al. Heart-lung transplantation: successful therapy for patients with pulmonary vascular disease. *N Engl J Med.* 1982;306:557–64.

239. Toronto Lung Transplant Group. Unilateral lung transplant for pulmonary fibrosis. *N Engl J Med.* 1986;314:1140–5.

240. Morrison DL, Maurer JR, Grossman RF. Preoperative assessment for lung transplantation. *Clin Chest Med.* 1990;2(2):207–15.

241. Maurer JR. Therapeutic challenges following lung transplantation. *Clin Chest Med.* 1990;11(2):279–90.

242. Snydman DR, Werner BG, Heinze-Lacey B. Use of cytomegalovirus immune globulin to prevent cytomegalovirus disease in renal transplant recipients. *N Engl J Med.* 1987;317:1049–54.
243. Prentice HG. Prophylaxis and treatment of cytomegalovirus infections in the bone marrow transplant recipient. *J Antimicrobial Chemother.* 1989;23(suppl E):23–30.
244. Egan TM, Cooper JD. Surgical aspects of single lung transplantation. *Clin Chest Med.* 1990;2(2):195–206.
245. Todd TRJ. Early postoperative management following lung transplantation. *Clin Chest Med.* 1990;2(2):259–67.
246. Theodore J, Starnes VA, Lewiston NJ. Obliterative bronchiolitis. *Clin Chest Surg.* 1990;2(2):309–21.
247. Shaw BW, Starzl TE, Iwatsuki S, Gordon RD. An overview of orthotopic transplantation of the liver. In: Flye MW, ed. Principles of organ transplantation. Philadelphia: W. B. Saunders Company; 1989:347–63.
248. Starzl TE, Demetris AJ. Liver transplantation: a 31 year perspective. *Curr Prob Surg.* 1990;17:55–116,123–78.
249. Samuel D, Bismuth A, Mathieu D et al. Passive immunoprophylaxis after liver transplantation in HBsAg-positive patients. *Lancet.* 1991;337:813–5.
250. Starzl TE, Demetris AJ, Van Thiel DV. Liver transplantation. *N Engl J Med.* 1989;321:1014–22,1092.
251. Tilney NL. Renal transplantation between identical twins: a review. *World Journal of Surgery.* 1986;10:381–8.
252. Tilney NL. Renal transplantation. *Curr Prob Surg.* 1989;26(9):607–69.
253. Blagg CR. Dialysis or transplantation? *JAMA.* 1983;250(8):1072–3.
254. Levinsky NG, Rettig RA. The Medicare end-stage renal disease program. *N Engl J Med.* 1991;324(16):1143–8.
255. Eggers PW. Mortality rate among dialysis patients in Medicare's end-stage renal disease program. *Am J Kidney Dis.* 1990;15(5):414–21.
256. Evans RW, Manninen DL, Garrison LP et al. The quality of life of patients with end-stage renal failure. *N Engl J Med.* 1985;312:553–9.
257. Pirsch JD, Sollinger HW, Kalayoglu M. Living unrelated renal transplantation: results in 40 patients. *Am J Kidney Dis.* 1988;12:499–503.
258. Frey W, Matas AJ. Renal transplantation. *Crit Care Clin.* 1990;6(4):899–910.
259. Terasaki PI, Takemoto S, Mickey MR. A report of 123 six-antigen matched cadaver kidney transplants. *Clinical Transplantation.* 1989;3:301.
260. Henry ML, Sommer BG, Ferguson RM. Triple drug therapy: an alternative regimen in renal transplantation. *Transplant Proc.* 1987;19(1):1920–1.

261. Landsberg D, Rae A, Chiu A et al. The effect of triple therapy on cyclosporine nephrotoxicity and hypertension in renal transplantation. *Transplant Proc.* 1989;21(2):3323-4.
262. Landsberg DN, Rae A, Chiu A et al. The use of triple therapy to minimize cyclosporine (CsA) nephrotoxicity in renal transplantation. *Transplant Proc.* 1989;21(1):1550-1.
263. Hodge E, Banowsky L, Novick A et al. Alternative immunosuppressive strategies in the management of recipients of living related renal transplants. *Transplant Proc.* 1989;21(1):1609-14.
264. Michael HJ, Francos GC, Burke JF et al. A comparison of the effects of cyclosporine versus antilymphocyte globulin on delayed graft function in cadaver renal transplant recipients. *Transplantation.* 1989;48(5):805-8.
265. Benvenisty AL, Cohen D, Stegall MD et al. Improved results using OKT3 as induction immunosuppression in renal allograft recipients with delayed graft function. *Transplantation.* 1990;49(2):321-7.
266. Matas AJ, Tellis VA, Quinn TA et al. Individualization of immediate posttransplant immunosuppression: the value of antilymphocyte globulin in patients with delayed graft function. *Transplantation.* 1988;45(2):406-9.
267. Novick AC, Ho-Hsieh H, Steinmuller D et al. Detrimental effect of cyclosporine on initial function of cadaver renal allografts following extended preservation: results of a randomized prospective study. *Transplantation.* 1986;42(2):154-8.
268. Rao KV. Mechanism, pathophysiology, diagnosis, and management of renal transplant rejection. *Med Clin North Am.* 1990;74(4):1039-57.
269. Butt KMH, Zielinski CM, Parsa I et al. Trends on immunosuppression for kidney transplantation. *Kidney Int.* 1978;8:S95-8.
270. Terasaki PI, Cecka Y, Cho S et al. A report from the UNOS Scientific Renal Transplant Registry. *Transplant Proc.* 1991;23(1):53-4.
271. Kelly WD, Lillehei RC, Merkel FK et al. Allotransplantation of the pancreas and duodenum along with the kidney in diabetic nephropathy. *Surgery.* 1967;67:827-37.
272. Squifflet JP, Moudry K, Sutherland DER. Is HLA matching relevant in pancreas transplantation? A registry analysis. *Transplant Int.* 1988;1:26-9.
273. Sutherland DER, Gillingham KJ, Moudry-Munns KC. Registry report on clinical pancreas transplantation. *Transplant Proc.* 1991;23(1):55-7.
274. Sutherland DER. Who should get a pancreas transplant? *Diabetes Care.* 1988;11:681-5.

275. Grundfest-Broniatowski S. Pancreas transplantation: state of the art. *Cleve Clin J Med.* 1990;57(6):564–70.
276. Sutherland DER, Gruber SA. Pancreas transplantation. *Crit Care Clin.* 1990;6(4):947–53.
277. Prieto M, Sutherland DER, Fernandez-Cruz I et al. Experimental and clinical experience with urine amylase monitoring for early diagnosis of rejection in pancreas transplantation. *Transplantation.* 1987;34:71–9.
278. Allen RDM, Wilson TG, Grierson JM et al. Percutaneous pancreas transplant, fine needle aspiration, and needle core biopsies are useful and safe. *Transplant Proc.* 1990;22:663–4.
279. Esmatjes E, Fernandez-Cruz L, Ricart MJ et al. Urinary c-peptide excretion in pancreas transplantation with urinary drainage. *Transplant Proc.* 1990;22(4):1598–9.
280. Perkins JD, Munn SR, Barr D et al. Evidence that the soluble interleukin-2 receptor level may determine the optimal time for cystoscopically directed biopsy in pancreaticoduodenal allograft recipients. *Transplantation.* 1990;49:363–6.
281. Tyden O, Reinholt F, Bohman S-O et al. Diagnosis of pancreatic graft rejection by pancreatic juice cytology. *Transplant Proc.* 1989;21:2780–1.
282. Fernstad R, Tyden G, Brattstrom C et al. Pancreas-specific protein: new serum marker for graft rejection in pancreas-transplant recipients. *Diabetes.* 1989;38(suppl 1):55–6.
283. Teule OJJ, Leunissen KML, Halders SGEA et al. Serial radionuclide determinations of graft perfusion in pancreas transplantation. *Transplant Proc.* 1989;21:2795–6.
284. Vahey TN, Glazer GM, Francis TR et al. MR diagnosis of pancreatic transplant rejection. *American Journal of Roentgenology.* 1988;150:337–60.
285. Gray DWR, Morris PJ. Transplantation of isolated pancreatic islets. In: Groth CG, ed. Pancreatic transplantation. Philadelphia: W. B. Saunders Company; 1988:363–83.
286. Skolnick A. Advances in islet cell transplantation: is science closer to a diabetes cure? *JAMA.* 1990;264(4):427–8.
287. Weir GC, Bonner-Weir S, Leahy JL. Islet mass and function in diabetes and transplantation. *Diabetes.* 1990;39:401–5.
288. Skerrett PJ. New transplant method evades immune attack. *Science.* 1990;249:1248.
289. Morris PJ, Gray DW, Sutton R. Pancreatic islet transplantation. *Br Med Bull.* 1989;456(1):224–41.
290. Lee KKW, Stangl MJ, Todo S et al. Comparison of short-term immunosuppressive therapy with cyclosporine and FK506 in small-bowel transplantation. *Transplant Proc.* 1990;22(6):2485–6.
291. Grant D, Wall W, Mimeault R et al. Successful small-bowel/liver transplantation. *Lancet.* 1990;335:181–4.

292. Lee KKW, Stangl MJ, Todo S et al. Successful orthotopic small bowel transplantation with short-term FK506 immunosuppressive therapy. *Transplantation.* 1990;22(suppl 1):78–9.
293. Watson AJM, Lear PA. Current status of intestinal transplantation. *Gut.* 1989;30:1771–82.
294. Grant D, Sommerauer J, Mimeault R et al. Treatment with continuous high-dose intravenous cyclosporine following clinical intestinal transplantation. *Transplantation.* 1989;48:151–2.
295. Tattersall C, Gebel H, Haklin M et al. Lymphocyte responsiveness after irradiation in canine and human intestinal allografts. *Curr Surg.* 1989;46(1):16–9.
296. Schroeder P, Goulet O, Lear P. Pancreas transplantation or insulin? *Lancet.* 1990;336:110–1.
297. Hansmann ML, Deltz E, Gundlach M et al. Small bowel transplantation in a child. *Am J Clin Pathol.* 1989;920:686–92.
298. Goulet O, Revillon Y, Jan D et al. Small bowel transplantation in children. *Transplant Proc.* 1990;22(6):2499–500.
299. Iwaki Y, Starzl TE, Yagihashi A et al. Replacement of donor lymphoid tissue in small-bowel transplants. *Lancet.* 1991;337:818–9.
300. Deitz E, Ulrichs K, Schack T et al. Graft-versus-host reaction in small-bowel transplantation and possibilities for its circumvention. *Am J Surg.* 1986;151:379–86.
301. Hurlbut D, Zhong R, Wang P et al. Intestinal permeability and bacterial translocation following orthotopic intestinal transplantation in the rat. *Transplant Proc.* 1990;22(6):2451.
302. Schrout WH. Current status of small-bowel transplantation. *Gastroenterology.* 1988;94:525–38.
303. Fabrega AJ, Lopez-Boado M, Gonzalez S. Problems in the longterm renal allograft recipient. *Crit Care Clin.* 1990;6(4):979–1005.
304. Kiok MC. Neurologic complications of pancreas transplants. *Neurol Clin.* 1988;6(2):367–76.
305. Van Thiel DH, Dindzans VJ, Gavaler JS et al. The postoperative problems and management of the liver transplant recipient. *Progress in Liver Diseases.* 1990;9:657–85.
306. Slavis SA, Novick AC, Steinmuller DR et al. Outcome of renal transplantation in patients with a functioning graft for 20 years or more. *J Urol.* 1990;144(1):20–2.
307. Braun WE. Long-term complications of renal transplantation. *Kidney Int.* 1990;37(5):1363–78.
308. Dunn DL, Najarian JS. Infectious complications in transplant surgery. In: Shires GT, Davis J, eds. Principles and management of surgical infection. Philadelphia: J. B. Lippincott; 1990:425–64.
309. Dunn DL. Problems related to immunosuppression: infection and malignancy occurring after solid organ transplantation. *Crit Care Clin.* 1990;6(4):955–77.

310. Peterson PK, Ferguson R, Fryd DS et al. Infectious diseases in hospitalized renal transplant recipients: a prospective study of a complex and evolving problem. *Medicine.* 1982;61:360–72.
311. Ramos E, Karmi S, Alongi SV et al. Infectious complications in renal transplant recipients. *South Med J.* 1980;73:751–4.
312. Rubin RH, Cosimi AB, Hirsch MS et al. Effects of antilymphocyte globulin on cytomegalovirus infection in renal transplant recipients. *Transplantation.* 1981;31:143–5.
313. Rubin RH, Cosimi AB. Therapy, both immunosuppressive and antimicrobial, for the transplant patient in the 1990s. In: Brent L, Sells RA, eds. Organ transplantation: current clinical and immunological concepts. London: Bailliere Tindall; 1989:71–9.
314. Simmons RL, Migliori RJ. Infection prophylaxis after successful organ transplantation. *Transplant Proc.* 1988;20(suppl 8):7–11.
315. Hughes WT. Comparison of dosages, intervals, and drugs in the prevention of pneumocystis carinii pneumonia. *Antimicrob Agents Chemother.* 1988;32(5):623–5.
316. Balfour HH, Chace BA, Stapleton JT et al. A randomized, placebo-controlled trial of oral acyclovir for the prevention of cytomegalovirus disease in recipients of renal allografts. *N Engl J Med.* 1989;320:1381–7.
317. Stratta RJ, Shaefer MS, Cushing KA et al. Successful prophylaxis of cytomegalovirus disease after primary CMV exposure in liver transplant recipients. *Transplantation.* 1991;51(1):90–7.
318. Dauber JH, Paradis IL, Dummer JS. Infectious complications in pulmonary allograft recipients. *Clin Chest Med.* 1990;11(2):291–308.
319. Markin RS, Stratta RJ, Woods GL. Infection after liver transplantation. *Am J Surg Pathol.* 1990;14(suppl 1):64–78.
320. Kusne S, Dummer JS, Singh N et al. Infections after liver transplantation: an analysis of 101 consecutive cases. *Medicine.* 1988;67(2):132–43.
321. Van Dorp WT, van Es LA, Thompson J et al. The effects of a maintenance immunosuppressive protocol after renal transplantation on infectious complications, comparing cyclosporine/prednisone, cyclosporine/azathioprine/prednisone, and conversion. *Transplantation.* 1991;51(1):193–7.
322. Hsu J, Griffith BP, Dowling RD et al. Infections in mortally ill cardiac transplant recipients. *J Thorac Cardiovasc Surg.* 1989;98(4):506–9.
323. Zenati M, Dowling RD, Dummer JS et al. Influence of the donor lung on development of early infections in lung transplant recipients. *J Heart Transplant.* 1990;9(5):502–9.
324. Porter GA, Bennett WM, Sheps SG et al. Cyclosporine associated hypertension. *Arch Intern Med.* 1990;150:280–3.
325. Scherrer U. Cyclosporine induced activation in hypertension after heart transplantation. *N Engl J Med.* 1990;323:693–9.

326. Loughran TP, Deeg HJ, Dahlbuy S et al. Incidence of hypertension after marrow transplant among 112 patients randomized to either cyclosporine or methotrexate as graft versus host disease prophylaxis. *Br J Haematol.* 1985;59:547–53.
327. Olivari MT, Antolick A, Ring WS. Arterial hypertension in heart transplant recipients treated with three-drug immunosuppressive therapy. *J Heart Transplant.* 1989;8:34–9.
328. Starling RC, Cody RJ. Cardiac transplant hypertension. *Am J Cardiol.* 1990;65:106–11.
329. Bennett WM, Porter GA. Cyclosporine-associated hypertension. *Am J Med.* 1988;85:131–3.
330. Jarowenko MV, Flechner SM, VanBuren CT et al. Influence of cyclosporine on posttransplant blood pressure response. *Am J Kidney Dis.* 1987;10:98–103.
331. Bantle JP, Boudreau RJ, Ferris TF. Suppression of plasma renin activity by cyclosporine. *Am J Med.* 1987; 83:59–64.
332. Myers BD, Sibley R, Newton L et al. The long-term course of cyclosporine-associated chronic nephropathy. *Kidney Int.* 1988;33:590–600.
333. Coffman IM, Carr DR, Yarger WF et al. Evidence that renal prostaglandins and thromboxane production is simulated in chronic cyclosporine nephrotoxicity. *Transplantation.* 1987;43:282–5.
334. June CH, Thompson CB, Kennedy MS et al. Correlation of hypomagnesemia with the onset of cyclosporine-associated hypertension in marrow transplant patients. *Transplantation.* 1986;4:47–51.
335. Miller LW, Pennington DG, McBride LR. Long-term effects of cyclosporine in cardiac transplantation. *Transplant Proc.* 1990;22(suppl 1):15–20.
336. Blum RL. Computer-assisted design of studies using routine clinical data: analyzing the association of prednisone and cholesterol. *Ann Intern Med.* 1986;104:858–68.
337. Becker DM, Chamberlain B, Swank R et al. Relationship between corticosteroid exposure and plasma lipid levels in heart transplant recipients. *Am J Med.* 1988;85:632–8.
338. Zimmerman J, Fainaru M, Eisenberg S. The effects of prednisone therapy on plasma lipoproteins and apolipoproteins: a prospective study. *Metabolism.* 1984;33:521–6.
339. Renlund DG, Bristow MR, Crandall BG et al. Hypercholesterolemia after transplantation: amelioration by corticosteroid-free maintenance immunosuppression. *J Heart Transplant.* 1989;8:214–20.
340. Taylor DO, Thompson JA, Hastillo A et al. Hyperlipidemia after clinical heart transplantation. *J Heart Transplant.* 1989;8(3):209–13.
341. Miller LW, McBride LR, Pennington DG. Safe withdrawal of steroids without use of induction therapy in cardiac transplantation. *J Am Coll Cardiol.* 1990;15(2):69. Abstract.

342. Ballantyne CM, Podet EJ, Patsch WP et al. Effects of cyclosporine therapy on plasma lipoprotein levels. *JAMA.* 1989;262(1):53–6.
343. Stamler JS, Vaughan DE, Rudd MA et al. Frequency of hypercholesterolemia after cardiac transplantation. *Am J Cardiol.* 1988;62(17):1268–72.
344. Superko HR, Haskell WL, DiRicco CD. Lipoprotein and hepatic lipase activity and high-density lipoprotein subclasses after cardiac transplantation. *Am J Cardiol.* 1990;66:1131–4.
345. Harris KPG, Russell GI, Parvin SD et al. Alterations in lipid and carbohydrate metabolism attributable to cyclosporin A in renal transplant recipients. *Br Med J.* 1986;292:16.
346. Kobashigawa JA, Murphy FL, Stevenson LW et al. Low-dose lovastatin safely lowers cholesterol after cardiac transplantation. *Circulation.* 1990;82(suppl 4):281–3.
347. Kuo PC, Kirshenbaum JM, Gordon J et al. Lovastatin therapy for hypercholesterolemia in cardiac transplant recipients. *Am J Cardiol.* 1989;64(10):631–5.
348. Corpier CL, Jones PH, Suki WN et al. Rhabdomyolysis and renal injury with lovastatin use. Report of two cases in cardiac transplant recipients. *JAMA.* 1988;260(2):239–41.
349. East C, Alivizatos PA, Grundy SM et al. Rhabdomyolysis in patients receiving lovastatin after cardiac transplantation. *N Engl J Med.* 1988;318(1):47–8.
350. Penn I. Cancers after cyclosporine therapy. *Transplant Proc.* 1988;20(suppl 1):276–9.
351. Penn I, Brunson ME. Cancers after cyclosporine therapy. *Transplant Proc.* 1988;20(suppl 3):885–92.
352. Penn I. Cancers following cyclosporine therapy. *Transplantation.* 1987;43:32–5.
353. Lanza RP: Malignant neoplasia in the immunocompromised patient. In: Cooper DKC, Lanza RP, eds. Heart transplantation. Hingham, MA: MTP Press; 1984:223–33.
354. Penn I. Cancers complicating organ transplantation. *N Engl J Med.* 1990;323(25):1767–9.
355. Penn I. The changing patterns of posttransplant malignancies. *Transplant Proc.* 1991;23(1):1101–3.
356. Nalesnik MA, Locker J, Jaffe R et al. Clonal characteristics of posttransplant lymphoproliferative disorders. *Transplant Proc.* 1988;20(suppl 1):280–3.
357. Hemmens VJ, Moore D. Photochemical sensitization by azathioprine and its metabolites. II. Azathioprine and nitroimidazole metabolites. *Photochem Photobiol.* 1986;43:257–62.
358. Edwards DI. Mechanisms of cytotoxicity of nitroimidazole drugs. *Prog Med Chem.* 1981;18:87–116.

359. Brumbaugh J, Baldwin JC, Stinson EB et al. Quantitative analysis of immunosuppression in cyclosporine-treated heart transplant patients with lymphoma. *J Heart Transplant.* 1985;4:307–11.
360. Bird AG, McLachlan M, Britton S. Cyclosporine A promotes spontaneous outgrowth in vitro of Epstein-Barr virus-induced B-cell lines. *Nature.* 1981;289:300–1.
361. Henle G, Henle W. The virus as the etiologic agent of infectious mononucleosis. In: Epstein MA, Achong BG, eds. The Epstein-Barr virus. New York: Springer-Verlag; 1979:297–310.
362. Klein G. The relationship of the virus to nasopharyngeal carcinoma. In: Epstein MA, Achong BG, eds. The Epstein-Barr virus. New York: Springer-Verlag; 1979:339–50.
363. Klein G. Lymphoma development in mice and humans: diversity of initiation is followed by convergent cytogenetic evolution. *Proc Natl Acad Sci USA.* 1979;76:2442–6.
364. Frizzera G, Hanto DW, Gajl-Peczalska KJ et al. Polymorphic diffuse B-cell hyperplasias and lymphomas in renal transplant recipients. *Cancer Res.* 1981;41:4262–79.
365. Hanto DW, Frizzera G, Gajl-Peczalska KJ et al. Epstein-Barr virus-induced B-cell lymphoma after renal transplantation: acyclovir therapy and transition from polyclonal to monoclonal B-cell proliferation. *N Engl J Med.* 1982;306:913–8.
366. Ferrara JL, Deeg HJ. Graft-versus-host disease. *N Engl J Med.* 1991;324:667–74.
367. Lehn PM. Gene therapy using bone marrow transplantation. *Bone Marrow Transplant.* 1987;1:243–58.
368. Lehn PM. Gene therapy using bone marrow transplantation: a 1990 update. *Bone Marrow Transplant.* 1990;5:287–95.
369. Welch GH and Larson EB. Cost effectiveness of bone marrow transplantation in acute nonlymphocytic leukemia. *N Engl J Med.* 1989;321:807–12.
370. Beatty PG, Clift RA, Michelson M et al. Marrow transplantation from related donors other than HLA identical siblings. *N Engl J Med.* 1985;313:765–71.
371. Beatty PG. The world experience with unrelated donor transplants. *Bone Marrow Transplant.* 1991;7:54–8.
372. Hows JM, Bradley BA. The use of unrelated marrow donors for transplantation. *Br J Haematol.* 1990;76:1–6.
373. Van Bekkum DW. Conditioning regimens for marrow grafting. *Semin Hematol.* 1984;21:81–90.
374. Garovoy MR, Melzer JS, Ascher N et al. Clinical transplantation. In: Sittes DP, Teit AI, eds. Basic and clinical immunology. East Norwalk, CT: Appleton and Lange; 1991:747–66.
375. Sullivan KM, Deeg HJ, Sanders J et al. Hyperacute graft versus host disease in patient not given immunosuppression after allogeneic marrow transplantation. *Blood.* 1986;67:1172–5.

376. Ash RC, Casper JT, Chitambar CR et al. Successful allogeneic transplantation of T-cell-depleted bone marrow from closely HLA-matched unrelated donors. *N Engl J Med.* 1990;322:485–94.

377. Atkinson K. Chronic graft-versus-host disease. *Bone Marrow Transplant.* 1990;5:69–83.

378. Fischer AC, Beschorner WE, Hess AD. Requirements for the induction and adoptive transfer of cyclosporine-induced syngeneic graft-versus-host disease. *J Exp Med.* 1989;169:1031–41.

379. Meyers JD. Infections in bone marrow transplantation. *Am J Med.* 1986;81:27–38.

380. Bodey GP, Buckley M, Sage YS et al. Quantitative relationship between circulating leukocytes and infection in patients with acute leukemia. *Ann Intern Med.* 1966;64:328–40.

381. Storb R, Prentice RL, Buckner CD et al. GVHD and survival in patients with aplastic anemia treated by marrow grafts from HLA identical siblings. *N Engl J Med.* 1983;308:302–9.

382. Piguet PF. Tumor necrosis factor and graft-vs-host disease. In: Burakoff SJ, Deek HJ, Ferrara J, et al, eds. Graft-vs-host disease: immunology, pathophysiology and treatment. New York: Marcel Dekker; 1990:225–76.

383. Aurer I, Ribas A, Gale RP. What is the role of recombinant colony stimulating factors in bone marrow transplantation? *Bone Marrow Transplant.* 1990;6:79–87.

384. Powles R, Smith C, Milan S et al. Human recombinant GM-CSF in allogeneic bone marrow transplantation for leukemia: double blind, placebo controlled trial. *Lancet.* 1990;336:1417–20.

385. Meyers JD, Flournoy N, Thomas ED. Nonbacterial pneumonia after allogeneic marrow transplantation: a review of ten years' experience. *Rev Infect Dis.* 1982;4:1119–32.

386. Meyers JD, Reed EC, Shepp DM et al. Acyclovir for prevention of cytomegalovirus infection and disease after allogeneic marrow transplantation. *N Engl J Med.* 1988;318:70–5.

387. Schmidt GM, Horak DA, Niland JC et al. A randomized, controlled trial of prophylactic ganciclovir for cytomegalovirus pulmonary infection in recipients of allogeneic bone marrow transplants. *N Engl J Med.* 1991;324:1005–11.

388. Bowden RA, Sayers M, Plownay N et al. CMV immune globulin and seronegative blood products to prevent primary CMV pneumonia after marrow transplantation. *N Engl J Med.* 1986;314:1006–10.

389. Atkinson K, Meyers JD, Storb R et al. Varicella-zoster virus infection after marrow transplantation for aplastic anemia or leukemia. *Transplantation.* 1980;29:47–50.

390. Rollins BJ. Hepatic venoocclusive disease. *Am J Med.* 1986;81:297–306.

391. Robbins RA, Linder J, Marlin G et al. Diffuse alveolar hemorrhage in autologous bone marrow transplant recipients. *Am J Med.* 1989;87:511–8.

Self-Study Questions

1. Which of the following immunosuppressive agents binds to the CD3 receptor, blocking the T cell's ability to be stimulated by foreign antigens?

   A. OKT3.
   B. Rapamycin.
   C. RS61443.
   D. Cyclophosphamide.

   1. A

2. Azathioprine is effective therapy for treating acute rejection following transplantation procedures.

   A. True.
   B. False.

   2. B

3. All heart transplant patients receive 500 mg of what immunosuppressive agent during the operative procedure?

   3. Methylprednisolone.

4. CsA whole-blood concentrations are usually maintained at higher levels for liver transplant patients than for BMT patients.

   A. True.
   B. False.

   4. A

5. Liver transplantation is most controversial in treating which of the following diseases?

   A. Acute liver failure.
   B. Hepatitis B virus.
   C. Liver carcinoma.
   D. Cystic fibrosis.

   5. C

6. There are no upper or lower age limits for heart transplant candidates.

   A. True.
   B. False.

   6. B

7. B

7. Acute heart or renal transplant rejection is initially treated with which therapy?

   A. ALG/ATG/OKT3 and/or prednisone.
   B. Steroid pulse and/or prednisone.
   C. CsA.
   D. Quadruple therapy.

8. B

8. Acute liver rejection is not effectively treated by intensifying immunosuppressive therapy.

   A. True.
   B. False.

9. 3 months.

9. Eighty percent of all infections in heart transplant patients occur within __________(period of time) after receiving high-dose immunosuppressive therapy.

10. C

10. What is the most common postoperative complication for kidney transplant patients?

    A. Hypertension.
    B. Hyperlipidemia.
    C. Allograft rejection.
    D. Viral infections.

11. A

11. Drugs used for preventing graft-versus-host disease in bone marrow transplant patients include methotrexate.

    A. True.
    B. False.

12. Usually steroids, with or without CsA and azathioprine.

12. What immunosuppressive drug is most commonly used to treat chronic graft-versus-host disease among bone marrow transplant patients?

13. Central venous catheters.

13. What is the major risk factor for Staphylococcus infections in bone marrow transplant patients during the period of neutropenia?

14. CMV (cytomegalovirus).

14. What is the leading cause of infectious mortality for allogeneic bone marrow transplant patients?

CHAPTER 10

Immunotherapy of Cancer

Suzanne M. Fields, Pharm. D.
Oncology Research Fellow
University of Texas Health Science Center
San Antonio, TX

Introduction

The many unanswered questions about the role of the immune system in combating cancer have led to extensive research into ways to manipulate the immune system for therapeutic effect. It is known that immunodeficient patients are predisposed to developing some types of malignancies. Perhaps vaccines will be able to prevent proliferation of cells inclined to become cancerous. The expanding knowledge of tumor cell immunology and cancer development has led to varied attempts to utilize the immune system for treating or preventing cancer cell growth.

The pharmacist's role in cancer immunotherapy can be significant. The areas of immunology and biotechnology are developing and changing rapidly. Additionally, many emerging products are prepared by recombinant DNA technology and will be very expensive. An appropriate balance between therapeutic effectiveness and cost containment will be an important consideration for cancer immunotherapy. Biologic agents can also be helpful in managing adverse effects. A working knowledge of the therapeutic effects and side effects of these agents will be critical for pharmacists involved in the care of the patient with cancer.

Learning objectives

After reading this chapter, the learner will be able to—

- Discuss the antitumor effects of interferon alfa.
- Discuss the side effects of interferon alfa.
- Discuss the antitumor effects of interleukin-2.
- Discuss the side effects of interleukin-2.
- Discuss the therapeutic effects of recombinant colony-stimulating factors.
- Discuss the side effects of colony-stimulating factors.

Chapter organization

This chapter describes tumor immunology and the role of the immune system in cancer development and treatment, including the function of tumor-associated antigens and antitumor immune mechanisms (e.g., natural killer cells). Tumor vaccines and immunostimulants (BCG and levamisole) used to manipulate the human immune system for the treatment of cancer are discussed briefly; most of this discussion focuses on the biologic response modifiers. Interferons, interleukins, colony-stimulating factors, and tumor necrosis factor are described in detail, with information about their antitumor mechanisms, method of administration, dosing, tumors against which each agent is used, and toxicities. The results of several studies are cited and referenced. The chapter finishes with a brief discussion of adoptive cellular immunotherapy and affinity column apheresis.

Tumor Immunology

Tumor cells are normal host cells that undergo malignant transformation and begin to divide uncontrollably, resulting in invasion of surrounding tissues or distant spread of disease. In the normal cell, growth and differentiation are regulated by genes known as proto-oncogenes. Genetic changes induced by viruses, chemical carcinogens, radiation, or other cellular mechanisms cause proto-oncogenes to be transformed into oncogenes, which stimulate neoplastic cell growth. If these newly transformed cells were recognized by the body as foreign, the body's natural immune system could play a role in the limitation of tumor development. Some malignant cells possess cell surface markers (tumor-associated antigens [TAAs]) that may help the immune system distinguish foreign cells from host cells. During the past decade, cancer immunology research has been greatly intensified in an attempt to treat malignancies by boosting the human immune system.

TAAs

The role of the immune system in cancer treatment was first investigated around the turn of the century, when it was discovered that laboratory rats developed a strong immune response against transplanted tumors. Following this discovery numerous attempts at host immunomodulation were made, but the results were quite disappointing. The observed immune response was attributed to the presence of normal histocompatibility antigens on cell surfaces rather than to the presence of specific TAAs. Cancer immunotherapy was virtually abandoned because researchers were unable to demonstrate TAAs on tumor cell surfaces and because the areas of cancer surgery and radiation therapy were developing rapidly. However, with the demonstration of TAAs on methylcholanthrene-induced sarcomas in laboratory mice by Foley and by Prehn and Main in the 1950s, the study of cancer immunotherapy was revived.[1,2]

Tumor-associated Surface Antigens

To produce an antitumor immune response the body must be able to distinguish host cells (self) from abnormal malignant cells (foreign). The presence of TAAs enhances the detection of malignant cells. However, many TAAs are present on the surface of normal cells as well as tumor cells. For example, oncofetal antigens such as carcinoembryonic antigen (CEA) and alpha-fetoprotein (AFP) are normally present in fetal and embryonic tissue during fetal development or during periods of cell differentiation in adults. Although these antigens are not immunogenic, they have been detected in the serum of patients with malignancies and other medical conditions. AFP levels are frequently elevated in patients with hepatomas, testicular carcinomas, and acute hepatitis and in pregnant women. CEA levels may be elevated in patients with adenocarcinoma of the gastrointestinal tract, pancreas, breast, and lung as well as in several nonmalignant conditions such as ulcerative colitis, alcoholic cirrhosis, pancreatitis, and emphysema. Heavy smokers have also been reported to have elevated CEA levels. Therefore, using the oncofetal antigens as a screening tool for malignancy is not very practical. Measuring CEA levels may be useful, however, for monitoring the clinical course in some patients with documented malignancies. Frequently patients exhibit a rise in the serum CEA level with disease recurrence before the recurrence is actually clinically detectable (e.g., colon cancer).[3]

CEA levels

Viral antigens located on the cell surface of tumors induced by both RNA and DNA viruses are another type of TAA. Viral antigens have been associated with malignancies such as Burkitt's lymphoma and nasopharyngeal carcinoma (Epstein-Barr virus), cervical carcinoma (human papilloma virus), hepatocellular carcinoma (hepatitis B virus), and T-cell leukemia and lymphoma (human T-lymphotropic virus type I). Viral TAAs are shared by all tumors that are induced by a single type of virus (immunologic cross-reactivity) and are able to induce both humoral and cell-mediated immune responses in humans. In contrast, cell surface antigens on chemically induced tumors are unique to each tumor, making it difficult to use immunotherapy in the diagnosis and treatment of these tumors.[4]

Viral TAAs

Tumor cells may also express tissue-specific antigens or differentiation antigens on the cell surface that are similar to the surface antigens expressed by normal cells during tissue differentiation.[4] Because these antigens also occur on normal cells, the body does not mount an immune response against cells expressing tissue-specific antigens. These antigens may, however, be used as targets for tumor-directed immunotherapy or as diagnostic markers. Prostate-specific antigen (PSA) and CA 125 are two tumor-derived markers that are useful for detecting and monitoring response in patients with prostate cancer and cancers originating in gynecologic tissues, respectively. Recent evidence suggests that measuring PSA concentrations is a useful addition to the screening process for prostate cancer and that serum PSA measurements are more accurate than rectal examination and ultrasonography for detecting prostate cancer.[5] Similar data exist for CA 125 levels in patients with ovarian cancer.[6] Serum CA 125 levels can aid in the diagnosis of ovarian cancer by distinguishing

PSA and CA 125

between a benign pelvic mass and a malignant mass. Changes in CA 125 concentrations have also correlated with disease recurrence, progression, and regression. The use of either of these markers to detect early-stage disease and to decrease mortality remains to be determined.

Antitumor Immune Mechanisms

Both humoral and cellular immune mechanisms are involved in the body's antitumor response. These mechanisms are discussed in detail in Chapters 1 and 2. Spontaneous tumor regression, increased frequency of tumor development in immunosuppressed hosts, and tumor infiltration with histiocytes, plasmacytes, lymphocytes, and eosinophils are all evidence for the involvement of the immune system in tumor cell kill.[7] The host effector mechanisms involved in tumor immunity include antitumor antibodies, complement, cytotoxic T cells, natural killer (NK) cells, killer (K) cells, macrophages, lymphokine-activated killer (LAK) cells, and antibody-dependent cellular cytotoxicity (ADCC).

Phagocytosis

Antitumor Antibodies and Complement. Although the humoral immune response against tumor cells is minimal, it may play a role in the host immune response. Tumor antigens stimulate the release of immunoglobulins (IgG and IgM), which bind to the surface of tumor cells. In the presence of complement, these antibodies destroy tumor cells via direct cell lysis or tumor opsonization and phagocytosis.[8] Antibody-coated target cells may also be eliminated from the body by ADCC mechanisms, which are discussed in a later section.

Cytotoxic T Cells. T lymphocytes contain antigen-specific receptors that recognize TAAs on the surface of tumor cells. These cells, however, recognize foreign antigens primarily in association with class I major histocompatibility complex (MHC) antigens, a fact that limits tumor cell lysis by T cells. T-cell-mediated killing can be intensified by the release of cytokines (e.g., interleukin [IL]-1, IL-2, IL-4, and interferon [IFN] gamma) from activated T cells that stimulate the activity of other effector cells of the immune system or have direct effects (e.g., IFN gamma).[9] For detailed discussion of MHC, see Chapter 3.

Natural Killer Cells. NK cells, also known as large granular lymphocytes, are lymphocytes found in the spleen, lymph nodes, bone marrow, and peripheral blood that can lyse various tumor cells. The exact mechanism by which NK cells kill tumor cells is still unknown. However, it may involve the release of cytotoxins from granules within the NK cells. NK cells may be stimulated by various agents, including interferon alpha (IFN alfa), interleukin-2 (IL-2), Bacillus Calmette-Guérin (BCG), tumor necrosis factor (TNF), and some chemotherapy agents. Prostaglandins, on the other hand, inhibit the activity of NK cells. NK cells also destroy tumor cells via ADCC because of the presence of crystallizable fragment (Fc) receptors on the cell membrane. There is also evidence that NK cells may help minimize the metastatic spread of tumor cells.[4,7-9]

Killer Cells. Both K and NK cells have been referred to as null cells because they lack either T- or B-cell surface markers. K cells differ from NK cells in that they require the presence of cell surface antibodies to destroy tumor cells. K cells express on the cell surface Fc and antibody receptors that bind to IgG antibodies, resulting in target cell lysis via ADCC mechanisms.[10]

Macrophages. Macrophages are cytotoxic effector cells that may be activated by various agents, including endotoxin, immune complexes, and lymphokines (IL-1 and macrophage-activating factors [MAFs], one of which is also known as gamma interferon [IFN gamma]). MAF is produced by antigen-stimulated T lymphocytes and attracts macrophages to the area of the tumor. These T lymphocytes also release migration inhibitory factor, which prevents the migration of macrophages away from the tumor-infiltrated area. Once macrophages are activated they selectively kill tumor cells via cell lysis and phagocytosis. The secretion of TNF by activated macrophages may also contribute to their cytotoxicity. Macrophages also express Fc receptors on their surfaces, enabling them to attack antibody-coated target cells.[4,8,11]

MAF

Lymphokine-activated Killer Cells. LAK cells are a heterogeneous population of cells, primarily NK cells and T cells that become cytotoxic in the presence of IL-2. These cells are found in peripheral blood, bone marrow, lymph nodes, and various other sites. LAK cells appear to be more selective for tumor cells than for normal cells. Furthermore, cells that are resistant to NK cells have demonstrated sensitivity to cytotoxic LAK cells.[7,11-14] In recent clinical trials, LAK cells stimulated in vitro by IL-2 have demonstrated activity in patients with metastatic disease.

Antibody-dependent Cellular Cytotoxicity. Some cytotoxic effector cells express Fc receptors on their surface (e.g., NK cells, K cells, granulocytes, and macrophages). These receptors are attracted to and bind to tumor antigens that have been coated with immunoglobulin antibodies, specifically IgG. Once the K cell is attached to the target cell via the Fc receptors, the tumor cell is then lysed by mechanisms that are poorly understood (Figure 10-1). ADCC may be initiated or stimulated by various cytokines, including IL-2, IL-1, TNF, granulocyte-macrophage colony-stimulating factor (GM-CSF), and macrophage colony-stimulating factor (M-CSF).[7]

Tumor Escape Mechanisms

Theories

Immune responses against tumor cells have been clearly demonstrated both in vitro and in vivo. However, these host defense mechanisms appear to be ineffective in preventing initiation and proliferation of many tumors. Several possible explanations for tumor cell evasion of the immune system have been proposed, one of which involves the kinetics of tumor cell growth. Low quantities of tumor cells may not be sufficient to stimulate a host immune response. As a result, resistant tumor cells may have time to develop before the tumor is large enough to be recognized by the immune system. This phenomenon has been called "sneaking through."[4,11] Two more explanations for tumor cell evasion are a tolerance to tumor antigens due to prior exposure and lost antitumor immunity resulting from lost tumor cell surface antigen (antigenic modulation). A fourth explanation is that tumor cell surface antigens are masked by certain molecules that appear on the surface of tumor cells, such as sialic acid-containing mucopolysaccharides. A fifth possibility is that tumor cells may secrete tumor antigens that form complexes with circulating antibodies. These complexes may then block Fc receptors on the surface of host effector cells or induce suppressor cells, resulting in suppression of cytotoxic T cells.[4] A final explanation for tumor cell evasion is that tumor cells may produce products that suppress the immune system. Prostaglandins and transforming growth factor beta (TGF beta) are two tumor products that inhibit the activity of immune effector cells.[4,11]

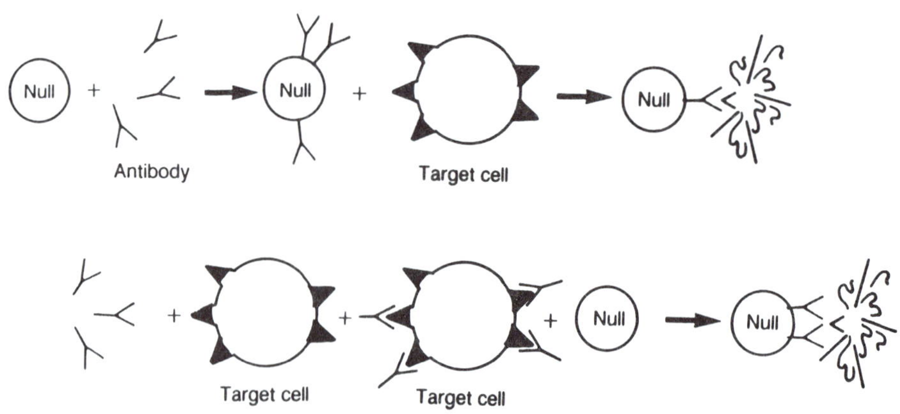

Figure 10-1. Antibody-dependent cellular cytotoxicity is due to the attachment of effector cells to aggregated antibody on target cells. This bestows on previously nonimmune reactive cells the capacity to react specifically with antigens on cells and kill them.

SOURCE: Reprinted with permission from Sell. Cell-Mediated Immunity in Vitro. In: Immunology, Immunopathology and Immunity. 4th ed. 1987:162.

In summary, tumor cells are normal cells that undergo malignant transformation and may be recognized by the host immune system as foreign because TAAs are present. Both humoral and cellular immune mechanisms are involved in the body's response to the tumor. However, there are also various mechanisms by which tumor cells evade destruction by immune effector cells. Increased understanding of the host immune response and of tumor cell evasion mechanisms may, in the future, allow malignancies to be treated by manipulating the host immune system.

Cancer Immunotherapy

Mechanisms for Manipulating the Immune System

The ability to differentiate normal cells from tumor cells on the basis of antigenic differences described thus far should permit tumor-directed therapy via immunotherapy. Unfortunately, in the studies conducted to date, immunotherapy has demonstrated minimal activity in patients with advanced disease. As a result, the role of immunotherapy in the treatment of malignancy may be in the adjuvant setting (microscopic disease only) or in combination with other treatment modalities (chemotherapy, radiation, or surgery).

Immunomodulation techniques

The human immune system can be manipulated to treat cancer through the following mechanisms: (1) vaccination of cancer patients with tumor cell preparations, (2) direct administration of biologic response modifiers (BRMs) or immunostimulants in an attempt to modulate the patient's immune system, (3) ex vivo manipulation of a patient's immune effector cells with BRMs to increase their cytotoxicity (adoptive cellular immunotherapy), and (4) ex vivo manipulation of a patient's plasma with affinity column apheresis (ACA) to remove blocking factors or add tumoricidal factors.

Tumor Vaccines

The rationale behind immunization and the use of various types of vaccines is discussed extensively in Chapter 7. Because TAAs are present on tumor cells, the use of vaccines in the treatment or prevention of cancer has been explored. Active immunization with viral antigens has been successful in preventing the development of virally induced tumors in animals (e.g., feline leukemia virus in cats and Marek's disease in chickens).[4] Administering the hepatitis B vaccine to humans may produce similar results because of the association between hepatitis B virus infections of the liver and hepatocellular carcinoma.

Autologous and allogeneic cells

Tumor vaccines may be produced from autologous tumor cells or allogeneic tumor cell lines in an attempt to attain active specific stimulation of the immune system. To increase the immunogenicity of the vaccine, the tumor cells may be altered with enzymatic, chemical, or radiation procedures. Concomitant administration of nonspecific immunostimulants (e.g., BCG) may also be used in an attempt to increase the immune response. More research is required before conclusions concerning the efficacy of tumor vaccines can be reached. Inherent problems in vaccine development include the need for an intact host immune system, the inability to affect large tumor cell masses, the inter- and intrapatient variation of TAAs, and the presence of similar surface antigens on both normal and tumor cells.[15]

Passive stimulation of the immune system via the administration of tumor-directed monoclonal antibodies (MoAbs) is also being investigated (see Chapter 11).

Immunostimulants

Nonspecific stimulation of the immune system with bacterial and viral agents, as well as other antigenic agents, has been investigated in the treatment of various malignancies. The antitumor activity of host immunomodulation was serendipitously discovered by Coley around the turn of the century when he observed regression of sarcoma in a patient following erysipelas.[7] After this observation he began to treat patients with "Coley's toxins," which were combinations of bacterial toxins, and some tumor regressions were reported. Numerous immunostimulants are currently under investigation for the treatment of cancer.

Nonspecific

BCG. BCG is a live attenuated strain of *Mycobacterium bovis* that nonspecifically stimulates the host immune system. Clinical trials have been conducted with BCG in patients with acute leukemia, melanoma, and colon, breast, renal cell, and bladder cancers. However, the only significant responses have been seen with direct intravesical BCG administration in the treatment of superficial bladder cancer. Cell-mediated inflammatory responses, alone or in combination with ADCC mechanisms, have been proposed as possible antitumor mechanisms of intravesical BCG. However, recent data suggest that T-cell-mediated immunologic mechanisms are primarily responsible for BCG's antitumor activity. Increased levels of various cytokines, including IL-l, IL-2, TFN, and IFN gamma, have been detected in patients' urine following intravesical BCG administration.[16,17] Criteria required for a tumor response include small tumor size, immunocompetence of the host, drug administration in close proximity to the tumor, and administration of adequate numbers of *Mycobacteria.*[18]

Efficacy

In a large trial conducted by the Southwest Oncology Group, intravesical BCG was shown to be more effective than intravesical doxorubicin in the treatment of superficial bladder carcinoma. Complete responses were achieved in 71% of patients treated with BCG versus 47% treated with intravesical doxorubicin.[19] Tumor recurrence occurred in 37% of the patients receiving doxorubicin and 15% receiving BCG, with the mean time to recurrence twice as long in the BCG group (22 months versus 10 months). In addition, patients with stage Ta and Tl tumors (high-risk patients) receiving BCG had less tumor recurrence than those receiving doxorubicin—57% versus 79%, respectively. Intravesical BCG administration was also superior to intravesical thiotepa and intravesical doxorubicin for the prophylaxis of disease progression and recurrence in superficial bladder carcinoma (percent recurrence: BCG = 13%, thiotepa = 36%, doxorubicin = 43%).[20]

Regimen

Currently, two BCG products are commercially available for the intravesical treatment of bladder carcinoma in situ: TheraCys-Connaught® and Tice BCG-Organon®. The regimen recommended by both manufacturers consists of induction therapy administered once a week for 6 weeks followed by maintenance therapy. Patients who do not respond to an initial 6-week course of treatment should receive a second 6-week course, because several studies have demonstrated responses in patients who receive a second course of therapy.[21-23] The maintenance regimen recommended by Connaught consists of one intravesical instillation 3, 6, 12, 18, and 24 months after the induction regimen. The Tice BCG should be administered monthly for 6 to 12 months.

Side effects

The most common side effects associated with BCG therapy (Table 10-1) usually occur after the third or fourth BCG dose and increase in severity with subsequent doses. Systemic symptoms usually begin 2 to 4 hours after BCG instillation and subside within 24 to 72 hours. Concurrent administration of diphenhydramine and antipyretics may palliate some of the systemic side effects.[24,25] Systemic BCG infections manifested by pneumonitis or granulomatous hepatitis have been reported in less than 1% of patients receiving intravesical BCG. Fatal disseminated mycobacterial infection and sepsis following BCG therapy have been reported in six patients to date.[26,27] As a result, it is recommended that BCG never be given at the time of surgical manipulation of the genitourinary tract, to patients who are immunosuppressed, or after a traumatic bladder catheterization. Antituberculous antibiotics should be administered at the first signs of systemic BCG infection.

Biohazards

BCG contains viable attenuated mycobacteria. Therefore, all of the materials used for drug preparation and administration should be immediately disposed of as biohazardous waste. Patients should be counseled to mix their urine with an equal volume of household bleach and

Table 10-1 Side Effects Associated with BCG Therapy

Irritable bladder symptoms
Dysuria
Frequency
Urgency
Gross hematuria
Cystitis
Flu-like syndrome
Fever
Malaise
Chills
Myalgias
Nausea and vomiting
Anorexia

allow it to sit for 15 minutes before flushing during the first 6 hours after drug administration. They should also be instructed to sit while voiding after BCG therapy.

Levamisole. Levamisole is an anthelmintic agent that was originally developed for veterinary and human use in the treatment of parasitic worms. However, in the past two decades the immunologic effects of levamisole have been described and clinical trials have been conducted in several malignant diseases. In the studies to date, levamisole has demonstrated the most clinical activity in the adjuvant treatment of colorectal cancer. The exact mechanism by which levamisole stimulates the host immune system is unknown and is probably quite complex. Levamisole appears to affect primarily the cells involved in cell-mediated immunity, because B lymphocytes and antibody production do not change after drug administration. Direct antitumor activity has also not been reported with levamisole.[28]

Colorectal cancer

Efficacy

Clinical trials conducted in the adjuvant treatment of colon cancer have demonstrated limited activity for single-agent levamisole.[29,30] However, the combination of levamisole and 5-fluorouracil has demonstrated significant clinical activity (Table 10-2). In a small European study, patients with colorectal cancer were randomized into three treatment groups: (1) supportive care only, (2) 5-fluorouracil only, and (3) levamisole plus 5-fluorouracil. After a minimum of 5 years of follow-up the patients receiving levamisole plus 5-fluorouracil had a significant survival advantage over the patients in the 5-fluorouracil group and the control group (32% disease recurrence versus 44% and 52%, respectively).[31]

Table 10-2 Clinical Trials of Levamisole Plus 5-Fluorouracil (5-FU) as Adjuvant Therapy for Colon Carcinoma

Reference	No. of Patients	Treatment	Disease Recurrence (%)
31[a]	45	Control	44
	42	5-FU	52
	44	5-FU/Levamisole	32
32[b]	315	Observation	49
	310	Levamisole	46
	304	5-FU/Levamisole	34

[a] Included patients with stage A, B, or C disease.

[b] Included only patients with stage C disease.

These results have since been confirmed in a large multicenter study in the United States.[32] In this study, patients with resected Dukes stage B2 or C colon cancer were randomized to observation alone, levamisole alone, or combination levamisole and 5-fluorouracil. At follow-up after 3 ½ years, 34% of the patients in the levamisole and 5-fluorouracil group had relapsed versus 46% in the levamisole-only group and 49% in the control group. As a result, the combination of fluorouracil and levamisole is now recommended as standard therapy for patients with resected Dukes stage C colon cancer. Because the number of patients with Dukes stage B colon cancer was much smaller than the number of patients with stage C, the data cannot be extrapolated to the treatment of stage B disease. The role of levamisole in the treatment of other stages of colorectal cancer remains to be determined.

Regimen and side effects

Levamisole is administered orally in a dose of 50 mg every 8 hours for 3 days every 2 weeks in combination with fluorouracil. Therapy should be started 3 to 5 weeks after surgery and continue for 1 year.[28,32] Side effects that have been reported with levamisole therapy include nausea, vomiting, metallic or altered taste, fever, malaise, dermatitis, mood elevation, insomnia, headache, and occasionally blood dyscrasias (granulocytopenia, leukopenia, and thrombocytopenia).[28,32]

Numerous other agents, including *Corynebacterium parvum,* bestatin, tuftsin, endotoxin, OK 432 viruses, and various chemicals are also being investigated as nonspecific stimulants of the host immune system. However, most of the data are preliminary, and none of these agents are available for commercial use.

Biologic Response Modifiers

Mechanisms

BRMs are natural or synthetic agents that modify the host's biologic response to tumor cells. On the basis of differences in their biologic effects, these agents can be divided into three major categories: (1) agents that modulate host immunologic mechanisms and lead to suppression of tumor cell growth, (2) agents that have direct antitumor effects, and (3) agents that modify the interaction between host and tumor via mechanisms other than immunologic or direct antitumor effects.[33] Many of the BRMs may have more than one mechanism of antitumor activity, and these mechanisms may vary depending on dose and schedule of administration. As a result, the exact mechanism responsible for BRM antitumor activity may be difficult to elucidate. However, the evolution of genetic engineering techniques now allows large-scale production of BRMs, and our understanding of the mechanisms of action and clinical utility of these agents is increasing rapidly.

Varied mechanisms

Interferons. The IFNs are a group of glycoproteins produced in response to viral infections or other IFN inducers. There are three types of IFN: alfa, beta, and gamma. IFN alfa and IFN beta are produced by a variety of cell types and cause similar biologic effects because of competitive binding at a common cell surface receptor. IFN gamma, on the other hand, binds to a distinct cell surface receptor and is produced by T lymphocytes. The IFNs create their biologic effects through a variety of different mechanisms including antiviral, antiproliferative, cytostatic, immunomodulatory, and differentiating effects.

The antitumor mechanisms of the IFNs may occur via direct or indirect effects on tumor cells. IFN has demonstrated direct antiproliferative effects both in vivo and in vitro.[34,35] These effects are due to lengthening of all phases of the cell cycle and suppression of the c-myc oncogene, which prevents cells from entering the division process. The IFNs also induce 2,5-A synthetase, protein kinase, and phosphodiesterase—three enzymes that inhibit RNA, DNA, and protein synthesis. Enzyme inhibition contributes to both the antiviral and the antitumor effects of the IFNs. The IFNs also exert various immunomodulatory effects that enhance their antitumor activity. After administration of IFN, patients have demonstrated enhanced NK, K, and LAK cell activity; increased T-cell cytotoxicity; and augmented macrophage activity via enhanced MHC class I expression. All the IFNs enhance MHC class I expression, but IFN gamma also enhances MHC class II antigen expression. As a result, IFN gamma demonstrates greater immunomodulatory activity than either IFN alfa or IFN beta.[34,36] All the antitumor effects of the IFNs depend on the timing, dose, route of administration, and duration of exposure to the biologic agent.

Dose and schedule

IFN may be administered intramuscularly, intravenously, or subcutaneously in a variety of doses and schedules. The antitumor effects appear to be dose responsive as hematologic malignancies respond to lower IFN doses (5 million units (MU) / m^2 three times weekly or 3 MU daily), and solid tumors respond to higher doses (6 MU to 35 MU). Continuous dosing daily or three times per week appears to be more effective than administering doses on intermittent schedules.[37] Patients with minimal disease demonstrate greatest responsiveness to IFN therapy. Presently, IFN alfa is approved by the Food and Drug Administration (FDA) for the treatment of hairy cell leukemia, Kaposi's sarcoma (KS), condylomata acuminata (genital warts), and chronic hepatitis C. IFN gamma is approved only for treating chronic granulomatous disease. However, the IFNs are also being used in clinical trials to treat numerous other malignancies (Table 10-3).

Applications

Hairy cell leukemia

IFN Alfa. IFN alfa was originally approved in 1986 for treating hairy cell leukemia. Following low doses of IFN (2 MU to 3 MU administered daily or three times weekly), objective response rates (normalization of complete blood counts) of approximately 70% and complete response rates of approximately 5% (normal blood counts and less than 5% hairy cells in the bone marrow) have been obtained in patients with hairy cell leukemia.[38,39] Furthermore, a prolongation in disease survival with fewer transfusion requirements and serious infections has occurred in patients who have only a partial response to therapy.[34,38] Peripheral blood and bone marrow counts

Table 10-3 Therapeutic Uses of Interferon Alfa

Hairy cell leukemia*
Kaposi's sarcoma*
Condylomata acuminata*
Chronic hepatitis C*
Chronic myelogenous leukemia
Chronic hepatitis B
Melanoma
Renal cell carcinoma
Multiple myeloma
Non-Hodgkin's lymphoma
Malignant glioma
Ovarian cancer
Carcinoid tumors
Cutaneous T-cell lymphomas

*Uses approved by the Food and Drug Administration.

begin to improve rapidly during the first 3 to 6 months after IFN administration. Improvements in both hematologic parameters may continue for as long as 1 year after IFN is started.[39,40]

In a recent small study, lower doses of IFN (0.2 MU/m^2 three times weekly) were determined to be relatively ineffective for treating relapsed hairy cell leukemia.[41] The use of minimal-dose maintenance therapy after initial higher dose therapy remains to be investigated. Optimal treatment duration also needs to be determined. Following 24 months of IFN therapy in 35 patients with hairy cell leukemia, disease progression occurred in approximately 50% of patients at a median of 10 months after the drug was discontinued.[42] Patients with a low platelet count at the completion of therapy experienced a high rate of disease progression. More studies examining optimal treatment regimens and risk factors predictive of disease recurrence are warranted.

Deoxycoformycin (pentostatin) is an antineoplastic agent that produces response rates ranging from 60% to 100% in patients with hairy cell leukemia. Because deoxycoformycin is non-cross-resistant with IFN alfa, a treatment regimen alternating cycles of the two agents could produce response rates higher than those obtained with either agent alone. However, preliminary data from 15 patients treated with an alternating regimen do not support this hypothesis.[43] None of the patients receiving the two-drug regimen obtained a complete response. However, all the patients did have an improvement in peripheral blood counts and at least 95% clearance of hairy cells from their bone marrow. Furthermore, all patients have remained free of disease progression for a median follow-up of 27 months. Prolonged follow-up of these patients is necessary to determine the true effects of alternating therapy with deoxycoformycin and IFN.

CML

Although not approved for the treatment of chronic myelogenous leukemia (CML), IFN alfa has produced impressive response rates in this disease. After a dose of 5 MU/m^2 per day, more than 70% of patients achieve a hematologic remission and 24% experience a durable, complete cytogenetic response (complete disappearance of the Philadelphia chromosome).[44] The median survival of CML patients after IFN therapy is 62 months, significantly longer than the survival rates obtained with chemotherapy. In a study conducted by the Cancer and Leukemia Group B, 55% of patients achieved a partial response, 18% achieved a complete response, and 13% achieved a complete cytogenetic response.[45] IFN therapy in CML appears to work best when started early in the disease course (before the accelerated phase) and when the patient has received no previous therapy. The median time to response in CML is 6 to 9 months after initiation of therapy, and the time to maximal cytogenetic response is greater than 24 months.

KS and HIV

Approximately 35% to 50% of patients with acquired immunodeficiency syndrome (AIDS)-related KS also experience an objective response to IFN therapy with fewer opportunistic infections and prolonged survival.[46-48] The recommended doses of IFN for KS are 18 MU to 36 MU three times weekly for IFN alfa-2a and 30 MU/m^2 three times weekly for IFN alfa-2b. Tumor response to IFN in KS appears to be dose related. However, many patients are unable to tolerate the side effects associated with high-dose therapy and require a dosage reduction. Tumor response may also be predicted by patient characteristics, because patients with less severe immune dysfunction, earlier stage disease, and fewer disease complications are most likely to respond to IFN. IFN suppresses the human immunodeficiency virus (HIV) in vitro and in vivo.[47,48] As a result, several studies have been conducted with the combination of zidovudine and IFN alfa in an attempt to potentiate antiviral activity and minimize toxicities.[49-51] Antitumor responses of 45% to 50% have been obtained with the combination regimen accompanied by decreased serum HIV p24 antigen levels and increased CD4+ lymphocyte counts. The dose-limiting toxicities in these studies included neutropenia, anemia, thrombocytopenia, and hepatotoxicity. IFN beta and IFN gamma have also been reported to produce antitumor and antiviral effects in patients with AIDS-related KS.[52,53] Further studies need to be conducted to determine the role of these agents in the treatment of KS.

Preventing hepatoma

As mentioned previously, patients with chronic hepatitis B or hepatitis C (non-A, non-B) are at increased risk for hepatoma. Because of its antiviral activity, IFN has demonstrated clinical activity in the treatment of hepatitis B and hepatitis C. Currently, IFN alfa is approved only for the treatment of hepatitis C. Numerous studies of IFN alfa therapy have been conducted in patients with chronic hepatitis C. In one large study 166 patients were randomized to receive (1) no treatment, (2) 3 MU of IFN alfa three times weekly for 24 weeks, or (3) 1 MU of IFN alfa three times weekly for 24 weeks.[54] Forty-six percent of patients receiving 3 MU and 28% receiving 1 MU had normalization of serum alanine aminotransferase levels versus only 8% of the untreated patients. The patients receiving 3 MU of IFN also demonstrated the most histologic improvement in paired liver biopsies. However, within 6 months of completing therapy, approximately 50% of patients in both treatment groups relapsed.

Patients in another study were randomized to IFN alfa at a dosage of 2 MU three times weekly or placebo for a 6-month period.[55] Forty-eight percent of the patients treated with IFN had a complete response (normalization of serum aminotransferase levels), and all but two patients demonstrated histologic improvement by liver biopsies. However, serum aminotransferase levels usually returned to pretreatment levels within 6 to

12 months of discontinuing the drug. The patients receiving placebo did not experience significant improvements in serum aminotransferase levels or liver biopsies.

The currently recommended dose of IFN alfa for chronic hepatitis C is 3 MU administered subcutaneously or intramuscularly three times a week for 24 weeks. Additional studies and prolonged follow-up after IFN therapy in patients with chronic hepatitis C are necessary to determine response duration and long-term benefits of therapy.

Hepatitis B

Although IFN is not approved for treating hepatitis B, several studies have been conducted in this area. In one controlled multicenter trial, patients were randomized to receive 6 weeks of prednisone followed by 5 MU of IFN daily for 16 weeks, placebo followed by 5 MU of IFN daily for 16 weeks, or observation with no treatment.[56] More than one third of the patients in both groups that received 5 MU of IFN demonstrated a sustained loss of hepatitis B viral replication. Responding patients also experienced improvement in serum aminotransferase levels and periportal necrosis. The most significant finding, however, was a complete disappearance of the hepatitis B surface antigen (HBsAg) in approximately 10% of the patients treated with IFN.

In another study, the duration of chronic hepatitis B remissions obtained in patients treated on four different IFN alfa protocols (various doses) was evaluated.[57] Overall, 23 patients (36%) responded initially to IFN therapy with loss of hepatitis Be antigen and improved serum aminotransferases. Furthermore, 65% of the responding patients also became negative for HBsAg after losing the hepatitis Be antigen. At a median follow-up of 4.3 years, only 3 of the 23 initial responders had relapsed. However, additional studies using IFN in the treatment of hepatitis B are warranted before FDA approval can be obtained.

Renal cell carcinoma

The role of IFN in the therapy of advanced renal cell carcinoma has been reviewed by Quesada.[58] The overall response obtained with various treatment regimens was 16%. It also appears that frequent administration schedules of IFN (e.g., daily or three times weekly) are more effective than cyclic schedules (e.g., 3- to 4-week rest intervals between doses). Prolonged drug administration over several months may be necessary to obtain a tumor response. Clinical characteristics of patients most likely to respond to IFN therapy include a performance status of better than 90%, prior nephrectomy, no prior therapy, and metastases confined to the lung and mediastinal lymph nodes. Further studies need to be conducted to determine the optimal IFN dose, the efficacy of IFN in combination with other biologic or chemotherapeutic agents, and the impact IFN has on survival in patients with metastatic renal cell carcinoma.

Melanoma

IFN has also been used to treat melanoma. Several phase I and II trials have been conducted with various doses of IFN and have produced overall response rates of 5% to 25% in patients with metastatic melanoma.[59,60] Although most responses were transient, responses obtained in four patients were long-term and lasted more than 22, 32, 36, and 41 months, respectively. Attempts to increase response rates using intralesional IFN administration and combination therapy with chemotherapeutic agents have been only marginally successful to date.[61-64] Concomitant administration of IFN and IL-2 has also been used to treat metastatic melanoma.

Multiple myeloma

Single-agent IFN therapy produces overall response rates of approximately 15% to 20% in patients with multiple myeloma that is refractory to standard therapy.[65-67] Response rates may be somewhat higher in patients who are treatment naive, but they are still lower than the response rates obtained with standard chemotherapy regimens. In an attempt to increase response rates, the combination of IFN therapy and chemotherapeutic agents is being investigated in clinical trials. An objective response rate of 71% was obtained in 30 patients with previously untreated multiple myeloma when IFN alfa was added to standard melphalan-prednisone therapy.[68]

In a recent phase III trial, patients receiving combined IFN, melphalan, and prednisone experienced greater tumor response than patients receiving only combined melphalan and prednisone (95% versus 68%, respectively).[69] Furthermore, the response duration and median survival were longer in the patients receiving IFN, melphalan, and prednisone combined.

Maintenance therapy with IFN after induction therapy with standard chemotherapy regimens has also been investigated. In this study, patients were randomized to maintenance treatment with IFN (3 million IU/m^2 three times weekly) or no treatment following disease stabilization with various standard induction regimens.[70] The patients receiving IFN maintenance therapy experienced longer response (26 months versus 14 months) and longer survival (52 months versus 39 months) than the control patients. These results need to be confirmed in additional studies.

Colorectal cancer

IFN alfa in combination with 5-fluorouracil has demonstrated significant activity in the treatment of advanced colorectal cancer. In the pilot study, 32 previously untreated patients were treated with 5-fluorouracil (5-day continuous infusion followed by weekly bolus therapy) in combination with IFN alfa (9 million IU administered subcutaneously three times per week).[71] Sixty-three percent of patients achieved a partial response, but three toxic deaths were associated with the treatment regimen. Unfortunately, the response rates were not reproducible in a second trial using the same dosage regimen. In this trial 15 of 45 patients experienced a partial response and one patient achieved a complete response, resulting in an overall response rate of 35%.[72] The toxicities associated with the treatment regimen were also greater than those reported in the pilot study. Randomized trials comparing (1) 5-fluorouracil and IFN combined, (2) 5-fluorouracil alone, and (3) 5-fluorouracil and leucovorin combined are currently being conducted to determine the role of this combination regimen in the management of patients with advanced colorectal cancer.

Therapy with IFN alfa has also produced partial responses in patients with non-Hodgkin's lymphoma, cutaneous T-cell lymphoma, malignant glioma, ovarian cancer, carcinoid tumors, and bladder cancer. Further trials need to be conducted to evaluate the utility of IFN therapy in these types of malignancies.

IFN gamma

IFN gamma was recently approved for treating chronic granulomatous disease. Fewer patients with chronic granulomatous disease developed serious infections while receiving IFN gamma (50 $\mu g/m^2$ three times weekly) than patients receiving placebo (22% versus 46%, respectively).[73] Furthermore, there were fewer serious infections in the IFN gamma group (20 infections) than in the placebo group (56 infections). The use of concomitant prophylactic antibiotics in some patients did not negate the beneficial effects of IFN gamma. As a result, it is now strongly recommended that patients with chronic granulomatous disease receive prophylactic IFN gamma to reduce the development of serious infections.

IFN gamma has demonstrated antitumor activity in various malignancies, including ovarian carcimona, renal cell carcinoma, melanoma, CML, and mycosis fungoides. Additional studies with IFN gamma alone and in combination with other BRMs or chemotherapeutic agents need to be conducted to determine its precise role in the treatment of cancer. Phase I studies with IFN beta are in progress, but it is too early to determine whether this agent has significant antitumor activity.

Toxicities

The toxicities experienced with IFN vary based on the type of IFN (alfa, beta, or gamma), dose and route of administration, and patient characteristics such as age and performance status.[34,74] The most common acute toxicity associated with IFN therapy is an acute flu-like syndrome consisting of fever, chills, headaches, myalgias, malaise, nasal congestion, dizziness, and tachycardia. The fevers associated with IFN alfa usually occur within 6 hours of drug administration and may persist for 4 to 8 hours. They occur most commonly with doses of 18 MU or more and may be ameliorated by administering acetaminophen. Instructing patients to administer their IFN dose at bedtime may also palliate some of the acute flu-like side effects. Antihistamines may help minimize the nasal congestion problems associated with IFN. Because patients develop tachyphylaxis to most of the acute symptoms of IFN with continued dosing, palliative agents should be necessary only for the first 7 to 10 days of therapy. However, patients who are receiving IFN on an intermittent schedule may not develop tolerance to the acute flu-like symptoms. Gradually escalating the IFN dose at first over a 7- to 10-day period may help minimize the acute toxicities of therapy. In contrast to the fevers associated with IFN alfa, the fever that follows IFN gamma peaks at 6 to 12 hours after drug administration and lasts longer. Furthermore, continuous daily administration of IFN gamma does not result in disappearance of the acute febrile response.

Patients receiving daily doses of 20 MU of IFN or more may also experience extreme fatigue that manifests as weakness, tiredness, or lack of desire and motivation. These symptoms may be worse in older patients or patients with a poor performance status. If the symptoms are severe enough, they may warrant dosage reductions or drug discontinuation. However, administering the dose on an intermittent schedule (e.g., two to three times weekly) may help to minimize the fatigue. Doses of IFN (10 MU or more) may also produce anorexia and weight loss in as many as 50% of patients. Gastrointestinal toxicities such as nausea, vomiting, diarrhea, and aberrant taste (metallic or salty) may further contribute to the anorexia and weight loss associated with therapy. Antiemetics and antidiarrheals may help minimize some of these side effects.[34,74]

IFN therapy may also be accompanied by various major organ toxicities. For example, extremely high doses of IFN (100 MU or more) may result in central nervous system toxicities including somnolence, lethargy, confusion, and mental slowing. Psychotic reactions and visual or auditory hallucinations have also been reported with IFN doses of 20 MU/m^2 or more. All these symptoms resolve when therapy is discontinued. Hematologic toxicities in the form of leukopenia, thrombocytopenia, and normocytic, normochromic anemia are also associated with IFN therapy but are rarely the dose-limiting toxicities. Elevations in serum glutamic-oxaloacetic transaminase (SGOT) and serum glutamic-pyruvic transaminase (SGPT) occur in approximately one third of patients receiving IFN alfa. With IFN gamma, patients may have elevated alkaline phosphatase and lactic dehydrogenase levels as well as SGOT and SGPT. Serum triglycerides may also be increased with IFN gamma. Finally, dermatologic toxicities are reported with IFN, including mild thinning or loss of hair, transient skin rashes, and excessive growth of eyelashes.[34,74]

The development of serum-neutralizing and -nonneutralizing antibodies after the administration of IFN has been reported. The formation and measurement of neutralizing IFN antibodies vary from patient to patient and may be influenced by several factors, including route of drug administration, duration of treatment and cumulative dose, tumor type, and antibody assay methodology.[75,76] There is some evidence that the IFN alfa-2a preparation may be more immunogenic than IFN alfa-2b. In 559 patients receiving IFN alfa-2a, 27.4% developed neutralizing antibodies while only 2.4% of 423 patients receiving IFN alfa-2b developed antibodies.[77,78] Variability in IFN doses and assay methodology as well as patient heterogeneity may influence these results. However, a more recent study conducted among patients receiving IFN for hepatitis used a single assay method to compare antibody development with IFN alfa-2a and IFN alfa-2b. In this study 20.2% of the patients treated with IFN alfa-2a developed neutralizing antibodies versus only 6.9% of the patients receiving IFN alfa-2b.[79] The clinical effect of neutralizing IFN antibody development remains controversial. However, some evidence suggests that antibody development is associated with decreased antitumor response.[34,42,75,80,81] The possibility of antibody development with prolonged drug administration in diseases such as hairy cell leukemia, CML, KS, and chronic hepatitis was thought to be a problem at first. However, a small study conducted recently demonstrated that the presence of IFN antibodies during long-term therapy is transient and that long-term effectiveness of IFN will probably not be affected by neutralizing antibody development in most patients.[82] Additional studies of antibody development and drug effectiveness need to be conducted to determine their true significance in IFN therapy.

Neutralizing antibodies

Interleukins. The ILs are a group of glycoproteins secreted primarily by activated lymphocytes and macrophages that are involved in the body's immune response. These agents exert their antitumor effects indirectly via complex interactions with host immune effector cells. Currently, 11 interleukins have been described, and some of the IL receptors have been defined. Both the primary cellular sources and the principal effects of these soluble cytokines are discussed in greater detail in Chapter 2. Recombinant DNA technology has allowed large-scale production of several IL products. Recombinant forms of IL-1, IL-2, IL-3, and IL-4 are currently being used in clinical trials, but IL-2 and IL-3 will probably be the first interleukins to become commercially available. IL-2 is discussed in detail in this section, and IL-1 and IL-3 are discussed in the section on colony-stimulating factors (CSFs).

rDNA products

T-cell growth factor

IL-2, also known as T-cell growth factor, is produced by T lymphocytes and stimulates lymphocytic proliferation (B, T, NK, and LAK cells).[83] IL-2 also increases the production of various other lymphokines, including TNF, IFN gamma, and GM-CSF, which further contributes to its tumoricidal activity. Figure 10-2 depicts the cell regulatory activities of IL-2. Numerous clinical trials have been conducted using various dosing schedules and routes of administration of recombinant IL-2. The patients had advanced-stage cancer and failed to respond to standard therapy or were untreatable with standard therapy. The two recombinant IL-2 products used in the clinical trials are aldesleukin (Proleukin®, Cetus Corporation) and teceleukin (Tecin®, Hoffmann-LaRoche). Originally the activity of the two

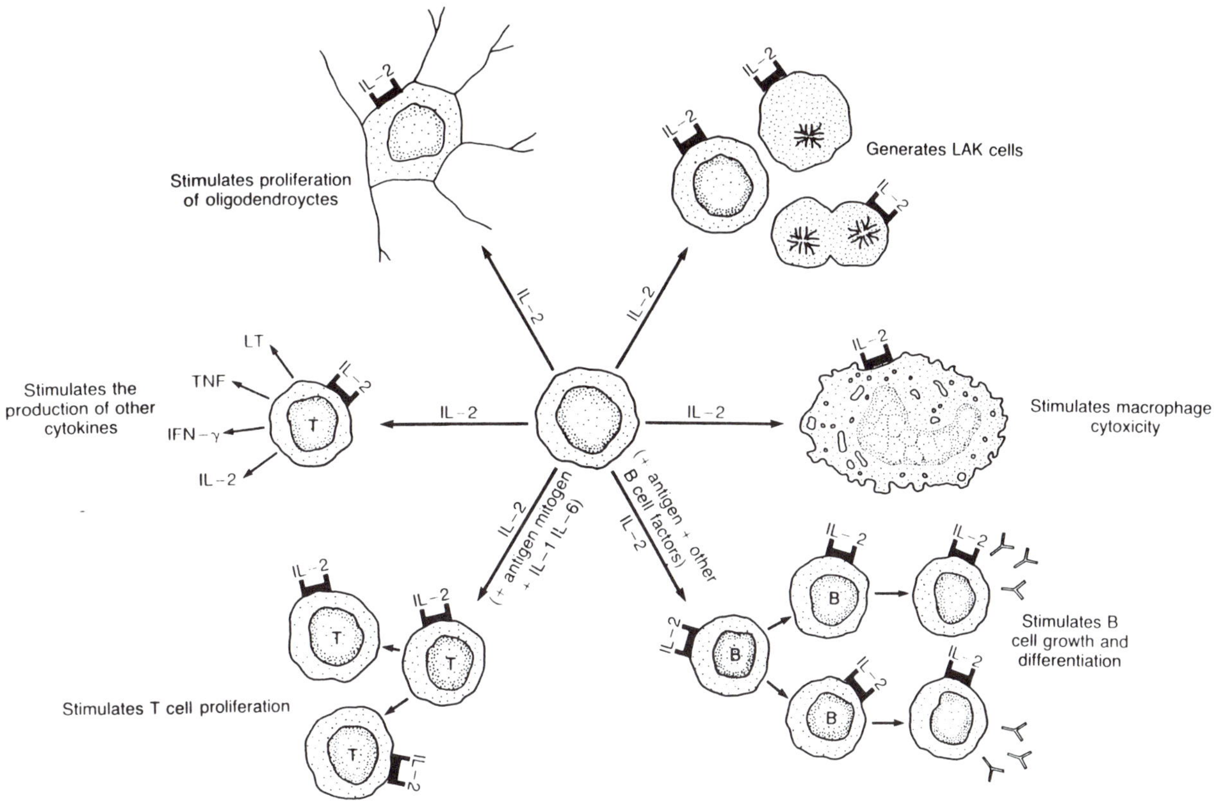

Figure 10-2. Biologic and regulatory activities of interleukin-2

SOURCE: Reprinted with permission from Bakwill FR. Cytokines in cancer therapy. Oxford: Oxford University Press; 1989:93.

different products was measured in Cetus units and Nutley units, respectively. However, in 1988 a standard international unit was authorized by the World Health Organization, and conversion factors for Cetus and Nutley units are available.

Study results

Table 10-4 summarizes the studies conducted with IL-2 therapy alone in patients with advanced malignancies.[84-97] The primary tumor types that have responded to therapy with recombinant IL-2 include renal cell carcinoma and melanoma. Objective responses of 20% to 30% have been reported, and a small subset of patients (less than 5%) has obtained a complete remission with IL-2 therapy. Efforts have been made to increase the clinical activity of recombinant IL-2 through drug administration localized to the tumor area or concomitant administration of chemotherapy agents or biologic agents. Low-dose IL-2 (200 U) injected perilymphatically produced complete or partial disappearance of tumor in six of eight patients with recurrent squamous cell carcinoma of the head and

Table 10-4 Selected Clinical Trials Using IL-2 Alone in Patients with Cancer

Treatment Regimen	No. of Evaluable Patients	CR (%)	PR (%)	Comment	Reference
.01 MU to 0.1 MU/kg[a]IVB every 8 hours or 1 MU to 6 MU/m^2[b]IVB every 8 hours	130	3	14	Responses in renal cell and melanoma only.	84
1 MU to 3 MU/m^2 per day[b] CI or IVB 4 days per week for 4 weeks	23	0	13	Responses in renal cell only.	85
10 MU/m^2[a] IVB three times weekly	41	2	10	All patients had renal cell carcinoma.	86
3 MU to 10 MU/m^2[a] CI for 24 hours weekly for 6 weeks	16	0	6	Response in renal cell only.	87
.01 MU to 1 MU/m^2[a] IVB weekly	17	0	0	Treatment duration ranged from 3 to 33 weeks.	88
1.5 MU to 3 MU/m^2[a] IVB 5 days per week for 4 weeks	26	0	12	Responses reported lymphoma, CLL, and melanoma only.	89
.001 MU to 30 MU/m^2[b] CI for 24 hours weekly for 4 weeks, then twice weekly for 4 weeks	33	0	6	Responses in melanoma only.	90
0.1 MU/kg[a] IVB every 8 hours for 14 doses	46	4	17	All patients had melanoma.	91
1 MU to 16.4 MU/m^2[a] for five doses in a 6-day period	31	0	13	All patients had melanoma. First dose intrasplenic, remaining four doses given IV at different intervals.	92
0.3 MU to 30 MU[b] IVB, CI, or SC weekly for 4 weeks	17	0	0	Pharmacokinetic study.	93
3 MU/m^2 per day[a]	42	6	13	All patients had renal cell carcinoma.	94
0.5 MU twice daily IV followed by 1 MU SC 6 days per week[c]	11	18	9	All patients had renal cell carcinoma. Prolonged IL-2 administration (21 to 240 days).	95
0.5 MU to 5 MU/m^2 per day[a] SC 5 days per week	15	0	0	All patients had renal cell carcinoma. One patient had a minor response.	96
.001 to 30 MU per m^{26} IM, IV, SC weekly	14	0	7	Response in patient with non-Hodgkin's lymphoma.	97

IVB = intravenous bolus; CI = continuous infusion; SC = subcutaneous; IM = intramuscular; CR = complete response; CLL = chronic lymphocytic leukemia; IV = intravenously

[a]Cetus Corporation IL-2.

[b]Hoffmann-LaRoche IL-2.

[c]IL-2 produced by Biogen, Inc., Switzerland.

neck.[98] Intraperitoneal administration of IL-2 with or without LAK cells is being investigated in patients with ovarian cancer, but the results are still quite preliminary.[99,100] Intraventricular administration of IL-2 (6 million IU) has resulted in clearance of tumor cells from the cerebrospinal fluid in nine patients with leptomeningeal carcinoma originating from metastatic melanoma and lung cancer.[101] Two studies have also been conducted on treatment of metastatic melanoma with dacarbazine (850 mg/m^2) in combination with IL-2 (Cetus Corporation) at a dose of 3 MU/m^2 per day continuous infusion.[102,103] The studies used different treatment schedules, but the overall response rates were similar with both regimens (25% and 22%). The beneficial effects of the combination regimen over IL-2 therapy alone remain to be determined in additional clinical trials. Studies with cyclophosphamide in combination with IL-2 are in progress to determine if this regimen will increase tumor responses.[84]

Combination trials

Combinations of IL-2 with IFN alfa or TNF demonstrated synergistic antitumor effects in murine models. As a result, IFN alfa doses of 3 MU to 6 MU/m^2 per day have been used in combination with 1 MU to 6 MU/m^2 of IL-2 (Hoffmann-LaRoche) to treat advanced cancer.[84] Seven complete responses (6%) and 25 partial responses (22%) have been reported. These responses occurred in patients with renal cell carcinoma, metastatic melanoma, and colorectal cancer. Two partial responses were reported in a small study conducted with the combination regimen in patients with head and neck cancer.[104] The results with IL-2 and IFN combined are promising and warrant additional studies. The responses obtained with IL-2 and TNF combined, however, have been somewhat disappointing. TNF in combination with IL-2 has been used to treat advanced cancer in 37 patients.[84] Three patients with renal cell carcinoma experienced a partial response to therapy while one patient with metastatic melanoma had a complete response. Clinical trials with IL-2 in combination with MoAbs are being conducted at the National Cancer Institute (NCI) and are discussed in Chapter 11.

IL-2 therapy has been administered via splenic artery perfusion in an attempt to stimulate LAK cell activity in vivo.[105] Patients demonstrated significant in vivo peripheral LAK cell generation and enhancement of inducible LAK and NK activity that persisted for 16 days after therapy was discontinued following splenic artery perfusion. One of 20 patients also demonstrated a partial regression of renal cell cancer with the regimen. LAK cells and tumor-infiltrating lymphocytes (TILs) stimulated in vitro with IL-2 have been administered concomitantly with IL-2 infusion. This process, commonly referred to as adoptive cellular immunotherapy (ACI), is discussed later in this chapter.

The use of IL-2 in the bone marrow transplant setting and in patients with HIV is under investigation. In vitro data and preliminary results obtained from a small phase I trial both suggest that IL-2 may be used after autologous bone marrow transplantation (BMT) to enhance immune function and stimulate a graft-versus-leukemia effect.[106,107] IL-2 plus zidovudine has been used to boost the immune system in asymptomatic HIV-infected individuals in order to prevent the spread of HIV in activated lymphocytes.[108] Additional studies are necessary to determine the utility of IL-2 in both of these treatment settings.

Toxicities

High-dose recombinant IL-2 therapy has been associated with a variety of toxic effects that are frequently quite serious and require intensive patient care management. These toxicities appear to be dose- and schedule-related, because the greatest toxicities are seen with high-dose continuous infusion therapy. Combination regimens using IL-2 therapy have also been associated with serious toxicities, but most of them may be attributed to IL-2.[109,110] The side effects of IL-2 therapy usually resolve spontaneously after therapy is discontinued.

Capillary leak syndrome

Toxicities associated with high-dose IL-2 therapy are listed in Table 10-5. One of the most common side effects that occurs with IL-2 therapy is a capillary or vascular leak syndrome.[110] Because of an increase in vascular permeability, patients may experience an accumulation of fluid in any organ system. Interstitial edema, fluid retention, and pulmonary lymphoid infiltrates frequently cause patients to require supplemental oxygen; 5% to 10% of patients may require ventilatory support.[110] The capillary leak syndrome may also cause a decrease in intravascular volume in many patients, leading to severe hypotension, which may be further compounded by the decrease in myocardial contractility that is associated with IL-2. As a result, most patients require blood pressure support with fluid supplementation and pharmacologic agents. However, one must be extremely careful with fluid supplementation in patients receiving IL-2 because of increased capillary permeability with fluid accumulation and renal abnormalities caused by impaired renal perfusion.

Table 10-5 Toxicities Associated with Interleukin-2 Therapy

Capillary leak syndrome
Interstitial edema
Fluid retention
Lymphoid infiltrates
Systemic symptoms
Fever
Chills
Rigors
Malaise

Table 10-5 (continued)

Dermatologic toxicities
Diffuse macular erythema
Desquamating rash
Burning, pruritus
Gastrointestinal toxicities
Nausea and vomiting
Diarrhea
Anorexia
Stomatitis
Neurologic toxicities
Hallucinations
Disorientation
Personality and behavior changes
Neuroendocrine toxicities
Elevated corticotropin, cortisol, prolactin, growth hormone
Hypothyroidism
Hematologic toxicities
Lymphopenia and lymphocytosis
Anemia
Thrombocytopenia
Eosinophilia
Bacterial sepsis
Hepatotoxicity
Intrahepatic cholestasis
Elevated liver function enzymes
Prolonged prothrombin time
Cardiotoxicity
Atrial and ventricular arrhythmias
Myocardial infarction
Decreased myocardial contractility
Nephrotoxicity
Prerenal azotemia
Oliguria

Several theories have been proposed as possible mechanisms for the capillary leak syndrome.[110] The first theory is that IL-2 has a direct effect on blood vessel integrity and results in increased vascular permeability. Another is that IL-2 causes the production or release of substances that have direct effects on vascular permeability. A third theory suggests that LAK cells, either stimulated in vivo or administered concomitantly, may be directly or indirectly responsible for the capillary leak syndrome. It may eventually be determined that a combination of these mechanisms contributes to the development of the capillary leak syndrome.

Systemic symptoms

Systemic symptoms, such as fever, rigors, chills, and malaise, usually occur 2 to 4 hours after IL-2 administration and are probably secondary to the release of various other cytokines including IL-1, IL-6, TNF, and IFN gamma.[110,111] These side effects may be minimized with the concomitant administration of acetaminophen, nonsteroidal anti-inflammatory agents, and meperidine for symptomatic relief. However, nonsteroidal anti-inflammatory agents must be administered cautiously in patients receiving IL-2, because they may increase the risk of renal function abnormalities.[110] Diffuse macular erythema, which may progress to a desquamating rash, has also been reported with IL-2 therapy.[112] Antipruritics such as diphenhydramine may help alleviate the burning and pruritus associated with IL-2 dermatologic toxicities. Gastrointestinal toxicities including nausea, vomiting, diarrhea, anorexia, and stomatitis commonly occur with IL-2 administration and may be managed with antiemetics, antidiarrheals, and topical oral anesthetics.

Neurologic

Neurologic toxicities manifested as hallucinations, disorientation, personality changes, and behavioral changes occur relatively frequently with IL-2 and warrant immediate discontinuation of the drug. These symptoms generally resolve after therapy is discontinued, but they may actually progress at first.[110,111] IL-2 also affects the neuroendocrine system, resulting in elevated levels of adrenocorticotropic hormone, cortisol, prolactin, and growth hormone.[113] Hypothyroidism has been reported in several patients when IL-2 was administered in combination with LAK cells.[110] Hematologic toxicities, including anemia, thrombocytopenia, eosinophilia, and initial lymphopenia followed by lymphocytosis, have all been associated with IL-2 therapy.[110,111] There is also some evidence that IL-2 may adversely affect neutrophil activity, resulting in increased patient susceptibility to infection.[114] As many as 10% to 30% of patients receiving IL-2 develop bacterial sepsis. The organisms that are cultured most frequently are *Staphylococcus aureus* and *S. epidermidis.* In an attempt to decrease the morbidity and mortality associated with IL-2 therapy, prophylactic antistaphylococcal antibiotics are now administered routinely during IL-2 treatment courses.

Colony-stimulating Factors. The hematopoietic CSFs are a group of growth factors that are essential for the proliferation, differentiation, maturation, and functional activity of various hematopoietic stem cells. The complex interactions of these agents and their precise role in the human immune system are discussed in Chapter 2. The CSFs that are currently manufactured via recombinant DNA technology are erythropoietin (EPO), GM-CSF, G-CSF, M-CSF, multipotential CSF (multi-CSF or IL-3), IL-1, IL-4, IL-5, and IL-6.[115] Of these, only EPO, GM-CSF, and G-CSF are commercially available. M-CSF, IL-1, IL-3, and IL-4 have only recently entered the clinical arena and their commercial availability is a few years away. The CSFs will have a major impact on cancer therapy; previously untreatable diseases may become treatable and toxicities associated with cancer therapy may be decreased with the use of these agents.

EPO

EPO, which is responsible for the proliferation and maturation of red blood cells (RBCs), was the first CSF approved by the FDA. Doses of 50 to 500 IU/kg three times weekly have been shown to decrease the number of transfusions required and increase the quality of life, with minimal side effects for patients with end-stage renal disease. EPO was also recently approved for treating anemia induced by zidovudine therapy in HIV-positive patients at a dose of 100 U/kg three times weekly. The use of EPO is also being investigated in numerous other treatment settings, including aplastic anemia, the anemia of chronic disease, myelodysplastic syndrome, and the anemia associated with malignancy.[116,117]

GM-CSF

GM-CSF stimulates the production and activity of neutrophils, basophils, eosinophils, monocytes, and early erythroid and megakaryocyte progenitor cells.[118] Recombinant GM-CSF has been derived from three different sources: bacteria (*Escherichia coli*), yeast (*Sacchoromyces cerevisiae*), and mammalian cells (Chinese hamster ovary [CHO] cells). The product manufactured by *E. coli* is nonglycosylated; the yeast product is partially glycosylated, and the CHO cell-derived product is fully glycosylated. Clinically significant differences in the therapeutic effectiveness and toxicity of the GM-CSF products based on recombinant techniques have yet to be established.[119] However, some preliminary evidence suggests that patients may develop antibodies to the yeast-derived GM-CSF product because the yeast sugars serve as haptens and the antibodies react with the unprotected glycosylation sites.[120] GM-CSF antibody development may cause decreased GM-CSF serum concentrations, possibly by increasing plasma clearance. A first-dose effect syndrome characterized by symptomatic hypoxia and hypotension has also been described following *E. coli*-derived GM-CSF in a small subset of patients.[121] The true incidence and mechanism of the first-dose effect of GM-CSF need to be determined.

G-CSF

G-CSF differs from GM-CSF in that it is more lineage specific and selectively stimulates neutrophil production and activity. Table 10-6 further describes the differences between the biologic effects of GM-CSF and G-CSF.[122] The currently available recombinant G-CSF product is derived from *E. coli* and is nonglycosylated. Both recombinant GM-CSF and G-CSF have been used in a variety of malignant and nonmalignant treatment settings, including leukopenia associated with AIDS or

Table 10-6 Comparison of Biologic Effects of G-CSF and GM-CSF

Proliferation/Differentiation	G-CSF	GM-CSF
Granulocytes		
Neutrophil	Effect	Effect
Eosinophil	No effect	Effect
Monocyte-macrophage	No effect	Effect
Neutrophil migration	Enhanced	Inhibited
True lymphokine (product of T cells)	No	Yes
Chromosomal localization	17q	5q
Detectable in serum	Yes	No

SOURCE: Reprinted with permission from Gabrilove JL. Introduction and overview of hematopoietic growth factors. *Seminars Hematology.* 1989; 26(suppl 2):3.

AIDS-related therapy, bone marrow failure secondary to myelodysplasia or aplastic anemia, idiopathic and congenital neutropenias, and leukopenia associated with cancer chemotherapy and bone marrow transplantation.[123] The only FDA-approved indication for recombinant GM-CSF is the acceleration of myeloid engraftment in patients undergoing autologous BMT for the treatment of non-Hodgkin's lymphoma, acute lymphoblastic leukemia, and Hodgkin's disease. The optimal route, dose, and schedule of administration of GM-CSF remain to be determined. The dose presently recommended by the manufacturer is 250 μg/m^2 per day for 14 to 21 days. Recombinant G-CSF received FDA approval for the treatment of neutropenia associated with myelosuppressive anticancer drugs at a recommended dose of 5 μg/kg per day. The optimal dosing regimen for the therapeutic effectiveness of G-CSF also remains to be determined.

BMT trials

Both GM-CSF and G-CSF have been administered in nonrandomized trials conducted in patients undergoing either autologous or allogeneic BMT. Several excellent review articles concerning the use of hematopoietic growth factors in BMT have been published.[124-126] Table 10-7 describes clinical trials conducted with GM-CSF after BMT.[127-136] Unfortunately, these were all relatively small nonrandomized studies, and the results were compared with historical controls. Overall, patients treated with recombinant GM-CSF experienced a decrease in the duration and degree of neutropenia compared with historical controls. However, the interval until the initial appearance of granulocytes in the peripheral blood following transplant was no shorter, indicating that early marrow progenitor cells are

Table 10-7 Selected Clinical Trials of GM-CSF Following Bone Marrow Transplantation

Number of patients		Days to neutrophils ≥ 0.5×10^9/L		Days to Neutrophils ≥ 1.0×10^9/L		Days Febrile		Infections (%)		Reference	GM-CSF Dose (per day)
Tx	Controls	Tx	Controls	Tx	Controls	Tx	Controls	Tx	Controls		
20	20	13	16	NR	NR	NR	NR	NR	NR	127	8 μg/kg/d
12	19	17	24.9	NR	NR	5.0	4.7	58	68	128	100–400 $\mu g/m^2$
6	86[a]	22	25	30	29	11	12	13	30	129	≤30 $\mu g/m^2$
8		14		22		6					≥60 $\mu g/m^2$
27	50[a]	NR	NR	16	21	5	10	18	NR	130	Group 1:
18	43[a]	NR	NR	21	25	11	10	22	NR		30–500 $\mu g/m^2$[b]
											Group 2:
											30–500 $\mu g/m^2$[c]
19	23[a]	15.8	19.2	NR	NR	NR	NR	16	35	131	2–32 μg/kg
5	27[a]	23	24	36	33	NR	NR	40	52	132	< 60 $\mu g/m^2$
16		23		30							≥60 $\mu g/m^2$
41	47	14	21	NR	NR	NR	NR	39	47	133	250 $\mu g/m^2$
17	13	NR	NR	19	23	NR	NR	NR	NR	134	250 $\mu g/m^2$
65	63	19	26	26	33	8	8	17	30	135	NR
41	47	14	21	17	30	4	2	47	39	136	NR
39	40	15	28	NR	NR	NR	NR	70[d]	38[d]	136	NR

NR = not reported; Tx = treatment.

[a]Historic controls.

[b]Did not receive methotrexate.

[c]Received methotrexate for graft-versus-host disease prophylaxis.

[d]Bacterial infections only.

not affected by recombinant GM-CSF or G-CSF.[137] Clinical trials are being conducted in which peripheral blood progenitor cells stimulated with GM-CSF or G-CSF either in vivo or ex vivo are administered concomitantly with bone marrow and a CSF in an attempt to decrease or eliminate the delay in initial granulocyte appearance.[138] The incidence of infection and severity of mucositis in BMT patients was also decreased when GM-CSF was administered after BMT.[128,129,131-133,138] G-CSF has been used in the BMT setting and has produced results comparable with those achieved with GM-CSF.[139-141] In addition, in one of the studies using G-CSF after autologous BMT for Hodgkin's disease, patients experienced a decrease in the severity (but not frequency) of regimen-related mucositis.[139] Issues that remain to be determined with the CSFs in the transplant setting include the following: whether the CSFs stimulate the proliferation of leukemia cells in patients with myeloid leukemias; whether the administration of CSFs in allogeneic transplants will stimulate graft failure or graft-versus-host disease; what effect ex vivo bone marrow purging has on the clinical activity of CSFs; and whether the decrease in duration of neutropenia and incidence of infection will translate into cost savings, decreased morbidity and mortality, or prolonged survival after BMT.

GM-CSF has also been used to stimulate hematopoiesis in patients with marrow graft failure after BMT.[142] Fifty-seven percent (21 of 37) of patients with marrow failure after autologous, allogeneic, or syngeneic BMT obtained an absolute neutrophil count of 500 or more within 2 weeks of treatment with GM-CSF doses ranging from 60 to 1000 $\mu g/m^2$ per day. None of the patients who received chemically purged bone marrow responded to the GM-CSF, whereas all the patients who received bone marrow purged with MoAbs responded to therapy with GM-CSF. The relationship between bone marrow purging and response to CSF therapy needs to be investigated further.

Neutropenia

The duration of neutropenia associated with various standard chemotherapy regimens has also been decreased after administration of recombinant GM-CSF and G-CSF. Table 10-8 summarizes most of the clinical trials conducted with G-CSF and GM-CSF in chemotherapy-induced neutropenia.[143-151] Overall, the duration of neutropenia is reduced by approximately 3 to 9 days when a CSF is administered after standard chemotherapy regimens. A decrease in the number of patient hospitalizations secondary to fever and neutropenia has also been reported in most studies. The incidence and severity of mucositis have also been decreased in patients receiving G-CSF after combination chemotherapy for transitional cell carcinoma of the urothelium.[147] The ability of patients to receive chemotherapy doses on schedule is another potential benefit of using CSFs, but this point has not been demonstrated on a regular basis in the trials conducted to date. The possibility of chemotherapy dose escalation with concomitant CSF administration also needs to be investigated. Further studies addressing these issues and their effects on patient response rates and cures are warranted.

The use of GM-CSF in AIDS patients resulted in an elevation of functional neutrophils and monocytes, but the leukocyte counts returned to baseline values when the drug was discontinued.[152] However, additional studies are needed to determine whether the effects of GM-CSF on neutrophils will result in decreased opportunistic infections. The administration of GM-CSF could also improve AIDS patients' tolerance to the hematologic toxicities associated with drugs used to treat their disease or opportunistic infections.[153-155] Furthermore, in vitro data suggest that GM-CSF may potentiate the antiviral effects of zidovudine.[156] However,

Table 10-8 Selected Clinical Trials of G-CSF and GM-CSF in Chemotherapy-induced Neutropenia

Type of Malignancy	G-CSF or GM-CSF Dose (per day)	Number of Patients		Duration of Neutropenia (days)		Reference
		Tx	Control	Tx	Control	
Various	20–60 μg/kg G-CSF	18	11	6	12	143
Acute leukemia	200 μg/m² G-CSF	48	50	20	28	144
Various	0.3–10 μg/kg G-CSF	31	ND	[a]	ND	145
Urogenital cancer	2 μg/kg G-CSF	32	38	1	6.7	146
Transitional-cell carcinoma of the urothelium	1–60 μg/kg G-CSF	22	NR	1[b]	NR	147
Small cell lung cancer	1–40 μg/kg G-CSF	12	ND	[c]	[d]	148
Sarcoma	4–64 μg/kg GM-CSF	12	12	3.5	7.4	149
Ovarian	1.5–6 μg/kg GM-CSF	9	6	[e]	[e]	150
Acute myeloid leukemia	250 μg/kg GM-CSF	18	39	22.5	25.2	151

ND = not done; NR = not reported; Tx = treatment.

[a]Only 9 of 31 patients developed neutropenia (absolute neutrophil count [ANC] <1,000). Median duration 3.7 days.

[b]Only 6 patients developed neutropenia (ANC <500). All patients were able to receive their complete chemotherapy course when treated with G-CSF.

[c]Eighty percent reduction in the period of absolute neutropenia following G-CSF.

[d]Patients served as their own controls.

[e]Neutropenia decreased significantly in the GM-CSF group.

because macrophages may be infected with HIV, stimulation of these cells by GM-CSF could result in disease progression. Although disease acceleration has not been reported in the clinical trials with GM-CSF, some patients in a single trial did experience an increase in p24 antigen levels when receiving GM-CSF alone during a treatment regimen alternating between GM-CSF plus zidovudine and GM-CSF alone.[157]

Myelodysplastic syndromes

Patients with myelodysplastic syndromes have experienced beneficial effects with GM-CSF and G-CSF in the form of an increased white blood cell (WBC) count, hematocrit, and platelet count.[119,123] Some patients may progress to acute leukemia because the CSF stimulates leukemic cell clones. This result may be difficult to separate from the natural course of the disease, however. The stimulation of leukemic cells may be beneficial in some treatment settings. When GM-CSF is administered before or along with chemotherapy, cell kill may be increased as blast cells in the resting phase of the cell cycle are recruited to the more vulnerable active phase of the cell cycle. A few studies have also been conducted with GM-CSF for treating aplastic anemia.[119,156] Drug-related increases in leukocyte counts have occurred only in patients with some residual bone marrow cellularity, while platelet and RBC counts remained the same. Aplastic anemia may best be managed with a combination of CSFs that have effects on RBCs, WBCs, and platelets. A final setting in which clinical trials have been conducted with G-CSF is the treatment of congenital or cyclic neutropenia.[123,156] In the studies to date, patients have experienced a significant and sustained increase in their neutrophil count and a decrease in subsequent infections.

Side effects

Both GM-CSF and G-CSF are relatively well tolerated by patients at the usual recommended doses. The primary side effects associated with G-CSF include bone pain, myalgias, and skin rash. In the phase II and III trials, approximately one fourth of patients experienced bone pain.[158] This bone pain was reported more frequently with higher doses (20 µg/kg per day and more) and could usually be controlled with non-narcotic analgesics. Transient hypotension after G-CSF administration was reported in approximately 4% of the patients in the phase III trials.

GM-CSF has been associated with more serious toxicities, especially at higher doses. At lower doses (10 µg/kg or less), mild side effects such as low-grade fever, myalgias, phlebitis or pain at the injection site, bone pain, headache, and nausea have been reported.[119,159] Most of these symptoms may be palliated with acetaminophen and supportive care measures. At higher doses (15 µg/kg or more), more serious toxicities have occurred. Pleural or pericardial effusions and ascites secondary to a capillary leak syndrome were reported in the early dose-ranging trials with GM-CSF.[131,149,160,161] Therefore, in patients with preexisting congestive heart failure, pleural effusions, or pericardial effusions, GM-CSF should be administered cautiously because these conditions may be aggravated during therapy. Other side effects that occur with higher dose therapy include severe myalgias and arthralgias, eosinophilia, and elevated liver function tests. Toxicities also appear to be greater with intravenous administration than with subcutaneous administration, especially if the rate of administration is rapid.

IL-1

IL-1 plays an important role in both the inflammatory process and the hematopoietic process.[119,162,163] After the administration of IL-1, patients experience acute symptoms consisting of fever, hypotension (dose-limiting toxicity), headache, myalgias, arthralgias, and tachycardia. IL-1 also produces hematologic responses such as elevated circulating neutrophil levels and prolonged elevated platelet counts. IL-1 has the unique ability to accelerate hematopoietic regeneration in normal cells that have been exposed to either radiation or chemotherapy. This phenomenon could be beneficial in preventing or decreasing both myelosuppression and mucositis in patients receiving radiation therapy. Preliminary results of a phase I and II trial indicate that IL-1 may have myeloprotective effects: patients receiving IL-1 plus fluorouracil had shorter and less severe neutropenia than patients receiving 5-fluorouracil alone.[164] Platelet effects have also been reported with IL-1. In one trial, patients experienced a 50% increase in their platelet counts that began 6 days after therapy and persisted for 18 more days.[165] Additional clinical trials using IL-1 are currently being conducted to determine whether the drug will be useful in patients with bone marrow failure.

IL-3/M-CSF

IL-3 (or multi-CSF) stimulates the differentiation of early progenitor cells, resulting in an increase in RBCs, platelets, monocytes, basophils, eosinophils, and mast cells. Currently, phase I and II clinical trials with IL-3 are being conducted in patients with chemotherapy- or radiation therapy-induced cytopenias, myelodysplastic syndromes, or aplastic anemia. Patients with normal bone marrow function and bone marrow failure secondary to chemotherapy or disease experienced almost a threefold increase in the circulating neutrophil counts.[166,167] A dose-dependent increase in platelet counts that was sustained for 2 to 3 weeks after therapy was also reported. When IL-3 was administered in combination with GM-CSF, the neutrophil response increased dramatically, but the platelet response did not change significantly. The adverse effects that have been reported with IL-3 include fever, headache, chills, and bone pain. Additional trials using IL-3 alone and in combination with GM-CSF need to be conducted to define optimal dosing regimens.

M-CSF stimulates the production and activity of monocytes and macrophages and the release of numerous cytokines (G-CSF, GM-CSF, IFN, IL-1, and TNF).[119] In animal models, M-CSF has demonstrated tumoricidal activity against melanoma and antimicrobial activity against bacteria and fungi. M-CSF also causes terminal differentiation of acute myelogenous leukemia cells in vitro.[168] On the basis of this activity, phase I trials are being conducted with M-CSF. In a phase I trial of M-CSF in patients with metastatic melanoma, one patient experienced an antitumor response. At all dosage levels patients experienced an increase in circulating monocytes and a transient decrease in platelet counts after M-CSF.[169] M-CSF has also shortened the duration of absolute neutropenia after BMT when compared with historical controls.[170,171] Significant antifungal activity has been reported with M-CSF in the BMT setting.[172] Additional studies with M-CSF are warranted.

Tumor Necrosis Factor. TNF is a cytokine that is produced and released by host effector cells during an immune response. Two different genes for TNF have been sequenced and produced via recombinant DNA technology: TNF alpha (also known as cachectin) and TNF beta or lymphotoxin.[173] Various biologic effects including inflammatory reactions, anorexia, and septic shock syndrome are elucidated by TNF because of immune cell activation and the release of other cytokines such as IL-1 and G-CSF.[174,175] TNF also produces antitumor effects via mechanisms that are not fully understood, but direct tumor cell cytotoxicity due to free-radical induction, DNA fragmentation, and nuclear membrane breakdown have all been proposed.[175] Several phase I and II clinical trials using various doses, schedules, and routes of administration of both recombinant TNF products have been conducted (Table 10-9).[176-181] Unfortunately, significant antitumor activity of TNF has not been reported in most of these studies. However, additional clinical trials using TNF in combination with other BRMs or chemotherapy agents are being conducted in an attempt to enhance the antitumor activity of recombinant TNF. The side effects reported in clinical trials with TNF reflect the biologic effects that have been described above and include fever, chills, rigors, headache, fatigue, hypotension, phlebitis, thrombocytopenia, leukopenia, hepatotoxicity, and altered lipid metabolism. The dose-limiting toxicities of TNF appear to be hypotension when bolus intravenous infusions are used and severe local reactions with subcutaneous injections.

Side effects

Adoptive Cellular Immunotherapy

ACI may be defined as the transfer of cells that have been boosted with BRMs in vitro to patients with cancer in an attempt to elicit an antitumor response.[4,15] Two primary techniques are currently being used in clinical trials with ACI. In the first method, peripheral blood leukocytes are removed from patients by apheresis and cultured in vitro with IL-2. The result is the generation of LAK cells. The LAK cells are then administered to the patient either intravenously or intraperitoneally, usually along with the concomitant administration of IL-2 to maintain cytotoxicity. The second method, for producing TILs, is similar, but the lymphocytes cultured in vitro with IL-2 are obtained from tumor specimens instead of from peripheral blood. This type of immunotherapy is extremely labor-intensive for both hospital and laboratory personnel and is also quite expensive.

Cultured cells

Clinical trials using ACI with a combination of IL-2 and LAK cells are described in Table 10-10.[182-190] Overall, objective response rates in the range of 20% to 25% have been obtained in the clinical trials; most responses occur in renal cell carcinoma, melanoma, and colon cancer. The fact that some patients with renal cell carcinoma and melanoma have achieved prolonged complete responses with combined IL-2 and LAK

Table 10-9 Selected Clinical Trials of Recombinant Human Tumor Necrosis Factor

Regimen	No. of Patients	Comment	Reference
5×10^4 to 3.0×10^5 U/m^2 per day continuous infusion for 5 days every 28 days	19	Dose-limiting toxicity leukopenia and thrombocytopenia.	176
1 to 200 μg/m^{2}IV bolus twice weekly alternating with 5 to 250 μg/m^{2}SC for 4 weeks	26	Only 13 patients completed the full treatment course. At doses ≥125 μg/m^2, SC administration caused severe local reactions.	177
4.5 to 645 μg/m^2 as a 24-hour infusion	50	Dose-limiting toxicity hypotension. Severe lethargy and fatigue at doses > 454 μg/m^2. One partial response in breast cancer.	178
5 to 200 μg/m^2 IV infusion days 1–5 every 2 to 3 weeks	27	Dose-limiting toxicity hypotension, rigors, phlebitis. One partial response in pancreatic cancer.	179
5 to 275 μg/m^2 IV infusion three times weekly	53	Dose-limiting toxicity hypotension, fatigue, nausea. One partial response in colon cancer.	180
1 to 200 μg/m^2 alternating IM and IV bolus twice weekly for 4 weeks	20	Two partial responses in renal cell and colon cancer. Relatively well tolerated.	181

IM = intramuscular; IV = intravenous; SC = subcutaneous.

Applications

therapy for more than 63 months is more significant because standard therapies have not done as well in the past. Both continuous infusion and intermittent bolus schedules have been used for IL-2 administration. The

Table 10-10 Selected Clinical Trials Using Interleukin-2 Plus Lymphokine-activated Killer Cells

Type of Malignancy	No. of Patients	Interleukin-2 Dose	Route	Response Rates (%) CR	PR	Ref.
Melanoma/renal cell	55	1 to 1.5 mg/m[2a]	Continuous infusion	4	5	182
Melanoma	32	0.1 MU/kg[a]	Bolus	3	16	183
Melanoma	33	1.25 mg/m^2 per day[a]	Continuous infusion	0	3	184
Various	27	0.1 MU/kg[a]	Bolus	0	7	185
	21	3 MU/m^2 per day[a]	Continuous infusion	0	10	
Renal cell	13	0.01 MU to 0.125 MU/kg for 24 hours[a]	Continuous infusion	0	46	186
Various	29	0.03 MU/kg[b]	Bolus	14	34	187
Various	40	1 MU to 7 MU/m^2 per day[a]	Continuous infusion	0	33	188
Renal cell	51	3 MU/m^2 per day[a]	Continuous infusion	10	18	94
Various	178	0.01 MU to 0.1 MU/kg[a]	Bolus	8	17	189
Various	83	0.1 MU/kg[a]	Bolus	5	12	190

MU = million units.

[a]Cetus Corporation IL-2.

[b]Amgen Corporation IL-2.

toxicities appear to be similar between the two regimens, but the intermittent bolus schedule produces a greater response rate in melanoma and renal cell carcinoma.[184] When combined IL-2 and LAK therapy is compared with IL-2 alone, the overall response rates and toxicities are similar. However, IL-2 plus LAK appears to produce more complete responses than IL-2 alone.[189] The combination of IL-2 and LAK has also been administered by direct intratumoral injection in patients with malignant glioma.[191-194] Tumor regressions have been reported with this regimen, but the effects of therapy on overall survival in patients with glioma remain to be determined.

The combination of IL-2 and TILs has also been used to treat advanced malignancies (Table 10-11).[195,196] In a promising study conducted at the NCI, an overall response rate of 55% was obtained in patients with metastatic melanoma, and one patient experienced a complete remission. Patients who failed with other IL-2 regimens responded to the combination IL-2 and TIL therapy.[189] The combination of IL-2 and TILs appears to be more effective than IL-2 and LAK therapy and produces toxicities similar

Table 10-11 Clinical Trials Using Interleukin-2 Plus Tumor-infiltrating Lymphocytes

Type of Malignancy	No. of Patients	Interleukin-2 Dose	Response Rates (%)		Reference
			CR	PR	
Various	28	1 to 3 x 10^6 U/m^2 per day	0	18	189
Melanoma	20	100,000 U/kg every 8 hours	5	50	190
Melanoma	50	100,000 U/kg every 8 hours	—	38*	183

CR = complete response; PR = partial response; U = units.

*Update of patients in reference 189. Overall response rate = 38%. CR and PR not stratified.

to IL-2 therapy alone. The data on TIL therapy are still extremely preliminary; alternative treatment regimens designed to enhance the response to TIL therapy are being investigated.

Applications

TILs modified by retroviral gene transduction have been used in five patients with metastatic melanoma in an attempt to optimize therapy and define the in vivo distribution and survival of TIL cells.[197] Three of the five patients experienced tumor regression after gene-modified TIL therapy, and the side effects were similar to those reported with combined TIL and IL-2 therapy. Futhermore, it appears that TIL cells survive in the circulation for almost 200 days and in tumor cells for as long as 2 months after administration. As a result, it may be possible to use TILs as vehicles for tumor-directed therapy or for introducing other genes to correct inherited genetic defects. Clinical experiments using TIL cells carrying retrovirally transduced TNF genes are now under way at the NCI.

Affinity Column Apheresis

An additional technique for immune system manipulation involves the use of ACA. In this procedure, a cancer patient's plasma is processed over an affinity column designed either to remove blocking factors of immune responses or activate tumor cytotoxic factors in the plasma.[15] Clinical trials to establish the role of ACA in cancer immunotherapy need to be conducted; the trials to date have produced variable results.

Summary

The immunotherapy of cancer encompasses a broad range of agents used to treat and prevent cancers as well as to treat side effects associated with anticancer therapy. Many of these agents are still under clinical study to determine optimum dose and regimen or to discover new therapeutic uses.

Tumor-associated antigens heighten the potential for selectively identifying cancer cells for destruction through the cellular and humoral immune systems. Vaccines, immunostimulants, biologic response modifiers, and affinity column apheresis have been and are currently under investigation for their antitumor effects.

Biologic response modifiers include the interferons (alfa, beta, and gamma), interleukins (IL-1, 2, 3, and 4), and colony-stimulating factors (erythropoietin; GM-CSF; G-CSF; and IL-1, 4, 5, and 6). Each agent may be used alone in therapy or in combination with other biologic or antineoplastic agents.

References

1. Foley EJ. Antigenic properties of methylcholanthrene-induced tumors in mice of the strain of origin. *Cancer Research.* 1953:13:835–7.
2. Prehn RT, Main JM. Immunity to methylcholanthrene-induced sarcomas. *JNCI.* 1957:18:769–78.
3. Martin EW, Minton JP, Carey LC. CEA-directed second-look surgery in the asymptomatic patient after primary resection of colorectal carcinoma. *Ann Surg.* 1985:202:310–7.
4. Abbas AK, Lichtman AH, Pober JS. Immunity to tumors. In: Wonsiewicz MJ, ed. Cellular and molecular immunology. Philadelphia: W. B. Saunders Company; 1991:336–52.
5. Catalona WJ, Smith DS, Ratliff TL et al. Measurement of prostate-specific antigen in serum as a screening test for prostate cancer. *N Engl J Med.* 1991:324:1156–61.
6. Berchuck A, Bast RC Jr. New directions in diagnosing, monitoring, and detecting epithelial ovarian cancer. *Advances in Oncology.* 1990:6:18–22.
7. Morton DL, Economou J. Cancer immunology and immunotherapy. In: Haskell CM, ed. Cancer treatment. 3rd ed. Philadelphia: W. B. Saunders Company; 1990:102–19.
8. Benjamin E, Leskowitz S. Tumor immunology. In: Immunology: a short course. New York: Alan R. Liss, Inc.; 1988:313–30.

9. Stevenson HC. Adoptive cellular immunotherapy of cancer: an overview. In: Stevenson HC, ed. Adoptive cellular immunotherapy of cancer. New York: Marcel Dekker, Inc.; 1989:1–18.
10. Sell S. The immune system. III. Development of lymphoid organs (ontogeny). In: Immunology, immunopathology and immunity. 4th ed. New York: Elsevier Science Publishing Company, Inc.; 1987:57–68.
11. Dawson M, Moore M. Tumor immunology. In: Roitt I, Brostoff J, Male D, eds. Immunology. 2nd ed. London: Gower Medical Publishing; 1989:18.1–18.18.
12. Borden EC, Sondel PM. Lymphokines and cytokines as cancer treatment. *Cancer.* 1990:65:800–14.
13. Parkinson DR. Interleukin-2 in cancer therapy. *Semin in Oncol.* 1988:15(suppl 6):10–26.
14. Vose BM. Immunomodulating agents. In: Byers VS, Baldwin RW, eds. Immunology of malignant disease. Lancaster: MTP Press Limited; 1987:70–82.
15. Stevenson HC, Tsang KY. Tumor immunology. In: Virella G, Goust JM, Fudenberg HH, eds. Introduction to medical immunology. 2nd ed. New York: Marcel Dekker, Inc.; 1990:513–33.
16. Bohle A, Nowc CH, Ulmer AJ et al. Elevations of cytokines interleukin-1, interleukin-2, and tumor necrosis factor in the urine of patients after intravesical bacillus calmette-guerin immunotherapy. *J Urol.* 1990:144:59–64.
17. Prescott S, James K, Hargreave TB et al. Radio-immunoassay detection of interferon-gamma in urine after intravesical Evans BCG therapy. *J Urol.* 1990:114:1248–51.
18. Droller MJ. Biologic response modifiers in genitourinary neoplasia. *Cancer.* 1987:60:635–44.
19. Lamm DL, Crissmann J, Blumenstein B et al. Adriamycin versus BCG in superficial bladder cancer: a Southwest Oncology Group study. *EORTC GU Group Monograph.* 1989:6:263–70.
20. Martinez-Pineiro JA, Leon JJ, Martinez-Pineiro L Jr et al. Bacillus calmette-guerin versus doxorubicin versus thiotepa: a randomized prospective study in 202 patients with superficial bladder cancer. *J Urol.* 1990:143:502–6.
21. Khanna OP, Son DL, Mazer H et al. Multicenter study of superficial bladder cancer treated with intravesical bacillus calmette-guerin or adriamycin. *Urology.* 1990:35:101–8.
22. Coplen DE, Marcus MD, Myers JA et al. Long-term follow-up of patients treated with 1 or 2, 6-week courses of intravesical bacillus calmette-guerin: analysis of possible predictors of response free of tumor. *Journal Urology.* 1990:144:652–7.
23. Sarosdy MF, Lamm DL. Long-term results of intravesical bacillus calmette-guerin therapy for superficial bladder cancer. *J Urol.* 1989:142:719–22.

24. Orihuela E, Herr HW, Pinsky CM et al. Toxicity of intravesical BCG and its management in patients with superficial bladder tumors. *Cancer.* 1987:60:326–33.
25. Lamm DL, Steg A, Boccon-Gibod L et al. Complications of bacillus calmette-guerin immunotherapy: review of 2602 patients and comparison of chemotherapy complications. *EORTC GU Group Monograph.* 1989:6:335–55.
26. Rawls WH, Lamm DL, Lowe BA et al. Fatal sepsis following intravesical bacillus calmette-guerin administration for bladder cancer. *J of Urol.* 1990:144:1328–30.
27. Deresiewicz RL, Stone RM, Aster JC. Fatal disseminated mycobacterial infection following intravesical bacillus calmette-guerin. *J of Urol.* 1990:144:1331–34.
28. Mutch RS, Hutson PR. Levamisole in the adjuvant treatment of colon cancer. *Clinical Pharmacy.* 1991:10:95–109.
29. Chlebowski RT, Nystrom S, Reynolds R et al. Long-term survival following levamisole or placebo adjuvant treatment of colorectal cancer: a Western Cancer Study Group trial. *Oncology.* 1988:45:141–3.
30. Arnaud JP, Buyse M, Nordlinger B et al. Adjuvant therapy of poor prognosis colon cancer with levamisole: results of an EORTC double-blind randomized clinical trial. *Br J Surg.* 1989:76:284–9.
31. Windle R, Bell PRF, Shaw D. Five-year results of a randomized trial of adjuvant 5-fluorouracil and levamisole in colorectal cancer. *Br J Surg.* 1987:74:569–72.
32. Moertel CG, Fleming TR, MacDonald JS et al. Levamisole and fluorouracil for adjuvant therapy of resected colon carcinoma. *N Engl J Med.* 1990:322:352–8.
33. Clark JW, Longo DL. Biologic response modifiers in cancer therapy. In: Magrath I, ed. New directions in cancer treatment. Berlin: Springer-Verlag; 1989:297–316.
34. Clark JW, Longo DL. Interferons in cancer therapy. Principles & Practice of Oncology Update 1987:4:1–16.
35. Nelson BE, Borden EC. Interferons: biological and clinical effects. *Seminars in Surgical Oncology.* 1989:5:391–401.
36. Peters M. Mechanisms of action of interferons. *Seminars Liver Disease.* 1989:9:235–9.
37. Spiegel RJ. Alpha interferons: a clinical overview. *Urology.* 1989:34(suppl 4):75–9.
38. Thompson JA, Fefer A. Interferon in the treatment of hairy cell leukemia. *Cancer.* 1987:59:605–9.
39. Cheson BD, Martin A. Clinical trials in hairy cell leukemia: current status and future directions. *Ann Intern Med.* 1987: 106:871–8.
40. Ratain MJ, Golomb HM, Bardawil RG et al. Durability of responses to interferon alfa-2b in advanced hairy cell leukemia. *Blood.* 1987:69:872–7.

41. Thompson JA, Kidd P, Rubin E et al. Very low dose α-2b interferon for the treatment of hairy cell leukemia. *Blood.* 1989:73:1440–3.

42. Berman E, Heller G, Kempin S et al. Incidence of response and long-term follow-up in patients with hairy cell leukemia treated with recombinant interferon alfa-2a. *Blood.* 1990: 75:839–45.

43. Martin A, Nerenstone S, Urba WJ et al. Treatment of hairy cell leukemia with alternating cycles of pentostatin and recombinant leukocyte-A interferon: results of a phase II study. *Journal Clinical Oncology.* 1990:8:721–30.

44. Talpaz M, Kantargian H, Kurzrock R et al. Interferon-alpha produces sustained cytogenetic responses in chronic myelogenous leukemia: Philadelphia chromosome-positive patients. *Ann Intern Med.* 1991:114:532–8.

45. Ozer H, Dear K, Testa J et al. Prolonged administration of subcutaneous alfa interferon induces major clinical and complete cytogenetic remissions in untreated Philadelphia chromosome positive (PH+) chronic myelogenous leukemia (CML). *ASCO Proc.* 1990:9:C21. Abstract 783.

46. Volberding PA, Mitsuyasu RT, Golando JP et al. Treatment of Kaposi's sarcoma with interferon alfa-2b (Intron^{R}A). *Cancer.* 1987:59:620–5.

47. DeWit R, Boucher CAB, Veenhof KHN et al. Clinical and virological effects of high-dose recombinant interferon-α in disseminated AIDS-related Kaposi's sarcoma. *Lancet.* 1988: 2(8622):1214–7.

48. Lane HC, Feinberg J, Davey V et al. Anti-retroviral effects of interferon-α in AIDS-associated Kaposi's sarcoma. *Lancet.* 1988:2(8622):1218–22.

49. Kovacs JA, Deyton L, Davey R et al. Combined zidovudine and interferon-α therapy in patients with Kaposi sarcoma and the acquired immunodeficiency syndrome (AIDS). *Ann Intern Med.* 1989:111:280–7.

50. Fischl MA, Uttamchandani RB, Resnick L et al. A phase I study of recombinant human interferon-α 2a or human lymphoblastoid interferon-αnl and concomitant zidovudine in patients with AIDS-related Kaposi's sarcoma. *Journal Acquired Immune Deficiency Syndromes.* 1991:4:1–10.

51. Krown SE, Gold JWM, Niedzwiecki D et al. Interferon-α with zidovudine: safety, tolerance, and clinical and virologic effects in patients with Kaposi sarcoma associated with the acquired immunodeficiency syndrome (AIDS). *Ann Intern Med.* 1990:112:812–21.

52. Miles SA, Wang H, Cortes E et al. Beta-interferon therapy in patients with poor-prognosis Kaposi sarcoma related to the acquired

immunodeficiency syndrome (AIDS): a phase II trial with preliminary evidence of antiviral activity and low incidence of opportunistic infections. *Ann Intern Med.* 1990:112:582–9.

53. Heagy W, Groopman J, Schindler J et al. Use of IFN-γ in patients with AIDS. *Journal Acquired Immune Deficiency Syndromes.* 1990:3:584–90.
54. Davis GL, Balart LA, Schiff ER et al. Treatment of chronic hepatitis C with recombinant interferon alfa: a multicenter randomized, controlled trial. *N Engl J Med.* 1989:321:1501–6.
55. DiBisceglie AM, Martin P, Kassianides C et al. Recombinant interferon alfa therapy for chronic hepatitis C: a randomized, double-blind, placebo-controlled trial. *N Engl J Med.* 1989:321:1506–10.
56. Perrillo RP, Schiff ER, Davis GL et al. A randomized, controlled trial of interferon alfa-2b alone and after prednisone withdrawal for the treatment of chronic hepatitis B. *N Engl J Med.* 1990:323:295–301.
57. Korenman J, Baker B, Waggoner J et al. Long-term remission of chronic hepatitis B after alpha-interferon therapy. *Ann Intern Med.* 1991:114:629–34.
58. Quesada JR. Role of interferons in the therapy of metastatic renal cell carcinoma. *Urology.* 1989:34(suppl):80–3.
59. Creagan ET, Ahmann DL, Frytak S et al. Three consecutive phase II studies of recombinant interferon alfa-2a in advanced malignant melanoma. Updated analyses. *Cancer.* 1987:59:638–46.
60. Legha SS, Papadopoulos MEJ, Plager C et al. Clinical evaluation of recombinant interferon alfa-2a (Roferon-A) in metastatic melanoma using two different schedules. *Journal Clinical Oncology.* 1987:5:1240–6.
61. Gundersen S, Flokkman A. Interferon in combination with vinblastine in advanced malignant melanoma: a phase I-II study. *Cancer.* 1989:64:1617–9.
62. Vorobiof DA, Falkson G, Voges CW. DTIC versus DTIC and recombinant interferon alfa 2b (rIFNα2b) in the treatment of patients with advanced malignant melanoma. *Proceedings American Society Clinical Oncology.* 1989:8:284. Abstract 1105.
63. Bajetta E, Negretti E, Giannotti B et al. Phase II study of interferon alpha-2a (rIFN alpha-2a) and dacarbazine (DTIC) in metastatic melanoma. *Proceedings American Society Clinical Oncology.* 1989:8:286. Abstract 1113.
64. VonWussow P, Block B, Hartmann F et al. Intralesional interferon-alpha therapy in advanced malignant melanoma. *Cancer.* 1988:61:1071–4.
65. Costanzi JJ, Cooper MR, Scarffe JH et al. Phase II study of recombinant alpha-2 interferon in resistant multiple myeloma. *Journal Clinical Oncology.* 1985:3:654–9.

66. Wagstaff JK, Loynds P, Scarffe JH. A phase II study of rDNA human alpha-2 interferon in multiple myeloma. *Cancer Treatment Report.* 1985:69:495–8.
67. Quesada JR, Alexanian R, Hawkins M et al. Treatment of multiple myeloma with recombinant alpha-interferon. *Blood.* 1986:67:275–8.
68. Cooper MR, Fefer A, Thompson J et al. Alpha-2 interferon/melphalan/prednisone in previously untreated patients with multiple myeloma: a phase I-II trial. *Cancer Treatment Report.* 1986:70:473–6.
69. Montuoro A, DeRosa L, DeBlasio A et al. Alpha-2a-interferon/melphalan/prednisone versus melphalan/prednisone in previously untreated patients with multiple myeloma. *British Journal Haematology.* 1990:76:365–8.
70. Mandelli F, Avvisati G, Amadori S et al. Maintenance treatment with recombinant interferon alfa-2b in patients with multiple myeloma responding to conventional induction chemotherapy. *N Engl J Med.* 1990:322:1430–4.
71. Wadler S, Wiernik PH. Clinical update on the role of fluorouracil and recombinant interferon alfa-2a in the treatment of colorectal cancer. *Semin Oncol.* 1990:17 (suppl 1):16–21.
72. Pazdur R, Ajani JA, Patt YZ et al. Phase II study of fluorouracil and recombinant alfa-2a in previously untreated advanced colorectal carcinoma. *Journal Clinical Oncology.* 1990:8:2027–31.
73. International Chronic Granulomatous Disease Cooperative Study Group. A controlled trial of interferon gamma to prevent infection in chronic granulomatous disease. *N Engl J Med.* 1991:324:509–16.
74. Quesada JR, Talpaz M, Rios A et al. Clinical toxicity of interferons in cancer patients: a review. *Journal Clinical Oncology.* 1986:4:234–43.
75. Figlin RA. Biotherapy with interferon-1988. *Semin Oncol.* 1988:15:3–9.
76. Koeller JM. Biologic response modifiers: the interferon alfa experience. *Am J Hospital Pharmacy.* 1989:46(suppl 2):S11–S15.
77. Jones GJ, Itri LM. Safety and tolerance of recombinant alfa-2b (Roferon-A) in cancer patients. *Cancer.* 1986:57(suppl 2):1709–15.
78. Spiegel RJ, Spicehandler JR, Jacobs SL et al. Low incidence of serum neutralizing factors in patients receiving recombinant alfa-2b interferon (Intron-A). *Am J Med.* 1986:80:223–7.
79. Antonelli G, Currenti M, Turriziani O et al. Neutralizing antibodies to interferon-α: relative frequency in patients treated with different interferon preparations. *J Infect Dis.* 1991:163:882–5.
80. Freund M, VonWussow P, Diedrich H et al. Recombinant human interferon (IFN) in chronic myelogenous leukemia: dose dependency of response and frequency of neutralizing anti-interferon antibodies. *British Journal Haematology.* 1989:72:350–6.

81. Steis RG, Smith II JW, Urba WJ et al. Resistance to recombinant interferon alfa-2a in hairy-cell leukemia associated with neutralizing anti-interferon antibodies. *N Engl J Med.* 1988:318:1409–13.
82. Steis RG, Smith II JW, Urba WJ et al. Loss of interferon antibodies during prolonged continuous interferon-α2a therapy in hairy cell leukemia. *Blood.* 1991:77(Feb 15):792–8.
83. Kintzel PE, Calis KA. Recombinant interleukin-2: a biological response modifier. *Clinical Pharmacy.* 1991:10:110–28.
84. Rosenberg SA, Lotze MT, Yang JC et al. Experience with the use of high-dose interleukin-2 in the treatment of 652 cancer patients. *Ann Surg.* 1989:210:474–84.
85. Sosman JA, Kohler PC, Hank J et al. Repetitive weekly cycles of recombinant human interleukin-2: responses of renal cell carcinoma with acceptable toxicity. *JNCI.* 1988:80:60–3.
86. Bukowski RM, Goodman P, Crawford D et al. Phase II trial of high-dose intermittent interleukin-2 in metastatic renal cell carcinoma: a Southwest Oncology Group study. *JNCI.* 1990:82:143–6.
87. Richards JM, Barker E, Latta J et al. Phase I study of weekly 24-hour infusions of recombinant human interleukin-2. *JNCI.* 1988:80:1325–8.
88. Atkins MB, Gould JA, Allegretta M et al. Phase I evaluation of recombinant interleukin-2 in patients with advanced malignant disease. *Journal Clinical Oncology.* 1986:4:1380–91.
89. Allison MAK, Jones SE, McGuffey P. Phase II trial of outpatient interleukin-2 in malignant lymphoma, chronic lymphocytic leukemia, and selected solid tumors. *Journal Clinical Oncology.* 1989:7:75–80.
90. Creekmore SP, Harris JE, Ellis TM et al. A phase I clinical trial of recombinant interleukin-2 by periodic 24-hour intravenous infusions. *Journal Clinical Oncology.* 1989:7:276–84.
91. Parkinson DR, Abrams JS, Wiernik PH et al. Interleukin-2 therapy in patients with metastatic malignant melanoma: a phase II study. *Journal Clinical Oncology.* 1990:8:1650–6.
92. Thatcher N, Dazzi H, Johnson RJ et al. Recombinant interleukin-2 (rIL-2) given intrasplenically and intravenously for advanced malignant melanoma: a phase I and II study. *British Journal Cancer.* 1989:60:770–4.
93. Thompson JA, Lee DJ, Cox WW et al. Recombinant interleukin 2 toxicity, pharmacokinetics, and immunomodulatory effects in a phase I trial. *Cancer Research.* 1987:47:4202–7.
94. Negrier S, Philip T, Stoter G et al. Interleukin-2 with or without LAK cells in metastatic renal cell carcinoma: a report of a European multicenter study. *European Journal Cancer Clinical Oncology.* 1989:25(suppl 3):S21–S28.

95. Marumo K, Muraki J, Ueno M et al. Immunologic study of human recombinant interleukin-2 (low-dose) in patients with advanced renal cell carcinoma. *Urology.* 1989:33:219–25.
96. Whitehead RP, Ward D, Hemingway L et al. Subcutaneous recombinant interleukin-2 in a dose escalating regimen in patients with metastatic renal cell adenocarcinoma. *Cancer Research.* 1990:50:6708–15.
97. Urba WJ, Steis RG, Longo DL et al. Immunomodulatory properties and toxicity of interleukin 2 in patients with cancer. *Cancer Research.* 1990:50:185–92.
98. Cortesina G, DeStefani A, Grovarelli M et al. Treatment of recurrent squamous cell carcinoma of the head and neck with low doses of interleukin-2 injected perilymphatically. *Cancer.* 1988:62:2482–5.
99. Stewart JA, Belinson JL, Moore AL et al. Phase I trial of intraperitoneal recombinant interleukin-2/1ymphokine-activated killer cells in patients with ovarian cancer. *Cancer Research.* 1990:50:6302–10.
100. Chapman PB, Kolitz JE, Hakes TB et al. A phase I trial of intraperitoneal recombinant interleukin-2 in patients with ovarian carcinoma. *Investigational New Drugs.* 1988:6:179–88.
101. Moser RP, Bruner JM, Grimm EA. Biologic therapy for brain tumors. *Cancer Bulletin.* 1991:43:117–26.
102. Stoter G, Shiloni E, Aamdal S et al. Sequential administration of recombinant human interleukin-2 and dacarbazine in metastatic melanoma: a multicentre phase II study. *European Journal Cancer Clinical Oncology.* 1989:25(suppl 3):S41–S43.
103. Shiloni E, Pouillart P, Janssens J et al. Sequential dacarbazine chemotherapy followed by recombinant interleukin-2 in metastatic melanoma: a pilot multicentre phase I-II study. *European Journal Cancer Clinical Oncology.* 1989:25(suppl 3):S45–S49.
104. Schantz SP, Clayman GL, Dimery I et al. Combination interleukin-2 and interferon-alpha in head and neck cancer. *Cancer Bulletin.* 1991:43:133–8.
105. Klasa RJ, Silver HKB, Kong S. In vivo induction of lymphokine-activated killer cells by interleukin-2 splenic artery perfusion in advanced malignancy. *Cancer Research.* 1990:50:4906–10.
106. Hauch M, Gazzola MV, Small T et al. Anti-leukemia potential of interleukin-2 activated natural killer cells after bone marrow transplantation for chronic myelogenous leukemia. *Blood.* 1990:75:2250–62.
107. Blaise D, Olive D, Stoppa AM et al. Hematologic and immunologic effects of the systemic administration of recombinant interleukin-2 after autologous bone marrow transplantation. *Blood.* 1990:76:1092–97.

108. Schwartz DH, Skowron G, Merigan TC. Safety and effects of interleukin-2 plus zidovudine in asymptomatic individuals infected with human immunodeficiency virus. *Journal Acquired Immune Deficiency Syndromes.* 1991:4:11-23.
109. Chang AE, Rosenberg SA. Overview of interleukin-2 as an immunotherapeutic agent. *Seminars Surgical Oncology.* 1989:5:385-90.
110. Siegel JP, Puri RK. Interleukin-2 toxicity. *Journal Clinical Oncology.* 1991:9:694-704.
111. Crum E. Biological-response modifier-induced emergencies. *Semin Oncol.* 1989:16:579-87.
112. Gaspari AA, Lotze MT, Rosenberg SA et al. Dermatologic changes associated with interleukin 2 administration. *JAMA.* 1987:258:1624-9.
113. Denicoff KD, Durkin TM, Lotze MT et al. The neuroendocrine effects of interleukin-2 treatment. *Journal of Clinical Endocrinology Metabolism.* 1989:69:402-10.
114. Klempner MS, Noring R, Mier JW et al. An acquired chemotactic defect in neutrophils from patients receiving interelukin-2 immunotherapy. *N Engl J Med.* 1990:322:959-65.
115. Metcalf D. Haemopoietic growth factors, 1. *Lancet.* 1989:1(8642):825-7.
116. Groopman JE, Molina JM, Scadden DT. Hematopoietic growth factors: biology and clinical applications. *N Engl J Med.* 1989:321:1449-59.
117. Metcalf D. Haemopoietic growth factors. 2. Clinical applications. *Lancet.* 1989:1(8643):885-7.
118. Robinson BE, Quesenberry PJ. Hematopoietic growth factors: overview and clinical applications. Part 2. *Am J Med Sci.* 1990:300(4):237-44.
119. Wallerstein R Jr, Deisseroth A. Hematopoietic growth factors in cancer treatment. Principles & Practice of Oncology Updates 1990:4:1-16.
120. Gribben JG, Devereux S, Thomas NSB et al. Development of antibodies to unprotected glycosylation sites on recombinant human GM-CSF. *Lancet.* 1990:335:434-7.
121. Lieschke GJ, Cebon J, Morstyn G. Characterization of the clinical effects after the first dose of bacterially synthesized recombinant human granulocyte-macrophage colony-stimulating factor. *Blood.* 1989:74:2634-43.
122. Gabrilove JL. Introduction and overview of hematopoietic growth factors. *Seminars Hematology.* 1989:26(suppl 2):1-4.
123. Golde DW. Overview of myeloid growth factors. *Seminars Hematology.* 1990:27(suppl 3):1-7.

124. Aurer I, Ribas A, Gale RP. What is the role of recombinant colony stimulating factors in bone marrow transplantation? *Bone Marrow Transplantation.* 1990:6:79–87.
125. Mertelsmann R, Herrmann F, Hecht T et al. Hematopoietic growth factors in bone marrow transplantation. *Bone Marrow Transplantation.* 1990:6:73–7.
126. Goldstone AH, Khwaja A. The role of haemopoietic growth factors in bone marrow transplantation. *Leukemia Research.* 1990:14:721–9.
127. Powles R, Smith C, Milan S et al. Human recombinant GM-CSF in allogeneic bone marrow transplantation for leukaemia: double-blind placebo-controlled trial. *Lancet.* 1990:336: 1417–20.
128. Devereaux S, Linch DC, Gribben JG et al. GM-CSF accelerates neutrophil recovery after autologous bone marrow transplantation for Hodgkin's disease. *Bone Marrow Transplantation.* 1989:4:49–54.
129. Nemunaitis J, Singer JW, Buckner CD et al. Use of recombinant human granulocyte-macrophage colony-stimulating factor in autologous marrow transplantation for lymphoid malignancies. *Blood.* 1988:72:834–6.
130. Nemunaitis J, Buckner CD, Appelbaum FR et al. Phase I/II trial of recombinant human granulocyte-macrophage colony-stimulating factor following allogeneic bone marrow transplantation. *Blood.* 1991:77:2065–71.
131. Brandt SJ, Peters WP, Atwater SK et al. Effect of recombinant human granulocyte-macrophage colony-stimulating factor on hematopoietic reconstitution after high-dose chemotherapy and autologous bone marrow transplantation. *N Engl J Med.* 1988:318:869–76.
132. Blazar BR, Kersey JH, McGlave PB et al. In vivo administration of recombinant human granulocyte/macrophage colony-stimulating factor in acute lymphoblastic leukemia patients receiving purged autografts. *Blood.* 1989:73:849–57.
133. Gorin NC, Coiffier B, Hayat M et al. RHU GM-CSF shortens aplasia duration after ABMT in non-Hodgkin's lymphoma: a randomized placebo-controlled double-blind study. *Bone Marrow Transplantation.* 1991:7(suppl 2):82.
134. Nemunaitis J, Singer JW, Buckner CD et al. Preliminary analysis of a randomized, placebo-controlled trial of rhGM-CSF in autologous bone marrow transplantation. *Proceedings American Society Clinical Oncology.* 1990:9:10. Abstract 34.
135. Nemunaitis J, Rabinowe SN, Singer JW et al. Recombinant granulocyte-macrophage colony-stimulating factor after antologous bone marrow transplantation for lymphoid cancer. *N Engl J Med.* 1991:324:1773–8.

136. Rabinowe SN, Nemunaitis J, Armitage J et al. The impact of myeloid growth factors on engraftment following autologous bone marrow transplantation for malignant lymphoma. *Seminars Hematology.* 1991:28:6-16.

137. Peters WP. The myeloid colony-stimulating factors: introduction and overview. *Seminars Hematology.* 1991:28(suppl 2):1-5.

138. Gianni AM, Bregni M, Stern AC et al. Granulocyte-macrophage colony-stimulating factor to harvest circulating haemopoietic stem cells for autotransplantation. *Lancet.* 1989:2(8663):580-5.

139. Taylor KM, Jagannath S, Spitzer G et al. Recombinant human granulocyte colony-stimulating factor hastens granulocyte recovery after high-dose chemotherapy and autologous bone marrow transplantation in Hodgkin's disease. *Journal Clinical Oncology.* 1989:7:1791-9.

140. Sheridan WP, Wolf M, Lusk J et al. Granulocyte colony-stimulating factor and neutrophil recovery after high-dose chemotherapy and autologous bone marrow transplantation. *Lancet.* 1989:2(8668):891-5.

141. Masaoka T, Takaku F, Kato S et al. Recombinant human granulocyte colony-stimulating factor in allogeneic bone marrow transplantation. *Experimental Hematology.* 1989:17:1047-50.

142. Nemunaitis J, Singer JW, Buckner CD et al. Use of recombinant human granulocyte-macrophage colony-stimulating factor in graft failure after bone marrow transplantation. *Blood.* 1990:76:245-53.

143. Neidhart J, Mangalik A, Kohler W et al. Granulocyte colony-stimulating factor stimulates recovery of granulocytes in patients receiving dose-intensive chemotherapy without bone marrow transplantation. *Journal Clinical Oncology.* 1989:7:1685-92.

144. Ohno R, Tomonaga M, Kobayashi T et al. Effect of granulocyte colony-stimulating factor after intensive induction therapy in relapsed or refractory acute leukemia. *N Engl J Med.* 1990:323:871-7.

145. Morstyn G, Campbell L, Lieschke G et al. Treatment of chemotherapy-induced neutropenia by subcutaneously administered granulocyte colony-stimulating factor with optimization of dose and duration of therapy. *Journal Clinical Oncology.* 1989:7:1554-62.

146. Kotake T, Miki T, Akaza H et al. Effect of recombinant granulocyte colony-stimulating factor (rG-CSF) on chemotherapy-induced neutropenia in patients with urogenital cancer. *Cancer Chemotherapy Pharmacology.* 1991:27:253-7.

147. Gabrilove JL, Jakubowski A, Scher H et al. Effect of granulocyte colony-stimulating factor on neutropenia and associated morbidity due to chemotherapy for transitional-cell carcinoma of the urothelium. *N Engl J Med.* 1988:318:1414-22.

148. Bronchud MH, Scarffe JH, Thatcher N et al. Phase I/II study of recombinant human granulocyte colony-stimulating factor in patients receiving intensive chemotherapy for small cell lung cancer. *British Journal Cancer.* 1987:56:809–13.
149. Antman KS, Griffin JD, Elias A et al. Effect of recombinant human granulocyte-macrophage colony-stimulating factor on chemotherapy-induced myelosuppression. *N Engl J Med.* 1988:319:593–8.
150. deVries EGE, Biesma B, Willemse PHB et al. A double-blind placebo-controlled study with granulocyte-macrophage colony-stimulating factor during chemotherapy for ovarian carcinoma. *Cancer Research.* 1991:51:116–22.
151. Bettelheim P, Valent P, Andreeff M et al. Recombinant human granulocyte-macrophage colony-stimulating factor in combination with standard induction chemotherapy in de novo acute myeloid leukemia. *Blood.* 1991:77:700–11.
152. Groopman JE, Mitsuyasu RT, DeLeo MJ et al. Effect of recombinant human granulocyte-macrophage colony-stimulating factor on myelopoiesis in the acquired immunodeficiency syndrome. *N Engl J Med.* 1987:317:593–8.
153. Grossberg HS, Bonnem EM, Buhles WC. GM-CSF with ganciclovir for the treatment of CMV retinitis in AIDS. *N Engl J Med.* 1989:320:1560.
154. Scadden DT, Bering HA, Levine JD et al. Granulocyte-macrophage colony-stimulating factor mitigates the neutropenia of combined interferon alfa and zidovudine treatment of acquired immune deficiency syndrome-associated Kaposi's sarcoma. *Journal Clinical Oncology.* 1991:9:802–8.
155. Miles SA, Mitsuyasu RT, Moreno J et al. Combined therapy with recombinant granulocyte colony-stimulating factor and erythropoietin decreases hematologic toxicity from zidovudine. *Blood.* 1991:77:2109–17.
156. Groopman JE, Molina JM, Scadden DT. Hematopoietic growth factors: biology and clinical applications. *N Engl J Med.* 1989:321:1449–59.
157. Pluda JM, Yarchoan Y, McAtee N et al. The use of an alternating regimen of AZT and subcutaneous (SC) GM-CSF in patients with severe HIV infection and leukopenia. In: Abstracts of the V International Conference on AIDS. Ottawa: International Development Research Centre, 1989:406. Abstract 329.
158. Amgen, Inc. Neupogen package insert. Thousand Oaks, CA. 1991 Feb.
159. Immunex Corporation. Leukine package insert. Seattle, WA. 1991 Mar and Hoechst-Roussel Pharmaceuticals, Inc. Prokine package insert. Somerville, NJ. 1991 Mar.

160. Steward WP, Austin R, Scarffe JH et al. Phase I study of recombinant DNA granulocyte-macrophage colony-stimulating factor (rGM-CSF). *British Journal Cancer.* 1988:57:258.
161. Lieschke GJ, Maher D, Cebon J et al. Effects of subcutaneously administered bacterially synthesized recombinant human granulocyte-macrophage colony stimulating factor in patients with advanced malignancy. *Ann Intern Med.* 1989:110:357–64.
162. Starnes Jr, HF. Biological effects and possible clinical applications of interleukin-1. *Seminars Hematology.* 1991:28(suppl 2):34–41.
163. Dinavello CA. Interleukin-1 and interleukin-1 antagonism. *Blood.* 1991:77:1627–52.
164. Crown J, Kemeny N, Jakubowski A et al. Phase I-II trial of recombinant human interleukin-1β (IL-1) in patients with metastatic colorectal cancer receiving 5-fluorouracil. *Blood.* 1989:74:(suppl):15a.
165. Tewari A, Buhles WC Jr, Starnes HF Jr. Preliminary report: effects of interleukin-1 on platelet counts. *Lancet.* 1990:336:712–4.
166. Hoelzer D, Seipelt G, Ganser A. Interleukin 3 alone and in combination with GM-CSF in the treatment of patients with neoplastic disease. *Seminars Hematology.* 1991:28(suppl 2):17–24.
167. Oster W, Frisch J, Nicolay U et al. Interleukin-3: biologic effects and clinical impact. *Cancer.* 1991:67:2712–7.
168. Bajorin DF, Cheung NKV, Houghton AN. Macrophage colony-stimulating factor: biological effects and potential applications for cancer therapy. *Seminars Hematology.* 1991:28(suppl 2):42–8.
169. Bajorin DF, Jakubowski A, Cody B et al. Recombinant macrophage colony stimulating factor (rhM-CSF): a phase I trial in patients with metastatic melanoma. *Proceedings American Society Clinical Oncology.* 1990:9:183. Abstract.
170. Peters WP, Kurtzberg J, Rao M et al. Effects of recombinant human macrophage colony stimulating factor (rHuM-CSF) on hematopoiesis following high dose chemotherapy and autologous bone marrow support. *Blood.* 1989:74(suppl):269a. Abstract.
171. Masaoka T, Shibata H, Ohno R et al. Double-blind test of human urinary macrophage colony-stimulating factor for allogeneic and syngeneic bone marrow transplantation: effectiveness of treatment and 2-year follow-up for relapse of leukaemia. *British Journal Haematology.* 1990:76:501–5.
172. Meyers JD, Buckner CD, Bianco JC et al. Phase I/II trial of recombinant human macrophage-colony stimulating factor (M-CSF) in patients with invasive fungal infection. *Blood.* 1990:76:158a. Abstract 625.
173. Cerami A. Cachectin/TNF and the immune response. *Advances in Oncology.* 1990:6:5–9.

174. Beutler B, Cerami A. Cachectin: more than a tumor necrosis factor. *N Engl J Med.* 1987:316:379–85.
175. Grunfeld C, Palladino MA. Tumor necrosis factor: immunologic, antitumor, metabolic, and cardiovascular activities. *Advances Internal Medicine.* 1990:35:45–72.
176. Sherman ML, Spriggs DR, Arthur KA et al. Recombinant human tumor necrosis factor administered as a five-day continuous infusion in cancer patients: phase I toxicity and effects on lipid metabolism. *Journal Clinical Oncology.* 1988:6:344–50.
177. Chapman PB, Lester TJ, Casper ES et al. Clinical pharmacology of recombinant human tumor necrosis factor in patients with advanced cancer. *Journal Clinical Oncology.* 1987:5:1942–51.
178. Spriggs DR, Sherman ML, Michie H et al. Recombinant human tumor necrosis factor administered as a 24-hour intravenous infusion. A phase I and pharmacologic study. *JNCI.* 1988:80:1039–44.
179. Creagan ET, Kovach JS, Moertel CG et al. A phase I clinical trial of recombinant human tumor necrosis factor. *Cancer.* 1988:62:2467–71.
180. Schiller JH, Storer BE, Witt PL et al. Biological and clinical effects of intravenous tumor necrosis factor-α administered three times weekly. *Cancer Research.* 1991:51:1651–8.
181. Blick M, Sherwin SA, Rosenblum M et al. Phase I study of recombinant tumor necrosis factor in cancer patients. *Cancer Research.* 1987:47:2986–9.
182. Gaynor ER, Weiss GR, Margolin KA et al. Phase I study of high-dose continuous-infusion recombinant interleukin-2 and autologous lymphokine-activated killer cells in patients with metastatic or unresectable malignant melanoma and renal cell carcinoma. *JNCI.* 1990:82:1397–1402.
183. Dutcher JP, Creekmore S, Weiss GR et al. A phase II study of interleukin-2 and lymphokine-activated killer cells in patients with metastatic malignant melanoma. *Journal Clinical Oncology.* 1989:7:477–85.
184. Dutcher JP, Gaynor ER, Boldt DH et al. A phase II study of high-dose continuous infusion interleukin-2 with lymphokine-activated killer cells in patients with metastatic melanoma. *Journal Clinical Oncology.* 1991:9:641–8.
185. Clark JW, Smith JW II, Steis RG et al. Interleukin 2 and lymphokine-activated killer cell therapy: analysis of a bolus interleukin 2 and a continuous infusion interleukin 2 regimen. *Cancer Research.* 1990:50:7343–50.
186. Wang J, Walle A, Gordon B et al. Adoptive immunotherapy for Stage IV renal cell carcinoma: a novel protocol utilizing periodate and interleukin-2-activated autologous leukocytes and continuous infusions of low-dose interleukin-2. *Am J Med.* 1987:83:1016–23.

187. Eberlein TJ, Schoof DD, Jung SE et al. A new regimen of interleukin 2 and lymphokine-activated killer cells. Efficacy without significant toxicity. *Arch Intern Med.* 1988:148:2571-6.
188. West WH, Tauer KW, Yannelli JR et al. Constant-infusion recombinant interleukin-2 in adoptive immunotherapy of advanced cancer. *N Engl J Med.* 1987:316:898-905.
189. Rosenberg SA. Adoptive cellular therapy in patients with advanced cancer. *Biologic Therapy of Cancer Updates.* 1991:1:1-15.
190. Hawkins MJ. PPO Updates IL-2/LAK. *Principles Practice Oncology.* 1989:3:1-14.
191. Jacobs SK, Wilson DJ, Kornblith PL et al. Interleukin-2 or autologous lymphokine-activated killer cell treatment of malignant glioma: phase I trial. *Cancer Research.* 1986:46:2101-4.
192. Barba D, Saris SC, Holder C et al. Intertumoral LAK cell and interleukin-2 therapy of human gliomas. *J Neurosurg.* 1989:70:175-82.
193. Lillehei KO, Mitchell DH, Johnson SD et al. Long-term follow-up of patients with recurrent malignant gliomas treated with adjuvant adoptive immunotherapy. *Neurosurgery.* 1991:28:16-23.
194. Yoshida S, Tanaka R, Takai N et al. Local administration of autologous lymphokine-activated killer cells and recombinant interleukin-2 to patients with malignant brain tumors. *Cancer Research.* 1988:48:5011-16.
195. Kradin RL, Lazarus DS, Dubinett SM et al. Tumor-infiltrating lymphocytes and interleukin-2 in treatment of advanced cancer. *Lancet.* 1989:1(8638):577-80.
196. Rosenberg SA, Packard BS, Aebersold PM et al. Use of tumor-infiltrating lymphocytes and interleukin-2 in the immunotherapy of patients with metastatic melanoma: a preliminary report. *N Engl J Med.* 1988:319:1676-80.
197. Rosenberg SA, Aebersold P, Cornetta K et al. Gene transfer into humans—immunotherapy of patients with advanced melanoma, using tumor-infiltrating lymphocytes modified by retroviral gene transduction. *N Engl J Med.* 1990:323:570-8.

Self-Study Questions

1. Which of the following is true of alfa interpheron therapy for AIDS-related Kaposi's sarcoma?

   A. Fewer than 20% of patients experience an objective response.
   B. Advanced KS patients are more likely to respond to therapy.
   C. Tumor response is unrelated to the dose.
   D. Interferon suppresses the human immunodeficiency virus in vitro and in vivo.

   Answer: 1. D

2. Interferons induce 2,5-A synthetase, protein kinase, and phosphodiesterase—which are associated with what types of antitumor effect?

   Answer: 2. Inhibit RNA, DNA, and protein synthesis.

3. Interferon alfa 2b appears to be more immunogenic than interferon alfa 2a.

   A. True.
   B. False.

   Answer: 3. B

4. What would be the purpose of administering interferon alfa at bedtime?

   Answer: 4. To minimize patient experience of side effects.

5. Interleukin-2 has proven effective in early clinical trials against which two cancers?

   Answer: 5. Renal cell and melanoma.

6. Interleukin-2 exerts its antitumor effects directly and indirectly by stimulating natural killer cell production and various other cytokines.

   A. True.
   B. False.

   Answer: 6. A

7. Why must nonsteroidal anti-inflammatory agents be administered with caution when palliating side effects to interleukin-2 therapy?

   Answer: 7. NSAIDs could increase the risk of renal function abnormalities.

8. C

8. Which is one of the most common toxicities associated with interleukin-2 antitumor therapy?

   A. Headache.
   B. Fungal sepsis.
   C. Capillary leak syndrome.
   D. Constipation.

9. A

9. Interleukin-1 can produce acute symptoms of fever, hypotension, headache, myalgia, arthralgias, and tachycardia.

   A. True.
   B. False.

10. B

10. Both granulocyte colony-stimulating factor (G-CSF) and granulocyte-macrophage colony-stimulating factor (GM-CSF) stimulate neutrophil production; however, GM-CSF is more selective and lineage specific.

   A. True.
   B. False.

11. D

11. Which of the following colony-stimulating factors is responsible for the proliferation and maturation of red blood cells?
   A. M-CSF.
   B. GM-CSF.
   C. IL-1.
   D. Erythropoietin.

12. A

12. Patients with myelodysplastic syndrome may experience disease progression to acute leukemia following GM-CSF administration, which could be beneficial in some cases.

   A. True.
   B. False.

CHAPTER 11

Monoclonal Antibodies

Karl Kwok, Pharm.D.
Clinical Pharmacist in Oncology
Pharmacy Services, University of Washington Medical Center, and
Clinical Associate Professor
Department of Pharmacy Practice, School of Pharmacy
University of Washington
Seattle, WA

Introduction

Our growing knowledge of the role of cell surface antigens has led to important advances in our understanding of disease as well as the development and purification of therapeutic agents.

Many tumor cells produce substances that are displayed on their cell surfaces or secreted into the serum. These compounds may be minimally present or completely absent in normal differentiated tissues and can make such tumor cells antigenically different from their normal counterparts. This cellular difference may be exploited by developing specific antibodies against such antigens. These antigens, known as tumor-associated antigens (TAAs), are made up of a number of different structures and are located primarily on the tumor cell surface. As shown in Figure 11-1, tumor cell antigens include activation antigens and normal cell antigens such as HLA-A and HLA-D/DR, modified blood group substances seen in some gastrointestinal and urologic tumors, epidermal growth factors encoded by oncogenes, human T lymphotropic virus, oncofetal antigens such as alpha-fetoprotein (AFP), carcinoembryonic antigen (CEA), and glycolipid antigens seen on melanoma cells.[1] The realization that TAAs unique to cancer cells may exist and that specific antibodies could be produced against these antigens has led the way for the concept of antibody-directed therapy in cancer management.

Heteroantisera have been used in treating cancers for many years with limited usefulness.[2] Recently, with the development of monoclonal antibody (MoAb) technology to produce large, reproducible quantities of antibodies with single specificity, there has been renewed interest in research on antibodies directed against tumor cells. MoAbs may be used to target tumor cells and to improve on the low therapeutic-to-toxic ratios currently seen with radiotherapy and chemotherapy. Many applications of MoAbs are still experimental, but their use is increasing and quite

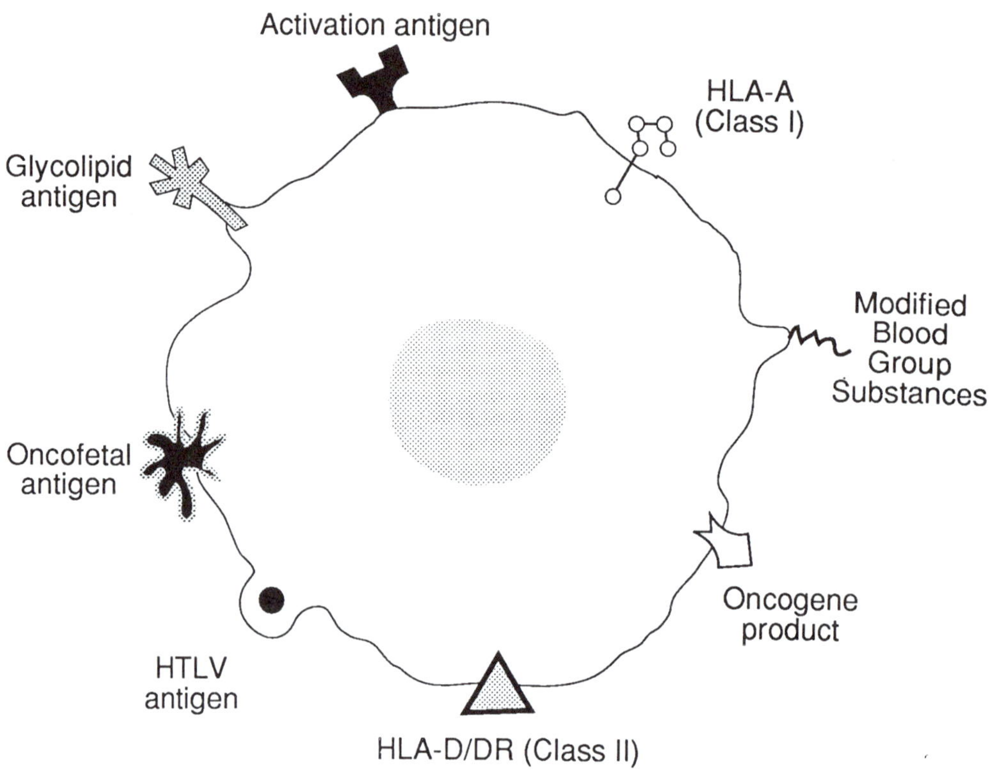

Figure 11-1. Antigens associated with human tumor cells

SOURCE: Reprinted with permission from Kagan JM, Fahely JL. Tumor immunology. Chapter 21. *JAMA*. 1987;258:2990. Copyright 1987, American Medical Association.

established in many areas of medicine. It is important for today's practitioner to become familiar with the origin and nature of MoAbs, because they have many applications in over-the-counter products and drug assay techniques. More important, MoAbs are establishing a role in the diagnosis, imaging, and treatment of cancer and other diseases.

Learning objectives

After reading this chapter, the reader will be able to—

- Discuss production techniques for creating monoclonal antibodies.
- Describe current applications of monoclonal antibody imaging and therapy.
- Discuss advantages of monoclonal antibody therapy.
- Discuss drawbacks to monoclonal antibody therapy.
- Describe cellular characteristics of individual monoclonal antibodies.

Chapter organization

This chapter begins with a brief discussion of the historical background on which MoAb technology is based. This discussion is followed by a detailed description of MoAb production techniques. Next, MoAb applications for early detection, imaging, and treatment of tumors are presented, including advantages and drawbacks associated with these techniques. Radioisotopes and immunotoxins are described, followed by a discussion of noncancer applications of MoAbs for cardiology, infectious diseases, and autoimmune diseases.

Suggested Preparation

Specific review reading is not absolutely required; however, reading Chapters 1, 2, 3, 6, and 10 may be beneficial.

Production of Monoclonal Antibodies

Historical Perspective

Animal antisera

Before the development of MoAbs, polyclonal antisera were produced by antigenic stimulation of animals—rabbits, goats, and horses. Next came blood extraction, isolation, and purification. Animals were bled over and over again to produce the antisera. This method provided useful diagnostic tools and was used therapeutically, but it had several limitations. The antibody quality varied with each lot, and the quantity of any single antiserum was limited to only a few grams. Most of the antisera produced by this method also contained many other antigen-nonspecific antibodies.

In 1974, Georges Kohler and Cesar Milstein[3] of the Medical Research Council in Cambridge, England, developed a procedure for potentially obtaining unlimited quantities of a pure antibody with single specificity. Their research into the somatic cell genetics of myeloma cells showed that malignant myeloma cells were capable of unlimited growth in vitro. Normal B lymphocytes that could secrete antibodies directed to a specific antigen did not survive long in cell cultures. Through their studies they originated the hybrid myeloma or hybridoma technique and produced MoAbs for the first time.

Hybrid myeloma

The first MoAbs were produced by fusing antibody-secreting B lymphocytes from the spleens of mice immunized with sheep red blood cells (RBCs) with cells of a mouse myeloma cell line, which had genetic deficiencies that did not allow it to grow under certain conditions. Equal numbers of spleen cells and myeloma cells were fused by using inactivated Sendai virus, and samples were grown in selective medium. Only the cells that inherited the features of both parents by fusion survived in the medium. These so-called hybridomas (contraction of *hybrid* and *myeloma*) could produce anti-sheep RBC antibodies while growing indefinitely in cell culture. An improved version of Kohler and Milstein's procedure is used by many scientists today to obtain virtually unlimited quantities of a pure antibody with single specificity.

MoAb Production

In MoAb production it is desirable to isolate the B lymphocyte that is producing the desired antibody. Normal B cells are not immortal; they die in cell cultures within several days. Myeloma cells, on the other hand, are neoplastic plasma cells that can grow in cell cultures and are considered immortal. Fusing an antibody-producing B cell with an immortal myeloma cell allows for the continuous production of a specific antibody. This fusion results in hybrid myeloma cells known as hybridomas. The hybridoma cell has the longevity of a myeloma cell and produces the antibody of a single specificity designated by the B lymphocyte's genes.

Cell fusion

General Procedures for Producing MoAbs. Procedures for producing murine MoAbs have been described by many investigators.[4,5] Minor modifications have been performed by different investigators to increase the yield and specificity of their MoAbs.[5-9] The overall scheme for the murine production of MoAbs is described in Figure 11-2.

Forming the Hybridoma. First, the desired antigen is injected into the mouse, stimulating the B lymphocytes that recognize the antigen. These B lymphocytes produce antibodies against the antigen. Many of the antibodies are directed against different epitopes. The mouse may be given additional antigen exposures to ensure a good yield of specific antibody-producing B lymphocytes. The mouse is sacrificed and the spleen is removed so that the lymphocytes from the spleen may be isolated. Only a few of the many B lymphocytes in the spleen are antigen specific and secrete the desired antibody. The lymphocytes are mixed with myeloma cells in the presence of polyethylene glycol. This step fuses the cellular membranes of the two cell types by making the membranes more adhesive.

Antibody stimulation

There are other techniques for fusion using viruses and electrical fields.[1,10] The fusion results in a mixture of cells of which only a small percentage are the desired hybridomas (those containing the cell contents of both parental cells). Other components of the cell mixture include lymphocyte-lymphocyte fused cells, myeloma-myeloma fused cells, unfused myeloma cells, and unfused lymphocytes, which die shortly.

Selecting the Hybridoma. The mixture contains a large number of unfused myeloma cells that compete with the hybridomas for nutrients. The viable unfused myeloma cells must be eliminated to select only the hybridomas. The mixture of spleen cells (lymphocytes), myeloma cells, and hybridomas is grown in a selective medium containing hypoxanthine,

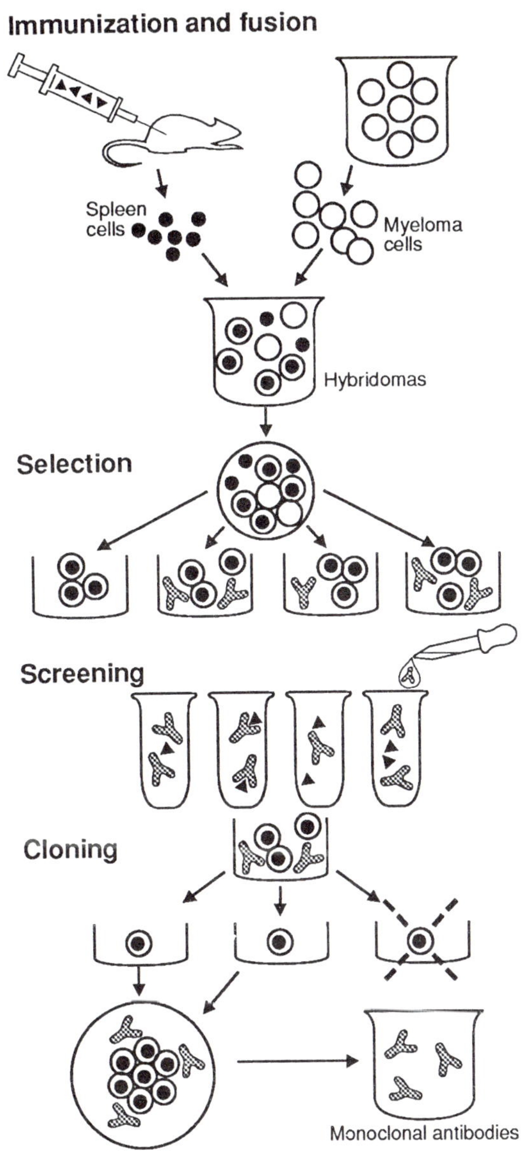

Figure 11-2. Production of murine monoclonal antibody

SOURCE: Reprinted with permission from Chisholm R. On the trail of the magic bullet. *High Technology Business.* 1983;3[Jan]:61.

HAT growth medium

aminopterin, and thymidine (HAT). Aminopterin blocks normal nucleic acid biosynthesis in cells. Hypoxanthine and thymidine can be used as substrates to produce nucleic acids via nucleotide salvage pathways in cells containing the enzymes hypoxanthine-guanine phosphoribosyl-transferase (HGPRT) or thymidine kinase (TK). The myeloma cell line chosen for fusion is a mutant lacking HGPRT and TK enzymes. The unfused myeloma cells die because they are able to use neither the substrate hypoxanthine nor the substrate thymidine to bypass the nucleic acid synthesis block caused by aminopterin. The hybridoma cells grow as the chromosomes from the lymphocytes provide the information for producing the enzymes HGPRT or TK. The unfused lymphocytes are eliminated because of naturally poor growth in vitro. The surviving hybridomas are grown as small colonies in separate wells of a culture dish.

Screening for the Desired Hybridoma. The cell cultures are allowed to grow for a few weeks (usually 2 to 3 weeks) and are then screened to select the hybridoma that is producing the desired antibody. There are many methods by which the specific hybridoma secreting the desired antibody can be identified. The most widely used methods are the radioimmunoassay (RIA) and enzyme-linked immunosorbent assay (ELISA) techniques, which are sensitive, quick, and easy to use (see Chapter 5). Other screening assays include flow microfluorimetry (also known as flow cytometry) and cytotoxicity.

RIA and ELISA

In the RIA and ELISA techniques the target antigen is chemically bound to the bottom of the testing tray in wells corresponding to the cultural wells of the hybridomas. The supernatant from each of the hybridoma cultures is added to corresponding antigen wells. Antibodies in the supernatant that are specific for the target antigen bind, but nonspecific antibodies are washed away. Radioactive or enzyme-labeled secondary antibodies specific for the primary antibodies are added to the wells, and the mixture is incubated and rewashed. The wells that show radioactivity or a color reaction contain the desired antibody. The corresponding wells of hybridoma cultures may be cloned to produce a clonal population of the hybridoma that produced the desired MoAb.

Cloning. The purpose of cloning is to ensure that all of the hybridoma cells are actually of one population. The various hybridomas in culture may secrete a mixture of antibodies that recognize different sites or epitopes on the target antigen. The hybridomas are diluted, and one cell is deposited into each well of a 96-well culture plate. The single cell grows into a colony of identical cells. Each of the single colonies is rescreened for specific antibody production. The hybridoma clone is selected according to its desired antibody specificity.

Large-scale Production of Monoclonal Antibodies. There are many methods for producing large quantities of desired MoAbs, and many more are being developed to provide for wide commercial applications of the antibodies.[11,12] The simplest production method is to grow the desired hybridoma in cell cultures and harvest the secreted antibodies from the supernatant. This method provides relatively low yields compared with

Culture techniques

other methods and is relatively expensive. However, it is useful for the production of antibodies for research purposes that require limited supplies.

Another method requires the hybridoma to be injected into the peritoneal cavities of mice. These hybridomas, which grow quickly because of their neoplastic properties, secrete antibodies into the peritoneal cavities and create ascitic fluid. In 10 to 21 days, 2 to 5 mL of ascitic fluid are harvested from each mouse. High concentrations of antibody are achievable in the ascitic fluid, approximately 5 to 15 mg/mL. This method usually produces 10 to 100 times the concentration of MoAbs obtainable from tissue culture. Hundreds to thousands of mice, however, are required to produce even 1 kg of MoAbs. Disadvantages of this method include contamination of the peritoneal fluid with other proteins besides the desired antibodies and the cost of harvesting from the large number of mice.[13]

In the early 1980s, the production requirements of MoAbs could generally be fulfilled by the cell culture or mouse ascites method that has been described, because early testing required amounts ranging from a few micrograms to a few grams per dose for therapeutic treatment of cancer. More recently, the need for large quantities of MoAbs has risen dramatically, requiring the production of hundreds of kilograms per MoAb, compared with the estimated total production of only 20 kg of MoAbs in 1986.

Bioreactors

A newer technique uses cell growth chambers consisting of a mass of hollow fibers packed longitudinally into cylindrical cartridges called bioreactors. Each of the fibers is a hollow tube with a 200-µm inner diameter and a semipermeable membrane. The cells are grown in the extracapillary volume among the fibers, and the fibers are used to deliver nutrients to the cells. Each of the bioreactors contains about 10 trillion cells. The hybridomas grow in high density and continuously produce MoAbs in concentrations of approximately 100 to 500 µg/mL in the media. MoAbs as relatively pure forms can be produced at a rate of several milligrams per day from an average-producing hybridoma cell line.

Storing Hybridomas. Hybridoma cells may be frozen and stored for future use. Cells stored in liquid nitrogen have been shown to be viable after several years. Because a hybridoma occasionally stops secreting antibodies, it is important that a parental seed stock of hybridomas be kept frozen. The frozen seed stock can then be retrieved and the cultures restarted.

Purification Procedures. MoAbs should be purified prior to in vivo use and commercial applications. MoAbs may be purified by precipitation with ammonium sulfate, gel filtration, electrophoresis, ion exchange, and affinity chromatography. Stability, affinity, activity, and formulation information should be obtained.

Specific Production Procedures. The production of monospecific antibodies proved useful for in vitro scientific study and biomedical research; thus, MoAb technology grew rapidly after it was introduced.

Currently, many of the applications of MoAbs are in the areas of in vitro and in vivo diagnosis and therapy.

HAMAs

Murine Production. Murine production of MoAbs is currently the predominant method of MoAb generation. Clinical trials involving the injection of MoAbs into humans have been under way for several years; most of the antibodies are derived from hybridomas of murine origin. These studies are defining the ability of a MoAb to reach and bind to its prospective antigen. When the MoAb is used alone, its inherent cytotoxicity can be determined along with its side effects. A major concern with the use of murine MoAbs is the potential adverse reaction that may be induced by the administration of a foreign (mouse) protein. The formation of human anti-murine antibodies (HAMAs) has been observed, and the continued administration of murine MoAbs has led to anti-murine antibody titers that may neutralize any therapeutic effect or lead to severe allergic reactions.[14]

Concerns over limitations of murine MoAbs have resulted in research to develop methods to improve the efficiency of the antibodies and decrease the antigenic nature of the molecules. These approaches include the production and use of human hybridomas to make human MoAbs, the generation of chimeric antibodies (antibodies with Fab and Fc regions of different species origin), the production and use of other hybrid MoAbs (such as bivalent antibodies and MoAb fragments), and recombinant DNA techniques to produce humanlike or humanized hybridomas.

Humanized hybridomas

Human Monoclonal Antibodies. The development of hybridoma methodology has been very successful in mice and rats; unfortunately, the strategies devised for these laboratory animals are not directly applicable to developing human hybridomas for producing human MoAbs.

Despite the potential advantages of reduced antigenicity of human versus murine antibody and increased effector activity with human MoAbs, the technology for producing them still lags behind murine MoAb technology. The standard method of fusing hyperimmunized spleen cells from the mouse or rat with mouse myeloma cells is not very feasible for producing human hybridomas. First, obvious ethical reasons prevent the introduction of many antigens into humans. Thus, fresh spleens for cell fusion are not usually available from selected hyperimmunized humans as they are from animals, and there is difficulty in selecting and obtaining the desired antigen-specific B lymphocytes.

Second, the derivation of a permanent human myeloma cell line has been more difficult than originally imagined. A number of HAT-sensitive human myeloma fusion partners have been developed and used to form hybridomas. However, human myeloma cell lines are usually unsatisfactory because of their slow-growing nature and low yield of hybrids.[15] Finally, human hybridomas are not easily grown in the ascites of tumor-bearing mice; thus, cell culture techniques to develop a clonable human hybridoma are needed.

Alternative approaches to the development of human MoAbs are being explored: (l) interspecies fusion with mouse myelomas to create mouse-human hybridomas,[16] (2) immortalization of B lymphocytes by Epstein-Barr virus (EBV) transformation,[17] (3) lymphoblastoid derivatives and development of more stable myeloid fusion partners,[18,19] (4) chimeric antibodies,[20,21] and (5) recombinant DNA techniques.[22] Most of these techniques have yielded usable MoAbs, but production limitations have prevented wide applications of any one methodology.

Interspecies hybridomas

Interspecies hybrids involve the fusion of human lymphocytes with mouse myeloma cells. The human lymphocytes must be derived from surgical patients who have had lymphatic tissue removed for therapeutic purposes and who may have been exposed to particular antigens. The technique results in relatively high fusion frequencies, and the resulting hybrids are capable of secreting high levels of human antibodies. The limitation encountered with the interspecies hybrids has been rapid loss of human chromosomes or altered gene expression resulting in unstable or decreased immunoglobulin production. The EBV technique uses in vitro EBV infection of human lymphocytes to induce polyclonal activation and immunoglobulin production. Antigen-specific cells can be preselected before transformation by EBV infection, or the EBV line may be cloned and then screened for antibody production. The production of human antibodies by this method has resulted in antibodies of the IgM class. Both amount and types of antibodies produced by this method are low. Other problems include the possibility of EBV being released into the culture and introduced into the patient.[17] True human hybridomas are being produced by combining human lymphocytes with human myeloma and lymphoblastoid cell lines. Desirable characteristics for hybridoma formation include high frequency of fusion with human lymphocytes, synthesis and secretion of adequate amounts of specific antibodies, and formation of stable hybrids. One of the limiting factors in producing human lymphocyte-human myeloma hybrids is the limited availability of human myeloma cell lines. The use of current human myeloma cell lines has been unsatisfactory and has forced many investigators to employ lymphoblastoid cell lines as fusion partners.[19]

Lymphoblastoid cell lines

Lymphoblastoid cell lines are typically EBV-containing nonmalignant B cells and may be superior to current human myeloma cell lines for the production of hybridoma cells. Lymphoblastoid fusion partners have relatively lower fusion frequencies and lower levels of immunoglobulin production than fusion partners from a murine myeloma cell line. Other methods using EBV hybridomas and genetic engineering techniques may eventually circumvent some of the problems described here. Investigators are continuing work on developing better fusion partners and on developing better methods for selecting antigen-specific B cells and providing them on a large scale.

Chimeric Antibodies. The desire to decrease antigenicity and improve efficacy of antibodies has led to the development of chimeric antibodies, immunoglobulin molecules created primarily by recombinant DNA techniques and gene transfection.[20,21,23-27] The process creates mouse-human antibodies consisting of mouse Fab or hypervariable regions and human Fc regions. The process for producing chimeric antibodies is summarized in Figure 11-3. Genes specifying the desired variable regions from the murine cell lines are spliced to the genes that code for the constant region of the human immunoglobulin. The chimeric gene containing the combined sequences of interest is spliced into an expression vector containing a selectable marker. The vector is transfected into the appropriate recipient cell line. The stable transfectants that synthesize the genes of interest are identified, selected, and amplified by growth in culture or in the ascitic fluid of tumor-bearing mice.

Gene transfection

Applications

Chimeric immunoglobulin molecules provide a new group of reagents with multiple potential applications.[28] Through recombinant DNA technology it would be possible to combine any murine variable region into a given Fc portion. Changing the Fc portion can alter the immunoglobulin's ability to bind to different proteins, to be multivalent, or to fix complement.

This technology has allowed researchers to overcome the problem that immunoglobulin produced by one hybridoma is of only one particular isotype. This, of course, is a problem only if the isotype expressed does not have the desired effector functions, such as complement fixation or binding of staphylococcal protein A, required for certain assays or cytotoxic effects.

Chimeric molecules with the encoded mouse Fab hypervariable regions and the human Fc portions should be much less antigenic than murine MoAbs. Their potential for adverse reactions is thus reduced and their potential for therapeutic effects increased.[28]

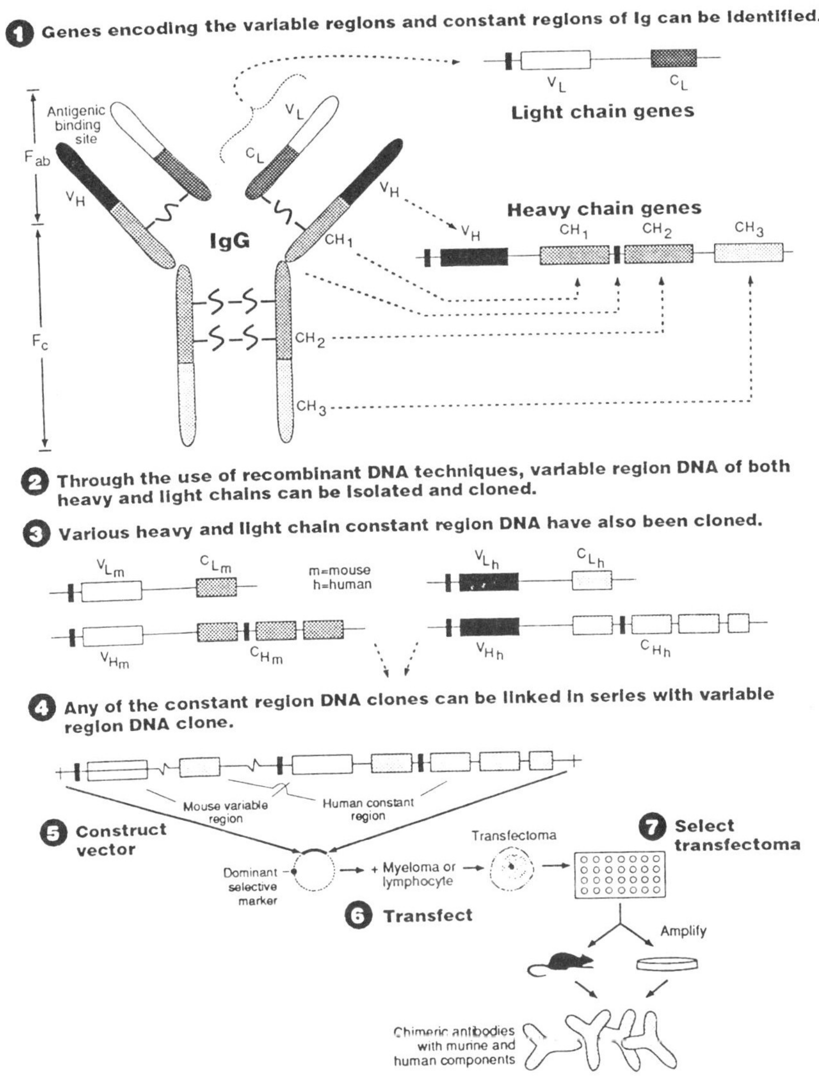

Figure 11-3. Production of chimeric antibody

SOURCE: Adapted with permission from Morrison SL. Transfectomas provide novel chimeric antibodies. *Science.* 1985;229:1203-4. Copyright 1985 by the AAAS.

The chimeric immunoglobulin can also be constructed so that the Fab is covalently bound to a nonimmunoglobulin protein.[25,26] The Fab may be bound to an enzyme so that detection of antigen-antibody binding may be noted with the addition of an appropriate substrate, or the Fab may be bound to a toxin and used as an immunotoxin. Chimeric antibodies have recently been taken one step further. Small regions located within the mouse Fab region have been isolated as the sections that actually bind antigen. These regions are known as hypervariable regions or complementarity-determining regions, because their amino acid sequence greatly differs from one antibody to another.

Researchers have cloned out the sequences for antigen-specific mouse hypervariable regions and placed these sequences into genes encoding for intact human immunoglobulin. The resulting chimeric antibody binds the antigen that the mouse antibody was directed against, but it is almost entirely human in composition.[29,30]

Two binding sites

Bivalent Antibodies. Bivalent antibodies are hybrids with two combining sites that can bind to different antigens. The bifunctional antibodies may be produced chemically or biologically.[31] Chemically, the antibody molecules are reduced to monovalent fragments, and the fragments of different antigenic specificity are mixed and then reoxidized to the bivalent form with dual specificity. The resulting antibodies can bind two different antigens simultaneously. Biologically, these antibodies may be produced by making second-generation hybridomas. This technique involves fusing two hybridomas so that the resulting cells produce antibody molecules with both specificities.

$F(ab')_2$

Some hybrid hybridomas can produce bispecific MoAbs that focus effector T-cell activity.[32] One of the Fab components of these antibodies is directed at a T-cell surface molecule and the other Fab component may be specific for a tumor. This capability allows very specific targeting of T-cell cytotoxicity in therapy of tumors. Alternatively, a bispecific antibody can be developed with one Fab that is specific for a drug or toxin and another Fab that is specific for a tumor. Recently a bispecific $F(ab')_2$ antibody has been developed to deliver saporin, a toxin, to lymphoma cells.[33]

Monoclonal Antibody Fragments. In the past decade the use of Fab and $F(ab')_2$ portions of MoAbs has included a broad range of immunologic and biochemical investigations. MoAb fragments have been used to study antigen-antibody binding where the absence of Fc-associated effector functions was desirable.

The Fab is monovalent, making it ideal for investigations where Fc function or cross-linking of antigen is not desirable (see Figure 11-4). The $F(ab')_2$ is bivalent and has substantially higher association constants to the antigen than the Fab. Uses of $F(ab')_2$ include comparisons with Fab and complete MoAb molecules to study the effects of receptor cross-linking on cellular activation. $F(ab')_2$ may be more desirable than Fab if a greater avidity to antigen is needed.

MoAb fragments are produced by proteolytic cleavage in the hinge region, which splits the immunoglobulin into fragments. Cleavage by papain produces the monovalent Fab of approximately 45,000 molecular weight; cleavage by pepsin, in the absence of reducing agent, produces the $F(ab')_2$ of approximately 100,000 molecular weight (see Figure 11-4). There are some advantages in using these MoAb fragments rather than whole antibodies. First, both fragments lack the Fc portion necessary for cytotoxic activity, an advantage when cytotoxic activity is neither necessary

Proteolytic cleavage

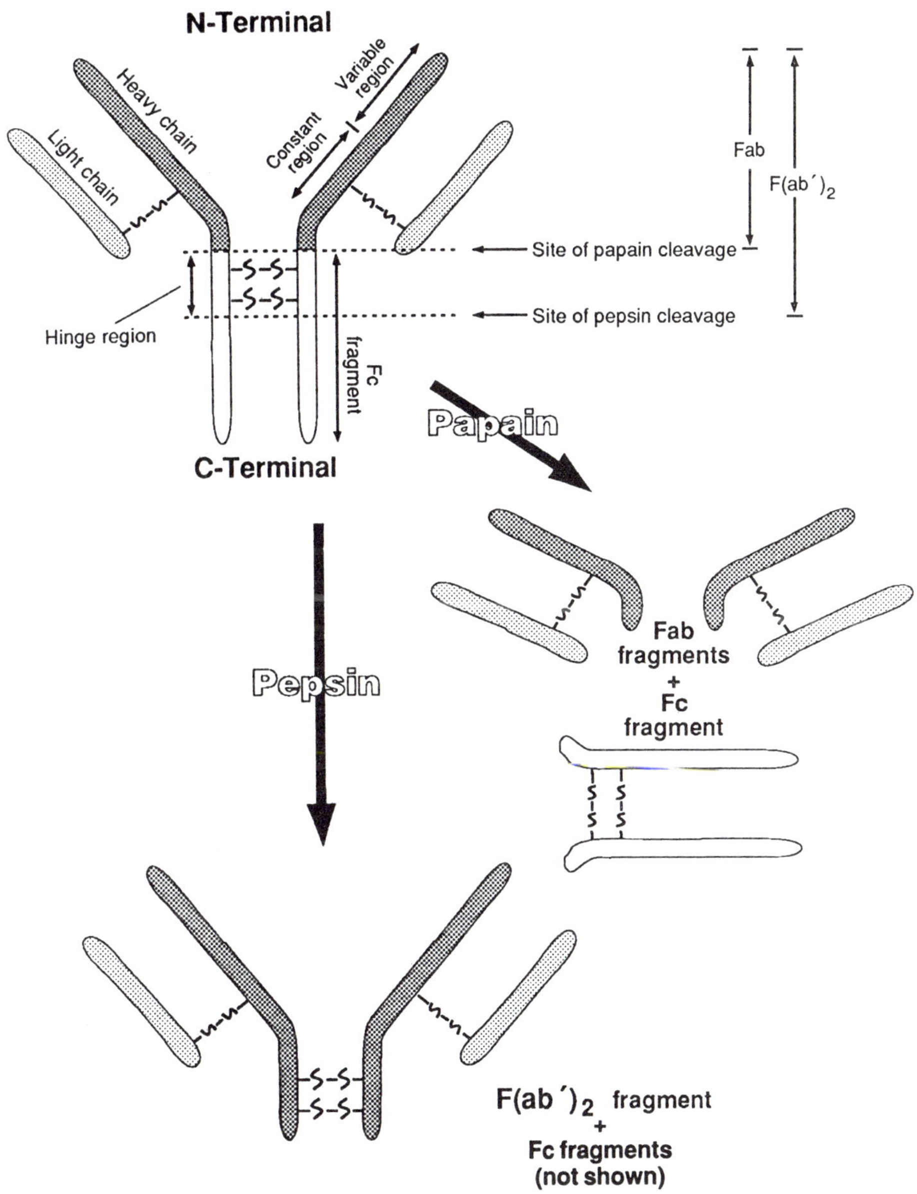

Figure 11-4. Schematic diagram of immunoglobulin molecule, with the cleavage sites for papain and pepsin for the production of Fab and $F(ab')_2$ fragments

nor desirable. Second, because of their lighter molecular weight, Fab and $F(ab')_2$ fragments may have better tissue penetration and biodistribution characteristics than intact MoAbs.[34-36] Third, MoAb fragments are cleared more quickly than the larger whole MoAb molecules.

Recombinant Molecules. Recombinant technology has made it possible to produce antibody fragments in the bacterium *Escherichia coli.* Monoclonal Fab fragments can be produced by extracting the genes that encode the heavy and light chains of the variable regions using polymerase chain reaction and incorporating the genes into a bacteriophage vector system.[37,38] MoAb fragments for ovarian cancer have been cloned into an *E. coli* expression system containing a portion of *Pseudomonas* exotoxin gene. They produced a recombinant single-chain immunotoxin that could bind and kill cells expressing an ovarian antigen.[39] Single-variable heavy chain genes called single-domain antibodies have also been cloned.[40] These antibody fragments have demonstrated affinity for the target antigen and may have advantages over traditional MoAbs by virtue of their shorter production time and good tissue penetration. Recombinant technology may provide the means by which antibodies or antibody fragments can be generated more cheaply from bacteria or plants such as tobacco[41] than from hybridomas.

Applications and Limitations of Monoclonal Antibodies in Oncology

Tumor cells express a number of surface antigens that are relatively specific for the neoplasm. MoAbs have been made against a variety of these TAAs.[42-44] Clinical trials are evaluating the usefulness of these antibodies in the diagnosis, imaging, and treatment of cancers.[45-47] Many of these MoAbs are used in vitro to detect the presence of circulating tumor antigens for the early detection of cancer. Some are labeled with radioactive isotopes and used in the imaging of tumors and metastatic disease. A number of MoAbs are undergoing early clinical trials for in vivo treatment of cancer. These trials are providing useful information on MoAbs—their relative specificity, pharmacokinetics, adverse reactions, efficacy, and possible limitations for wide clinical applications.

Tumor Antigen and Antibody Selection

A number of factors must be considered when tumor antigens and appropriate MoAbs are selected. The common requirement for tumor targeting is to select MoAbs that react specifically with antigens that are present in high levels on tumor cells but are not expressed in most normal tissues. Specificity is a critical feature for potential applications of MoAbs.

Specificity

However, absolute specificity is neither necessary nor always desired; specificity limited to one particular antigen may limit the application of that MoAb for the detection, imaging, and treatment of TAAs in other patients who have the same type of tumor but lack that specific antigen.

In the ideal situation using a MoAb for in vivo treatment or imaging, an antigen would be expressed exclusively on the surface of tumor cells, in high density, in both primary and metastatic lesions. The antigen would be neither secreted nor shed from the cell surface and would not undergo modulation. These antigen characteristics are different for in vitro diagnostic applications of MoAbs; here, shedding and secretion of tumor antigen make serum monitoring easier. Thus, the usefulness of a given MoAb depends on its desired application and on whether the targeted antigen can be found only on the cell surface or is also secreted in the serum.

The choice of MoAbs depends on a number of factors that may have an impact on their biodistribution, their ability to target tumor cells, and their ability to elicit some therapeutic effect. One selection factor is the antibody class type (e.g., IgG versus IgM) and subclass (e.g., IgG2a versus IgG3), and another is whether the MoAb should be used as a whole molecule or digested into fragments such as Fab or $F(ab')_2$. Finally, the antibody should be selected for its avidity to the target cells, thus determining its degree of binding.

Use of Monoclonal Antibodies for Assaying Tumor Serum Markers

Much of the work with MoAbs concerns their use in diagnosing, imaging, and treating cancers. In recent years, immunocytochemical techniques have been increasingly used to study cell surface antigens on bone marrow and peripheral blood samples. These studies have provided information on white blood cell populations and their differentiation, and they are extremely valuable in diagnosing and classifying hematologic malignancies.

AFP and CEA

MoAbs may be used as reagents for the immunochemical staining and diagnosing of neoplasms in pathologic specimens. Specific tumors are also known to shed different characteristic antigens into the host circulation (see Chapter 10). These TAAs may allow for relatively noninvasive early detection of the cancer. Two recognized TAAs with widespread clinical applications are AFP and CEA. AFP is an important marker for detecting and monitoring nonseminomatous germ cell tumors. Serum elevations of CEA have been primarily due to colon and gastrointestinal carcinomas. MoAbs have been prepared against AFP and CEA epitopes.

Other anti-TAA MoAbs are being tested for potential applications.[48-50] A drawback to the clinical application of some of these MoAbs is their potential cross-reactivity with similar antigens found on normal cells. Continued research will lead to the development of MoAbs of greater specificity, resulting in improved tumor detection and fewer cross-reactions with normal tissues and, thus, in increased efficiency of these MoAbs for early detection of cancer.

Use of Monoclonal Antibodies for Tumor Imaging

The use of antibodies in tumor imaging is not a new concept. Isotope-labeled polyclonal antibodies have been used in the past to visualize and localize tumors.[51] Progress in directing MoAbs to specific cell surface antigens on tumors should make it possible to use radiolabeled MoAbs to define tumor location, size, and extent.[52,53] Periodic injections of isotope-labeled MoAbs should provide information on the progression of the disease and the effectiveness of treatment. A number of MoAbs and MoAb fragments, primarily labeled with indium 111 (^{111}In) or technetium 99m (^{99m}Tc), are undergoing clinical trials in this country. The available MoAbs used for imaging are directed at melanomas and breast, colon, and lung cancers.[36,54-58] Others are being developed to target malignancies such as neuroblastoma, lymphoma, and ovarian and gastrointestinal tumors.[53,59-62]

Therapy evaluation

Initial trials have determined the relative safety of using these radiolabeled MoAbs; essentially no adverse reactions or toxicities have been observed. Further trials are under way to assess the efficacy of the labeled MoAbs in detection of tumors and determine the optimum dose to be used, as well as to generate data relating to biodistribution, clearance, and image enhancement.[52,63-68] Further trials are under way to correlate results using MoAbs with results obtained by surgery or biopsy to identify persistent or metastatic disease.[69,70] Such imaging scans may in the future eliminate the need for exploratory surgery or help oncologists determine prognoses and plans for additional medical treatments. Concerns remain about the nonspecific binding of the MoAbs to normal tissues and about nonspecific organ distribution (primarily in the liver, spleen, kidneys, and the highly vascularized tissues), as well as about nonbinding to known tumor. Before routine clinical use is practical, MoAb fragments used for targeting will have to be carefully selected; better conjugation methods and better choices of isotopes for the desired applications also need to be made.

Concerns

In vivo imaging with MoAbs is the first step in developing therapeutic efforts with MoAbs. The imaging tool allows investigators to determine the specificity of the MoAb for the intended tumor antigen and to overcome some of the limitations of in vivo use before using MoAbs that carry potentially harmful, highly active radioisotopes or cytotoxic ligands.

Strategies for in Vivo Use of Monoclonal Antibodies

Mechanisms

In vivo use of MoAbs for treating cancer currently involves a number of general strategies, including the application of MoAbs for (l) direct immunologic destruction of the tumor cell, (2) targeting molecules that are critical for growth or differentiation of tumor cells, and (3) delivering antitumor agents.

Early trials of MoAbs for treatment involved the application of unconjugated antibodies. Studies in animal tumor models have demonstrated that passive administration of unmodified MoAbs can prevent tumor growth and lead to the regression of some established tumors.[71,72] The antitumor effects are believed to be mediated by host immune mechanisms involving the direct killing of tumor cells by complement activation or opsonization and elimination or MoAb-directed killing of target cells by immune-effector cells (antibody-dependent cellular cytotoxicity [ADCC]) (Figure 11-5). Immune effector cells include killer cells, natural killer cells, macrophages, and neutrophils. Another possible mechanism of the antitumor effects of MoAbs includes the direct binding to or blockage of a vital growth receptor on the tumor cells. Finally, the MoAbs may indirectly stimulate the production of host antibody against tumor antigens.

Most murine MoAbs do not seem to be potential mediators of tumor killing in the presence of either immune cells or complement, since they cannot fix human complement. Mouse MoAbs of certain subclasses such as IgM and IgG3 can fix complement. The use of human or humanized MoAbs may overcome these limitations.

Many different growth factors (e.g., colony-stimulating factors [CSFs], interleukins) are responsible for the growth and differentiation of cells (see Chapters 2 and 10). Tumor cells seem to be immortal and may be stimulated by some autostimulatory growth factors. MoAbs directed at these factors or their receptors may interrupt the growth of the tumor. MoAbs have been prepared against epidermal growth factor receptors and can inhibit the growth of epidermal carcinomas.[73,74] The MoAbs that have been prepared against bombesin, a potential autocrine growth factor for small cell carcinomas of the lung, have also inhibited tumor growth.[75]

Clinical Trials with Unmodified Monoclonal Antibodies

Applications

Most clinical trials with unmodified MoAbs in humans involve the use of murine MoAbs in phase I or II trials to determine dosing, adverse effects, and host response. Some of the MoAbs used and responses to them are listed in Table 11-1. The early trials concentrated on treating leukemia, lymphoma, melanoma, and gastrointestinal carcinomas. Although some

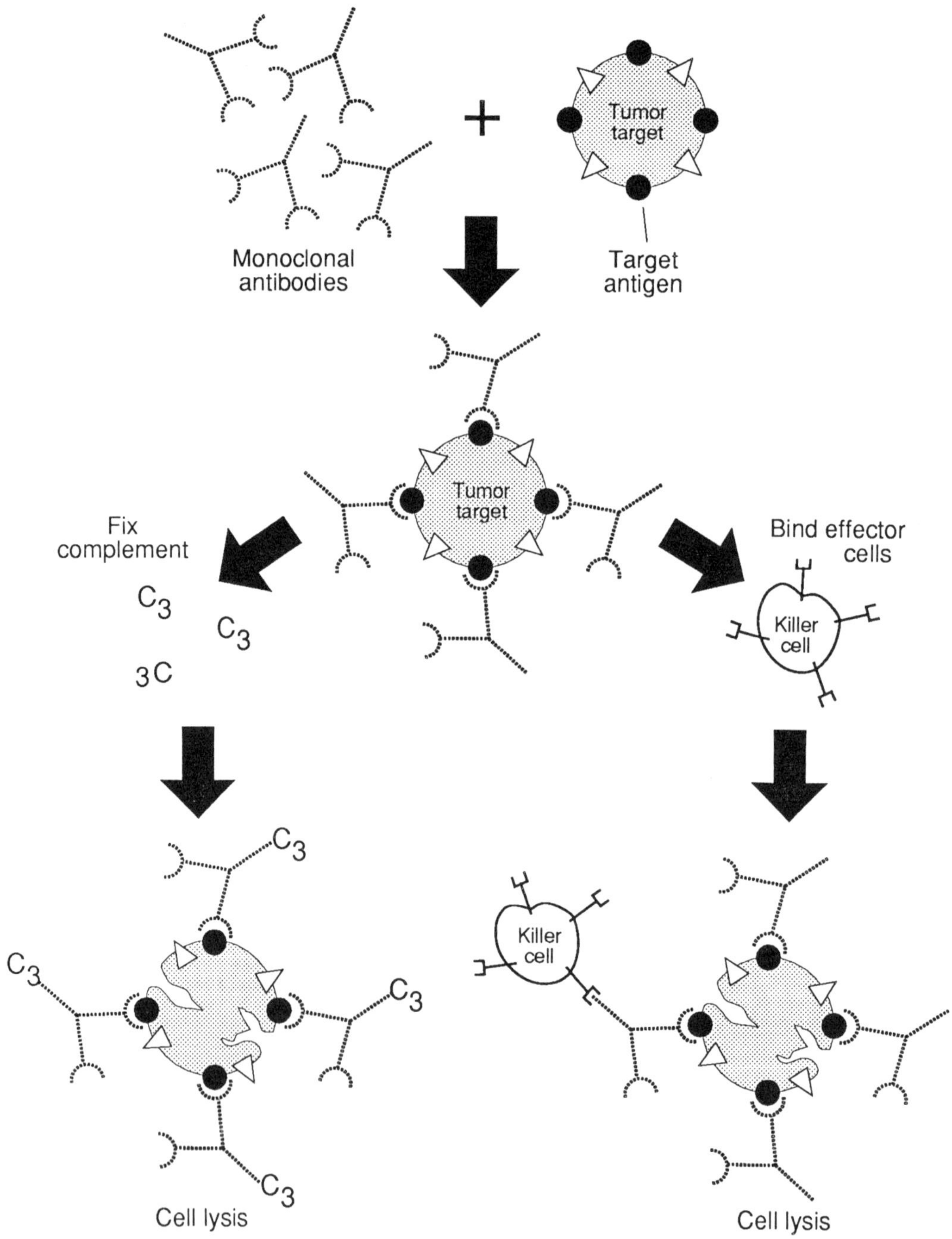

Figure 11-5. Antibody-dependent cellular cytotoxicity (ADCC)

SOURCE: Adapted with permission from Lowder JN. The current status of monoclonal antibodies in the diagnosis and therapy of cancer. *Current Problems in Cancer.* 1986;10:503.

Table 11-1 Results of Clinical Trials with Monoclonal Antibodies (MoAbs) Against Human Tumors

Tumor	MoAb/Class	Evaluable Patients	Response
ALL	J5	4	0/4
T-ALL	Leu-1, others	6	1/6
AML	Several	3	0/3
CLL	T101/IgG2a	23	2/23
CTCL	T101/IgG2a, Leu-1	35	15/35
CTCL	^{131}I-T101	6	6/6
T-cell	T101	5	1/5
B-lymphoma	Anti-idiotype	10	5/10
	^{131}I-MB-1/IgG1	2	2/2
	AB89	1	0/1
Ovarian (IP)	^{131}I-HMFG1, -HMFG2, -AUAI, -H17E2	24	8/24
GI	17-1A/IgG2a	40	5/40
Melanoma	R24/IgG3	21	6/21
	96.5-RTA/IgG2a (ricin)	22	5/22
	96.5/IgG2a	5	0/5
	9.2.27/IgG2a	8	0/8
	48.7/IgG1	4	0/4

SOURCE: Adapted with permission from Scheinberg DA, Houghton AN. Current status of antitumor therapy with monoclonal antibodies. *Oncology.* 1987;1:34.

ALL = acute lymphocytic leukemia; T-ALL = T-cell acute lymphocytic leukemia; AML = acute myelogenous leukemia; CLL = chronic lymphocytic leukemia; CTCL = cutaneous T-cell lymphoma; IP = intraperitoneal; GI = gastrointestinal.

therapeutic responses with MoAbs used for immunocytotoxic effects in therapy have been reported, virtually all responses have been transient.[76]

Dosing

Doses employed in most of these trials have been in the range of 1 to 500 mg per patient given as a single dose three times a week or daily for a week. Most of the doses have been delivered via slow intravenous bolus or slow infusions. With infusion rates greater than 5 to 10 mg per hour, pulmonary toxicity manifested as dyspnea and wheezing has been observed. The cause of the dyspnea appears to be associated with leukoagglutination and trapping in the lungs after antibody therapy.[77] Some studies have used 24- to 50-hour infusions to limit administration rate toxicity.[77,78]

Toxicities

In general, toxicity was minimal in the lower doses and slower infusion rates but increased with higher doses. Some of the more frequent toxicities observed with unmodified MoAbs were chills, fevers, flushing, urticaria, headaches, rigors, myalgias, pruritus, dyspnea, wheezing, nausea, vomiting, diarrhea, hypotension, and facial edema. Most of these toxicities were generally tolerated. Rare toxicities occurring in individual patients were anaphylactoid reactions, serum sickness, and facial palsy.

The degree of toxicity appears to depend on the amount of antibody-targeted intravascular antigen provided as free or tumor-attached binding sites. Lysis of tumor cell contents in the bloodstream may also play a role. Pretreatment with acetaminophen and diphenhydramine seems to mitigate the symptoms associated with the reactions. Parenteral diphenhydramine, meperidine, and prochlorperazine have also been used to alleviate specific problems.[77-79] Another consideration is the presence or amount of HAMA.

Anti-CD5

Early human trials using unconjugated MoAbs have involved primarily leukemia and lymphoma in small numbers of patients. These studies demonstrated that murine MoAbs may be given safely, and some therapeutic response may be elicited. Miller et al. used MoAb Leu-l (anti-CD5) to treat T-cell leukemia.[80] They were able to decrease the leukemic cell count transiently in the peripheral blood of a patient. These drops in peripheral leukemic cell counts were brief, lasting only several hours before the leukemic cell numbers returned to pretreatment levels. A proposed mechanism of leukemia cell clearance includes the removal of antibody-coated leukemic cells from the peripheral blood by the reticuloendothelial system. Other small trials with unconjugated MoAbs in acute myelogenous and lymphocytic leukemias demonstrated either no or transient responses. The MoAb T101 (anti-CD5) has been used in a number of T-cell tumors including chronic lymphocytic leukemia and cutaneous T-cell lymphoma.[81-84] Tumor regression occurred in a number of patients, but the response was again transient.[77,79,83,85] These studies confirmed the binding of T101 antibodies to circulating and bone marrow cells, lymph node cells, and cutaneous skin nodules.[86]

Anti-idiotype MoAb

Miller et al. employed another approach to targeting MoAbs for treating lymphomas.[87] As an alternative to a MoAb that recognizes a general TAA, a MoAb targeted against the idiotype region of a specific patient's B-cell lymphoma was developed (Figure 11-6). This MoAb or anti-idiotype antibody is specific for the variable region of the surface immunoglobulin on the lymphoma cells of that patient. These trials have achieved objective responses lasting 1 to 6 months; one patient had a sustained, complete

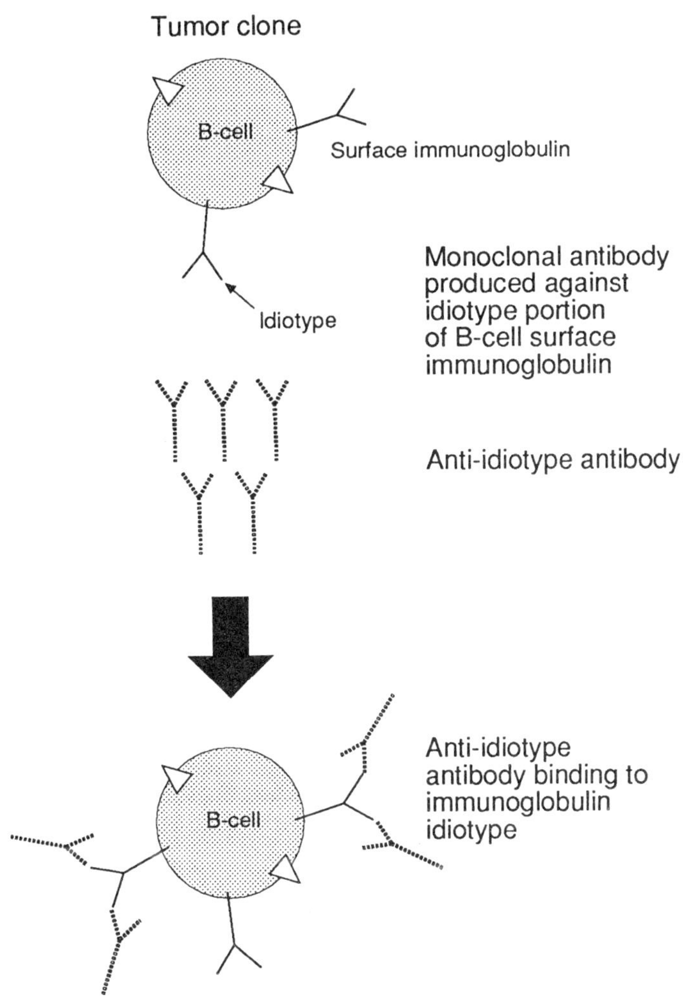

Figure 11-6. Antibody directed against surface immunoglobulin of neoplastic B-cell lymphomas—"anti-idiotype antibodies"

remission of more than 4 years.[88] The mechanism for the response is unclear. The anti-idiotype antibody could possibly act as an antigen, however, and stimulate a human immune response against the anti-idiotype antibody, which may then boost the patient's own antibody response to the antigenically similar tumor.[89] Since the application of directed anti-idiotype MoAb therapy is generally considered patient specific, it is not usually effective for other patients, whose B-cell lymphomas express different idiotypes on the tumor surface. There are, however, some anti-idiotype MoAbs that work against other patient cells, suggesting that some idiotypes on the tumor share a common determinant or a "public" idiotype. Anti-idiotype antibody therapy has been tried in a number of clinical trials for the treatment of B-cell lymphoma.[90] A recent trial used anti-idiotype antibodies in combination with interferon alfa in an attempt to improve the therapeutic outcome. The interferons can increase expression of some TAAs and have a different mechanism of action than MoAbs that may augment their activity. Brown et al.[91] showed that 2 of 11 patients achieved a complete remission and 6 had partial remission, with tumor regression often continuing months after the completion of the treatment phase. The production of a T-cell anti-idiotype antibody by Janson et al.[92] raises the possibility of using anti-idiotype antibody therapy for T-cell diseases.

A number of phenomena were identified in these trials that may be responsible for decreasing MoAb activity. First, since these trials used murine MoAbs, the body could recognize these proteins as foreign and make its own antibodies against the mouse antibodies after several injections. These HAMAs usually developed 2 to 3 weeks after initial murine MoAb exposure. With subsequent therapy the HAMA could bind up the murine MoAbs before they reached their target cells, decreasing clinical effectiveness and possibly exposing the patient to an antibody-induced allergic or anaphylactic reaction.[14,93]

Antigenic modulation

Another observed phenomenon is known as antigenic modulation, in which the surface antigen targeted by the MoAb disappears from the cell surface[94] (Figure 11-7). The modulation may result from the cell's internalizing or shedding of the antigen. This response may occur rapidly; surface antigens may disappear within 2 hours after administration of the MoAb and reappear on the cell surface 24 hours later. If the tumor cell internalizes the antigen, the tumor can escape targeting by the MoAb. However, this property may be exploited therapeutically with cytotoxic-conjugated MoAbs, in which internalization of the toxic antibody-antigen complex leads to cell death.

Other problems recognized in the early trials include lymphoma cells that escape targeting via phenotypic alteration of the idiotype, and the presence of blocking antigens in the peripheral circulation.[95,96] These blocking antigens are often seen in lymphomas in which neoplastic cells secrete their surface antigens.

An in vivo MoAb cytotoxic immune response to tumor cells has been observed in a few patients. Most of these responses have been only transient and are believed to be the result of either complement activation or ADCC. Research is being conducted to examine unconjugated MoAbs further, select more specific antigens, produce better antibodies, and devise methods of dealing with problems noted in the studies.

Recent attempts to augment the effects of unmodified MoAbs to increase ADCC function involved the use of MoAbs with cytokines such as interleukin-2 (IL-2) to activate killer cell cytotoxicity.[97-99] Other attempts

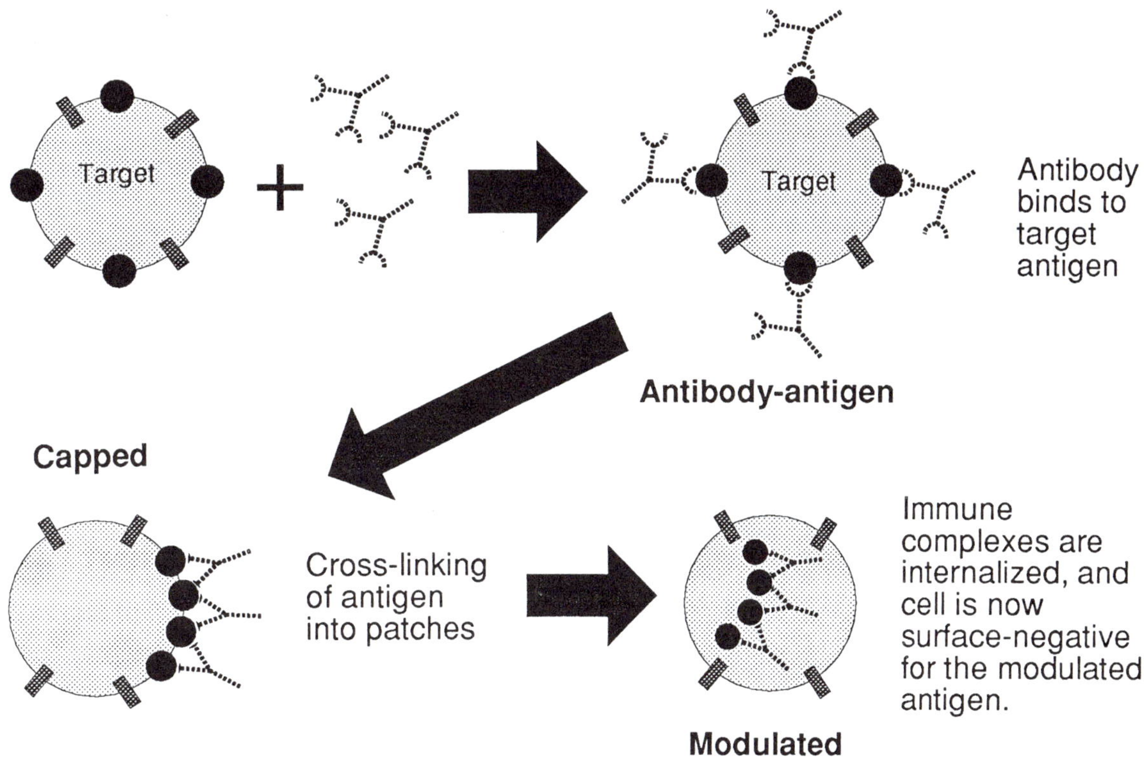

Figure 11-7. Antigenic modulation

SOURCE: Adapted with permission from Lowder JN. The current status of monoclonal antibodies in the diagnosis and therapy of cancer. *Current Problems in Cancer.* 1986;10:505.

include the use of granulocyte-macrophage colony-stimulating factor (GM-CSF), which can augment the cytotoxic capacity of mononuclear cells in ADCC.[100] Clinical trials will determine the effectiveness of this approach with the unmodified MoAbs.

Because of the limited efficacy of unconjugated MoAbs and dependent Fc-mediated cytotoxicity, another approach to the treatment of cancer is being explored: use of MoAbs to carry and deliver radioisotopes, toxins, chemotherapy agents, or liposome-filled drugs to the tumor cells. This technique is aimed at increasing the generally low therapeutic-to-toxic ratio currently experienced by radiotherapy and systemic chemotherapy with MoAb immunoconjugates.

Applications with Monoclonal Antibody Immunoconjugates

There are some general requirements for conjugating various toxic agents to antibodies. Primarily, the antibody in the conjugated form should retain its antigen-binding capacity to maintain specificity for targeted tissue. The agents should also be covalently linked and stable to prevent random distribution of the cytotoxin. However, linkage to the antibody should not inhibit activity of the agent and should allow the agent to be liberated at its site of action. The conjugated MoAb or the cytotoxic agents should not accumulate in nontargeted tissues and should follow normal clearance from the body.

Radioisotope Conjugates. One of the earliest immunoconjugates used was a radioisotope conjugated to an antibody. Radioisotopes are a vital part of the development of MoAbs because of their use as research tools in clinical assays and for in vivo applications of imaging and therapy of cancer.[52,101-103] Conjugation with radioisotopes is often done before other cytotoxic conjugation to demonstrate the specificity of the MoAb for the tumor antigen and to reveal the biodistribution of the MoAb conjugate.

Advantages

Advantages of radioisotopes as conjugates for therapy include cytotoxic activity without being internalized into the cells, the ability to cause cytotoxicity over a large area by the ionizing radiation, and the decreased dependency of each of the tumor cells to express the targeted tumor antigen. The range of the toxicity to nearby tumor cells and normal cells depends on the isotope and its type of radiating energy. These characteristics of radioisotope MoAb conjugates might be useful in treating larger tumors in which not all cell surfaces are directly exposed to the blood supply or when surface antigen loss or lack of antigen expression is encountered in certain cells within a tumor.

Toxicity

On the other hand, these characteristics may be a disadvantage because of indiscriminate toxic effects to nearby healthy tissue, especially at nonspecific sites where the MoAb conjugate might be retained (e.g., lung, spleen, liver). Therefore, dosimetry studies are important for determining ratios between radiation doses received by targeted tissues and doses received by nonspecific organs.[104] The prior administration of unconjugated nonspecific MoAbs may reduce the indiscriminate collection of MoAb conjugates by vital organs.

Goal

The goal of using MoAb-radioisotope conjugates in vivo is to achieve the maximum specific and minimum nonspecific localization of the isotope. In the development of a radioisotope conjugate, decisions must be made about the isotope and the isotope conjugation method, the form of antibody, the method of delivery, the disease of interest, and the intended purpose of the conjugated antibody. In treating cancer, the targeted tumor antigen should be specific for tumors that are sensitive to radiation therapy.

Production techniques

Techniques for the covalent conjugation of radioisotopes and other drugs and toxins are evolving. Attaching large moieties to antibodies always risks the loss of activity in the variable region of the molecule. The most common methods of conjugation depend on the presence of such amino acid side chains on the MoAb as lysine, aspartic acid, glutamic acid, and tyrosine. Carbodimides, anhydrides, active esters, and oxidizing substances are used to promote the stable binding of the moiety and the MoAb.

Isotope selection

The choice of isotope is important. Short-half-life isotopes are best for in vivo use, but fresh isotopes have to be coupled to the antibody before every treatment. Current methods employ covalent conjugation of a chelating agent such as diethylenetriamine penta-acetic acid to the antibody.[105,106] The chelated antibody conjugate is stable and can be stored for long periods without loss of activity.[107] The radioisotope conjugate is formed by adding the radioisotope to the chelated antibody, resulting in a very tight bond. Activation can be performed with a freshly generated isotope shortly before treatment.

For imaging purposes, the choice of radioisotopes is usually short-half-life isotopes that emit gamma rays that can exit the body and be detected ex vivo. A commonly used radioisotope is ^{111}In, which emits two photons per disintegration. Isotopes that emit alpha and beta radiation are more useful for treatment: these massive particles penetrate only several cells beyond the site of decay, thereby helping to limit radiation-induced cellular toxicity to the area of antibody binding. The most commonly used isotope is iodine 131 (^{131}I); it emits beta radiation and some gamma radiation. Although ^{131}I is the least expensive radioisotope and easiest to use, it has poor emission characteristics. The emission characteristics of other radioisotopes range from good emission with ^{111}In to excellent emission with ^{123}I and ^{99m}TC. Radioisotopes generally have short half-lives. Problems with stable chelates on the antibodies may exist; the iodines are easily dehalogenated in vivo.

Other radioisotopes currently of therapeutic interest are the beta emitters yttrium 90,[108] rhenum 186,[109] and scandium 47 as well as the alpha emitters bismuth 212, lead 212,[110,111] and ^{123}I.

Antibody form selection

The form of antibody may also be important.[112] Antibody fragments should have several potential advantages over intact antibodies. Indeed, fragments such as Fab and F(ab')$_2$ should clear the blood substantially faster than the whole antibody.[36,113-115] Such rapid clearance eliminates the blood pool background for imaging and reduces the toxicity of therapy.[116] The lack of Fc receptor in fragments should eliminate nonspecific binding. The smaller size also facilitates more rapid diffusion out of the vascular space and might be less immunogenic. Most studies with radioisotope conjugates have been done with intact MoAbs. The theoretical advantages of fragment conjugates are only beginning to be explored.

MoAbs conjugated to radioisotopes (most commonly ^{131}I) have been evaluated in animal systems using human tumor xenografts in nude mice models. These studies demonstrated specific tissue uptake of MoAb conjugates, with the ratio of radioactivity anywhere from 4 to 90 times higher in tumor to liver and 2 to 25 times higher in tumor to blood. Regression of the tumor xenografts could be induced with sufficient dose.

Trial results

Therapeutic trials in humans are being conducted with radioisotope conjugates.[117] In one trial using ^{131}I-labeled T101 MoAb for cutaneous T-cell lymphoma, tumor regression was seen in all six patients treated. The dose-limiting toxicity was related to bone marrow, causing thrombocytopenia and granulocytopenia. Carrasquillo et al.[118] have studied the therapeutic effects of ^{131}I-conjugated antimelanoma Fab fragments. Doses of 374 to 861 mCi delivered an estimated 3,800 to 8,500 rad to the tumor and produced responses in two of three patients. Patients treated with lower doses had no response. Kalofonos et al.[119] have studied the therapeutic effects of an ^{131}I-conjugate MoAb directed against the epidermal growth factor receptor in treating 10 patients with grades III and IV brain gliomas. One patient remained in remission for 3 years, and six others showed signs of clinical improvement. These initial results are encouraging for the therapeutic application of radioimmunoconjugates.

Iodine and other radioisotopes may be rapidly cleaved from amino acid residues on degraded MoAbs, leading to decreased tumor uptake and increased nonspecific tissue doses. Nonspecific uptake of the radioactive iodine by the thyroid gland can be partially blocked by pretreating these patients with saturated solution of potassium iodide. Flooding the reticuloendothelial system (RES) with unlabeled antibody may decrease nonspecific localization of radioisotope conjugates in the liver and spleen. The onset of hematologic toxicities is generally delayed, and patients may become profoundly neutropenic and thrombocytopenic.[120] An adjunctive measure to alleviate such marrow dysfunction is to rescue the patient with stored autologous bone marrow or CSFs.

Immunotoxin Conjugates. Toxin conjugates, or immunotoxins, are compounds formed by chemically linking antibodies to naturally occurring toxic polypeptides that inactivate protein synthesis.[121-125] The toxin may be a whole toxin of plant or bacterial origin, a subunit of a toxin, or a class of plant proteins known as hemitoxins. Table 11-2 lists examples of these types of toxins.

Mechanism

In its natural state, a toxin usually consists of an enzymatically cytotoxic A peptide chain and a B peptide chain that binds to galactose residues on the cell surface. The B chain binds to the cell surface and may facilitate the translocation of the A chain through the cell membrane into the cytosol. The A chain then inactivates protein synthesis by one of two methods

Table 11-2 Available Toxins to Conjugate with Monoclonal Antibodies

Category	Examples
Plant hemitoxins	Pokeweed antiviral protein
	Gelonin
	Saporin
	Momordica charanthia inhibitor
Plant toxins	Ricin
	Abrin
	Modecin
Bacterial toxins	Diphtheria toxin
	Pseudomonas exotoxin A
Toxin subunits	Ricin A chain
	Abrin B chain
Toxin fragments	Diphtheria toxin fragment A

SOURCE: Adapted with permission from Frankel AE, Houston LL, Issell BF. Prospects for immunotoxin therapy in cancer. *Annu Rev Med.* 1986;37:129.

depending on the origin of the toxin. Bacterial toxins (diphtheria and *Pseudomonas* exotoxin A) disrupt protein synthesis by ribosylating elongation factor 2, whereas the plant toxins (ricin, abrin, and modecin) inactivate protein synthesis by inactivating the 60S subunit of ribosomes. Once in the cytoplasm, a single molecule of this extremely potent toxin can produce cell death.

Whole toxins are toxic to both tumor and normal cells. The A chain subunit may be obtained from whole toxin by reducing the interchain disulfide bond and separating the subunits. The A chain subunit is essentially inactive unless attached to the cell surface and internalized. The objective of preparing conjugates of antibodies with toxin A chains is to modify the binding patterns of toxins to cells so that they will attach to and kill only the designated targeted tumor cells.[125,126] (The proposed action of an immunotoxin is shown in Figure 11-8.)

Specificity

Several issues must be addressed before constructing immunotoxins. A MoAb that is very specific for the target cell must be selected; this MoAb should also be capable of efficiently internalizing and delivering the toxin to its intracellular target. Not all tumor cells are capable of internalizing MoAb conjugates. The nature of the antibody-toxin linkage is crucial because, once internalized, the toxin must be separated from the antibody to function properly. If nonspecific toxicity is to be prevented, this separation should not occur until the conjugate reaches the cell and is internalized. Innovative conjugation systems have been developed that incorporate an acid-labile ligand that cleaves inside the acidic environment of the lysosome after the conjugate has been phagocytosed.

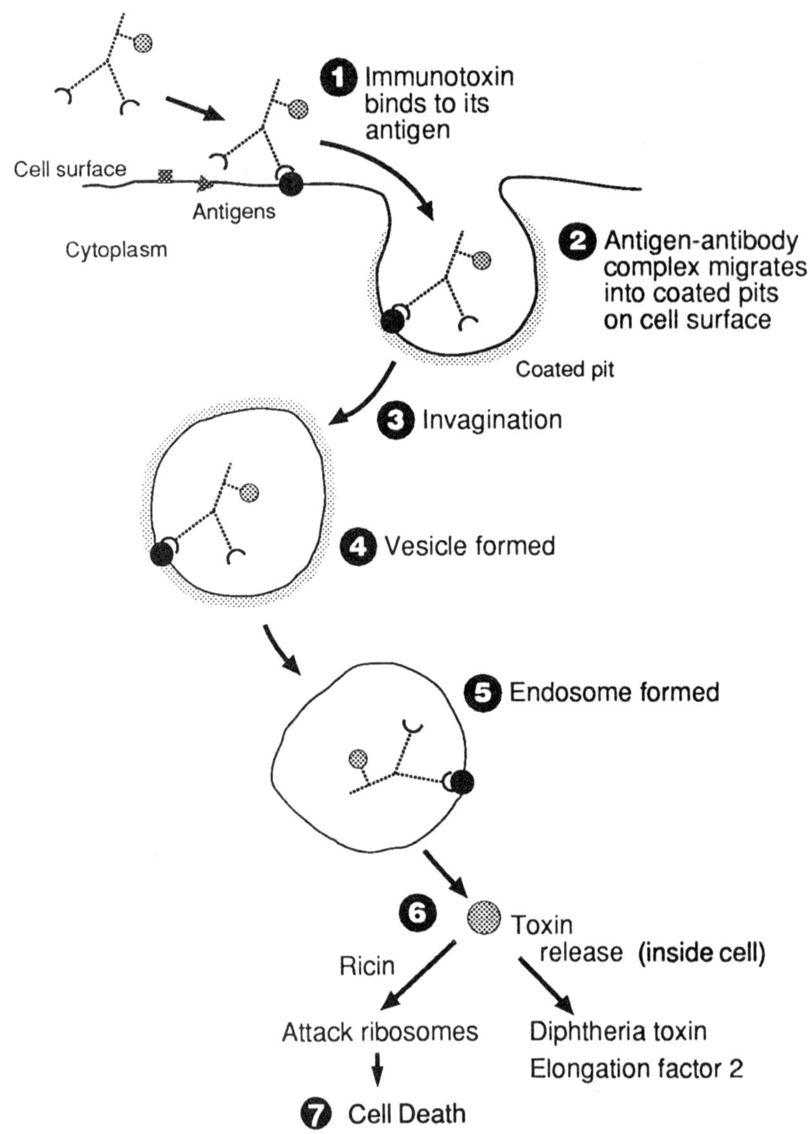

Figure 11-8. Proposed action of immunotoxin

Source: Adapted with permission from Frankel AE, Houston LL, Issell BF. Prospects for immunotoxin therapy in cancer. *Ann Rev Med.* 1986;37:132.

Applications

There are several possible levels of clinical immunotoxin applications. Immunotoxins may be used in (l) ex vivo therapy (e.g., against specific cancer cells to purge them from autologous bone marrow)[127]; (2) intracavitary therapy (e.g., in ovarian carcinoma for intraperitoneal therapy of minimal residual disease)[128]; and (3) in vivo, for systemic therapy to attack circulating tumor cells, metastatic tumors, and solid tumor disease[129] or cells involved in graft-versus-host disease (GVHD).

Ricin

Ricin, derived from castor beans, is the toxin currently receiving attention for ex vivo and in vivo applications.[129-135] When the A chain of ricin, which inhibits protein synthesis, is conjugated to a MoAb, toxicity should be limited to only those tumor cells specifically targeted by the MoAb. Because the conjugate lacks the ricin B chain, which allows intact ricin to bind to nearly all cells, any free A chains released from killed cells or disattached from MoAbs should not be toxic to other cells.

Ex Vivo Applications of Immunotoxin Conjugates. A number of investigators are studying ex vivo applications of ricin immunotoxin in bone marrow transplantation (BMT) therapy.[130,136] The transplantation of the pluripotent stem cells in bone marrow is a proven method of restoring hematopoiesis after supralethal chemotherapy. The major impediments to the use of marrow transplant are (1) the presence of donor T cells that can cause GVHD in allogeneic specimens and (2) the possible reinfusion of tumor cells in autologous marrow transplants.

Trials

Filipovich and coworkers[137,138] used a cocktail of anti-T-cell antibodies conjugated to ricin in attempting to deplete T cells from allogeneic marrow before transplantation. The donor marrows of 14 patients undergoing allogeneic transplants for leukemia were pretreated with ricin-conjugated anti-T-cell antibodies. Only two cases of grade II GVHD occurred, many fewer than would normally be expected. There were no deaths due to GVHD; however, there were two cases of marrow rejection (or failure to engraft) resulting in eventual patient death. Anti-T-cell immunotoxins appear to offer an effective means of T-cell depletion ex vivo before bone marrow reinfusion. However, biologic problems such as stem cell depletion, failure to engraft, rejection, and relapse must be addressed in future clinical trials.[139]

Ex vivo use of immunotoxin to deplete residual cancer cells in autologous bone marrow is under investigation. Ramsay and coworkers[136] used two anti-T-cell ricin conjugates (T101-ricin, TA-ricin) to purge autologous marrow grafts in T-cell leukemia and lymphoma patients. The marrow of six patients was pretreated with the immunotoxin and reinfused after a marrow conditioning regimen of high-dose cyclophosphamide and total body irradiation. Four of these patients relapsed. Other trials are under way to evaluate the efficacy of this technique of immunotoxin and unconjugated MoAb therapy in patients undergoing autologous BMT therapy for hematopoietic and solid tumors.[136,140-142]

Trials

In Vivo Applications of Immunotoxin Conjugates. In vivo investigations have primarily involved animals; human trials are just beginning and recently reviewed.[143] In animal trials, Krolick et al. treated mice with BCLl B-cell tumors using immunotoxins.[134] The immunotoxins were ricin-A conjugated to polyclonal anti-idiotype and antidelta antibody. Results showed that immunotoxins prolonged survival of these BCLl B-cell tumorous mice. In a human trial, Spitler et al.[135] used antimelanoma antibodies coupled with the ricin A chain. Some clinical responses have been seen, with several persistent regressions.

Perhaps the most encouraging in vivo use of an immunotoxin is in the treatment of steroid-resistant acute GVHD. Orthozyme-CD5® plus (XomaZyme H65®) is an immunotoxin with ricin-A conjugated to a murine MoAb directed against the CD5 antigen. This antigen is expressed primarily on mature T lymphocytes. In a multicenter trial of 34 steroid-resistant GVHD patients, 16 of the 32 evaluable patients had either a complete or a partial response.[144] These patients received doses between 0.05mg/kg and 0.33mg/kg per day for up to 14 days in this dose-escalation trial. The highest incidence of response occurred with skin lesions (73%); the incidence of improvement or response with gastrointestinal and liver GVHD was 45% and 28%, respectively. This study suggests that this immunotoxin may be an effective immunosuppressive agent for treating acute GVHD. Other nonimmunotoxin MoAbs such as anti-IL-2 receptor antibody (B-B10) and antibody B-C7 against tumor necrosis factor (TNF) alpha are also undergoing trials in the treatment of patients with steroid-resistant acute GVHD.[145]

Clinical trials in the treatment of malignancies to date have had only mixed findings of some partial response or transient falls in circulating tumor cells.[146] Toxicities have been dose related and similar: capillary leak syndrome, low serum albumin, and weight gain. Rarely has pulmonary edema been reported. A more serious toxicity of profound sensory motor peripheral neuropathy was noted in three patients treated for breast cancer with a ricin-A immunoconjugate.[147] So that MoAbs used in immunotoxin conjugates may have a greater role in tumor therapy, research is needed (1) to better understand the cross-reactivity of MoAbs to normal cells and the design of the toxins and (2) to find the best delivery method.

Antineoplastic Drug Conjugates. The concept of attaching an antineoplastic drug to antibodies for therapeutic use is not new. Chlorambucil had been conjugated to polyclonal goat antibodies for investigational therapeutic use well before MoAbs were developed.[148,149] The combination of antineoplastic agents with MoAbs should direct the drug to the specifically targeted tumor cells, improving the therapeutic-to-toxic ratio compared with the shotgun approach of systemic chemotherapy. The requirements for conjugating drugs to MoAbs are as before: (l) conjugates should be stable enough to prevent indiscriminate release of drugs and exposure to normal tissue but be able to act once they reach the targeted cell; (2) conjugation should neither interfere with the specificity of the antibody nor reduce the effectiveness of the drug; and (3) conjugates may or may not have the same mechanisms of action, side effects, or pharmacokinetics as their individual components. A number of trials are under way to evaluate these antineoplastic conjugates to MoAbs.[150,151] The most common agents used as conjugates are antimetabolites and such antibiotics as doxorubicin and daunorubicin.[152-157]

Specifications

Several studies using various antineoplastic conjugates have demonstrated cytotoxicity in cell cultures and in animal tumors.[156,158,159] From the animal studies it is not clear what doses of conjugates are necessary; however, it appears that more drug per antibody is needed to kill the cell than with immunotoxins. This problem of drug potency may be approached by increasing the amount of active drug per milligram of immunoglobulin or using agents with higher intrinsic potencies on a molar basis, such as the vinca alkaloids. Ford et al.[150] have studied a small number of patients with advanced colorectal or ovarian cancers. These patients were treated with a polyclonal anti-CEA antibody conjugated to vindesine. While there were no therapeutic responses to the conjugate, this study demonstrated the safety of administering the conjugate and its ability to localize in tumor cells. A new cis-platinum (CDDP) immunoconjugate has been produced and will provide potentially new treatment opportunities for CDDP-sensitive tumors.[160] Research efforts concentrate on identifying a potent drug that can be properly conjugated to the desired MoAb. Other trials with antineoplastic drug conjugates are being published.[161]

Liposomal Conjugates. One of the most interesting approaches in targeting drugs to specific areas in the body is the use of liposomes.[162-165] Liposomes are typically composed of some combination of phosphatidylcholine, cholesterol, phosphatidylglycerol, or other glycolipids or phospholipids. Liposomes may be filled with almost any drug before administration. Liposomes typically concentrate the drug in cells of the RES of the liver and spleen, and they reduce drug intake in the heart, kidney, and gastrointestinal tracts. The application of liposome-associated doxorubicin reduces cardiotoxicity,[166] and liposome-associated amphotericin-B reduces nephrotoxicity and other adverse effects.[167-169]

RES concentration

If attached to MoAbs, liposomes may be targeted to specific tissues, and uptake by the cells of the RES may be avoided. Antibodies can be coupled to liposomes either directly by a covalent link or by means of protein A, which binds to the Fc fragment of an immunoglobulin. Health et al.[170]

demonstrated the ability of liposomes targeted with anti-H2K antibody to bind and deliver encapsulated methotrexate-gamma-aspartate to L929 fibroblasts. The antibody-delivered drug's ability to inhibit the growth of L929 fibroblasts was increased tenfold over systemic administration of the drug. The liposome-targeted drug is more toxic to the cells than either targeted drug or liposome drug alone. Clinical trials using liposomal conjugates are just beginning.[171]

Prodrug conversion

Antibody-enzyme Conjugates. A new approach in applying MoAbs to cancer therapy is to use MoAbs to deliver enzymes to tumor cell surfaces. The chosen enzyme conjugate would be able to convert relatively noncytotoxic drug precursors into active drugs. The prodrug is then activated at the tumor site and can penetrate the nearby tumor cells.[172] MoAb conjugates to the enzyme alkaline phosphatase (AP) have been developed and used to convert the prodrug etoposide phosphate into etoposide; the prodrug mitomycin phosphate has also been converted into mitomycin alcohol in both in vitro and in vivo models.[173] Antitumor responses were observed in animals treated with the MoAb-AP conjugated to carboxypeptidase G2 enzyme, which has been used for the prodrug activation of nitrogen mustard 1 to form active benzoic acid mustard 2.[174] Antibody enzyme conjugates may overcome the limitations of other MoAb conjugates, which require antibody internalization, release of immunotoxin or drug once in the cell, low potency of the many cytotoxins, tumor heterogeneity, and physiological barriers. However, the MoAb-enzyme conjugates may have a new set of limitations—immunogencity, availability of similar enzymes in normal cell tissue, insufficient clearance of the conjugates, and nonspecific uptake into cells—all of which can reduce the therapeutic tumor-to-host ratios. Careful selection of antibodies and enzymes and development of designer chimeric antibodies, recombinant molecules, and prodrugs will bring these new antibody-enzyme conjugates to clinical trial.

Limitations of Monoclonal Antibodies

While MoAb technology advanced in the past decade, limitations remain associated with the production and effective applications of MoAbs.[175] Many of these limitations are being identified in studies. Limitations may be divided into two general classes: those that affect the production of MoAbs and those that affect the application of MoAbs and conjugates in therapy.

Limitations on Production. Myeloma immortality is not perfect, and some of the hybridomas do not grow indefinitely. The loss of immortality may be associated with chromosomal shedding from the cell to reach a stable chromosome number after fusion, involving the potential loss of a vital chromosome. Selecting hybridomas that will produce and secrete desired antibodies indefinitely is still a trial-and-error process. There are also limitations in the production of large quantities of MoAbs. Newer technologies are required to increase production. Furthermore, specificity of MoAbs is not absolute, for many antigens found on tumor cells can be located on normal cells. Improved selection techniques for a specific and unique tumor antigen may increase the specificity of the antibody prepared against it.

Quantity and quality

Another limitation is that the binding of MoAbs to antigens may not initiate the desired responses. Carefully screening available antibodies, antibody classes or subclasses, and fragments for their reactions to antigen may help select for antibodies yielding the desired effects. Newer biotechnologic techniques may make it possible to create designer MoAbs.[6,7,37,176,177]

Although the production of human hybridomas and human MoAbs is a desired option, there are a number of technical difficulties. For instance, very few myeloma cell lines can produce human hybridomas. These hybridomas typically do not produce the quantity of MoAbs that can be obtained with murine hybridomas. An obvious problem is that selected antigens, such as tumor cells, cannot be injected into humans to obtain the necessary transformed B lymphocytes. It is also difficult to harvest human B cells in the state of optimum differentiation needed for cell fusion. Many methods are being devised to improve on the development of human hybridomas and other methods of human MoAb production. These methods are discussed in the MoAb production section in this chapter.

Limitations in Applications of Monoclonal Antibodies. The following limitations were observed during in vitro and in vivo clinical applications; possible solutions to these problems are also discussed.

HAMA

The Human Anti-murine Antibody Response. Most MoAbs in current clinical use are of murine origin. Studies have shown that these foreign proteins may be administered safely at first, but HAMA development has also been demonstrated.[178-180] The presence of HAMA is detectable approximately 7 to 30 days after the initial dose of murine antibody. HAMA can be made against both the constant and variable regions of the murine antibody. Controlled suppression of the host response against the murine antibody is important for the success of prolonged in vivo MoAb therapy. HAMA can consume the infused murine MoAbs and prevent them from binding to the target antigens, reducing any therapeutic effects. HAMA binding to the murine MoAbs may elicit an allergic-type response, increasing toxicity to the patient. Possible approaches to decreasing the production of HAMA include the concurrent administration of immunosuppressive drugs to decrease production of HAMA,[181] plasmapheresis to remove HAMA before treatment,[182] induction of immunologic tolerance, alteration of dose and schedule of subsequent doses, and use of human MoAbs [183] or chimeric antibodies[184] to reduce immunoglobulin antigenicity.

Binding of Free Tumor Antigens. The targeted antigen can be secreted or shed into the extracellular fluid by the tumor. Free tumor antigens would be valuable in increasing the sensitivity of assays to detect tumor markers. However, in treatment these free tumor antigens can bind up the MoAb or MoAb conjugates, consuming the antibodies or preventing the desired distribution of the MoAbs to tumor cells. The excess free tumor antigens have been associated with shortened half-life of the infused MoAbs because of an increased clearance of the complex.[185] As with HAMA, the formation of large amounts of immune complexes of free tumor antigen and MoAb may produce toxicity. Possible solutions to this problem include plasmapheresis before therapy to reduce the level of free tumor antigens, scheduling multiple MoAb treatments, and using large doses to overcome free tumor antigen binding.

Possible solutions

Antigenic Modulation. Antigenic modulation (the disappearance of antigen from the surface of cells targeted with MoAb) was observed in many patients within a few minutes to 2 hours after exposure to the antibody. The modulation appears to be temporary; antigen reappears on cell surfaces within 24 to 36 hours. The modulated cell is targeted-surface-antigen negative, making it resistant to serotherapy by the specific MoAb. This property may not be a limitation in the setting of immunoconjugates, in which it is desirable to have the conjugate gain entrance into the cell. Not all antigens modulate, nor do all antibodies cause modulation.

Problematic Biodistribution and Localization. Administered MoAbs do not always distribute and concentrate in the targeted tissues. The MoAbs can be concentrated by the RES, exposing these organs to toxicity. Tumors located in tissue distal from the circulatory system may not be accessible to the MoAbs, thus rendering them less susceptible to the antibody therapy. Approaches for overcoming such problems include selecting and using antibody classes or subclasses, or antibody fragments, that will give a more desirable distribution. Moreover, administering cold unlabeled antibodies to saturate nonspecific uptake sites before administering cytotoxic MoAbs may enhance binding of the targeted cells.

Lack of Surface Antigen. Subpopulations of the tumor may lack the surface antigen targeted by the MoAb because of tumor heterogeneity and may escape therapy. This lack may be overcome by using MoAb cocktails[186] for different tumor antigens on the tumor cell or by using radioisotope conjugates that may kill the cells within the radiation fields.

MoAb cocktails

MoAb localization to the tumor may also be improved by changing to subcutaneous administration (for example, in melanoma)[186] or interperitoneal administration (in ovarian cancer).[187]

These are some of the major limitations currently identified and some possible solutions. Ongoing studies will examine these limitations and methods of managing them in the next several years. New problems with the use of MoAbs will undoubtedly be discovered; however, MoAbs will also be applied more widely as these limitations are overcome and techniques are developed for increasing the efficacy while reducing the toxicities of MoAb therapy.

Other Applications of Monoclonal Antibodies in Medicine

More uses are being found for MoAbs in all areas of science and medicine. The primary areas of application are as research tools, chemical reagents, industrial purifiers, and both diagnostic and therapeutic agents in animals and humans.

Protein purification

Specific MoAbs make excellent reagents and biologic tools for assaying, purifying, and detecting proteins. As research tools, MoAbs can recognize specific amino acid sequences of polypeptides, allowing for the detection of minor antigenic determinants in cells, viruses, and polypeptides. MoAbs have been used to define regions of immunogenic determinants on a protein and to elucidate the essential amino acid sequences that can serve as synthetic vaccines. MoAbs have been labeled with fluorescein and used to sort out cells with selected surface-binding proteins. MoAbs are also used in purifying protein molecules. MoAbs can be placed on an affinity column; mixtures containing the target protein are then passed through the column. The desired protein molecule binds specifically to the MoAb while the impurities are washed through. The protein may then be isolated from the column. Many proteins, including AFP and interferon, can be purified by means of MoAbs.[188,189] This procedure is also used to purify factor VIII (see Chapter 5).

The area of greatest interest is the use of MoAbs in diagnosing and treating diseases. This section examines applications of MoAbs in clinical medicine for diagnosis, assay, imaging, and tissue typing and possible treatment applications in cardiology, infectious diseases, and autoimmune diseases.

Diagnostic and Drug Assays

AIDS

MoAbs are employed today primarily as in vitro diagnostic reagents. Several hundred diagnostic tests have been developed and are being marketed, ranging from tests for detecting antibodies against human immunodeficiency virus type 1 (HIV-1) in patients with acquired immunodeficiency syndrome (AIDS) to over-the-counter home pregnancy tests.[190,191] One of the early diagnostic uses of MoAbs in health care was the quantitative measurement of CD4+ and CD8+ T-lymphocyte ratios in the blood for assessing immune-compromised individuals and patients with other disease states. Commercial MoAb diagnostic kits are now available for tumor markers, pregnancy tests, drug assays, and tissue and blood typing and for such infectious diseases as chlamydia, herpes simplex, gonorrhea, hepatitis B, and bacterial infections.

The diagnostic use of MoAbs relies on ability to detect the desired specific antigen. In general, most of the tests involve placing pure antibody in a test solution to which a sample of biologic fluid can be added. If the target antigen is present in the sample, an antibody-antigen reaction takes place. The techniques used to detect this reaction (see Chapter 5) are RIA, ELISA, and agglutination inhibition.

Monoclonal Antibody-based Diagnostic Tests

Home tests

The largest market for MoAb use is currently the self-care market. The number of MoAb home testing kits used as aids to diagnosis has rapidly increased, largely because of advances in MoAb technology.

Pregnancy Tests. The first publicly available MoAbs were developed for pregnancy testing. Many companies are now manufacturing MoAb diagnostic assays for pregnancy and for ovulation.[191] Home pregnancy tests detect human chorionic gonadotropin (HCG) in the patient's urine.

False-positives

Most older pregnancy tests used an agglutination-inhibition methodology and pooled antibodies of animal origin. These antibodies react to the alpha subunit of the HCG molecule. Other hormones, including luteinizing hormone (LH), follicle-stimulating hormone, and thyroid-stimulating hormone, also contain the alpha subunits of the same amino acid sequence as HCG; therefore, the tests may give false-positive reactions when these hormones are elevated. To minimize the cross-reactivity, the sensitivity of the home test is reduced. The accuracy rate of the older tests ranges from 97% to 99%, assuming proper use of the test kits. Drug interactions have been reported with the older kits. Methyldopa, levodopa, carbidopa, methadone, antidepressants, and anticonvulsants may inhibit agglutination.

The newer pregnancy tests use MoAbs that react with the beta subunit found only on HCG. The problem of cross-reactivity with other hormones is eliminated with these MoAb kits. The newer kits use enzyme assays that are unaffected by vibration and sunlight, and color changes that indicate positive results are stable, allowing results to be further interpreted by a physician or pharmacist. The manufacturers of these kits report 99% accuracy with positive results, and some can be read within a minute after use.

Newer tests

Ovulation Tests. Being able to predict ovulation allows a woman to identify periods when she is fertile. This ability facilitates conception by enabling intercourse or intrauterine insemination and in vitro fertilization to be properly timed. MoAb-based tests are available to detect the surge in LH that precedes ovulation.[192] Because MoAbs used in these tests are specific for the beta subunit of the LH molecule, cross-reactivity with other hormones is unlikely. A number of test kits are available that use enzyme immunoassay.

The MoAb ovulation tests offer semiquantitative determinations of the LH level in the urine. Testing, using the morning urine, starts in advance of likely ovulation and is continued daily until ovulation occurs, as indicated by an increase in color intensity. Some kits include a dipstick that has been coated with an antibody directed to the alpha subunit of LH and a test solution that contains a MoAb-enzyme complex that is specific for the beta subunit of LH. If LH is present in the added urine, the alpha subunit of LH binds to the dipstick. The test solution, which recognizes the beta subunit of the bound LH, is then added, forming a sandwichlike complex on the dipstick. After the dipstick has been rinsed, a color substrate in the test is added that reacts with the enzyme bound to the stick, imparting a blue color. The intensity of the blue color reflects the amount of LH in the urine sample. A kit contains either six or nine tests. The prediction rate of ovulation increases with the number of tests performed. Limitations include administration of exogenous hormones (estrogen-progestin combinations) that can alter LH levels and interfere with testing; the tests also detect exogenous LH contained in the menotropins, and the test is affected by the administration of danazol, which suppresses LH production.

Limitations

Detection of Anti-Rh Factors. MoAbs have long been available for detecting the presence of Rh factors. One product detects the presence of anti-Rh factors. The antibody can be used to determine whether the pregnant woman has potentially dangerous Rh antibody against an Rh-positive fetus. The antibody may also be administered prophylactically to an Rh-negative woman who is carrying an Rh-positive fetus to avoid the risk of hemolytic anemia in the newborn.

Drug Assays. A number of standard laboratory methods have been determined for monitoring drug levels: high-pressure liquid chromatography, RIAs, and enzyme-multiplied immunoassay technique. MoAbs are also available for drug assays. MoAb-based assays are very specific and highly sensitive. Currently, they are used to detect digoxin, phenobarbital, and theophylline; assays for many other drugs will soon be available. The use of MoAbs in drug assays has opened the door to home testing of serum and saliva drug levels. A number of kits are now available for office use by physicians to monitor drug therapy. These office kits are similar to the quantitative immunoassays used in many laboratories. MoAbs for different drugs are replacing many of the polyclonal reagents formerly used in larger drug-assaying systems.

Sensitive and specific

Infectious Disease Diagnosis. MoAb-based kits for detecting bacterial infections, viral infections, and fungal infections are being developed.[193] There are many MoAbs available against these microorganisms. Most of the currently available kits and laboratory studies use immunofluorescence (IF) methods to detect antigen-antibody reactions. MoAbs directed against agents of sexually transmitted diseases are beginning to appear on the market. Panels of MoAbs have been prepared that distinguish *Neisseria gonorrheae, Chlamydia trachomatis,* and herpes simplex viruses (HSVs) 1 and 2 from one another and from common organisms.[193-196] Often a panel of several MoAbs directed at different antigenic components of the organism is used in the test to capture the majority of different isolates of an organism. Each of the antibodies reacts with a single specificity to identify a particular antigenic determinant of one of the organisms. Alternatively, one could, through careful selection, prepare a specific MoAb that would identify major outer proteins in all of the serovars (immunotypes) of the organism.

Trachomatis can be diagnosed by direct fluorescein-conjugated MoAbs.[197,198] The IF slide test identifies *Chlamydia* bodies in scrapings of genital secretions; other diagnostic IF methods can be used for rapid confirmation of organisms in tissue culture. The IF slide test compares favorably in sensitivity and specificity with tests using tissue cell culture: approximately 92% and 97%, respectively. The MoAb IF test is easier to perform, quicker, and less expensive than standard tissue culture techniques. IF slide test results are obtained in 30 minutes, whereas cell cultures take 6 days. Other bacterial diagnostic assays are being developed. MoAbs are also available for detecting viral antigens.[199-203] A rapid laboratory diagnosis of cytomegalovirus (CMV) infections by a direct IF method using a MoAb directed against CMV-infected cells is available.[200] The antibody produces dense IF with prominent lobular staining within the nucleus. A new diagnostic assay developed for CMV infections measures the presence of CMV-immediated early antigens in peripheral blood leukocytes during active CMV infection.[201] MoAbs and restriction

CMV

endonuclease digestion have been used for distinguishing HSVs 1 and 2. Other MoAbs directed at viral antigens, including those of hepatitis, are being developed, which will be useful for screening blood to prevent post-transfusion hepatitis.

AIDS, malaria, PCP

The largest area of diagnostic monoclonal assay development has been the detection of antibodies in the serum of patients who have been exposed to HIV-l, which is responsible for AIDS. Most of these tests use ELISA methodology to detect the presence of anti-HIV antibodies rapidly.[203,204] The assays are being used to screen donated blood and to make initial diagnosis of HIV infections. A number of confirmation assays are being developed using MoAbs against viral elements such as p24 core antigen.

MoAbs developed for other infectious organisms raise the possibility of developing diagnostic assays for these organisms; a MoAb against *Rickettsia rickettsii* is one example.[194] MoAb immunoassays for *Plasmodium falciparum* are being examined for use to screen blood donors for malaria.[205] MoAbs are being used to detect *Pneumocystis carinii* in sputum, providing a rapid and less invasive technique for the diagnosis of *P. carinii* pneumonia. Pools of MoAbs with specificity for different viruses are used to diagnose respiratory infections such as parainfluenza, influenza A and B, respiratory synetial virus, and adenovirus.[206]

Imaging. MoAbs have proven useful in vitro as diagnostic assays for drugs, infections, and diseases. The in vivo use of MoAbs for imaging is a powerful application. MoAbs may be covalently linked with radioisotopes or contrast agents for in vivo administration, for ex vivo detection by a gamma camera, or for a magnetic resonance imaging scanner to localize damaged tissues or tumors.[207-209] Imaging with labeled MoAbs provides useful information regarding differential diagnosis, extent of disease or damage, and the progression or resolution of the disease. Initial applications of MoAb-targeted imaging have been mainly in oncology, cardiology, and infectious diseases.

The use of MoAb-targeted imaging requires overcoming several limitations.[210] The potential sources of problems include background interference or trapping of conjugated MoAbs, the type of ligands or coupling techniques needed to attach the dye or radioisotope to the MoAbs, the type of imaging material, and the pharmacokinetics of the MoAbs and imaging agents. The trapping or nonspecific binding of the conjugated MoAb is important for the resolution and accuracy of the image. Trapping and nonspecific binding can occur during the initial infusion, as the body breaks down the bonds between the conjugated isotope and MoAbs, and as the antibody is cleared. This trapping can increase the background interference or decrease the resolution of the image. Carefully selecting the

MoAb and type of ligand to strengthen the bonds between antibody and isotope minimizes this limitation.

MoAbs may be conjugated and labeled with a number of different isotopes and contrast agents. The most common labels are ^{111}In, ^{131}I, and ^{99m}Tc. The choice of conjugate is important; previously most MoAbs were linked to ^{111}In, but there is increasing use of ^{99m}Tc with new chelation and linkage chemistries. Technetium has advantages, because most gamma cameras are calibrated in the photon range of ^{99m}Tc, and it is less expensive than other agents. Researchers are concerned with the relatively short half-life of ^{99m}Tc (6 hours) versus the longer half-life of ^{111}In (2.7 days), which permits imaging over a longer period. Technetium-labeled MoAbs have been able to provide clear images without background in about 3 hours. The type of conjugated isotope determines the type of equipment needed to visualize the image.[211-212]

The last issue, which must be addressed before development and release of MoAbs for imaging purposes, is that the specific conjugation of MoAbs to isotopes may change the binding affinity of the antibody and the pharmacokinetics of either MoAb or isotope alone.

Cardiac Imaging Techniques. Cardiac imaging techniques with MoAbs have arisen from the development of antibodies to thrombus, fibrin, and myosin.[209] Cardiac myosin can be detected after cardiac injury and cellular death. The antimyosin MoAbs and MoAb fragments have been labeled with either ^{99m}Tc or ^{111}In to detect zones of acute myocardial necrosis and to determine the size of the infarction.

Antimyosin MoAbs

Clinical trials note that an overall sensitivity for the diagnosis of acute infarction has been greater than 90% with little or no localization of the antibodies in regions of previous infarctions.[213,214] Diagnostic scan with ^{111}In antimycosin Fab antibodies can provide a diagnosis of subacute as well as acute myocardial necrosis.[215] The antimyosin MoAb-labeled imaging tool is useful in differentiating between severe ischemia and irreversible necrosis. Other trials are ongoing to yield a noninvasive approach to the diagnosis of myocarditis or cardiomyopathy.[216]

Antifibrin and antiplatelet

The antifibrin MoAbs[217,218] and antiplatelet MoAbs[219,220] are useful in delineating thrombi in both arteries and veins, and they are under investigation for detecting deep venous thrombosis[221] and thrombi in organs with high blood pool activity.[222] The choices of (1) MoAb antiplatelet versus antifibrin, (2) types of antibody fragments, and (3) radionucleotide are still controversial. Both types of antibodies have been suitable for imaging thrombis, and labeled Fab fragments are more advantageous than whole molecules because the lower molecular weight improves antibody penetration into the thrombus. The absence of Fc portion decreases immune reaction and improves clearance of these antibodies. Future applications of these antibodies might include early detection of atherosclerotic plaque, monitoring of clot resolution after therapy with thrombolytics, and other noninvasive imaging techniques.

Infectious Disease Imaging Techniques. The possible applications of MoAbs in the imaging of infectious diseases are numerous. Many MoAbs are already available that are directed toward different types of microorganisms. Current interest is in the imaging of deep-seated infections, which allows the location of the infection to be identified; it may also allow the organism or organisms to be identified without the use of invasive surgical procedures.[223]

Uses of MoAbs for Tissue Typing. The importance of identifying surface structures on cells that play a major role in the acceptance or rejection of transplanted tissues has been apparent for some time. Polyclonal antisera have been used to identify these surface structures. The use of MoAbs will aid in more specifically defining these molecules and their roles in graft tolerance. MoAbs will also aid in the phenotyping of normal cells (such as lymphocytes) within the body and identifying the roles that these cells play in the maintenance of homeostasis.

Graft rejection

HLA Typing. The major histocompatibility complex—in humans, called human leukocyte antigen (HLA)—is important for the transplantation of organs, tissues, and bone marrow.[224] (See Chapter 3.) The HLA complex is located on chromosome 6 and is responsible for encoding self antigens. Tissue typing to determine HLA antigens can help to increase the chances of tissue engraftment and organ acceptance.

The HLA antigens were among the first human structures recognized by MoAbs. Many reagents have since been produced for recognizing HLA antigens. MoAbs to these antigens have given immunologists tools to analyze the structure, function, and role of the HLA antigens in diseases.[224] The role of MoAbs used for HLA typing is growing. However, because many of the existing MoAbs for HLA antigens are not cytotoxic, they cannot be used with existing serology methods, which involve assays that often identify the lysis of cells as their end point.

Blood Typing. There are more than 300 antigenic determinants on the surface of the human RBC membrane. Those antigens, which are genetically linked, are grouped together to form the blood group systems. (The term *blood type* refers to the antigenic phenotype, which is the serologic expression of the inherited blood group genes.) Twenty-one blood groups are currently recognized. The antigens were first recognized by the analysis of the alloantibodies produced as a result of transfusions or pregnancy. Blood typing is important for avoiding the transfusion of antigen-incompatible blood and the early detection and prevention of hemolytic disease of the newborn. (See Chapter 3.)

MoAbs are used to study the function and structures of these antigens. MoAbs directed at blood groups A and B have been produced by hybridoma techniques.[225] Other blood group antigens have been isolated and studied; purified sources are relatively abundant. MoAb affinity chromatography can be used to purify the antigens. The antigens could then be used to further immunize mice to produce reagents for blood typing. One role of MoAbs will thus be to provide unlimited quantities of reagents useful for blood bank typing.

Classification of Lymphocyte Subpopulations. As a research tool, MoAbs have been invaluable in identifying human lymphocyte subpopulations.[226] MoAbs have enhanced the understanding of the structures and functions of the subclasses of both B and T lymphocytes. A familiar use of MoAbs is the classification of subpopulations of T lymphocytes. The OKT (Ortho) series of MoAbs was first discovered by Reinherz, Kung, and Goldstein.[227] OKT antibodies recognize antigens on the cell surface of the T lymphocytes. Mature T cells are all detected by the MoAb OKT3, which recognizes the CD3 antigen. The MoAb OKT4 primarily binds helper/inducer T cells at the CD4 antigen, and the MoAb OKT8 binds cytotoxic/suppressor T cells at the CD8 antigen. Other MoAbs of the OKT series may bind tissues and cells other than T cells. Other MoAbs have been produced that also recognize specific subpopulations, for example, Leu-3 (Becton Dickinson) for the helper/inducer T cells. These MoAbs are placed in categories called clusters of differentiation (CDs). Thus, the CD4 cluster is a group of MoAbs that recognizes the CD4 antigen primarily found on helper/inducer T cells.

OKT MoAbs

MoAbs can be used to determine the proportions and absolute numbers of T cells and T-cell subsets. The ratio of helper cells to suppressor cells (CD4+ to CD8+) in peripheral blood is of significance in many disease states. A clinical use of ratios of CD4+ to CD8+ is in the diagnosis of immunodeficiency syndromes, AIDS in particular. In patients with AIDS, the number of helper T cells in circulation is diminished. The helper T cells may be detected by anti-CD4 MoAbs, and the T suppressor cells may be detected by anti-CD8 MoAbs. The diagnosis of AIDS may be supported with a decrease in the ratio of helper T cells to suppressor T cells. The ratios of CD4+ to CD8+ also are altered in a number of various other disease processes, such as infectious diseases, autoimmune diseases, allergies, aging, and transplantation.

Immunohistology. MoAbs are also useful for classifying leukemias and lymphomas. The antibody reagents can distinguish between T- and B-cell leukemias and can also provide information on T-cell malignancies. T-cell malignancies of early differentiated T cells bind OKT10 or OKT9 or both; more mature T-cell malignancies, such as cutaneous T-cell lymphomas, bind OKT4 MoAbs. The type of acute lymphocytic leukemia may also be determined by MoAbs.

Potential Nontumor Therapeutic Uses of Monoclonal Antibodies

The early focus of MoAb research was often on cancer immunotherapy, but the potential for the use of MoAbs in other areas has been recognized as well. The clinical applications of immunosuppressive therapy with MoAbs OKT3[228] and newer MoAbs[229] for the prophylaxis and treatment of transplant rejection is discussed in depth in Chapter 9. The potential therapeutic applications in infectious disease, cardiology, and autoimmune disorders are discussed here.

Infectious Disease Therapy. MoAbs have been produced against a variety of viruses,[230-232] bacteria,[233-235] and parasites.[194,236] Applications for these MoAbs are being seen in the areas of diagnosis, imaging, and treatment or prevention of infectious diseases.[230,237] Uses in diagnosis and imaging have been reviewed elsewhere.[193]

Viral strains

One of the early applications of MoAbs was in defining antigenic sites on viruses (e.g., influenza, measles, rabies). These MoAb reagents were capable of distinguishing among the strains of viruses isolated in different parts of the world. By means of a panel of MoAbs, the differences and similarities of these viruses can be determined and vaccines produced. These studies on viruses, as well as studies on bacteria and parasites, will have implications for the use of MoAbs in the treatment and prevention of infectious disease in clinical medicine and will also provide information on the structures and biology of the microorganisms.

MoAbs have been used in the study of specific parasitic diseases. MoAbs against various stages of malarial parasites can induce protective immunity. Protective MoAbs have been produced against merozoites of *Plasmodium yoelii, P. knowlesi,* and *P. falciparum.* In studies with mice infected with *P. yoelii,* injections of MoAbs specific for *P. yoelli* reduced the level of infection (although extent of control over the infection was not the same for all mice infected). MoAbs against *P. falciparum* are capable of inhibiting parasite reinvasion and intraerythrocytic development in vitro. Passive protection has been demonstrated with MoAbs to the promastigote stage of *Leishmania mexicana* and to the schistosomula of *Schistosoma mansoni.* Thus, MoAbs against specific antigens on these parasites may be useful as reagents to treat these infections passively.[238]

In addition to providing passive immunity, these MoAbs may be sources for the production of vaccines for active immunization.[239,240] An antibody has a specific antigen-binding site unique to itself within its variable region. This site on the immunoglobulin is known as its idiotype. The idiotype consists of an antibody's unique amino acid sequence and the configuration of its antigen-binding site. Anti-antibodies may be produced against the idiotype and other parts of the antibody. The antibodies formed against the idiotype are known as anti-idiotype antibodies. Any given anti-idiotype antibody can be structurally similar to the antigen against which the MoAb was originally developed. In other words, the anti-idiotype is an internal image of the original antigen. This anti-idiotype antibody should thus be antigenic (i.e., capable of inducing immunity). For example, an anti-idiotype antibody could be produced against the idiotype of a MoAb specific for a parasite,[238] and this anti-idiotype antibody would then be used as a vaccine to induce immunity (Figure 11-9). This technique would be advantageous over the current method of purifying antigens and producing them in large quantities, because the anti-idiotype antibody would serve as a nonpathogenic antigen. This method of vaccine production is now undergoing research.[233]

Anti-idiotypes

MoAbs have a number of potential applications in bacteriology in both diagnosis and treatment of bacterial infections. Some of these applications are classifying bacterial species, serotyping within species, serodiagnosing bacterial infections (including use for passive immunity as with parasites), immunizing, and treating sepsis. MoAbs as reagents will eventually replace

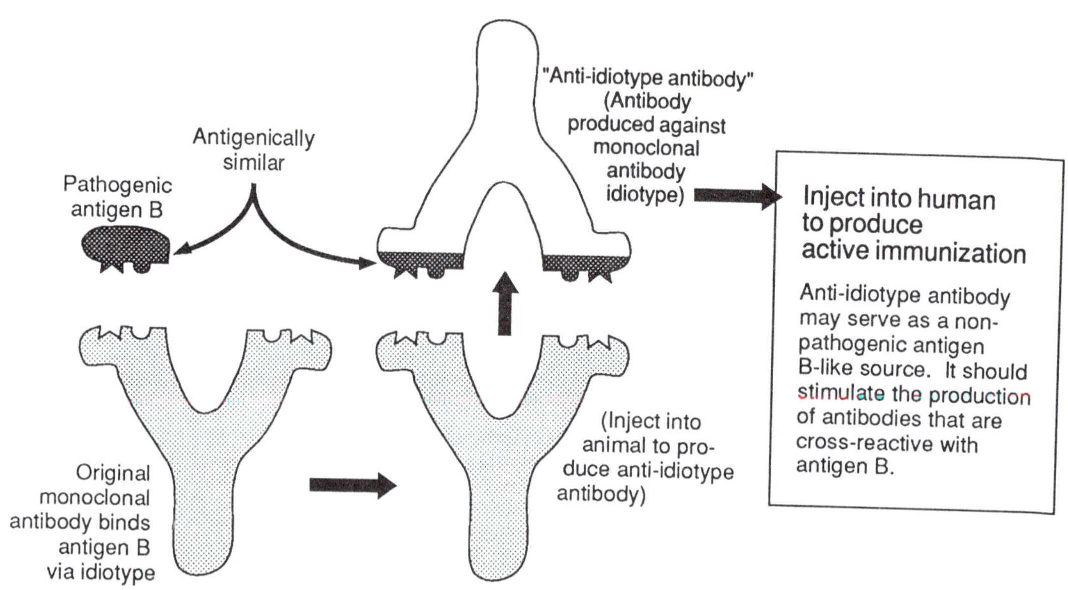

Figure 11-9. Anti-idiotype antibody for active immunization

the current polyclonal antisera used in serology because of their advantages in cost, convenience, specificity, reproducibility, and unlimited availability. In serodiagnosis, MoAbs would be useful in identifying specific bacterial antigens in sputum or cerebrospinal fluid. As part of therapy, human MoAbs have been prepared against the C fragment of tetanus toxin and have been shown to protect mice from 10 times the LD50 of tetanus toxin in mice.[241] This capability may have future applications in the treatment of human tetanus toxin exposures.

Septic shock

Perhaps the area of greatest therapeutic interest is the use of MoAbs to treat Gram-negative bacteremia and septic shock.[234] The sepsis syndrome seems to be the result of the release of endotoxins from the bacterial cell wall. The lipid A component of the lipopolysaccharide (LPS) molecule appears to be responsible for most endotoxic activities. Animal studies[242-244] and human studies[245,246] have shown the effectiveness of immunoglobulins in providing some protective activity against septic shock and death. A recent international multicenter study examined the efficacy of adjunctive treatment with a human IgM MoAb targeted against LPS known as HA-lA (Centoxin®).[247] Patients in a double-blinded trial received either 100 mg of HA-lA MoAb as a single infusion for 15 to 20 minutes or a placebo of albumin. The patients who had documented bacteremia and received the HA-lA MoAb had a lower mortality rate at day 28 (30% versus 49%). The incidence of adverse effects was similar. Ziegler et al. concluded that HA-lA is safe and effective for treating patients with sepsis and Gram-negative bacteremia. In another placebo-controlled trial a murine IgM MoAb, E5,[248] with reactivity to the lipid A portion of LPS, was studied in patients with suspected Gram-negative sepsis. The patients received either two 2-mg/kg intravenous doses of E5 MoAb 24 hours apart or placebo in addition to standard antibiotics and supportive care. Improved survival was seen in patients who received E5 MoAb when they were evaluated at day 14, whether they were bacteremic or not. Mortality was also reduced in the 30-day evaluation of patients with Gram-negative sepsis but without shock. The authors concluded that IgM E5 MoAb is safe and effective. Of the patients who received E5 MoAb, less than 2% developed adverse reactions. Two developed rashes, one had an anaphylactoid reaction, and one developed hypotension. However, more than 40% of the patients did develop an asymptomatic humoral immune response to the murine immunoglobulin as assessed by HAMA titers.

Trials

Further trials to evaluate the most effective time for administration, dosage, and the number of doses of HA-lA, E5, and other MoAbs to endotoxins will determine the ability of these MoAbs to limit mortality due to sepsis.

The pathogenesis of septic shock also involves the release of cytokines, including TNF and IL-l, in response to endotoxin and other mediators.

MoAbs have been prepared against these cytokines.[249] Several MoAbs directed against TNF are now in clinical trials. A phase I trial with MoAb (CB0006) to TNF alpha in humans found it to be safe and without acute side effects.[250] Future trials will determine the efficacy and role of anti-TNF antibodies in the treatment of septic shock.

Other approaches, such as an IL-1 receptor antagonist produced by recombinant DNA techniques, are also being studied.[251] Soluble forms of IL receptors have been developed as well.

MoAbs are being prepared for a variety of other infectious organisms, including HSV,[252] and group B *Streptococcus.*[253] Trials are under way to evaluate the protective activity of these antibodies.

Cardiac Disease Therapy. The therapeutic role of MoAbs in cardiovascular medicine is starting to widen.[254] MoAbs may play a role in imaging infarctions and thrombi, as immunosuppressives in cardiac transplantation, and as fibrinolytic or antithrombolic agents. The use of monoclonal myosin-specific Fab for imaging myocardial infarction is under clinical trial and has been discussed in the section on imaging techniques.[255,256] MoAb OKT3 has been used to manage acute rejection in cardiac transplant patients[257-259] and for prophylaxis against rejection.[260] Other applications of MoAbs now being explored include detecting intravascular thrombi and targeting fibrinolysis by means of a fibrin-specific antibody-urokinase complex; they can also serve as antithrombolic agents by inhibiting platelet aggregation.[261]

Imaging

One of the most widely used drugs in cardiac therapy is digoxin; however, digitalis intoxication is also one of the most frequently reported adverse drug reactions. Management of digitalis overdose has traditionally consisted of supportive measures. The use of digoxin-specific polyclonal antibodies in treating digoxin overdose is an established therapeutic alternative.[262] Digoxin-specific polyclonal antibodies have been prepared from sheep, and digoxin-immune Fab fragments are now available to treat digoxin or digitoxin intoxication. The current product, while not a MoAb, is a good example of how MoAbs can be targeted to specific drugs. MoAbs have been prepared against digoxin and have been shown to reverse digoxin intoxication in animals.[263]

Toxin reversal

The digoxin-immune Fab fragment known by the proprietary name Digibind® (Burroughs Wellcome) is prepared from antibodies produced by sheep in response to immunization with a digoxin albumin conjugate. The polyclonal antibodies are digested with papain and purified to produce the digoxin-specific Fab fragment. The Fab fragment is used because the goal of therapy is to bind the drug, thereby inactivating it. The constant portion of the immunoglobulin, which contains the Fc receptor (useful for binding to cell receptor sites or to complement to initiate cytotoxic effects), is discarded. The Fab has a number of desirable properties over an intact molecule. Because of their molecular size, Fab molecules may be distributed more quickly, in larger volumes, and with a shorter half-life; and when administered intravenously, Fab particles are probably less antigenic than whole molecules.[264]

Transplants

The murine MoAb OKT3, which is reactive for the CD3 surface antigen of T lymphocytes, has proved effective in managing organ transplant rejection and preventing rejection in renal and cardiac transplantation. Gilbert et al.[265] treated refractory cardiac allograft rejection in seven patients. Each patient received 5 mg of OKT3 MoAb by intravenous push daily for 10 to 14 days. OKT3 binds to the CD3 surface antigen on T lymphocytes, blocking cytotoxic T-lymphocyte-mediated cell lysis and other T-cell functions. Four of the patients had a complete response and two patients had a partial response as shown by biopsy. One of the patients, who died secondary to cardiogenic shock due to accelerated rejection, had received only one dose of OKT3. Adverse effects were generally tolerated; symptoms were worse during the first 2 days of therapy. The most common adverse effects were pyrexia and headache, nausea, and diarrhea. OKT3 has also been used prophylactically with other immunosuppressive agents to prevent acute cardiac rejections and to treat a patient with biopsy-proved myocarditis.[265]

Fibrin-specific MoAbs

Fibrin-specific MoAbs are being developed to target thrombi. A MoAb labeled with ^{111}In specific for fibrin has been injected into dogs to localize pulmonary and coronary thrombosis.[266,267] If in vivo applications are feasible, this antibody may be useful for delineating the presence and location of thrombi in arteries and veins and for detecting fibrin deposits in ulcerated atherosclerotic plaques. A further application of such an antibody would be to target fibrin for fibrinolysis with such fibrinolytic agents as streptokinase, urokinase, or tissue-type plasminogen activator.[268] Reduced urokinase has been coupled to the fibrin-specific MoAb 64C5. In an in vitro fibrinolytic assay, the MoAb conjugate with urokinase increased the efficiency of plasmin lysis a hundredfold. If these effects can be demonstrated in vivo, the dose of urokinase required for effective lysis of a thrombus will result in only minimal fibrinogenolysis, the major impediment to widespread application of this form of therapy.

Autoimmune Disease Therapy. MoAbs have long been recognized as useful research tools in the study of autoimmune diseases.[269,270] MoAbs to human T cell surface antigens are useful for studying the T cells, their subpopulations, and their functions. There are a number of clinical disorders (e.g., systemic lupus erythematosus, Sjögren's syndrome, juvenile rheumatoid arthritis, multiple sclerosis) associated with disorders of T lymphocytes. MoAbs are also being used to study the nature of such autoimmune diseases as myasthenia gravis,[271] type I diabetes,[272] and autoimmune thyroid diseases.[273] Potential exists for applying MoAbs in the therapy of such autoimmune diseases as myasthenia gravis,[274] systemic lupus erythematosus,[275] rheumatoid arthritis,[276] and systemic vasculitis.[277]

Summary

Monoclonal antibodies are produced by fusing antibody-specific B lymphocytes to an immortal myeloma cell. The MoAb can be produced in cell cultures, mouse ascites, and bioreactors. A single MoAb is cloned to produce a colony of identical cells that can be frozen for storage.

Murine MoAbs are dominantly produced; however, HAMAs have been identified in patient serum, leading researchers to seek ways of producing human or human-like MoAbs. Human MoAbs are difficult to produce, primarily due to the lack of sufficient human myeloma cell lines and desired lymphocytes. Hybrid MoAbs have been created, however, and include interspecies MoAbs, EBV-transformed MoAbs, lymphoblastoid derivatives, chimeric antibodies, and those produced by recombinant DNA techniques. These hybrid MoAbs are less antigenic than murine MoAbs but not as easy to produce.

MoAb fragments are created by cleaving the immunoglobulin molecule at the hinge region, resulting in Fab and $F(ab')_2$ fragments. Recombinant DNA fragments are produced by combining genes that encode for the heavy and light chains or the variable regions. MoAb fragments may prove to be more effective and have fewer side effects than whole MoAbs.

MoAbs can be used for detecting, imaging, and treating cancerous cells. Specificity is crucial for MoAb effectiveness; the ideal situation is a MoAb specific for antigens found in abundance on the tumor cells but not on normal cells. MoAbs affect tumor cells either by directly destroying the neoplasm, destroying growth molecules, or transporting cytotoxic agents to the cancer cells. MoAbs generally have few serious side effects. Murine MoAbs, however, can produce anaphylactic responses.

Conjugated MoAbs may be more toxic. Radioisotopes can have indiscriminate toxic effects on healthy tissue and have been known to produce hematologic toxicities. Immunotoxins may be produced from bacterial or plant toxins. Studies have been conducted for ex vivo, interactive, and in vivo therapy.

MoAb applications may be limited by complications arising from production techniques or therapy. Specificity is difficult to attain and antigens often modulate, making MoAbs ineffective. Subpopulations of the tumor may have insufficient antigens present or may be too distant from the circulatory system for the MoAb to be completely effective. Human myeloma cells are also difficult to obtain, and the alternate murine MoAb has been known to produce HAMA in patients.

In addition to antitumor therapy, MoAbs can be used for diagnostic tests and assays—ranging from pregnancy tests and drug assays to diagnosis of infectious diseases and imaging. MoAbs are also used in treating infectious, cardiac, and autoimmune diseases.

References

1. Kagan JN, Fahey JL. Tumor immunology. *JAMA.* 1987;258:2988–92.
2. Rosenberg SA, Terry WD. Passive immunotherapy of cancer in animals and man. *Advances in Cancer Research.* 1977;25:323–88.
3. Kohler G, Milstein C. Continuous cultures of fused cells secreting antibody of predefined specificity. *Nature.* 1975;256:495–7.
4. Milstein C. Monoclonal antibodies. *Cancer.* 1982;49:1953–7.
5. Diamond BA, Yelton DE, Scharff MD. Monoclonal antibodies: a new technology for producing serologic reagents. *N Engl J Med.* 1981;304:1344–9.
6. DePinho RA, Feldman LB, Scharff MD. Tailor-made monoclonal antibodies. *Ann Intern Med.* 1986;104:225–33.
7. Schonherr OT, Houwink EH. Antibody engineering: a strategy for the development of monoclonal antibodies. *Antonie van Leeuwenhoek.* 1984;50:597–623.
8. Beverley PCL, ed. Methods in hematology: monoclonal antibodies. Edinburgh: Churchill Livingstone; 1986.
9. Schook LB, ed. Monoclonal antibody production techniques and applications. New York: Marcel Dekker; 1986.
10. Zimmerman U, Vienken J. Electric field-induced cell fusion. *Journal of Membrane Biology.* 1982;62:165–85.
11. Charles M. Fermentation scaleup: problems and possibilities. *Trends in Biotechnology.* 1985;3:135–7.
12. Posillico EG. Microencapsillation technology for large scale antibody production. *Biotechnology.* 1986;4:114–7.
13. Levy JA, Lee HM, Kawahata RT et al. Purification of monoclonal antibodies from mouse ascites eliminates contaminating infectious mouse type C viruses and nucleic acids. *Clinical and Experimental Immunology.* 1984;56:114–20.
14. Schroff RW, Steven HC. Human immune responses to murine monoclonal antibodies. In: Foon KA, Morgan AC, eds. Monoclonal antibody therapy of human cancer. Boston: Martinus Nijhoff Publishing; 1985:121–38.

15. Abrams PD, Knost JA, Clark G et al. Determination of the optimal human cell lines for the development of human hybridomas. *J Immunol.* 1983;131:1201–4.
16. Ostberg L, Pursch E. Human X (mouse X human) hybridomas stably producing human antibodies. *Hybridoma.* 1983;2:361–7.
17. Campling BG, Cole SPC, Atlaw T et al. The EBV hybridoma technique and its applications. In: Strelkauskas AJ, ed. Human hybridomas: diagnostic and therapeutic applications. New York: Marcel Dekker; 1987:3–22.
18. Glassy M, Handley H, Hagiwara H et al. UC-729-6: ahuman lymphoblastic B-cell line useful for generating antibody secreting human/human hybridomas. *Proc Natl Acad Sci USA.* 1983;80:6327–31.
19. O'Hare MJ, Edwards PAW. Human monoclonal antibodies and LICR-LONHMy2 system. In: Strelkauskas AJ, ed. Human hybridomas: diagnostic and therapeutic applications. New York: Marcel Dekker; 1987:47–64.
20. Morrison SL. Transfectomas provide novel chimeric antibodies. *Science.* 1985;229:1202–7.
21. Jones PT, Dear PH, Foote J et al. Replacing the complementarity determining regions in a human antibody with those from a mouse. *Nature.* 1986;321:522–5.
22. Edwards PAW, O'Hare MJ. The production of human monoclonal antibodies. In: Beverley PCL. Methods in hematology: monoclonal antibodies. Edinburgh: Churchill Livingstone; 1986:60–96.
23. Morrison SL, Johnson MJ, Herenberg LA et al. Chimeric human antibody molecules: mouse antigen-binding domains with human constant region domains. *Proc Natl Acad Sci USA.* 1984;81:6851–5.
24. Boulianne GL, Hozumi N, Shulman MJ. Production of functional chimeric mouse/human antibody. *Nature.* 1984;312:643–6.
25. Neuberger MS, William GT, Fox RO. Recombinant antibodies possessing novel effector functions. *Nature.* 1984;312:604–8.
26. Hartman N, Gill LL, De Winter RFC et al. Generation of a recombinant mouse-human chimeric monoclonal antibody directed against carcinoembronic antigen. *International Journal of Cancer.* 1989;44:424–33.
27. Sun LK, Curtis P, Rakowicz-Szulczynska E et al. Chimeric antibody with human constant regions and mouse variable regions directed against carcinoma associated antigen 17-1A. *Proc Natl Acad Sci USA.* 1987;84:214–8.
28. Liu AY, Robinson RR, Hellstrom KE et al. Chimeric mouse-human IgGl antibody that can mediate lysis of cancer cells. *Proc Natl Acad Sci USA.* 1987;84:3439–43.
29. Riechmann L, Clark M, Waldmann H et al. Reshaping human antibodies for therapy. *Nature.* 1988;332:323–7.

30. Junghans RP, Waldmann TA, Landolfi NF et al. Anti-Tac-H, a humanized antibody to the interleukin-2 receptor with new features for immunotherapy in malignant and immune disorders. *Cancer Research.* 1990; 50:1495-1502.
31. Perez P, Hoffman RW, Titus JA et al. Specific targeting of human peripheral blood T cells by heteroaggregates containing anti T-3 crosslinked to antitarget cell antibodies. *Journal of Experimental Medicine.* 1986;163:166-78.
32. Staez UD, Bevan MJ. Hybrid hybridoma producing a bispecific monoclonal antibody that can focus effector T-cell activity. *Proc Natl Acad Sci USA.* 1986;83:1453-75.
33. Glennie MJ, Brennand DM, Bryden F et al. Bispecific F(ab')$_2$ antibody for the delivery of saporin in the treatment of lymphoma. *J Immunol.* 1988;141:3552-670.
34. Buchegger F, Haskell CM, Schreyer M et al. Radiolabeled fragments of monoclonal antibodies against carcinoembryonic antigen for the localization of human colon carcinoma grafted into nude mice. *Journal of Experimental Medicine.* 1983;158:413-27.
35. Mach JP, Carrel S, Forni M et al. Tumor localization of radiolabeled antibodies against carcinoembryonic antigen in patients with carcinoma: a critical evaluation. *N Engl J Med.* 1980;303:5-10.
36. Delaloye B, Bischof-Delaloye A, Buchegg F et al. Detection of colorectal carcinoma by emission computerized tomography after injection of I-123 labeled Fab or F(ab')$_2$ fragments from monoclonal anti-carcinoembryonic antigen antibodies. *J Clin Invest.* 1986;77:301-11.
37. Orland I, Gussow DH, Jones PT et al. Cloning immunoglobulin variable domains for expression by polymerase chain reaction. *Proc Natl Acad Sci USA.* 1989;86:3833-7.
38. Huse WD, Sastry L, Iverson SA et al. Generation of a large combinatorial library of the immunoglobulin repertoire in phage lambda. *Science.* 1990;246:1275-81.
39. Chaudhary VK, Batra JK, Gallo MG et al. A rapid method of cloning functional variable region antibody genes in *Escherichia coli* as single chain immunotoxins. *Proc Natl Acad Sci USA.* 1990;82:1066-70.
40. Ward ES, Gussow D, Griffiths AD et al. Binding activities of a repertoire of a single immunoglobulin variable domains secreted from *Escherichia coli. Nature.* 1989;341:544-6.
41. Hiatt A, Cafferkey R, Bowdish K. Production of antibodies in transgenic plants. *Nature.* 1989;342:76-8.
42. Koprowski H, Herlyn M, Steplewski Z et al. Specific antigen in serum of patients with colon carcinoma. *Science.* 1981;212:53-5.
43. Steplewski Z, Chang TH, Herlyn M et al. Release of monoclonal antibody-defined antigens by human colorectal carcinoma and melanoma cells. *Cancer Research.* 1981;41:2723-7.

44. Herlyn M, Sears HF, Steplewski Z et al. Monoclonal antibody detection of a circulating tumor associated antigen: presence of antigen in sera of patients with colorectal, gastric and pancreatic carcinoma. *J Clin Immunol.* 1982;2:135–40.
45. Morgan AC, Foon KA. Monoclonal antibody therapy of cancer: preclinical models and investigations in humans. In: Heberman RB, ed. Cancer immunology: innovative approaches to therapy. Boston: Martinus Nijhoff Publishers; 1986:177–200.
46. Lowder JN, Levy R. Monoclonal antibodies: therapeutic and diagnostic uses in malignancy. *West J Med.* 1985;143:810–8.
47. Levy R, Miller RA. Biological and clinical implications of lymphocyte hybridomas: tumor therapy with monoclonal antibodies. *Annu Rev Med.* 1983;34:107–16.
48. Smith LH, Teng NN. Clinical applications of monoclonal antibodies in gynecological oncology. *Cancer.* 1987;60:2068–74.
49. Colcher D, Hand H, Wunderlich D et al. Monoclonal antibodies to human mammary carcinoma associated antigens and their potential uses for diagnosis, prognosis, and therapy. *Immunodiagnostics.* 1983:215–58.
50. Papsidero LD, Croghan GA, Asirwatham J et al. Immunohistochemical demonstration of prostate-specific antigen in metastases with the use of monoclonal antibody F5. *Am J Patho.* 1985;121:451–4.
51. DeLand FH, Goldberg DM. Diagnosis and treatment of neoplasms with radionuclide-labeled antibodies. *Seminars of Nuclear Medicine.* 1985;25:2–11.
52. Larson SM. Radiolabeled monoclonal anti-tumor antibodies in diagnosis and therapy. *Journal of Nuclear Medicine.* 1985;26:538–45.
53. Moldofsky PJ, Sears HF, Mulhern CB et al. Detection of metastatic tumor in normal sized retroperitoneal lymph nodes by monoclonal antibody imaging. *N Engl J Med.* 1984;311:106–7.
54. Larson SM, Carrasquillo JA, Krohn KA et al. Diagnostic imaging of malignant melanoma with radiolabeled antitumor antibodies. *JAMA.* 1983;249:811–2.
55. Foster CS, Neville AM. Monoclonal antibodies to the human mammary gland. *Human Pathology.* 1984;15:502–13.
56. Halpern SE, Dilman RO, Witztum KF et al. Radio-immunodetection of melanoma utilizing ^{111}In-96.5 monoclonal antibody: a preliminary report. *Radiology.* 1985;155:493–9.
57. Larson SM, Carrasquillo JA, McGuffin RW et al. Use of ^{131}I-labeled, murine Fab against a high molecular weight antigen of human melanoma: preliminary experience. *Radiology.* 1985;155:487–92.
58. Rainsbury RM. Localization of human breast carcinomas by radiolabeled monoclonal antibodies. *Br J Surg.* 1984;71:805–12.

59. Horne T, Granowska M, Dicks-Mireaux C et al. Neuroblastoma imaged with 123-I-meta-iodo-benaylguanidine and with ^{123}I-labeled monoclonal antibody, UJ13A, against neural tissue. *Br J Radiol.* 1985;58:476–80.
60. Leyden MJ, Thompson CH, Lichtenstein M et al. Visualization of metastases from colon carcinoma using an iodine 131-radiolabeled monoclonal antibody. *Cancer.* 1986;57:1135–9.
61. Allum WH, MacDonald F, Anderson P et al. Localization of gastrointestinal cancer with a ^{131}I labeled monoclonal antibody to CEA. *British Journal of Cancer.* 1986;53:203–10.
62. Pateisky N, Philipp K, Skodler WD et al. Radio-immunodetection in patients with suspected ovarian cancer. *Journal of Nuclear Medicine.* 1985;26:1369–76.
63. Weinstein JN, Eger RR, Covell DG et al. The pharmacology of monoclonal antibodies. *Annals of the New York Academy of Science.* 1987;507:199–210.
64. Koizumi K, DeNardo GL, DeNardo SJ et al. Multicompartmental analysis of the kinetics of radioiodinated monoclonal antibody in patients with cancer. *Journal of Nuclear Medicine.* 1986;27:1243–54.
65. Hantowich DJ, Griffin TW, Kosciuczyk C et al. Pharmacokinetics of an indium-111-labeled monoclonal antibody in cancer patients. *Journal of Nuclear Medicine.* 1985;26:849–58.
66. Murray JL, Rosenblum MG, Lamki L et al. Clinical parameters related to optimal tumor localization of indium-111-labeled mouse antimelanoma ZME-018. *Journal of Nuclear Medicine.* 1987;28:25–33.
67. Nelp WB, Eary JF, Jones RF et al. Preliminary studies of monoclonal antibody lymphoscintigraphy in malignant melanoma. *Journal of Nuclear Medicine.* 1987;28:34–41.
68. Sicardi AG. Tumor immunoscrintigraphy by means of radiolabeled monoclonal antibodies. Multicenter studies of the Italian National Research Council. Special project "Biomedical Engineering." *Cancer Research.* 1990;50(Feb suppl):899s–903s.
69. Beatty JD, William LE, Yamauchi D et al. Presurgical imaging with indium-labeled anticarcioembryonic antigen for colon cancer staging. *Cancer Research.* 1990;50:922–6.
70. Ellis G, Ferguson M, Yamanak D et al. Monoclonal antibodies for the detection of occult carcinoma cells in bone marrow of breast cancer patients. *Cancer.* 1989;63:2509–14.
71. Berstein ID, Tam MR, Nowinski RC. Mouse leukemia: therapy with monoclonal antibodies against a thymus differentiation antigen. *Science.* 1980;207:68–71.
72. Scheinberg DA, Strand M. Leukemic cell targeting and therapy by monoclonal antibody in a mouse model system. *Cancer Research.* 1982;42:44–9.

73. Masui H, Kawamoto T, Sato JD et al. Growth inhibition of human tumor cells in thymic nude mice by anti-epidermal growth factor receptor monoclonal antibody. *Cancer Research.* 1984;44:1002–7.
74. Brady LW, Woo DV, Karlsson U et al. Radioimmunotherapy of human glioma using I-125-labeled monoclonal antibody to epidermal growth factor receptor. *Proceedings of the American Society of Clinical Oncology.* 1988;7:82. Abstract 319.
75. Cuttitta F, Carney DN, Mulshine J et al. Bombesin-like peptides can function as autocrine growth factors in human small cell lung cancer. *Nature.* 1985;316:823–6.
76. Harris DT, Mastrangelo MJ. Serotherapy of cancer. *Seminars in Oncology.* 1989;16:180–98.
77. Foon KA, Schroff RW, Bunn RA et al. Effects of monoclonal antibody therapy in patients with chronic lymphocytic leukemia. *Blood.* 1984;64:1085–93.
78. Dillman RO, Dillman JB, Cutter M et al. Toxicity and efficacy of 24 hour infusion of T 101 monoclonal antibody in chronic lymphocytic leukemia. *Proceedings of the American Society of Clinical Oncology.* 1985;4:230.
79. Dillman RO, Beauregard JC, Halpern SE et al. Toxicities and side effects associated with intravenous infusions of murine monoclonal antibodies. *Journal of Biological Response Modifiers.* 1986;5:73–84.
80. Miller RA, Maloney DG, McKillop J et al. In vivo effects of murine hybridoma monoclonal antibody in a patient with T-cell leukemia. *Blood.* 1981:78–86.
81. Goodman GE, Beaumier P, Hellstrom I et al. Pilot trial of murine monoclonal antibodies in patients with advanced melanoma. *Journal of Clinical Oncology.* 1985;3:340–52.
82. Miller RA, Levy R. Response of cutaneous T-cell lymphoma to therapy with hybridoma monoclonal antibody. *Lancet.* 1981;2:226–9.
83. Ritz J, Scholossman SF. Utilization of monoclonal antibodies in treatment of leukemia and lymphomas. *Blood.* 1982;59:1–11.
84. Dillman RO, Shawler DL, Sobol RE et al. Murine monoclonal antibody therapy in patients with chronic lymphocytic leukemia. *Blood.* 1982;59:1036–45.
85. Foon KA, Schroff RW, Mayer D et al. Monoclonal antibody therapy in chronic lymphocytic leukemia and cutaneous T cell lymphoma: preliminary observations. In: Boss BD, Langman R, Trowbridge I, et al., eds. Monoclonal antibodies and cancer. Orlando, FL: Academic Press; 1983:39–52.
86. Shawler DL, Beauregard J, Halpern SE et al. Tissue distribution and serum kinetics of T101 monoclonal antibody during passive anticancer therapy. *Clinical Immunology and Immunopathology.* 1986;41:43–54.

87. Miller RA, Maloney DG, Earnke R et al. Treatment of B-cell lymphoma with monoclonal anti-idiotype antibody. *N Engl J Med.* 1982;306:517-22.
88. Lowder JN, Meeker T, Maloney AC et al. Anti-idiotype monoclonal antibody therapy of human B lymphocytic malignancy. *Proceedings of the 20th Annual Meeting of the American Society of Clinical Oncology.* 1984;3:250. Abstract.
89. Koprowski H, Herlyn D, Rubeck M et al. Human anti-idiotype antibodies in cancer patients is the modulation of immune response beneficial for the cancer patient. *Proc Natl Acad Sci USA.* 1984;81:216-20.
90. Brown SL, Miller RA, Levy R. Antiidiotype antibody therapy of B-cell lymphoma. *Seminars in Oncology.* 1989;16:199-210.
91. Brown SL, Miller RA, Horning SJ et al. Treatment of B-cell lymphomas with anti-idiotype antibodies alone and in combination with alpha interferon. *Blood.* 1989;73:651-61.
92. Janson CH, Tehrani M, Mellstedt H et al. Anti-idiotypic monoclonal antibody to T-cell chronic lymphatic leukemia. *Cancer Immunology and Immunotherapeutics.* 1989;28:225-32.
93. Dillman RO. Human antimouse and antiglobulin responses to monoclonal antibodies. *Antibody, Immunoconjugates, and Radiopharmaceuticals.* 1990;3:1-15.
94. Shawler DL, Miceli MC, Wormsley SB et al. Induction of in vitro and in vivo antigenic modulation by the anti-human T cell monoclonal antibody T101. *Cancer Research.* 1984;44:5921-7.
95. Meeker T, Lowder J, Cleary MI et al. Emergence of idiotype variants during the treatment of B-cell lymphoma with anti-idiotype antibodies. *N Engl J Med.* 1985;312:1658-65.
96. Nadler LM, Stashenko P, Hardy R et al. Serotherapy of a patient with a monoclonal antibody directed against a human lymphocyte-associated antigen. *Cancer Research.* 1980;40:3147-54.
97. Masucci G, Wershall P, Nielsen J et al. Lymphokine activated killer (LAK) cells in antibody-dependent cellular cytotoxicity (ADCC) using Mab 17-1A: a combination of potential usefulness in tumor therapy. *Hybridoma.* 1989;8:507-16.
98. Tong AW, Lee JC, Wang RM et al. Augmentation of lymphokine activated killer cell cytotoxicity by monoclonal antibodies against human small cell lung carcinoma. *Cancer Research.* 1989;49:4103-8.
99. Eisenthal A, Cameron BB, Uppenkamp I et al. Effects of combined therapy of lymphokine-activated killer cells, interleukin-2 and specific monoclonal antibody on established melanoma lung metastases. *Cancer Research.* 1988;48:7140-5.
100. Masucci G, Wershall P, Raghammar P et al. Granulocyte monocytecolony-stimulating factors augments the cytotoxic capacity of lymphocytes and monocytes in antibody-dependent cellular

cytotoxicity. *Cancer Immunology and Immunotherapeutics.* 1989;29:288-92.

101. Bloomer WD, Lipsztein R, Dalton JF. Antibody-mediated radiotherapy. *Cancer.* 1985;55:2229-33.
102. Pectaside D, Stewart S, Courtenay-Luck N et al. Antibody-guided irradiation of malignant pleural and pericardial effusion. *Br J Cancer.* 1986;53:727-32.
103. Keenan AM, Harbert JC, Larson SM. Monoclonal antibodies in nuclear medicine. *Journal of Nuclear Medicine.* 1985;26:531-7.
104. Humm JL. Dosimetric aspects of radiolabeled antibodies for tumor therapy. *Journal of Nuclear Medicine.* 1986;27:1450-97.
105. Esteban JM, Schlom J, Gansow OA et al. New method for the chelation of indium-111 to monoclonal antibodies: biodistribution and imaging of athymic mice bearing human colon carcinoma xenografts. *Journal of Nuclear Medicine.* 1987;28:861-70.
106. Mears CF. Chelating agents for the binding of metal ions to antibodies. *Nuclear Medicine Biology.* 1986;13:311-5.
107. Krejcarek GE, Tucker KL. Covalent attachment of chelating groups to macromolecules. *Biochemical and Biophysical Research Communications.* 1977:581-5.
108. Hantowich DJ, Virzi F, Doherty PW. DTPA-coupled antibodies labeled with yttrium-90. *Journal of Nuclear Medicine.* 1985;26:503-9.
109. Schroff HP, Weiden PL, Appelbaum J et al. Rhenium-186 labeled antibody inpatients with cancer: report of a pilot phase 1 study. *Antibody, Immunoconjugates, and Radiopharmaceuticals.* 1990;3:99-111.
110. Strand M, Scheinberg DA, Gansow OA et al. Monoclonal antibody conjugates for diagnostic imaging and therapy. In: Bous BD, Langman R, Trowbridge I, et al, eds. Monoclonal antibody and cancer. Orlando, FL: Academic Press; 1983:125-31.
111. Kozak RW, Atcher RW, Gansow OA et al. Bismuth-212-labeled anti-Tac monoclonal antibody: particle emitting radionuclides as modalities for radioimmunotherapy. *Proc Natl Acad Sci USA.* 1986;83:474-8.
112. Goodwin DA. Pharmacokinetics and antibodies. *Journal of Nuclear Medicine.* 1987;28:1358-62.
113. Moldofsky PJ, Powe J, Mulhern CB et al. Metastatic colon carcinoma detected with radiolabeled $F(ab')_2$ monoclonal antibody fragments. *Radiology.* 1983;149:549-55.
114. Wilbanks AB, Peterson LA, Miller S et al. Localization of mammary tumors in vivo with I-131-labeled Fab fragments of antibodies against mouse mammary epithelium (MME) antigens. *Cancer.* 1981;48:1768-75.

115. Ford CHJ, Cason AG. Antibody mediated targeting in the treatment and diagnosis of cancer: an overview. *Cancer Chemotherapy and Pharmacology.* 1986;17:197-208.
116. Wahl RL, Parker CW, Philpott GW. Improved radioimaging and tumor localization with monoclonal F(ab')$_2$. *Journal of Nuclear Medicine.* 1983;24:316-25.
117. Lashford LS, Davies AG, Richardson RB et al. A pilot study of 131-I monoclonal antibodies in the therapy of leptomeningeal tumors. *Cancer.* 1988;61:857-68.
118. Carrasquillo JA, Krohn KA, Beaumier P et al. Diagnosis of and therapy for solid tumors with radiolabeled antibodies and immune fragments. *Cancer Treatment Report.* 1984;68:317-28.
119. Kalofonos HO, Pawlikowska TR, Hemingway A et al. Antibody guided diagnosis and therapy of brain gliomas using radiolabeled monoclonal antibodies against epidermal growth factor receptor and placental alkaline phosphatase. *Journal of Nuclear Medicine.* 1989;30:1636-45.
120. Bertram JH, Gill PS, Levin AM et al. Monoclonal antibody T101 in T-cell malignancies: a clinical, pharmacokinetic and immunologic correlation. *Blood.* 1986;68:752-61.
121. Frankel AE, Houston LL, Issell BF. Prospectives for immunotoxin therapy in cancer. *Ann Rev Med.* 1986:37:125-42.
122. Vitetta ES, Uhr JW. Immunotoxins. *Annual Review of Immunology.* 1985;3:197-212.
123. Neville DM Jr. Immunotoxins for in vivo therapy: where are we? *Annals of the New York Academy of Science.* 1987;507:155-64.
124. Marsh JW, Neville DM Jr. Development of an immunotoxin with in vivo efficacy for murine systems. *Annals of the New York Academy of Science.* 1987;507:165-77.
125. Raso V, Watkins SC, Slayter II et al. Intracellular pathways of ricin A chain cytotoxins. *Annals of the New York Academy of Science.* 1987;507:172-86.
126. Vitetta ES, Krolick KA, Miyama-Inaba M et al. Immunotoxins: a new approach to cancer therapy. *Science.* 1983;219:644-50.
127. Bregni M, De Fabritiis P, Raso V et al. Elimination of clonogenic tumor cells from human bone marrow using a combination of monoclonal antibody: ricin A chain conjugates. *Cancer Research.* 1986;46:1208-13.
128. Epenetos AA, Hooker G, Krausz T et al. Antibody-guided irradiation of malignant ascites in ovarian cancer: a new therapeutic method possessing specificity against cancer cells. *Obstet Gynecol.* 1986:68(suppl):71-4.
129. Gilliland DG, Steplewski Z, Collier RJ et al. Antibody directed cytotoxic agents: use of monoclonal antibodies to detect the action of toxin A chains to colorectal carcinoma cells. *Proc Natl Acad Sci USA.* 1980;77:4539-43.

130. Muirhead M, Martin P, Torok-Storb B et al. Use of antibody-ricin A chain conjugate to deplete neoplastic cells from human bone marrow. *Blood.* 1983;62:327–32.
131. Donay L, Gorin N, Lopez M et al. Evidence for absence of toxicity of T 101 immunotoxin on human hematopoietic progenitor cells prior to bone marrow transplantation. *Cancer Research.* 1985;45:438–43.
132. Youle RJ, Neville DM. Anti-Thy 1.2 monoclonal antibody linked to ricin is a potent cell-type-specific toxin. *Proc Natl Acad Sci USA.* 1980;77:5483–586.
133. Fodstad 0, Koalheim G, Godal A et al. Phase I study of the plant protein ricin. *Cancer Research.* 1984:44:862–5.
134. Krolick KA, Uhr JW, Slavin S et al. In vivo therapy of a murine B cell tumor (BCLl) using antibody ricin A chain immunotoxins. *Journal of Experimental Medicine.* 1982;155:1797–809.
135. Spitler LE, del Rio M, Khentigan A et al. Therapy of patients with malignant melanoma using a monoclonal anti-melanoma antibody/ricin A chain immunotoxin. *Cancer Research.* 1987;47:1717–23.
136. Ramsay NK, Kersey JH. Bone marrow purging using monoclonal antibodies. *Journal of Clinical Immunology.* 1988;8:81–8.
137. Filipovich AH, Youle R, Neville D et al. Ex vivo treatment of donor bone marrow with anti-T cell immunotoxins for prevention of graft-versus- host disease. *Lancet.* 1984;1:469–72.
138. Filipovich AH, Vallera D, Youle R et al. Ex vivo depletion with immunotoxins in allogenic bone-marrow transplantation: the pilot clinical study for prevention of graft-versus-host disease. *Transplantation Proceedings.* 1985;17:442–4.
139. Byers V, Henslee J, Antin J et al. Safety and therapeutic response to a pan-t-lymphocyte monoclonal antibody ricin A chain in graft versus host disease (GVHD). *Proceedings of the American Society of Clinical Oncology.* 1988;7:190. Abstract 734.
140. Ramsay N, LeBein T, Nesbit M et al. Autologous bone-marrow transplantation for patients with acute lymphoblastic leukemia in second or subsequent remission: results of bone marrow treated with monoclonal antibodies BA-1, BA-2, and BA-3 plus complement. *Blood.* 1986;66:508–13.
141. Baumgartner C, Imbach P, Luthy A et al. Autologous bone marrow transplantation for stage IV abdominal non-Hodgkins lymphoma after in vitro purging with anti-y 29/55 monoclonal antibody and complement. In: Boss BD, Langman RE, Trowbridge IS, et al, eds. Monoclonal antibody and cancer. Orlando, FL: Academic Press; 1983:73–9.
142. Gorin NC, Dousay L, Paporte JP et al. Autologous bone marrow transplantation with marrow decontamination by immunotoxin T 101

in the treatment of leukemia and lymphoma: first clinical observation. *Cancer Treatment Reports.* 1985;69:953–9.

143. Press OW. Immunotoxins. *Biotherapy.* 1991;3:65–76.
144. Byers VS, Henslee PJ, Kernan NA et al. Use of anti-pan T-lymphocyte ricin A chain immunotoxin in steroid resistant acute graft-versus-host disease. *Blood.* 1990;75:1426–32.
145. Herve P, Bordigoni P, Cahn JY et al. Use of monoclonal antibodies in vivo as a therapeutic strategy for acute GVHD in matched and mismatched bone marrow transplantation. *Transplantation Proceedings.* 1991;23:1692–4.
146. Hertler AA, Frankel AE. Immunotoxins: a clinical review of their use in the treatment of malignancies. *Journal of Clinical Oncology.* 1989;7:1932–42.
147. Gould BJ, Borowitz MJ, Groves ES et al. Phase I study of an anti-breast cancer immunotoxin by continuous infusion: report of a targeted toxic effect not predicted by animal studies. *JNCI.* 1989;81:775–81.
148. Ghose T, Norvell ST, Guclu A et al. Immunochemotherapy of human malignant melanoma with chlorambucil-carrying antibody. *European Journal of Cancer.* 1975;11:321–6.
149. Ghose T, Norvell ST, Guclu A et al. Immunochemotherapy of cancer with chorambucil carrying antibody. *Br Med J.* 1972;26:495–9.
150. Ford CHJ, Newman CE, Johnson JR et al. Localization and toxicity study of a vindesine-anti-CEA conjugate in patients with advanced cancer. *British Journal of Cancer.* 1983;47:35–42.
151. Takashi T, Yamaguchi T, Kitamura K et al. Clinical application of monoclonal antibody-drug conjugates for immunotargeting chemotherapy of colorectal carcinoma. *Cancer.* 1988;61:881–8.
152. Lagueux J, Page M, Delorme F. Daunorubicin-albumin copolymer targeting to leukemic cells in vitro and in vivo. *Seminars in Oncology.* 1984;11:59–63.
153. Page M, Delorme F, Lafontaine F et al. Chemotherapy with daunorubicin-anti-CEA conjugates in human colon adenocarcinoma grafted in nude mice. *Seminars in Oncology.* 1984;11(suppl 3):56–58.
154. Arnon R, Sela M. In vitro and in vivo efficacy of conjugates of daunomycin with anti-tumor antibodies. *Immunology Review.* 1982;62:5–27.
155. Primm MV, Jones JA, Price MR et al. Tumor localization of monoclonal antibody against a rat mammary carcinoma and suppression of tumor growth with adriamycin-antibody conjugates. *Cancer Immunology, Immunotherapy.* 1982;12:125–34.
156. Dillman RO, Shawler DL, Johnson DE et al. Preclinical trials with combination and conjugates of T101 monoclonal antibody and doxorubicin. *Cancer Research.* 1986;46:4886–91.
157. Greenfield RS, Dauesa A, Edson HA et al. Optimization of immunotherapy with adriamycin (hydrazone)-immunoconjugates in

human B-lymphoma xenografts. *Antibody, Immunoconjugates, and Radiopharmaceuticals.* 1991;4:107–19.

158. Garnett MC, Baldwin RW. An improved synthesis of a methotrexate albumin-T791/36 monoclonal antibody conjugate cytotoxic to human osteogenic sarcoma cell lines. *Cancer Research.* 1986;46:2407–12.
159. Mueller BM, Reisfeld RA, Silveria MH et al. Pre-clinical therapy of human melanoma with morpholino-doxorubicin conjugated to monoclonal antibody directed against an intergrin on melanoma cells. *Antibody, Immunoconjugates, and Radiopharmaceuticals.* 1991;4:99–106.
160. Koch B, Baum W, Beck E et al. In vitro activity of immunoconjugates between cis-platinum and monoclonal antibodies. *Antibody, Immunoconjugates, and Radiopharmaceuticals.* 1991;4:121–32.
161. Schneck D, Butler F, Dugan W et al. Phase I studies with a murine monoclonal antibody vinca conjugate (KSI14-DAVLB) in patients with adenocarcinoma. *Antibody, Immunoconjugates, and Radiopharmaceuticals.* 1989;2:93–100.
162. Papahadjopoulos F, Gabizon A. Targeting of liposomes to tumor cells in vivo. *Annals of the New York Academy of Science.* 1987;507:64–74.
163. Klausner A. Will 1988 be the year of the liposome? *Biotechnology.* 1988;6:20. Editorial.
164. Perez-Soler R. Liposomes as carriers of antitumor agents: towards a clinical reality. *Cancer Treatment Reviews.* 1989;16:67–82.
165. Konno H, Suzuki H, Tadakuma T et al. Antitumor effect of adriamycin entrapped in liposomes conjugated with anti-human alphafetoprotein monoclonal antibody. *Cancer Research.* 1987;47:4471–7.
166. Rahman A, Fumagalli A, Goodman A et al. Potential of liposomes to ameliorate anthracycline-induced cardiotoxicity. *Seminars in Oncology.* 1984;11(suppl 3):45–55.
167. Lopez-Berestein G, Fainstein V, Hopfer R et al. Liposomal amphotericin B for the treatment of systemic fungal infections in patients with cancer: a preliminary study. *J Infect Dis.* 1985;151:704–10.
168. Shirkhoda A, Lopez-Berestein G, Holbert JM. Hepatosplenic fungal infection: CT and pathologic evaluation after treatment with liposomal amphotericin B. *Radiology.* 1986;159:349–53.
169. Lopez-Berestein G, Bodey GP, Frankel LS et al. Treatment of hepatosplenic candidiasis with liposomal-amphotericin B. *Journal of Clinical Oncology.* 1987;5:310–7.
170. Health TD, Montgomery JA, Piper JR. Antibody-targeted liposomes: increase in specific toxicity of methotrexate-gamma-aspartate. *Proc Natl Acad Sci USA.* 1983;80:1377–81.

171. Hege KM, Paleke DL, Waldman TA et al. Comparison of antiTac and anti-transferrin receptor conjugated liposomes for specific drug delivery to adult T-cell leukemia. *Blood.* 1989;74:2043–52.

172. Senter PD. Activation of prodrugs by antibody-enzyme conjugates: a new approach to cancer therapy. *FASEB Journal.* 1990;4:188–93.

173. Senter PD, Schreiber GJ, Hirschberg DL et al. Enhancement of in vitro and in vivo tumor activities of phosphorylated mitomycin-c and etoposide derivatives by monoclonal antibody-alkaline phosphatase conjugates. *Cancer Research.* 1989:49:5789–92.

174. Bagshawe KD, Springer CJ, Searle F et al. A cytotoxic agent can be generated selectively at cancer sites. *British Journal of Cancer.* 1988;58:700–3.

175. Pinsky CM. Monoclonal antibody process is slow but sure. *N Engl J Med.* 1986;315:704–5.

176. Morrison SL, Wims L, Wallick S. Genetically engineered antibody molecules and their application. *Annals of the New York Academy of Science.* 1987;507:187–98.

177. Mayforth RD, Quintans J. Designer and catalytic antibodies. *N Engl J Med.* 1990;323:173–8.

178. Shawler DL, Bartholomew RM, Smith LM et al. Human immune response to multiple injections of murine monoclonal IgG. *J Immunol.* 1985;135:1530–5.

179. Schroff RW, Foon KA, Beatty SM et al. Human anti-murine immunoglobulin responses in patients receiving monoclonal antibody therapy. *Cancer Research.* 1985:45;879–85.

180. Chatenoud L, Joker M, Villemain F et al. The human antibody response to the OKT3 monoclonal antibody is oligoclonal. *Science.* 1986;232:1406–8.

181. Orats R, Speyer J, Eernz J et al. Immunotoxin and cyclophosphamide in malignant melanoma. *Proceedings of the American Society of Clinical Oncology.* 1988;7:253. Abstract 981.

182. Zimmer AM, Rosen ST, Spies SM et al. Radioimmunotherapy of patients with cutaneous T-cell lymphoma using an iodine-131-labeled monoclonal antibody: analysis of retreatment following plasmapheresis. *Journal of Nuclear Medicine.* 1988;29:174–80.

183. Steis RG, Carrasquillo A, McCabe R et al. Toxicity, immunogenicity, and tumor radioimmunodetecting ability of two human monoclonal antibodies in patients with metastatic colorectal carcinoma. *Journal of Clinical Oncology.* 1990;8:476–90.

184. Buchsbaum DJ, Brucbacker PG, Hanna DE et al. Comparative binding and preclinical localization and therapy studies with radiolabeled human chimeric and murine 17-1A monoclonal antibodies. *Cancer Research.* 1990; 50:993–9.

185. Meeker TC, Lowder JN, Maloney DG et al. A clinical trial of anti-idiotype therapy for B-cell malignancy. *Blood.* 1985;65:1349-63.
186. Wahl RL, Lieber TM, Headington J et al. Lymphoscintigraphy in melanoma: initial evaluation of a low protein dose monoclonal antibody cocktail. *Cancer Research.* 1990;50:941-8.
187. Stewart JSW, Hird V, Snook D et al. Intraperitoneal radioimmunotherapy of ovarian cancer, pharmacokinetic, toxicity and efficacy of I-131 labeled monoclonal antibodies. *International Journal of Radiation Oncology and Biophysics.* 1989;16:405-13.
188. Secher DS, Burke DC. A monoclonal antibody for large scale purification of human leukocyte interferon. *Nature.* 1980;285:446-50.
189. Tsung YK, Milkunsky A, Alpert E. Derivation and characterization of a monoclonal hybridoma antibody specific for human alphafetoprotein. *Journal of Immunologic Methods.* 1980;39:363-8.
190. Denis F, Leonard G, Mounier M et al. Efficacy of five enzyme immunoassays for antibody to HIV in detecting antibody to HTLV-IV. *Lancet.* 1987;1:324-5.
191. Batzer FR. Test kits for ovulation and pregnancy. *Contemporary OB/GYN.* 1986;28:7-16.
192. Baker HWG, Burger HG, Kovals GT et al. Timing of ovulation by determination of the urinary luteinizing hormone surge with an enzyme-linked monoclonal antibody dipstick (Ovustick). *Australian and New Zealand Journal of Obstetric Gynecology.* 1986;26:79-83.
193. Nowinski RC, Tam MR, Goldstein LC et al. Monoclonal antibodies for diagnosis of infectious diseases in humans. *Science.* 1983;219:637-44.
194. Lange JV, Walker DH. Production and characterization of monoclonal antibodies to *Rickettsia rickettsii. Infection and Immunity.* 1984;46:289-94.
195. Tam MR, Stamm WE, Handsfield H et al. Culture-independent diagnosis of chlamydia trachomatis using monoclonal antibodies. *N Engl J Med.* 1984;310:1146-50.
196. DeYoung HG. The greening of biotechnology. *High Technology.* 1984;4:59-67.
197. Bell TA, Kuo C, Stamm WE et al. Direct fluorescent monoclonal antibody stain for rapid detection of infant chlamydia trachomatis infections. *Pediatrics.* 1984;74:224-8.
198. Kiviat N, Peterson M, Kinney-Thomas E et al. Cytologic manifestations of cervical and vaginal infections. II. Confirmation of chlamydia trachomatis infection by direct immunofluorescence using monoclonal antibodies. *JAMA.* 1985;253:997-1000.
199. Guenthner SH, Linnemann CG Jr. Indirect immunofluorescence assay for rapid diagnosis of influenza virus. *Laboratory Medicine.* 1988;19:581-3.

200. Schuster EA, Benke JS, Tegtmeier GE et al. Monoclonal antibody for rapid laboratory detection of cytomegalovirus infections: characterization and diagnostic application. *Mayo Clinic Proceedings.* 1985;60:577-85.
201. Van de Berg AP, von Son WJ, Jiwa NM et al. Recent advances in the diagnosis of active cytomegalovirus infection after organ transplantation. *Transplant Proceedings.* 1990;22:226-8.
202. Sarngadharan MG, Popovic M, Bruch L et al. Antibodies reactive with human T-lymphocytropic retroviruses (HTLV-111) in the serum of patients with AIDS. *Science.* 1984;224:506-8.
203. Lawrence J. Diagnostic test for HIV infection. *Infections in Surgery.* 1987;6:339-44, 368.
204. Dopel SH, Porstmann T, Grounow R et al. Application of human monoclonal antibody in a rapid competitive anti-HIV ELISA. *Journal of Immunologic Methods.* 1989;116:229-33.
205. Dubarry M, Luilier M, Malot N et al. Enzyme immunoassay for detection of malarial antigens in human plasma by *Plasmodium falciparum* monoclonal antibodies. *American Journal of Tropical Medicine.* 1990;43:116-23.
206. Stout C, Murphy MD, Lawrence S et al. Evaluation of a monoclonal antibody pool rapid diagnosis of respiratory infections. *Journal of Clinical Microbiology.* 1989;27:448-52.
207. Mach J, Chatal J, Lumbroso J et al. Tumor localization in patients by radiolabeled monoclonal antibodies. *Cancer Research.* 1983;43:5593-600.
208. Murry J, Rosenblum N, Sobol R et al. Radioimaging in malignant melanoma with ^{131}I-labeled monoclonal antibody. *Cancer Research.* 1985;45:2376-80.
209. Berger HJ. Myocardial imaging new radiotracers aid diagnosis. *Diagnostic Imaging.* 1987;9:78-89.
210. Halpern SE, Dillman RO, Hagen PL. The problems and promise of monoclonal antitumor antibodies in diagnostic imaging. *Diagnostic Imaging.* 1983;5:40-7.
211. Carrasquillo JA, Mulshine JL, Bunn PA et al. Indium-111 T101 monoclonal antibody is superior to iodine-131 T101 in imaging of cutaneous T-cell lymphoma. *Journal of Nuclear Medicine.* 1987;28:281-7.
212. Eary JF, Schroff RW, Abrams PG et al. Successful imaging of malignant melanoma with technetium-99m-1abeled monoclonal antibodies. *Journal of Nuclear Medicine.* 1989;30:25-32.
213. Khaw BA, Yasuda T, Gold HK et al. Acute myocardial infarct imaging with indium-111-labeled monoclonal antimyosin Fab. *Journal of Nuclear Medicine.* 1987;28:1671-8.
214. Khaw BA, Strauss HW, Moore R et al. Myocardial damage delineated by indium-111 antimyosin Fab and technetium-99m pyrophosphate. *Journal of Nuclear Medicine.* 1987;28:76-82.

215. Tamaki N, Yamada T, Matsumor IA et al. Indium-111-antimyosin antibody imaging for detecting different stages of myocardial infarction comparison with technetium-99m-pyrophosphate imaging. *Journal of Nuclear Medicine.* 1990;31:136–42.
216. Williamdec G, Palacio I, Yasuda T et al. Antimyosin antibody cardiac imaging: its role in diagnosis of myocarditis. *Journal of the American College of Cardiology.* 1990;11:97–104.
217. Alavi A, Gupta N, Dalevsky HI et al. Detection of thrombophlebitis with ^{111}In-labeled anti-fibrin antibody: preliminary results. *Cancer Research.* 1990;50(suppl):958s–961s.
218. Rosenbrough SF, Mcalee JG, Grossman ZD et al. Thrombus imaging: a comparison of radiolabeled GC4 and T2GlS fibrin specific monoclonal antibodies. *Journal of Nuclear Medicine.* 1990;31:1048–54.
219. Oster ZH, Srivastava SC, Som P et al. Thrombus radioimmunoscintigraphy: an approach using monoclonal antiplatelet antibody. *Proc Natl Acad Sci USA.* 1985;82:3465–8.
220. Peter AM, Lavender LD, Needham SG et al. Imaging thrombus with radiolabel monoclonal antibody to platelets. *Br Med J.* 1986;293:1525–7.
221. Jung M, Kletter K, Dudczak R et al. Deep vein thrombosis: scintigraphic diagnosis with In-111 label monoclonal antifibrin antibodies. *Radiology.* 1989;173:469–75.
222. Oster ZH, Som P, Zamora PO. Mesenteric vascular occlusion: a diagnostic method using a radiolabeled monoclonal antibody reactive to platelet. *Radiology.* 1989;171:653–6.
223. Kovacs JA, Ng VL, Hasur H et al. Diagnosis of *Pneumocystis carinii* pneumonia improved detection in sputum with use of monoclonal antibodies. *N Engl J Med.* 1988;318:589–93.
224. McMichael AJ. Monoclonal antibodies to HLA antigens: new approaches to the study of structure, genetics and function. In: McMichael AJ, Fabre JW, eds. Monoclonal antibodies in clinical medicine. London: Academic Press; 1982:335–64.
225. Raubitcheck A, Senyk G, Larrick J et al. Human monoclonal antibodies against group A red blood cells. *Vox Sanguinis.* 1985;48:305–8.
226. Whiteside TL. Monoclonal antibodies in tissue section diagnosis. In: Gordon DS, ed. Monoclonal antibodies in clinical diagnostic medicine. Tokyo: Igaku-Shou; 1985:19–43.
227. Kung PC, Goldstein G, Reinherz EL et al. Monoclonal antibodies defining distinctive human T-cell surface antigens. *Science.* 1979;206:24–79.
228. Hooks MA, Wade C, Millikan WJ. Muromonab CD-3: a review of its pharmacology, pharmacokinetics, and clinical use in transplantation. *Pharmacotherapy.* 1991;11:26–37.

229. Friend PJ. Immunosuppression with monoclonal antibodies. *Current Opinions in Immunology.* 1990;2:859–63.
230. Emanuel D, Peppard J, Chenimi J et al. The diagnostic, prophylactic, and therapeutic uses of monoclonal antibodies to human cytomegalovirus. *Transplantation Proceedings.* 1987;19(suppl 7):132–7.
231. Emanual D, Gold J, Colacino et al. A human monoclonal antibody to cytomegalovirus (CMV). *J Immunol.* 1984;133:2202–5.
232. Foung SK, Perkins S, Koropchak C et al. Human monoclonal antibodies neutralizing varicella zoster virus. *J Infect Dis.* 1985;52:280–5.
233. Steinitz M, Tamir S, Goldfarb A. Human antipneumococci antibody produced by an Epstein-Barr virus (EBV) immortalized cell line. *J Immunol.* 1984;132;877–82.
234. Teng NNH, Kaplan HS, Herbert JM et al. Protection against gram-negative bacteremia and endotoxemia with human monoclonal IgM antibodies. *Proc Natl Acad Sci USA.* 1985;82:1790–4.
235. Hunter K Jr, Fisher G, Hemming V et al. Antibacterial activity of a human monoclonal antibody against *Haemophilus influenzae* type B capsular polysaccharide. *Lancet.* 1982;2:798-9.
236. Udomsangpetch R, Lungren K, Berzins K et al. Human monoclonal antibodies to Pfl55: a major antigen of malaria parasite *Plasmodium falciparum. Science.* 1986;231:57–9.
237. Engleberg NC, Eisenstein BI. The impact of new cloning techniques on the diagnosis and treatment of infectious diseases. *N Engl J Med.* 1984;311:892–901.
238. David JR. The immunology of parasites. In: Braunwald E, Isselbacher KJ, Petersdorf RG, et al, eds. Harrison's internal medicine 11th ed. New York: McGraw-Hill; 1987:771–3.
239. Steinitz M, Tamir S, Frodin JE et al. Human monoclonal anti-idiotypic antibodies. *J Immunol.* 1988;141:3516–22.
240. Hiernaux JR. Idiotypic vaccines and infectious diseases. *Infection and Immunity.* 1988;56:1407–13.
241. Fremark BD, Ozer H. Construction of a stable protective human monoclonal antibody to the C fragment of tetanus toxin. In: Strelkauskas AJ, ed. Human hybridomas: diagnostic and therapeutic applications. New York: Marcel Dekker; 1987:81–94.
242. Morrison DC, Silverstein R, Bright SW et al. Monoclonal antibody to mouse lipopolysaccharide receptor protects mice against lethal effects of endotoxin. *J Infect Dis.* 1990;162:1063–8.
243. Pier GB, Thomas D, Small G et al. In vitro and in vivo activity of polycolonal and monoclonal human immunoglobulins G, M, and A against *Pseudomonas aeruginuosa* lipopolysaccharide infections. *Immunology.* 1989;57:174–9.
244. Salles MF, Mandine E, Zalisz R et al. Protective effects of murine monoclonal antibodies in experimental septicemia *E. coli* antibodies

protect against different serotypes of *E. coli*. *J Infect Dis.* 1989;159:641–9.

245. Ziegler EJ, MuCutchan JA, Fierer J et al. Treatment of gram-negative bacteremia and shock with human antiserum to mutant of *Escherichia coli. N Engl J Med.* 1982;307:1225–30.
246. Dunn D, Priest BP, Condie RM. Protective capacity of polyclonal and monoclonal antibodies directed against endotoxin during experimental sepsis. *Arch Surg.* 1988;123:1389–93.
247. Ziegler EJ, Fisher CJ, Spring CL et al. Treatment of gram-negative bacteremia and septic shock with HA-1A human monoclonal antibody against endotoxin. *N Engl J Med.* 1991;324:429–36.
248. Gorelick K, Seannon PJ, Hannigan J. Randomized placebo-controlled study of E-5 monoclonal antiendotoxin antibody. In: Borrebaek CAK, Larrick JW, eds. Therapeutic monoclonal antibodies. New York: Stockton Press; 1990:259–61.
249. Hinshaw LB, Temkamp-Olson P, Chang ACK et al. Survival of primates in LD100 septic shock following therapy with antibody to tumor necrosis factor (TNF-alpha). *Circulatory Shock.* 1990;30:279–92.
250. Excey AR, Cohen J, Burman W et al. Monoclonal antibody to TNF in severe septic shock. *Lancet.* 1990;335:1275–7.
251. Ohisson K, Bjork P, Bergenfeblt M et al. Interleukin-1 receptor antagonist reduces mortality from endotoxin shock. *Nature.* 1990;348:550–2.
252. Mester JC, Glorioso JC, Rouse BT. Protection against zosteriform spread of herpes simplex virus by monoclonal antibodies. *J Infect Dis.* 1991;163:263–9.
253. Hill HR, Gonozales LA, Knappe WA et al. Comparative protective activity of human monoclonal and hyperimmune polyclonal antibody against group B streptococci. *J Infect Dis.* 1991;163:792–8.
254. Haber E. In vivo diagnostic and therapeutic uses of monoclonal antibodies in cardiology. *Ann Rev Med.* 1986;37:249–61.
255. Khaw BA, Gold HK, Yasuda T et al. Acute myocardial infarct imaging with technetium-99m-DPTA-antimyosin Fab. *Circulation.* 1982;66:272. Abstract.
256. Katus HA, Yasuda T, Gold HK et al. Diagnosis of acute myocardial infarction: detection of circulating cardiac myosin light chains. *Am J Cardiol.* 1984;54:964–70.
257. Kremer AB, Barnes L, Hirsch RL et al. Orthoclone OKT3 monoclonal antibody reversal of hepatic and cardiac allograft rejection unresponsive to conventional immunosupressive treatments. *Transplantation Proceedings.* 1987;19(suppl 1):54–7.
258. Gilbert EM, Dewitt CW, Eiswirth CG et al. Treatment of refractory cardiac allograft rejection with OKT3 monoclonal antibody. *Am J Med.* 1987;82:202–6.

259. Gilbert EM, Eiswirth CC, Renlund RL. Use of orthoclone OKT3 monoclonal antibody in cardiac transplantation: early experience with rejection prophylaxis and treatment of refractory rejection. *Transplantation Proceedings.* 1987;19(suppl 1):45–53.

260. Starnes VA, Oyer PE, Stinson EB et al. Prophylactic OKT3 use as induction therapy for heart transplantation. *Circulation.* 1989;80(suppl 3):79s–83s.

261. Coller BS, Scudder LE, Berger HJ et al. Inhibition of human platelet function in vivo with a monoclonal antibody. *Ann Intern Med.* 1988;109:635–8.

262. Wenger TL, Butler VP, Haber E. Treatment of 63 severely digitalis-toxic patients with digoxin-specific antibody fragments. *Journal of American Colleges of Cardiology.* 1985;5(suppl A):118a–123a.

263. Lechat P, Mudgett-Hunter M, Margolies M et al. Reversal of lethal digoxin toxicity in guinea pigs using monoclonal antibodies and Fab fragments. *Journal of Pharmacology and Experimental Therapeutics.* 1984;229:210–3.

264. Rose DR, Seaton BA, Petsko GA et al. Crystallization of the Fab fragment of a monoclonal anti-digoxin antibody and its complex with digoxin. *Journal of Molecular Biology.* 1983;165:203–6.

265. Gilbert EM, O'Connell JB, Hammon ME et al. Treatment of myocarditis with OKT3 monoclonal antibody. *Lancet.* 1988;1:759.

266. Hui KY, Haber E, Matsueda GR. Monoclonal antibodies to a synthetic fibrin-like peptide bind to human fibrin but not to fibrinogen. *Science.* 1984;222:1129–32.

267. Hui KY, Haber E, Matsueda GR. Immunodetection of human fibrin using monoclonal antibody-64C5 in an extracorporeal chicken model. *Thrombosis Haemostasis.* 1985;54:524–7.

268. Bode C, Matsueda GR, Hui KY et al. Antibody-directed urokinase: a specific fibrinolytic agent. *Science.* 1985;229:765–7.

269. Chiorazzi N. Human monoclonal antibodies as probes to study autoimmune and allergic disorders. *Biotechnology.* 1986;4:210–7.

270. Morimoto C, Schlossman SF, Reinherz EL. Use of monoclonal antibodies in the study of autoimmunity and immunodeficiency: In: Hayes BF, Eisenbarth GS, eds. Monoclonal antibodies: probes for the study of autoimmunity and immunodeficiency. Orlando, FL: Academic Press; 1983:116.

271. Lindstrom J. Use of monoclonal antibodies in the study of myasthenia gravis. In: Hayes BF, Eisenbarth GS, eds. Monoclonal antibodies: probes for the study of autoimmunity and immunodeficiency. Orlando, FL: Academic Press; 1983:259–98.

272. Eisenbarth GS, Jackson R, Srikanta S. Type I diabetes: autoimmunity and immunodeficiency. In: Hayes BF, Eisenbarth GS, eds. Monoclonal antibodies: probes for the study of autoimmunity

and immunodeficiency. Orlando, FL: Academic Press; 1983:197-219.

273. Kohn LD, Yavin E, Yavin Z. Autoimmune thyroid disease studied with monoclonal antibodies to the thyrotropin receptor. In: Hayes BF, Eisenbarth GS, eds. Monoclonal antibodies: probes for the study of autoimmunity and immunodeficiency. Orlando, FL: Academic Press; 1983:221-58.
274. Christadoss P, Dauphinee M. Immunotherapy for myasthenia gravis: a murine model. *J Immunol.* 1986;136:2437-40.
275. Schoenfeld Y, Raugh J, Massicotte H et al. Polyspecificity of monoclonal lupus autoantibodies produced by human/human hybridomas. *N Engl J Med.* 1983;24:414-20.
276. Billingham MEJ, Hicks C, Carney S. Monoclonal antibodies and arthritis. *Agents and Action.* 1990;29:77-87.
277. Mathieson PW, Cobbold SP, Hale G et al. Monoclonal antibody therapy in systemic vasculitis. *N Engl J Med.* 1990;323:250-3.

Suggested Reading

Baldwin RW, Byers VS, eds. Monoclonal antibodies for cancer detection and therapy. New York: Academic Press; 1985.

Beverley PCL, ed. Methods in hematology: monoclonal antibodies. Vol 13. Edinburgh: Churchill Livingstone; 1986.

Borreback CAK, Larrick JW, eds. Therapeutic monoclonal antibodies. New York: Stockton Press; 1990.

Burchiel SW, Rhodes BA, Friedman BE, eds. Tumor imaging: the radioimmunochemical detection of cancer. New York: Masson Publishing USA; 1982.

Harkomer S, Scannon P, Mischak RP et al. Phase I study of a murine monoclonal anti-lipid A antibody in bacteremic and nonbacteremic patients. *Antimicrobial Agents and Chemotherapy.* 1988;32:710-6.

Kupchick HZ, ed. Cancer diagnosis in vitro using monoclonal antibodies. New York: Marcel Dekker; 1988.

Riechmann L, Clark M, Waldmann H et al. Reshaping human antibodies for therapy. *Nature.* 1988;332:323-7.

Strelkauskas AJ, ed. Human hybridomas: diagnostic and therapeutic applications. New York: Marcel Dekker; 1987.

Verhoeyen M, Milstein C, Winter G. Reshaping human antibodies: grafting an antilysozyme activity. *Science.* 1988;239:1534-6.

Vogel CW, ed. Immunoconjugates: antibody conjugates in radioimaging and therapy of cancer. New York: Oxford University Press; 1987.

Self-Study Questions

1. B

1. Monoclonal antibodies are produced by injecting the desired antigen into a mouse, then isolating and purifying the antibodies from the serum.

    A. True.
    B. False.

2. B

2. What two types of cells are used to create an antibody-secreting hybridoma cell?

    A. B lymphocyte and B lymphocyte.
    B. B lymphocyte and myeloma.
    C. Myeloma and myeloma.
    D. Virus and myeloma.

3. C

3. Early trials of MoAb T101 used against leukemia resulted in which of the following outcomes?

    A. No drop in leukemic cell counts.
    B. Insignificant drops in leukemic cell counts for a small percentage of patients.
    C. Transient drops in leukemic cell counts for most patients.
    D. Sustained complete remission in a small percentage of patients.

4. D

4. Which of the follow tumor types is currently imaged with MoAb technology?

    A. Hairy cell leukemia.
    B. Renal cell carcinoma.
    C. Liver.
    D. Colon.

5. B

5. Murine MoAbs are less antigenic and more effective than chimeric antibodies.

    A. True.
    B. False.

6. B

6. Which of the following is an advantage of Fab MoAb fragments?

    A. They are more cytotoxic.
    B. They have better tissue penetration.
    C. They can bind to two different antigens.
    D. They have greater antigen specificity than whole MoAbs.

7. Which of the following MoAbs has been associated with thrombocytopenia?

   A. Bivalent.
   B. T-101.
   C. Tc-99.
   D. Radioisotope conjugate.

   7. D

8. Covalent conjugation of radioisotopes to cytotoxic drugs requires the binding of fresh isotopes to the antibody before every treatment.

   A. True.
   B. False.

   8. A

9. Bacterial toxins used to produce immunotoxic conjugates inactivate protein synthesis by inactivating the 60S subunit of ribosomes.

   A. True.
   B. False.

   9. B

10. Explain why free A chains released from ricin conjugated to a MoAb should not kill nontumor cells.

    10. The B chain is lacking, and it is the B chain that binds ricin to other cells.

Glossary

ABO system: The major blood grouping system in humans.

Acquired immunity: Immunity that develops as a result of exposure to an antigen.

Active immunization: Inducing immunity against harmful agents by exposure to antigens (also known as vaccination).

Adoptive immunotherapy: The transfer of active immunologic reagents to a tumor-bearing host (such as cells with antitumor reactivity, to mediate antitumor effects).

Adjuvant: Material, usually an aluminum salt, capable of nonspecifically enhancing an immune response.

Affinity: The strength of attraction between one binding site on the antigen or epitope and a single binding site on the antibody; an expression of strength of binding between two entities.

Affinity chromatography: A method used to isolate pure proteins by coupling either antibody or antigen to an inert solid phase such as dextran beads in a column. A solution containing the antigen or the antibody of interest is run through the column where the specific antigen or antibody may bind and be eluted from the column in a concentrated pure form.

Agammaglobulinemia: A deficiency of all classes of serum immunoglobulins.

Agglutination: The process by which particles (e.g., red blood cells, bacteria) complex to form clumps, as effected by specific immunoglobulins.

AIDS-related complex: A term encompassing a variety of conditions, including unexplained weight loss, oral candidiasis, unexplained fever, extrainguinal lymphadenopathy, oral hairy leukoplakia, unexplained night sweats, herpes zoster, and unexplained diarrhea.

Allele: An alternate form of a gene at a given locus.

Allergen: An antigen that is capable of causing an allergic reaction.

Allergy: An immunologic hypersensitivity.

Alloantigens: Allelic forms of antigens present in some, but not all, individuals in a given species.

Allogeneic: Molecules or cell types within a species that have identical functions but are antigenically distinct.

Allograft: Grafted tissue of genetically dissimilar individuals of the same species.

Alpha-fetoprotein: An embryonic globulin, similar to serum albumin, which can be detected in the serum of adults with particular tumors (i.e., primary liver cancer).

Anaphylaxis: An immediate allergic reaction mediated by IgE-sensitized mast cells.

Anergy: Diminished cell-mediated reactivity as shown by the inability to react to a battery of common skin test antigens.

Antibody: An immunoglobulin that is produced by mature B cells or plasma cells in response to antigenic stimulus and is capable of binding with a specific antigen.

Antibody affinity: A measure of the strength of the bond between a single antigen-combining site (Fab) and an antigenic determinant.

Antibody avidity: A measure of the antigen-antibody binding strength that is dependent on the affinity to the epitope and the effective number of binding sites on the antibody. Avidity is enhanced by the number of bonds formed and is usually much greater than affinity.

Antibody-dependent cellular cytotoxicity: A means of destroying target cells by coating them with antibody that attracts Fc-receptor-bearing immune effector cells (killer cells, natural killer cells, macrophages, neutrophils).

Antigen: A substance capable of reacting with products of the specific immune system.

Antigen-binding sites: Locations on the antibody molecule that combine specifically with the corresponding antigenic determinant.

Antigenic modulation: A phenomenon occurring when cells lose or internalize their surface antigens after interactions with the immune system.

Antigen-presenting cell: A specific type of cell (e.g., a macrophage, dendritic cell, B cell) that stimulates T lymphocytes by displaying processed antigen to them in conjunction with major histocompatibility complex class II molecules.

Antiglobulin test: *See* **Coombs' test**.

Anti-idiotype antibodies: Antibodies directed against the surface determinants of the antigen-combining site of other antibodies.

Antilymphocyte globulins: Antibodies that are directed against lymphocytes, usually used as an immunosuppressive agent. Commonly produced by hyperimmunizing animals with human lymphocytes.

Antiserum: Serum from any animal that contains antibodies against a specific antigen.

Antithymocyte globulins: Polyclonal antibodies that are directed against human thymus lymphocytes, typically used as an immunosuppressive agent. Commonly produced by hyperimmunizing horses with human thymocytes.

Antitoxin: An antibody or antiserum prepared in response to a toxin or toxoid.

Ascites: Serous fluid that collects in the peritoneum of an animal; this fluid may contain antibodies produced by an injected hybridoma.

Atopy: The state of being allergic to normal environmental antigens.

Attenuated: Made less virulent.

Attenuated vaccine: A preparation composed of live microbes of low virulence that can induce immunity against highly virulent microbes.

Autoantibody: An antibody to normal self antigens.

Autoantigen: A host's self-antigen.

Autoimmunity: An immune response to autoantigens.

Autologous antigen: An antigen that is found in the host and that does not normally elicit an immune response; also called a self antigen.

Avidity: The total binding strength between antigen and the entire antibody (multiple Fab sites). *See* **Antibody avidity**.

Azathioprine: A purine analog converted to 6-mercaptopurine in vivo, useful as an immunosuppressant.

B lymphocytes: Cells derived from the bone marrow in mammals that are the precursors of plasma cells, which respond to antigen stimulation by producing antibodies.

Bacille Calmette-Guérin: A strain of live, attenuated mycobacterium that may induce resolution of some local tumors, probably through enhanced macrophage- or T-cell-mediated activity.

Beta 2 microglobulin: A protein associated with HLA class I antigens.

Biologic response modifiers: A heterogeneous group of substances that, in a specific or nonspecific manner, promote immune interactions with malignant cells.

Blotting: A technique of transferring DNA, RNA, or protein separated in gels onto a reactive membrane such as nitrocellulose.

Bursa of Fabricius: Lymphoid tissue found in the hind gut of birds that is responsible for B-lymphocyte maturation.

Cachectin: A monokine, also referred to as tumor necrosis factor, which is an endogenous pyrogen and catabolic substance.

Carcinoembryonic antigen: An antigen normally found in the fetal gut but that may be present in the serum of patients with cancer (primarily colon and lung) as well as in patients with inflammatory conditions and smokers.

Cell-mediated immunity: Specific immunity dependent principally on the presence of T lymphocytes.

Chemotaxis: The chemical attraction of phagocytic cells to the site of inflammation or infection; the attraction of living protoplasm to chemical stimuli.

Chimeric antibody: An antibody made up of fragments from different species (e.g., an antibody with mouse Fab and human Fc segments).

Class I genes: Genes of the major histocompatibility complex responsible for compatibility of tissues and organs (also known as histocompatibility or transplantation genes); HLA-A, -B, and -C loci encode for the class I HLA molecules in humans.

Class II genes: Genes of the major histocompatibility complex that participate in the immune response (also known as Ir genes); HLA-D loci encode for the class II HLA molecules in humans.

Class III genes: Genes of the major histocompatibility complex that contribute to the complement system and tumor necrosis factor.

Clone: A group of genetically identical cells derived from a single original cell.

Clusters of differentiation: A nomenclature system that categorizes cell surface molecules of human leukocytes; also used to categorize monoclonal antibodies according to the antigens they recognize.

Colony-forming unit granulocyte-monocyte: A term used to describe the in vitro production of a colony of cells of granulocytic and monocytic lineage within a semisolid medium such as methylcellulose.

Colony-stimulating factors (CSFs): A group of substances that increase production and activity of various types of hematologic cells; granulocyte-macrophage CSF stimulates granulocytes and macrophages; granulocyte CSF stimulates primarily granulocytes (neutrophils).

Complement: A group of plasma proteins that may induce cell lysis when stimulus initiates their sequential activation.

Complementarity-determining regions: Regions within the variable portion of a receptor, such as immunoglobulin, that have been identified as playing a major role in the actual binding of the receptor to antigen. Also known as hypervariable regions.

Complement fixation test: A test used to detect the presence of antibody or antigen. In the test, the test antibody is mixed with the antigen and a small amount of active complement. If the specific antibody is present, an antibody-antigen complex forms and fixes the complement; if no antibody is present, the active complement remains and may be detected by the addition of antibody-sensitized red blood cells (RBCs). The RBCs lyse if complement is available, representing a negative screen for the antibody in question.

Congenic strain: Separate strains of animals with identical genotypes except for a difference at a single genetic locus.

Conjugate: A product obtained by joining two or more dissimilar molecules (e.g., radioisotopes, drugs, or toxins covalently coupled to an antibody).

Coombs' test (antiglobulin test): A hemagglutination test that detects antibodies to red blood cell (RBC) antigens. The direct Coombs' test detects antibodies located on the RBC surface, and the indirect Coombs' test detects antibodies in the serum against antigens on the RBC membrane; both require the addition of a second antibody such as antiglobulin.

Cytokines: A generic term for soluble substances produced by cells to communicate with other cells to trigger or suppress cellular activity after interaction with antigen. *See also* **Soluble mediators** (synonym).

Cytotoxicity: The process of killing cells.

Delayed hypersensitivity: A specific inflammatory immune reaction elicited by an antigen and mediated by primed T cells; does not usually appear until 24 hours after contact with antigen.

Determinant: A three-dimensional site on an antigen to which antibody is specifically able to become attached by its antigen-binding site. A single antigen may have several antigenic determinants (epitopes).

Diapedesis: The movement of blood cells, including phagocytes, through the walls of the blood vessel into the tissue.

Double immunodiffusion technique (Ouchterlony): A gel-based immunoprecipitation method used to distinguish antigens in mixtures. Both the antigen and the antibody are placed in holes punched into the gel and allowed to diffuse toward each other. At the equivalence point of the antigen and antibody, precipitation arcs are formed in one of three basic patterns of identity.

Effector cells: Cells (lymphocytes, phagocytes) that directly function to achieve the end result, as opposed to regulatory cells.

Electrophoresis: The separation of molecules in an electrical field, usually within a gel.

Env: The gene that encodes for the envelope protein of human immunodeficiency virus.

Enzyme-linked immunosorbent assay: An immunoassay in which antibody or antigen is detected by the binding of an enzyme coupled to either anti-immunoglobulin or antibody specific for the antigen.

Enzyme-multiplied immunoassay technique: A quantitative competitive immunoassay that uses an enzyme detection system. The enzyme-coupled antigen retains its enzymatic activity when unbound but loses its activity when bound to the antibody. The enzyme activity is inversely proportional to the amount of antibody-antigen binding.

Epitope: A single antigenic determinant; the smallest structural portion of an antigen to which antibody can specifically attach by its antigen-binding site.

Fab: Fragment of antigen binding—the single antigen-binding site of an antibody formed by the cleaving of the antibody to fragments with papain.

F(ab')$_2$: A dimeric fragment that contains two antigen-binding sites formed by the cleaving of the antibody to fragments with pepsin.

Fc: Crystallizable fragment—The portion of an immunoglobulin that binds to macrophages, lymphocytes, and mast cells via Fc receptors. Also carries sites for fixation of complement.

Fc receptors: Receptors that are located on cells and that are capable of binding the Fc portion of an immunoglobulin.

Ficoll-Hypaque® gradient: A liquid-density separation medium used to isolate cells on the basis of their densities. The gradients are used primarily to isolate lymphocytes.

Flow microfluorometry: Cell sorting by means of a flow microfluorimeter or flow cytometer, a device that uses laser and monoclonal antibody technology. Antibodies labeled with fluorescent markers are incubated with the cells of interest. Cells that have the antigenic target for the antibody are labeled with the fluorescent marker. These labeled cells can be separated from the other cells according to fluorescence detected on the cell surface.

Fluorescence: Absorption of light at one wavelength and the emission of light at another wavelength.

Fluorescence immunoassay: An immunoassay technique that uses fluorescent-labeled antibodies or antigens to detect the presence of the antibody-antigen complex.

Fusion: A technique by which the cellular membranes of two or more cells are combined to form one cell; the resulting hybrid cell contains many of the chromosomes of the fusion partners.

Gag: The gene that encodes for the core protein of human immunodeficiency virus.

Gamma globulin: Immunoglobulins that migrate within the gamma region during electrophoresis.

Gene: A unit of DNA that encodes for a single polypeptide chain.

Graft-versus-host disease: A pathologic reaction that is caused by the transplantation of competent donor T cells into an incompetent host, that is, one unable to reject them. This reaction occurs when the donor cells attack the host.

Graft-versus-leukemia effect: The decreased incidence of leukemic relapses seen in patients receiving allogeneic transplants in comparison with autologous transplants.

Granulocytopenia: Decreased numbers of granulocytic cells (neutrophils, eosinophils, basophils) in the peripheral blood.

Group-specific: Common to all the members of a group of viruses.

Haplotype: The set of genes present on any one chromosome; inherited as a unit. Each somatic cell will have two haplotypes: one of paternal origin and one of maternal origin.

Haptens: Small molecules that are not immunogenic unless conjugated to a larger carrier molecule.

HAT: Acronym for a selective cell culture medium containing hypoxanthine, aminopterin, and thymidine; used in monoclonal antibody technology to select for fused myeloma and B-lymphocyte cells (hybridomas).

Helper T cell (T4+, CD4+): A subclass of T cells responsible for stimulating other T cells and B cells; also called helper T lymphocytes.

Hemagglutination: The agglutination of red blood cells (RBCs). This technique is used in a number of tests to detect antibody-antigen reactions. The antigen may be either located on the surface of the RBC or chemically linked to the RBC surface. The test is performed by the addition of these RBCs to wells titrated with the antibody of interest.

Hematopoiesis: The formation and development of blood cells.

Hematopoietic growth factor: *See* **Colony-stimulating factor.**

Hemolytic disease of the newborn: A disease of newborns characterized by anemia and jaundice; due to incompatibilities of the Rh phenotype of mother and fetus (also known as erythroblastosis fetalis).

Human immunodeficiency virus: Believed by most investigators to be the cause of acquired immunodeficiency syndrome.

Human antimurine antibody response: Antibody response produced in humans against infused immunogenic murine antibodies (usually monoclonal antibodies); also called human antibodies to mouse antibodies, or human antimouse antibodies.

Human leukocyte antigens: The major histocompatibility antigens in humans.

Humoral immunity: Specific immunity mediated principally by immunoglobulins, which are secreted from plasma cells; found in plasma, lymph, and other tissue fluids.

Hybridoma: A cell or cell line obtained by the fusion of two different cells. A B-cell hybridoma results from the fusion of a B lymphocyte and a tumorous plasma cell and is capable of secreting antibody and prolonged survival. A hybridoma cell contains chromosomes from each of the fusion partners.

Hyperchimeric antibody: A monoclonal antibody in which the hypervariable regions are of a nonhuman source (such as mouse) while the rest of the antibody structure is of a human framework. Also known as a humanized antibody.

Hypergammaglobulinemia: An excess of gamma globulin in the blood.

Hypervariable region: Subsections within the variable region of an antibody responsible for the antigen specificity of the antibody. Denoted for the high variance of amino acid sequences between antibodies of different specificity. (*See also* **Complementarity-determining regions.**)

Idiotypes: Surface determinants in the variable domain of antibodies that are typically the binding sites for the target antigen.

Immune complexes: Antigen-antibody complexes.

Immunization: The process of inducing active or passive specific immunity by administering antigenic substances or antigen-specific antibodies.

Immunoblotting: A technique used to identify blotted proteins by incubating the blot with labeled antibody or antigen. The antibody binds to antigens on the blot, the location of which can be detected by autoradiography or enzyme-induced color changes. Also known as Western blotting.

Immunodeficiency: A partial or total deficiency of either cellular immunity, humoral immunity, or both.

Immunoelectrophoresis: A qualitative gel-based technique, in which the mixture of antigens is first separated in an electric field according to the charge of the antigens and then precipitated with antiserum from a trough lying parallel to the separated antigens.

Immunoglobulin: A glycoprotein consisting of heavy chains and light chains linked together, often synthesized in response to the presence of a foreign substance. *See also* **Antibody**.

Immunomodulator: An agent capable of enhancing, suppressing, or restoring an immune system either directly or indirectly.

Immunoradiometric assay: A noncompetitive radioisotope immunoassay technique used to measure antigen. Excessive radiolabeled antibodies are added to a plastic plate containing bound antigen. The antigen is bound by the antibody; then free radiolabeled antibodies are removed. The quantity of antigen is proportional to the radioactivity of the remaining bound antibodies.

Immunotoxin: The conjugate of an antibody and a naturally occurring toxic substance, such as ricin.

Interferon: A glycoprotein that exerts virus-nonspecific but host-specific antiviral activity.

Interleukin: A soluble factor released from leukocytes or other cells with defined biologic effects. Protein composition and DNA sequence of encoding gene are defined. (See Chapter 2 for specific interleukins.)

J chain: Joining chain normally found in polymeric immunoglobulins (IgM and IgA).

K cell: Killer cell, responsible for antibody-dependent cellular cytotoxicity.

Kupffer cells: Mononuclear phagocytes that are fixed within the sinusoids of the liver.

Leukotrienes: Lipoxygenase metabolites of arachidonic acid with multiple biologic activities.

Levamisole: Antihelminthic drug with possible immunostimulant effects.

Linkage-associated antigens: Surface antigens, each of which is commonly associated with one or more specific diseases.

Lipopolysaccharide: Any compound in which lipid is linked to polysaccharide. Often refers to an endotoxin derived from the cell wall of gram-negative bacteria.

Liposome: A spherical microstructure consisting of concentric phospholipid bilayers. Liposomes are hollow in the center and may be filled with drugs.

Locus: Position on the chromosome where a specific gene is found.

Lymphokine-activated killer cells: A type of lymphocyte that develops an increased antitumor effect when stimulated by interleukin-2.

Lymphokines: Soluble secretory products of lymphocytes that stimulate or suppress the activity of other cells.

Lymphopoiesis: The development of lymphatic tissue.

Lymphoreticular malignancies: Lymphomas and lymphocytic leukemias.

Lymphotoxin: A lymphokine that effects the lysis of certain nonlymphocytic target cells such as fibroblasts. Also known as tumor necrosis factor beta.

Lysosomes: Intracellular organelles containing digestive enzymes (lysozymes).

Lysozyme: A muramidase capable of hydrolyzing structural bonds in the cell walls of certain bacteria, particularly gram-positive cocci.

Macrophage: A phagocytic cell found in tissue and believed to be derived from blood monocytes. May act as an antigen-presenting cell.

Major histocompatibility complex (MHC): A collection of structural genes associated with transplantation, immune response, and the complement system. In humans, the MHC is also known as the human leukocyte antigen complex. *See* **Human leukocyte antigens**.

Microcytotoxicity test: A test to assess histocompatibility in which antisera are used to measure the presence of antigens on donor and recipient lymphocytes.

Mitogen: A substance that induces proliferation of lymphocytes.

Mixed lymphocyte culture: A technique used for determining the compatibilities of one individual's lymphocytes with another's by measuring the amount of proliferation induced when the lymphocytes are cultured together.

Mixed lymphocyte reaction: The in vitro proliferative response of lymphocytes after exposure to lymphocytes of differing haplotypes.

Modulation: The disappearance of cell surface receptors after combining with specific antibodies.

Monoclonal antibodies (MoAbs): Homogeneous antibodies produced by a single clone. MoAbs can be of any class of antibodies; however, most murine MoAbs are of the IgG or IgM class.

Monocytes and macrophages: Mononuclear phagocytic cells.

Monokines: Substances such as interleukin-1 and tumor necrosis factor, which are secreted by monocytes and macrophages.

Mononuclear phagocyte system: Mononuclear phagocytic cells found primarily in the reticular connective tissue of immune and other organs. *See also* **Reticuloendothelial system**.

Mucositis: Inflammation of the mucosal membrane.

Mucus: A clear, viscid secretion of mucous membranes consisting of mucin, epithelial cells, and leukocytes.

Muramyl dipeptide: A substance derived from myobacterial cell walls, used as an immunostimulant, similar to bacille Calmette-Guérin.

Myeloma cell line: A category of tumorous plasma cells with the sustained ability to grow in culture.

Natural killer cells: Lymphocytes that preferentially kill virally infected or malignant cells in the absence of prior immunization.

Neuroleukin: Neurotropic factor that promotes the survival of various neurons.

Neutralization: Process in which antibody either with or without complement neutralizes the infectivity of microorganisms such as viruses.

Nude mice: A hairless strain of mice that congenitally lack a thymus and have a marked deficiency in T lymphocytes but do possess natural killer cells.

Oncofetal antigens: Cell surface markers that are normally present on fetal, but not adult, tissue and that can be found on malignant cells.

Oncogene: A gene of mammalian or viral origin that is capable of causing neoplastic transformation of cells.

Ontogeny: The development of the individual organism.

Opsonin: A substance that binds to antigens and enhances phagocytosis by macrophages and neutrophils (e.g., complement and antibodies).

Opsonization: The process by which particles, microorganisms, or immune complexes become coated with complement or antibodies that make them more easily phagocytosed.

Orthotopic: Occurring at the normal place in the body.

Ouchterlony: *See* **Double immunodiffusion technique.**

Panning: An isolation technique that uses plastic plates sensitized with antigen (or antibody). A mixture of cells may be incubated on these plates and components containing receptors for the antigen (or antibody) will bind and thus be isolated from the mixture.

Passive immunization: Inducing immunity by introduction of protective agents (e.g., preformed antibodies or specific cells) derived from extrinsic sources into a nonimmune host.

Phagocytes: Cells that are capable of phagocytosis.

Phagocytosis: The process whereby cells ingest and digest solid substances such as bacteria and foreign particles.

Phagosome: A vesicle that forms around a particle within the phagocyte that engulfed the particle.

Phenotype: A description of all the alleles detected in a given individual.

Phytohemagglutinin: A lectin extracted from red kidney beans, capable of agglutinating certain erythrocytes; often used as a mitogen for T lymphocytes.

Plasma cell: The mature B lymphocyte, which is capable of secreting antibody.

Pluripotent cell: A primitive cell that has the potential to differentiate into any mature, functional cell.

Polyclonal activation: Activation of many clones of nonspecific lymphocytes.

Polymerase chain reaction: A process that enables the amount of a particular DNA sequence or gene to be greatly amplified.

Precipitin reactions: The reaction of antigen and antibody in which cross-linking and precipitation of the complex occurs.

Prostaglandins: Cyclo-oxygenase metabolites of arachidonic acid with many biologic activities.

Proto-oncogene: A normal gene that is usually involved in cellular growth or regulation and that, when altered or mutated, can become an oncogene.

Radial immunodiffusion: A gel-based immunoprecipitation technique in which immunodiffusion occurs with only a single component and the other reactant is fixed in the gel. The antibody-antigen complex results in the formation of a ring of precipitation that can be quantitated.

Radioimmunoassay: A technique used to detect antibody-antigen reaction; one of the components of the reaction is radiolabeled with a radioisotope.

Radioimmunosorbent test: A radioimmunoassay technique used to detect IgE in the serum.

Regulatory cell: A cell that has the primary function of stimulating or suppressing the production or activation of other cells such as effector cells.

Reticuloendothelial system: A term, perhaps inaccurate, used to describe the mononuclear phagocyte system, a collection of cells that share the common function of phagocytosis and digestion of particulate material.

Retrovirus: A virus that carries genetic material (reverse transcriptase) capable of transcribing viral RNA to DNA.

Rheumatoid factor: An antibody directed at human IgG that is present in patients with rheumatoid arthritis and other connective tissue diseases.

Rh system: A blood grouping system based on Rh antigens.

Rosetting: A method of isolating lymphocytes by allowing them to associate with red blood cells (usually sheep RBCs) in the form of a cluster with the lymphocyte as the central cell. There are three main rosetting types: erythrocyte rosettes, erythrocyte-antibody rosettes, and erythrocyte-antibody-complement rosettes.

Serologic typing: A method of detecting cell surface antigens by using antisera.

Serotherapy: Administration of antisera or specific immunoglobulins that are targeted for a specific antigen (also see passive immunization).

Soluble mediators: Secreted regulatory proteins, including all proteins or glycoproteins—such as interleukins, interferons, and cytokines—that mediate immune function.

Specificity: Selective reactivity; the ability to distinguish among different determinants or sections of antigens.

Stem cell: A cell capable of self-replication and differentiation into various kinds of secondary cells.

Suppressor T cell (T8+, CD8+): A subclass of T cells responsible for suppressing the immune response to a stimulus; also called suppressor T lymphocytes.

Swine flu: The name given to a type of influenza that broke out in 1976 and stimulated a nationwide vaccination program.

Syngeneic: Genetically identical (as in identical twins or inbred strains of animals).

T-cell receptor: A molecule on the surface of T lymphocytes specifically capable of recognizing antigen in association with major histocompatibility complex molecules. Consists of two polypeptide chains (alpha and beta, or gamma and delta) associated with the CD3 complex.

T lymphocytes: Cells that are derived from the bone marrow and that differentiate within the thymus; they play a major role in the activity of the cell-mediated immune system. *See also* **Helper T cell** and **Suppressor T cell.**

Tolerance: An immunologic response of nonreactivity to a particular antigen, although responses to other antigens are normal.

Toxoid: A pharmacologically inactive toxin preparation that retains the ability to stimulate production of antitoxin.

Transfection: The process by which a DNA segment may be introduced into another cell, incorporated, and read to produce a protein.

Transfectoma: A continually renewing cell (e.g., a hybridoma or a myeloma cell) that has been transfected with a foreign DNA segment.

Tumor necrosis factor (TNF) alpha: A substance that is capable of killing tumorous cells and eliciting inflammatory responses and is produced by host monocytes and macrophages; also referred to as cachectin. (For TNF-beta, *see* **Lymphotoxin.**)

Type-specific: Distinct for each virus within the group.

Vaccination: Active immunization with modified attenuated or killed microorganisms to provide resistance and to prevent infectious disease (also known as active immunization).

Vaccine: A product consisting of attenuated or killed microbial agents used as an antigen to provide immunity.

Variolation: Injection of live smallpox virus from disease pustules to protect against smallpox.

Virion: Formed virus particle.

Virulence: The degree of pathogenicity of various strains of organisms.

Western blot: An immunoblotting method used for identifying specific proteins recognized by antibodies.

Wheal-and-flare: A cutaneous reaction in response to an injected antigen consisting of a raised edematous lesion surrounded by erythema.

Xenogeneic: Derived from tissues of individuals of different species (*see* **Allogeneic**).

About the Authors

Jeffrey C. Delafuente, M.S., is associate professor and associate chairman for education in the Department of Pharmacy Practice at the College of Pharmacy and associate professor at the College of Medicine, Division of Clinical Immunology, Rheumatology, and Allergy at the University of Florida at Gainesville. He earned his B.S. and M.S. in pharmacy from the University of Florida, where he completed a residency specialization in clinical pharmacy and a research fellowship in clinical immunology at the College of Medicine. Delafuente is a frequent author of journals and book chapters on pharmacotherapy and immunotherapeutics. He has presented at the local, state, and national levels on pharmacotherapy with special attention to geriatrics and immunology. He authored *Therapeutics in the Elderly* and has developed related educational materials in nontraditional media. He is active in local, state, and national academic and pharmacy associations.

Suzanne M. Fields, Pharm.D., is clinical instructor and oncology pharmacy fellow at the University of Texas Health Science Center at San Antonio. She earned her B.S. in pharmacy and Pharm.D. at the University of North Carolina at Chapel Hill. She completed an ASHP residency in oncology at Audie L. Murphy Memorial Veterans' Hospital. Fields has coauthored articles and book chapters on oncology therapeutics and clinical pharmacology. She presents locally and nationally on cancer-related subjects and is active in several professional associations.

Jeanne T. Flynn, Pharm.D., is manager of professional services at Amgen, Inc. She earned her B.S. in pharmacy from the University of Illinois Health Sciences Center and her Pharm.D. from the University of Texas Health Sciences Center. She completed her ASHP oncology residency at Audie L. Murphy Memorial Veterans' Hospital. Flynn's presentations and publications have focused on immunotherapy and antineoplastic therapy. She is presently involved with professional information services and clinical development of Amgen's granulocyte colony-stimulating factor.

Jim Koeller, M.S., is clinical associate professor at the University of Texas at Austin's College of Pharmacy; clinical associate professor of the Department of Medicine and Pharmacology at the University of Texas Health Science Center at San Antonio; and oncology clinical specialist at Audie L. Murphy Memorial Veterans' Hospital. He earned his B.S. and M.S. in pharmacy at the University of Wisconsin Hospital, where he completed an ASHP residency. Koeller is a frequent contributor of articles about clinical research and has coauthored several book chapters about antineoplastic agents. His presentations have been made to regional, national, and international audiences on anticancer therapy, pain management, and computerized pharmacy management practices. He is an active member of regional and national pharmacy associations and previously served as chairman of ASHP's SIG on Oncology Pharmacy Practice.

Karl K. Kwok, Pharm.D., is clinical associate professor at the University of Washington's School of Pharmacy and clinical pharmacist of oncology service at the University of Washington Medical Center. He earned his B.S. in pharmacy from Oregon State University and his Pharm.D. from the University of Washington. Kwok's presentations and publications have reported on immunologic research and pharmacologic considerations in cancer chemotherapy. He is active in local, state, and national pharmacy associations.

Kathleen D. Lake, Pharm.D., is program director, Division of Cardiothoracic Transplantation and Research at the Minneapolis Heart Institute Foundation and clinical assistant professor at the University of Minnesota College of Pharmacy. She earned her B.S. in pharmacy and Pharm.D. from the University of Minnesota. Lake is a frequent presenter to local, state, and national audiences about immunosuppressive drugs and support therapy for transplant patients. Her written work in her field includes book chapters on cardiothoracic transplantation in *Pharmacotherapy: A Pathophysiologic Approach* (second edition) and *Cardiothoracic Transplantation*. She is an active member of several professional associations and presently serves as secretary of the Board of Regents for the American College of Clinical Pharmacy.

Timothy R. McGuire, Pharm.D., is assistant professor of pharmacy practice at the University of Nebraska Medical Center. He earned his B.S. in pharmacy at the University of Washington in Seattle and his Pharm.D. at the Philadelphia College of Pharmacy and Science. He completed a residency in clinical pharmacy at the Seattle Veterans Administration Medical Center and an ASHP oncology pharmacotherapy fellowship at the University of Florida at Gainesville. McGuire has written extensively on the subject of cyclosporine and bone marrow transplant patients and has published articles and a book chapter on cancer-related subjects. He is an active member of national professional organizations.

Karen I. Plaisance, Pharm.D., is associate professor of clinical pharmacy at the University of Maryland School of Pharmacy. She earned her B.S. in pharmacy from the University of Washington and her Pharm.D. from the State University of New York at Buffalo. She completed a 2-year fellowship in infectious diseases and pharmacokinetics at Hartford Hospital's Department of Pharmacy Services. Plaisance's publications focus on pharmacokinetics and human immunodeficiency virus (HIV) infection. She has presented to regional, national, and international audiences on antibiotic, antifungal, and antimicrobial agents and HIV infection. She is active with local and national professional associations.

Bonnie D. Purdy, Pharm.D., is a Clinical Pharmacy Specialist in acquired immunodeficiency syndrome and infectious disease at Albany Medical Center Hospital and adjunct assistant professor at Albany College of Pharmacy. She earned her Pharm.D. at the University of Maryland, where she completed a residency in infectious disease and pharmacokinetics. Purdy's presentations and publications have focused on pharmacotherapy for HIV-infected patients. She is an active member of state and national pharmacy associations.

Kelly A. Scott, Pharm.D., is an oncology clinical pharmacist and residency preceptor at Good Samaritan Hospital and Medical Center, Portland, Oregon. She earned her Pharm.D. from the University of the Pacific and completed an ASHP residency at Good Samaritan Hospital and Medical Center. Scott's presentations and publications have focused on immunotherapy, pain management, and chemotherapy. She is an active member of state and national pharmacy associations.

Joseph A. Tami, Pharm.D., is director of the Bone Marrow Transplantation Laboratory; research assistant professor for the Department of Medicine, Division of Hematology; and assistant clinical professor for the Department of Pharmacology at the University of Texas Health Science Center. He earned his B.S. in genetics at the University of California at Davis and his Pharm.D. at the University of Southern California. He completed a general residency at the University of Kentucky Medical Center and fellowship in immunology and oncology at the University of Texas Health Science Center and Audie L. Murphy Memorial Veterans' Hospital. Tami's publications have addressed a wide range of immunotherapy issues, including monoclonal antibody therapy, hybridomas, and lymphokine-activated killer cell applications. He is the principal investigator of a clinical study on the use of biologic response modifiers in immunotherapy and is active in local and national professional associations.

Index

A

I

R